MODERN
DRUG USE

MODERN DRUG USE

An Enquiry on Historical Principles

RONALD D. MANN
MD, MRCGP, FCP

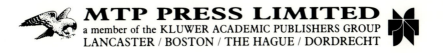

MTP PRESS LIMITED
a member of the KLUWER ACADEMIC PUBLISHERS GROUP
LANCASTER / BOSTON / THE HAGUE / DORDRECHT

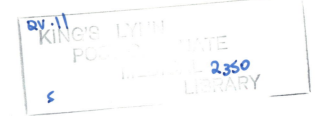

Published in the UK and Europe by
MTP Press Limited
Falcon House
Lancaster, England

British Library Cataloguing in Publication Data

Mann, R. D.
   Modern drug use.
   1. Drugs—History
   I. Title
   615'.1'09   RS61

   ISBN 0-85200-717-5

Published in the USA by
MTP Press
A division of Kluwer Boston Inc
190 Old Derby Street
Hingham, MA 02043, USA

Library of Congress Cataloging in Publication Data

Mann, Ronald D. (Ronald David), 1928–
  Modern drug use.

  Bibliography: p.
  Includes index.
  1. Pharmacology—History.   2. Drugs—History.
I. Title.
RM41.M36   1984   615'.1'09   84–14386
ISBN 0-85200-717-5

Copyright © 1984 Ronald D. Mann

Typesetting by Georgia Origination, Liverpool
Printed by Butler and Tanner, Frome and London

Contents

Acknowledgements

The reading programme for this book has been guided by Garrison and Morton's *A medical bibliography* in both its third edition of 1970 and its 1983 edition by Leslie T. Morton; an equally indispensable means of instruction has been Fielding H. Garrison's *An introduction to the history of medicine* in its fourth edition of 1929. Without these two works an approach to the present subject from an historical point of view would have provided great difficulty.

I am greatly indebted to the facilities of the Royal Society of Medicine, London: Mr David Stewart, Librarian to the Society, has been at all times helpful, has shared his fine knowledge of the great resources of the Library, and has given permission for the publication of the Withering letter *The Spasmodic Asthma*... and the reply of June 8, 1786 by B. P. van Lelyveld; I also wish to express my sincere thanks to Mr Stewart's staff, who have attended with great kindness to the demands of an extensive reference list, and to the staff of the Society's house and the Domus Medica. I have particularly appreciated access to the Osler bequest to the Society and the Minute Books and records of its Section of the History of Medicine. It is a great pleasure to express appreciation to those who have permitted all of these materials to be studied under conditions of both comfort and courtesy.

I have been much assisted by being given access to the collections of the Library of the Wellcome Institute for the History of Medicine, London, and I wish to express my warmest thanks to the staff of that Library and especially to Mr Robin Price, Deputy Librarian, who has shown great interest in this study. I am also most grateful to both Mr William Schupbach, Curator, Iconographic Collections, for the provision of a number of important illustrations; and to Mrs Christine English, who has kindly undertaken the translation of sections of the Latin of Scribonius Largus.

Many of the illustrations in the present work are derived from the seemingly endless resources of the Wellcome Institute library and the Royal Society of Medicine library. In most instances the relevant source, unless from the work of the author, has been acknowledged in the captions. I would, however, like to express my keen appreciation of the practical help and interest of the Audiovisual Unit of the Royal Society of Medicine; this Unit, now of expanded proportions, has been of the greatest assistance in illustrating this work and lectures based upon it.

Amongst the other specialist librarians who have been of help and advice I wish to record my gratitude to: Mr Sandy Roger, Librarian to the Royal College of Physicians and Surgeons of Glasgow, for the provision of material on Joseph Jackson Lister; Mr G. D. Hargreaves and Miss Gray of the University Library of St Andrews for the provision of copies of sections of Markham's *Memoir* of 1874, and Mr F. P. Richardson, Librarian to the Law Society, London, who responded very helpfully to an enquiry regarding the writ *De leproso amovendo*.

It has seemed important to see this subject, to the greatest extent possible, within its social context. In this attempt a number of librarians responsible for general collections have been of great assistance. I have been much helped by Mrs Gillian Deakin and the staff of the Public Library at Midhurst, Sussex. At that library many uncommon and difficult references have been obtained for me and it is important to note the manner in which our public library resources remain capable of supporting serious study. Mr Hugh Harmer, of the Chichester Public Library, has given helpful access to his valuable collection of material on Sussex and Dr Mary Hobbs has very kindly made available parts of the early written material in the possession of the Dean of Chichester Cathedral. The Librarian of the Kungliga Biblioteket at Stockholm has provided requested material on John d'Arderne and both Mr E. Kahn, Librarian of the Jews College, Finchley, and Miss Sonja L. Sopher, Paintings Conservator of the Cleveland Museum of Art, Ohio, have responded helpfully to specific enquiries.

A reference in the text to Samuel George Shattock (1852–1924) will be noticed. Shattock, for many years associated with St Thomas's Hospital, London, was one of the first to give his whole time to the study and teaching of pathology. His grandson, Dr Francis M. Shattock, presently Head of the Department of International Community Health at the Liverpool School of Tropical Medicine, responded with great kindness to my enquiries regarding his grandfather's studies on the histopathology of certain human remains of Ancient Egypt. Sadly, it would seem that Shattock's valuable material on this subject was destroyed when St Thomas's lost its histology records due to enemy action in 1940/41 – and for this information I am indebted to Professor J. R. Tighe of the Department of Histopathology at Shattock's old hospital.

My interest in the studies of Brian J. Ford on Leeuwenhoek and early microscopy was aroused by Mr Ford's paper on *Revelation and the single lens* (1982). Subsequently, Mr Ford has been generous with additional information and it is a great pleasure to express my appreciation. I am also particularly grateful to Dr Derrick Baxby, of the Department of Medical Microbiology of the Royal Liverpool Hospital, for interesting and helpful comments on smallpox vaccination and the history of Jenner's vaccine – subjects upon which Dr Baxby has recently written important and full-length studies.

I have been privileged to discuss the conclusions arising from this present *Enquiry* with Sir James Black FRS, now Director of Therapeutic Research, The Wellcome Research Laboratories. For this enjoyable and very valuable discussion I am deeply grateful. Few things are more important than the exchange of comment and criticism in what is intended to be a contribution to debate upon a subject of the greatest importance, and I much appreciate the hospitality of Sir James to me on this occasion.

I would like to express a word, in concluding these acknowledgements, to Dr Helen Townsend, my colleague of a number of years in the pharmaceutical industry and its clinical pharmacology. I have to thank Dr Townsend for certain translations from the French but record with pleasure rather than any formality my gratitude for her professional endeavours and support.

My sincere thanks are also due to Mr David Bloomer, Managing Director, MTP Press Limited for his encouragement during the process of writing this book and to Mr Philip Johnstone, my editor.

Finally, my wife has catalogued the reference material for this book, maintained this rather considerable collection in good order, and shared in the growth of the study; my daughter has played her part, and one is grateful to express, to one's own family, a singular appreciation.

Note

The conclusions of this *Enquiry* represent personal deductions and opinions; they are not necessarily those of any authority consulted during this study nor are they, as far as is known, those of the pharmaceutical houses or government departments with which the author is or has been associated. This study was written during a period, free from external obligation, and employed for the purpose. With the volume in press a few references have been updated and the final section (Conclusion) added; this section contains only information in the public domain – it serves to emphasize and recapitulate views previously expressed – nevertheless, the permission of Dr J. Griffin, in respect of permission to publish this concluding section, is acknowledged.

Within the context of this work certain tables relating to side-effects and apparent adverse reactions experience with licensed medicinal drugs are presented. These tables are abbreviated forms of the computer print-outs of the Licensing Authority. These tables and their interpretation are the responsibility of the author only.

Botanical names in this text are usually those of the period of the subject of discussion; as botanical names have, in some instances, changed over the period since the early classifications, these names should be interpreted accordingly.

The letter by William Withering (*'The Spasmodic Asthma...'*) and the reply by B. P. van Lelyveld (*'Think only, my dear Magellan...'*), both of which form part of the Osler bequest to the Royal Society of Medicine and are previously unpublished, are now reproduced by courtesy of the Librarian of the Royal Society of Medicine, which Society retains the world-wide copyright of these documents.

List of Illustrations

Introduction

Aureolus Theophrastus Bombastus von Hohenheim (1493–1541), commonly called Paracelsus, was both one of the most original medical thinkers of the sixteenth century and was the man who made opium (as laudanum), arsenic, copper sulphate, iron, lead, mercury, potassium sulphate, and sulphur part of the pharmacopoeia. A man of many parts, but a pioneer chemist, Paracelsus can be regarded as the originator of a body of work which was the precursor of chemical pharmacology and therapeutics. To no small extent he stands, therefore, as a father figure of the modern pharmaceutical industry.

Today's physician who wants to look at that industry since the days of Paracelsus and weigh the great gains against the problems soon encounters difficulties. To diminish them, this *Enquiry* approaches its subject from historical principles. This gives increased perspective to questions asked late in the book – these questions being prompted by medical practice outside the industry and some twenty years of drug development activity within it.

In antiquity medicines often seem to have been used as part of magic and primitive man thought disease to be due to supernatural forces which he could influence. The legacy remains – and in trying to sort out what is rational in our use of drugs today we have to separate our small bits of science from the ancient magic and from modern commercial pressures and conditioning.

Knowledge of drugs may have arisen from the use of foods prepared for the sick; what is certain is that such knowledge became codified early and, in Ancient Greece, Dioscorides (fl. AD 54–68) recorded some 500 plant drugs. The Arabian apothecaries added many more and throughout the Byzantine ages and the Renaissance information continued to accumulate.

The first printed English herbal, a small quarto volume, was produced anonymously by the London printer, Rycharde Banckes, in 1525. *The grete herball . . .*, printed in London by Peter Treveris, followed a year later and formed the first of a series of a new type of larger, profusely illustrated books based on splendid works printed on the Continent. The growth of knowledge was such that in sixteenth century England the beautiful herbal of William Turner (1510–1568), himself often called 'The Father of English Botany', ran to three volumes, the first part of the complete edition of 1568 being dedicated to Queen Elizabeth.

Without doubt the most popular of all the English herbals was that of John Gerarde (1545–1612), sometime Master of the Barber-Surgeons' Company; Gerarde's *The herball or generall historie of plantes*, printed in London in 1597, has 1392 numbered pages excluding its index and related material. A second 'very much enlarged and amended' edition was brought out in 1633 by Thomas Johnson (*c.* 1600–1644), a prominent member of the Society of Apothecaries; this volume, of 1631 numbered pages, by adding some 800 new species, provided 2850 plant descriptions.

The last of the great English herbalists was John Parkinson (1567–1650) who, like Turner, Gerarde and Johnson, maintained a garden in which he grew numbers of rare and fine species. Apothecary to James I, Parkinson's *Theatrum botanicum: The theater of plants...*, of 1640, occupied much of the long life of this distinguished old gardener and botanist. Apart from prefatory material this book provides 1755 pages describing nearly 3800 plants. Acknowledged as 'one of the pillars of English botany'[2] the lavish proportions of this work show that there was no real way of evaluating the contents of such books – and the presence of so many remedies suggests that few, if any, were effective.

These several herbals were written when there were no general practitioners of medicine: for there were none, as we would recognize them now, in either Shakespeare's day or the few decades that followed. The physicians, of course, already existed and had been incorporated as a College by Henry VIII in 1518 but the apothecaries grew from within the Grocers' Company and were not freed from it until 1617 (the year after Shakespeare's death) when James I gave the young Society of Apothecaries their Charter. In their turn the general practitioners arose from the Apothecaries who, in 1703 and against great opposition, finally established their right to give medical advice as well as compound and sell remedies. Even at this stage the apothecaries with medical interests had to wait roughly another century before being allowed to charge for their advice. It may be of interest to us today that throughout that century, still not far distant, the common man's 'doctor' who did *not* prescribe at each consultation could guarantee that he would not make a living. Perhaps today's ritual act of prescription has one of its firmest roots in the practices of the eighteenth century.

The Industrial Revolution and the vast changes in social organization in the last quarter of the eighteenth and the first half of the nineteenth centuries led to a growing demand for medical care. This demand gave increased scope to those who could provide what was needed and the new situation showed itself in the Apothecaries Act of 1815 – which so strengthened the Society that it became responsible for the standard of medical practice throughout the country. It is as well that, in the event, these great powers were judiciously and wisely used. We have much to be thankful for in the way that this Society reacted when its great day came. Nevertheless, it was not until the process of medical reform was almost completed by the Medical Act of 1858 that the apothecaries who practised medicine were finally able to leave their shops and become general medical practitioners, akin to those of today. The mid-nineteenth century apothecaries whose interests had remained in the compounding and provision of remedies and medicines then joined forces with the better chemists and druggists of the day to found, in 1841, the Pharmaceutical Society of Great Britain.

We are now so used to thinking of all medical men and women as being university graduates that, despite the long history of the older universities, we are apt to forget that it was not until 1836 that the University of London was enabled to confer medical degrees. It was not until almost 1870 that the, by then, time-honoured system of medical education by apprenticeship finally withered away, to be replaced by full-time undergraduate tuition for all medical students. Previously, among medical people, such university education had been enjoyed by few, apart from the physicians. Even today, when all medical practitioners in Britain are university-trained, the diversity of medical qualifications puzzles American colleagues: in Britain, in witness to this complex history, registerable medical qualifications include not only the medical and surgical degrees of a recognized university but also the conjoint diploma of the Royal Colleges of Physicians and Surgeons and the Licence of the Society of Apothecaries.

The change in the nature and degree of usefulness of the medicines available for use by the medical practitioners of all countries has, of course, been even more recent. In 1910 scientific medicine recognized only three drugs: mercury in syphilis, quinine in malaria, and emetine in amoebic dysentery, as being specific. Of the non-specific, symptomatic remedies – those useful but unable to attack the underlying cause of the disease – aspirin, atropine, cocaine, digitalis, male fern, and morphine were among the most notable – and smallpox vaccine was the most important. Looking back over the long history of the use of medicinal drugs – a history as ancient or older than the earliest civilizations of Egypt and Mesopotamia – it is remarkable that hardly any of the pure and potent drugs of today is older than the First World War.

The period since 1911, when Ehrlich's 'Salvarsan' (compound number 606 in his synthetic series) was first used in the treatment of human syphilis, has therefore seen all of the antibiotics, all of the chemotherapeutic agents, and virtually all of the medicines of modern therapeutics, discovered and developed. The rapidity of the change is amazing – its benefits, and its hazards, things which are fresh with us. If we look back at the translation of the Pharmacopoeia of the Royal College of Physicians of London of 1787, we look at something totally strange. If we look at the first British Pharmacopoeia of 1864 – much less than a century later – we look at something still largely botanical. If we look at the fifth British Pharmacopoeia, of 1914, published in the year of the beginning of the First World War, we still look at something the contents of which leave us listing the few diseases we could treat usefully.

The period of that latter Pharmacopoeia signalled the great change. In the year of 'Salvarsan' Lloyd George's Insurance Act of 1911 produced a situation which fairly soon swamped the then available means of drug supply. The resources of the private pharmacist and the small pharmaceutical company soon became unable to meet the demand. Fairly rapidly the growing commercial resources became the great providers of medicines. In 1922, their resources out-stripped, the Society of Apothecaries finally closed their own pharmacy shop, long established in their premises in Blackfriars Lane, so ending 300 years of pharmaceutical practice.

It would seem that a still greater force than the provision of an insured population brought about the great change. It may be that the existence of an insured or affluent population, and perhaps even some degree of what some would consider the exploitation of such a population, is needed for the rapid growth of the pharmaceutical houses. But this seems to be only a small part of the truth: an industry selling nothing but the strange contents of the eighteenth and nineteenth century pharmacopoeias would have achieved very little. The main reason for the growth of the pharmaceutical industry – and the great centre of interest – has been the provision of effective drugs for conditions that were, until very recently, serious and life-threatening forms of disease.

Although the rate of change may, of itself, have inflamed controversy it seems curious that the industry which has played so large a part in the modern provision of health care should be treated with widespread suspicion. That it is so treated now seems axiomatic: powerful agencies of government have arisen to concern themselves with the efficacy, safety, and quality of drugs; other governmental means are used in an attempt to control the price of drugs; the medical profession and public share concerns regarding the incidence and severity of drug-induced, iatrogenic disease, and the ethics of human experimentation and the economics of the pharmaceutical industry are the sources of a diverse number of studies.

Historically, there is one sense in which the rational pattern of the thought of Newton narrows into the growth of modern medical science, and then narrows again to delineate the worthwhile use of drugs. We can perhaps pick out the wood from the trees in each of the present controversies by following some such historical principle. Preserving that point of view, beginning with a brief review of the early use of drugs, we can follow the changes as the modern pharmacopoeia evolved and consider some of the medicines now included in the World Health Organization's 'Model List of Essential Drugs'. We can also look at the way new drugs are developed today and how that process is regulated by the agencies of government. In doing this we will notice how little the process is influenced by either the prescriber or patient.

In recent years the rate of innovation of major new drugs of real importance seems to have slowed down. This raises the possibility that the regulatory process may have had a harmful effect. During the same period problems with drugs, some of which have had to be withdrawn from the market, seem to have become more noticeable. This might imply that the drug regulatory agencies are setting their standards too low; it also suggests that the prescribers of drugs judge the benefit-to-risk considerations badly. These different possibilities seem worthy of much discussion – bearing in mind that the conquests of disease, when successful, are soon forgotten and the problems that remain, and the price to be paid for success, become all the more obvious.

Some of the residual problems are likely to be overcome if the innovative end of the pharmaceutical industry receives the understanding and help that it merits. But the problems that remain and the price to be paid will carry forward many of the present questions. Is the education of the doctor and the patient adequate for present needs? Are the ethics of patient-care well enough worked out for the next few decades? Has the industry damaged itself with its self-imposed secrecy regarding scientific data and its overemphasized marketing energies? Finally, is an alternative pathway for drug registration needed for the coming century, or for the immediate present?

1

The Ancient World

Prehistory

The first medical activity of which the bones of antiquity provide a record is trephination. Skulls of the New Stone Age, which in the Near East began about 9000 years BC, show that our prehistoric forefathers sometimes survived this operation in which an opening was made through the vault of the skull. An example, from Jericho, and of about 2200 BC, is shown in Figure 1. The subject

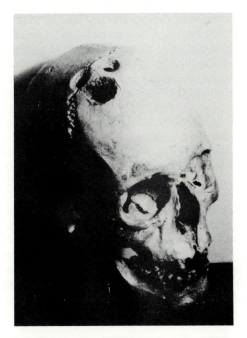

Figure 1   A trepanned skull from about 2200 BC, Jericho. [*Wellcome Institute library, London.*]

was fairly extensively reported by Just Marie Lucas-Championnière (1843–1913) in his *Trépanation néolithique, trépanation pré-Colombienne, trépanation des Kabyles, trépanation traditionnelle*[3] published in Paris in 1912 – this eminent French surgeon being of interest as having been one of the first to adopt the principles of Listerism, and having written the first authoritative work on antiseptic surgery after introducing the practice of antisepsis into France.

In neolithic times these circular or square holes in the skull can have been produced only by using a pointed flint or a flint knife or scraper to drill a ring of small holes and remove a disc of bone or, as seems to have been more common, scraping away at the skull until a piece of bone could be lifted out without damage to the meninges. These skulls are far older than the dawn of the art of writing some 5500 years ago and it is remarkable that few indeed of them show signs of injury or evidence of any other practical reason why this difficult and dangerous operation should have been undertaken: they must be taken to show the considerable lengths to which primitive man, driven by some strange motive of his own, was prepared to go.

A differential diagnosis is provided by Figure 2 which represents skulls, used as holy relics, from the tombs of the eleventh century Anglo-Saxon bishops of Wells. In two cases holes have been cut in the backs of these skulls, probably to make religious amulets from the cut-out roundels[4]. Apart from their location in the skulls (and such pieces of bone could hardly be removed in primitive times from the living) these holes show no sign of new bone formation at their edges, whereas, as shown in Figure 1, many of the Stone and Bronze Age skulls exhibit new bone formation, sometimes closing the trephination; this establishes that some of those who underwent this operation survived to grow new bone.

Why, under such conditions, was it undertaken? The practice is usually said to provide evidence that primitive man believed in the supernatural as a cause of disease and trepanned the skull to let the demon of such disease escape. It seems likely that much primitive medicine arose from equally primitive religion and that many medical practices had their origin in magic. The roundels from the Anglo-Saxon skulls in Figure 2 were presumably intended to transfer sanctity with them. It is also possible (though this is little more than a guess) that trephination was, in prehistoric times, undertaken as a treatment for epilepsy. This illness continued to be known even in the days of classic Greece as the 'divine disease'. Although it shows no feature of divinity that we would now recognize, few things could, to primitive man, look more like demonic possession than the aura, tonus, clonus and recovery of the epileptic fit.

Whatever the exact truth, there is little doubt that these trephined skulls form part of the evidence suggesting that early in his history man looked to some sort of supernatural force for the cause of disease. In seeking a cure he thought that, by intercession, he could influence those same supernatural forces.

Folk medicine has always been, and still is, full of such ideas. It also embodies items of everyday wisdom arising from maternal, hunting, and domestic experience. Some of the early knowledge of plant medicines may have arisen in the same way: from noting what seemed especially helpful in the feeding of the sick.

The practical element may though have been small. Many ideas on medicines seem to have arisen from what we would call magic and a good deal of primitive

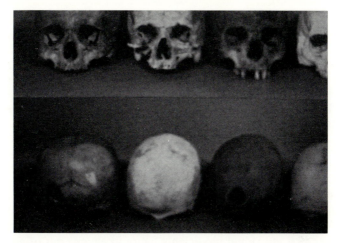

Figure 2 Skulls from the tombs of the eleventh-century Anglo-Saxon bishops of Wells.

medicine arose from early forms of religion. Thus, such medicine had its benign, sensible, practical elements; its bigger proportion of magic, awe and witchcraft – and its ideas of demonic possession and the power of the supernatural. Evidently, these proportions varied from time to time and place to place.

Ancient Egypt

Man slowly emerged from his primitive beginnings to found the oldest Western civilization that we know in the Valley of the Nile roughly sixty centuries ago. James Henry Breasted (1865–1935), later to make a vitally important study of the Edwin Smith Surgical Papyrus, in his *A History of the Ancient Egyptians*[5], says that in the Nile Delta, 'civilization rapidly advanced, and the calendar year of 365 days was introduced in 4241 BC, the earliest fixed date in the history of the world as known to us.'

The religion of the early Egyptians included the worship of the sun (chiefly at On, the Delta city known to the Greeks as Heliopolis) and the moon – the measurer of time, which furnished the god Thoth, god of reckoning, letters, wisdom, and much of medicine. Early in the history of the nation there arose a kind of state religion in which the Pharaoh himself played a supreme part. In parallel with this there gradually evolved a complex and detailed practice of providing for the dead.

From the medical point of view this particular religious practice is of great importance for in no other land, either ancient or modern, has the same attention been given to providing for the dead in their eternal sojourn and voyage as was given in Ancient Egypt. These beliefs form the basis of the great monuments of the Dynasties and Kingdoms of Egypt and provide the grave relics of her successive epochs; they account also for the human remains forming much of our evidence of the diseases of those times.

3

Early in the thirtieth century BC we reach the beginnings of the era of the pyramid builders with the start of the Old Kingdom whose first prominent figure was Zoser, founder of the Third Dynasty. The accession of Zoser was followed by the predominance of the city of Memphis and his success seems to have been due in no small degree to the wise and provident counsel of Imhotep, one of his chief advisers. Breasted, in a passage[6] which caught the attention of William Osler (1849-1919), says of Imhotep that, 'In priestly wisdom, in magic, in the formulation of wise proverbs, in medicine and architecture, this remarkable figure of Zoser's reign left so notable a reputation that his name was never forgotten, and two thousand five hundred years after his death he had become a god of medicine, in whom the Greeks, who called him Imouthes, recognized their own Asklepios.' The reign of Zoser marked the beginning of extensive building in stone and in the desert behind Memphis there stands the monument, 190 feet high, often called 'the terraced pyramid', which is the first great stone structure of history. It is a monument which reminds us not only of Zoser but also of Imhotep, the first individual physicianly figure to emerge out of antiquity, and whose personality became the guide and mentor of medicine in Egypt.

With the passage of time it came to be believed that in their long journey in the afterlife the dead were threatened by many dangers and disasters – and that against these they could be protected by magical formulae. Frequently, such warnings and remedies were written, for the use of the dead, on the inside of the coffin. By the time of the Middle Kingdom, of Dynasties Eleven and Twelve and the period reaching for about 200 years both before and after the year 2000 BC, these formulae were becoming so numerous that the inside of the coffin itself provided inadequate space for them. Thus, from the early days of the First Period of the Empire, beginning about 1580 BC, they were often written on papyrus and placed in the tomb.

Gradually, the best of these texts became used more and more often and were collected together in the so-called 'Book of the Dead'. As more time passed a statuette was sometimes placed in the tomb to do the work, and take the risks, that would otherwise fall to the lot of the deceased. Sometimes a sacred beetle or scarabaeus was cut from stone and inscribed with a charm which could serve the special purpose of protecting the dead from giving witness to his own evil. In the end the 'Book of the Dead' came to contain scenes of judgement – at times complete with the desired verdict of acquittal.

Many of these mortuary relics remain, bearing their own testimony. But the great medical papyri, some of which date from the zenith of the Ancient Egyptian civilization, are even more informative. As is known from Clement of Alexandria (Titus Flavius Clemens; c.150-c.215), who is cited by John Dixon Comrie (1875-1939) in a widely-read article of 1909[7], these great papyri were preceded by the sacred books of Thoth, preserved in the temples and known as the Hermetic Books; of these, 42 in number, 36 were concerned with philosophy and six with medicine. Although at one time carried in the sacred processions by the priest-physicians, these books have all been lost: we must assume that they recorded the remedies learnt over the centuries and the rudiments of pathology gathered in the frequent examination of the dead.

The oldest of the extant papyri is that known as the Kahun and dating from about 1900 BC; it is therefore of the period of the Middle Kingdom. It is located in

London where it was published by Francis Llewellyn Griffith (1862–1934) in his *The Petrie Papyri: Hieratic Papyri from Kahun and Gurob (Principally of the Middle Kingdom)*, of 1898[8]. The Kahun Papyrus consists of only three pages and is in somewhat poor condition; it deals mainly with some aspects of the diseases of women and pregnancy.

The great papyri which provide so much of our knowledge of Ancient Egypt come from a slightly later period and take us back to the early days of the New Empire, roughly 3500 years from our own time. This is the zenith of the civilization of Egypt, the period of the Eighteenth Dynasty, in the sixteenth century BC. Such was the glory of Egypt that Comrie[9] recounts that:

> Her Pharaohs exacted tribute, and her armies marched unhindered from the Libyan desert to the Euphrates, and in this state of external peace and domestic felicity there was opportunity for intercourse with outside nations, – the dwellers in Greece and Crete, for great advance in the technical arts, and for sending forth exploring expeditions which brought back treasure and strange animals from the . . . sources of the Nile.
>
> This period is to be placed two centuries and a half before that epoch familiar to us for the Exodus of Israel from Egypt. To it belong some of the chief literary and monumental remains of this country, and during it the Egyptians attained to a level of thought and of executive skill which they did not at any time surpass, save under Greek influence in the Ptolemaic period, more than a thousand years later.

The first of the vastly important papyri is the Edwin Smith Papyrus of about 1600 BC. It is now in New York and was published in a magnificent edition by James Henry Breasted as *The Edwin Smith Surgical Papyrus: Published in Facsimile and Hieroglyphic Transliteration with Translation and Commentary*[10]. The original papyrus was acquired by the accomplished Egyptologist, Edwin Smith (1822–1906) in Luxor in 1862. It forms an astonishing document providing 17 columns of hieratic writing with four columns on the verso. The main text provides a well-organized surgical dissertation describing 48 typical cases and giving cosmetic formulations on the verso.

From the physician's point of view the Ebers Papyrus, of about 1550 BC, is perhaps the most important papyrus of all. Now at Leipzig, it was acquired by Georg Ebers (1837–1898) and, by him, was published in the sumptuous facsimile entitled *Papyros Ebers: Das Hermetische Buch über die Arzeneimittel der Alten Ägypter in Hieratischer Schrift*, published in Leipzig in 1875[11]. The much-reduced title page of this beautiful work is shown in Figure 3 and the prescriptions from the second page of the Papyrus, but taken from the facsimile of Ebers, are illustrated in Figure 4.

The original seems to represent a complete medical text derived from a number of much earlier sources. It provides 108 columns (although the scribe has numbered them 110). The text starts with three general 'recitals', or incantations, to increase the efficacy of some of the remedies; these are followed by some hundreds of recipes grouped according to the presenting illness or problem. Altogether there are 829 prescriptions, a few of which are duplicated. Some of the illnesses mentioned cannot be exactly identified and the translators have had to make intelligent suppositions; in a similar way many of the ingredients of the

PAPYROS EBERS

DAS HERMETISCHE BUCH

ÜBER

DIE ARZENEIMITTEL DER ALTEN ÄGYPTER

IN

HIERATISCHER SCHRIFT.

HERAUSGEGEBEN, MIT INHALTSANGABE UND EINLEITUNG VERSEHEN

VON

GEORG EBERS.

MIT HIEROGLYPHISCH-LATEINISCHEM GLOSSAR

VON

LUDWIG STERN.

MIT UNTERSTÜTZUNG DES KÖNIGLICH SÄCHSISCHEN CULTUSMINISTERIUM.

ERSTER BAND.

EINLEITUNG UND TEXT, TAFEL 1—LXIX.

LEIPZIG,

VERLAG VON WILHELM ENGELMANN.

1875.

Figure 3 Georg Ebers. Title page from: *Papyros Ebers: Das Hermetische Buch über die Arzeneimittel der Alten Ägypter in Hieratischer Schrift.* (1875), Vol. I. [*Royal Society of Medicine library, London.*]

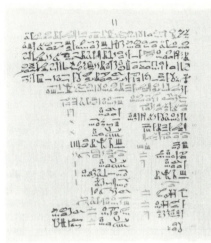

Figure 4   Georg Ebers. Prescriptions on the second page of the Ebers Papyrus.

different prescriptions remain unknown. The text ends with an account of diseases of women, some anatomical monographs and, finally, some comments on surgical diseases.

In the original the so-called hieratic writing has been used, the characters being exceptionally beautiful and clear; headings and such items are given in red ink, whereas the rest of the text is black. The writing is from right to left, the two-coloured system providing a text which is easy to follow and a design antecedent to the rubric of the mediaeval manuscripts and our finely printed books. The original papyrus was 20.23 m long and 30 cm high. The document is dated from part of a calendar with a king's name on the reverse.

An unexpected and interesting feature is that, despite the massive number of remedies for the diseases of internal medicine, there is virtually no account of the diseases themselves. It is as if the patient presents with a complaint, the nature of which is obvious to him, and the physician provides a remedy for it. Exactly the same thing is to be observed in the market-places of simple communities today. Many of the remedies are, therefore, intentionally symptomatic. A few syndromes are described but it is clear that this approach is in its infancy: the physician treated cough, unwanted expectoration, or wheezing without the knowledge or means to differentiate bronchitis, pneumonia or phthisis.

A considerable list of possibly active drugs is provided in the text, along with many inert and strange materials. Comrie[12] gives the following list of well-known substances as appearing in the Ebers Papyrus and other medical papyri:

> Sulphate, oxide, and other salts of lead used as astringents and demulcents; pomegranate and acanthus pith as vermifuges; sulphate and acetate of copper; magnesia, lime, soda, iron and nitre; oxide of antimony, sulphide of mercury;

peppermint, fennel, absinth, thyme, cassia, coriander, carraway, juniper, cedar wood oil, turpentine and many other essential oils; gentian and other bitters; mandrake, hyoscyamus, opium with other hypnotics and anodynes; linseed, castor oil, squills, colchicum, mustard, onion, nasturtium, tamarisk, frankincense, myrrh, yeast. Besides these are many drugs, especially essential oils, which probably were valuable remedies, but of which the names, being highly technical, are impossible, so far, to translate.

Among external applications were – the knife, the actual cautery, niassage, ointments, plasters, poultices, suppositories, enemata, inhalations, and the vaginal douche and fumigation.

Such a list less than fully prepares one for the prescriptions themselves. These can readily be studied in the very accessible translation of Bendix Ebbell whose *The Papyrus Ebers: The Greatest Egyptian Medical Document* was published in 1937[13]; Ebbell prepared his translation from the hieroglyphic transcript[14] of Walter Wreszinski (*Der Papyrus Ebers: Umschrift, Übersetzung und Kommentar*). In looking at a small number of the translated prescriptions we came across the Egyptian methods of pharmaceutical measurement – always, it would appear, measures of volume or capacity, and not weight, even for dry materials. One of the most common such measures was the 'ro', or mouthful, now the spoonful that provides about 15 ml. (In the following quotations from Ebbell's text the standard measure of quantity is shown by a vertical stroke and some words left untranslated.)

From the recitals at the beginning of the Papyrus; this one was to be used when drinking a remedy:

> Recital on drinking a remedy: Come remedy! Come thou who expellest (evil) things in this my stomach and in these my limbs! The spell is powerful over the remedy. Repeat it backwards! Dost thou remember that Horus and Seth have been conducted to the big palace at Heliopolis, when there was negotiated of Seth's testicles with Horus, and he shall get well like one who is on earth. He does all that he may wish like these gods who are there. – Spoken when drinking a remedy. Really excellent, (proved) many times!

Three examples from the large number given of remedies to open the bowels:

> fresh dates |, northern salt |, *šbbt*-fluid, | are mixed with water and placed in a *mḥt*-vessel; powder of senna is added to it, boiled together and put into a box or a *bȝw*-vessel; is eaten by the man when finger-warm and swallowed with sweet beer.
>
> Another: colocynth 4 ro, honey 8 ro, are ground fine, eaten by the man and swallowed with sweet beer.
>
> Another: malachite |, is ground fine, put into bread-dough, made into 3 pills and swallowed by the man and gulped down with sweet beer.

From the prescriptions for killing roundworm:

> To kill roundworm (Ascaris lumbricoides): root of pomegranate 5 ro, water 10 ro, remains during the night in the dew, is strained and taken in 1 day.
>
> Another: Upper Egyptian barley 5 ro, northern salt 2½ ro, water 10 ro, likewise.

8

Another: juice of acacia 5 ro, water 10 ro, remains during the night in the dew, is strained and taken in 1 day.

To expel pains caused by roundworm or tapeworm:

Another to expel pains caused by roundworm or tape-worm (tænia): powder of hyoscyamus |, the best of ' *mꜣw* |, goose-fat |, are mixed together, strained and eaten for 4 days.

To expel pains caused by tape-worm: juice of acacia |, leaves of *iꜣjw* |, '*fꜣ* |, *dꜣjś* |, are pounded together and the belly of a woman or a man is bandaged with it.

Examples from those to control fever, purulency, the rose (? erysipelas), and an ointment for the latter:

Another to expel evil fever: alum |, red ochre |, fruit of tamarisk |, natron |, salt |, are mixed together and given against it.

Another to clear out purulency: hyoscyamus 2 ro, dates 4 ro, beer *śḥr* 10 ro, fruit of sycamore 4 ro, wine 5 ro, ass's milk 20 ro, are boiled, strained and taken for 4 days.

Another to clear out purulency in the belly and eradicate the root of the rose (?) in the belly of a man or woman: powder of roasted manna 8 ro, colocynth 4 ro, sweet powder 4 ro, powder of dates 4 ro, goosegrease 8 ro, honey 8 ro, are ground together and eaten in 1 day.

Another ointment: *śʿt*-cake of roasted barley, roasted flax (?), roasted ammi, *śpdw*-stone, milk of (a woman) who has borne a male (child), fresh balanites-oil, are boiled and (it) is anointed herewith for 7 days.

Three prescriptions from those concerned with the urinary tract:

The beginning of remedies to remove retention of the urine, when the hypogastric region is painful: wheat 4 ro, dates 8 ro, toasted manna 8 ro, water 24 ro, are ground, strained and taken for 4 days.

Another to cause a child to evacuate an accumulation of urine which is in his belly: an old letter boiled with oil, his belly is rubbed, until his urination is in order.

Another to bring in order the urine of a child: pith which is in a reed, is rubbed out all through with a *ḥꜣw*-bowl of sweet beer in coagulation and is drunk by the woman; it is given to the child in a hin-vessel.

And two medicines to alleviate asthma:

Another: figs 4 ro, sebesten 4 ro, grapes 4 ro, sycamore-fruit 4 ro, frankincense ½ ro, cumin ½ ro, fruit of juniperus 2 ro, wine 2½ ro, goosegrease 4 ro, sweet beer 5 ro, are ground, mixed together, strained and taken for 4 days.

Another: '*mꜣw* 5 ro, fresh bread 2½ ro, yellow ochre 1 ro, fruit of juniperus 4 ro, oil 5 ro, northern salt 8 ro, are mixed together, strained and taken for 4 days.

9

A possibly useful recipe and a probably harmful one from the section on diseases of the eyes:

> Another for night-blindness in the eyes: liver of ox, roasted and crushed out, is given against it. Really excellent!

> Another for blindness: pig's eyes, its humour is fetched, real stibium |, red ochre |, lees of honey |, are ground fine, mixed together and poured into the ear of the man, so that he may be cured immediately. Do (it) and thou shalt see.

A further inappropriate one for the eyes:

> Another for not letting hair grow in the eye, after it has been pulled out: fly's dirt |, red ochre |, urine |, are pounded and applied to this place of the hair, after it has been pulled out.

Two examples concerned with the hair:

> Another to make the hair of a bald-headed person grow: fat of lion |, fat of hippopotamus |, fat of crocodile |, fat of cat |, fat of serpent |, fat of ibex |, are mixed together, and the head of a bald person is anointed therewith.
> Another to make the hair grow for spotted baldness: burnt quills of hedgehog with oil, the head is anointed therewith for 4 days.

An example suggesting that ideas on wound healing were limited to producing union by second intention:

> Remedy for a wound the first day: grease of ox – or ox-beef – until it (i.e. the wound) suppurates; but if it suppurates (too) much, then thou shalt bandage it with sour barleybread, until it is dried thereby; then thou shalt again bandage it with grease, until it suppurates. But if it closes (i.e. an incrustation is formed) over its effluency, then thou shalt bandage it with grease of ibex, turpentine, *thwj,* is ground.

Finally, three examples, from the many given, of remedies to improve the skin:

> Another to improve the skin: honey |, red natron |, northern salt |, are ground together, and the body is rubbed therewith.
> Another to beautify the body: powder of alabaster |, powder of natron |, northern salt |, honey |, are mixed together with this honey, and the body is anointed therewith.
> Another to expel wrinkles of the face: gum of frankincense |, wax |, fresh balanites-oil |, rush-nut |, are ground fine, put in viscous fluid and applied to the face every day. Make (it) and thou shalt see.

These several sets of examples, chosen mainly from those prescriptions with few untranslated words, inadequately represent a long, complex text – itself a moderately early translation. The original text is almost certainly that compiled by a scribe from a number of sources for an individual practitioner: its sources

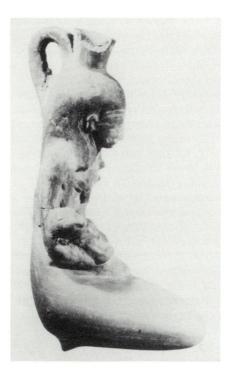

Figure 5   Jar in which was kept 'the milk of a woman who had borne a male child'. (Isis, with her son from Osiris after his death.) [*From: Paul Ghalioungui, Magic and medical science in Ancient Egypt. London, Hodder and Stoughton, (1963).*]

may range from the recipes used by the finest physicians of the day to those of the market-place. There are items, usually ingredients, that would seem appropriate to us: senna is used as a bowel evacuant, hyoscyamus to relieve the pain of smooth muscle spasm, and the list (already quoted) of Comrie included iron, opium, castor oil, colchicum, yeast, and other items likely to be of use – had the knowledge of their properties been available. Liver was used in the treatment of night-blindness without any knowledge of vitamins.

Such rational elements in this long list of remedies seem few and far between – but some of them may not be obvious to us because we may miss useful, active substances by being unfamiliar with some of the botany.

There is clearly a great deal of what we must call magic: the milk of a woman who has carried a male child is used as a specific ingredient, more than once mentioned, and it is thought that there were special vessels, as shown in Figure 5, in which this milk was kept. These jars are in the shape of a young woman (Isis) nursing on her lap a child, probably a weakling (the son of Isis by Osiris after his death). Many other items are clearly expected to be effective because of this reasoning by attribute and association.

The recitals and spells which are present are almost always there to intensify the healing virtue of the remedy. It is as if the bulk of diseases are thought to be due to physical causes, to be tackled by natural means, augmented by religious reference. It is perhaps what might be expected from a people who believed that by actions taken in the natural world the departed could be helped and preserved in the afterlife. Seldom, apart from epilepsy, does there seem to be obvious belief in frank demonic possession or resort to exorcism.

Despite all this, few can forget reading Ebbell, and these strange prescriptions, for the first time. The dichotomy between a long civilization, capable of great art, architecture, culture, and social order – and this very primitive pharmacology, is not readily forgotten. There are later translations and later papyri, but before considering these (briefly, for they make no fundamental difference to our first impression) we can look at the identity of some of the diseases treated in those distant days of the rise and splendour of Egypt.

Much of our knowledge comes from the mummies of Egypt and arises, like the beginnings of anatomical knowledge, from the ritual by which the dead were preserved for the afterlife. The brilliance of Greek scientific enquiry, reaching its peak in the sixth to fourth centuries before Christ, achieved nothing, as far as the knowledge of anatomy is concerned, in its native land. It was the Egyptian tradition of opening the dead which permitted the later dissections of the cadaver in Alexandria and, had it not been for the distinctive beliefs of the Ancient Egyptians in the need to preserve the body for survival after death, they would neither have begun a crude knowledge of anatomy nor left us the mummified remnants of their pathology.

However, this anatomical knowledge was nothing but an accident and the result of techniques used in mummification: the Egyptian embalmer was purely a sacerdotal technician deriving his knowledge from his ritual. In his article *Ancient Egypt and the Origin of Anatomical Science*[15] Alexander James Cave notes that the Egyptians had specific names for the 'heart, lung, kidney, bladder, stomach, bowel, uterus, vagina, diaphragm, spinal cord, brain, cerebral convolutions, and meninges'; he observes that they wrote these terms with animal determinatives, showing that they recognized the similarities between human and animal anatomy. Cave adds, before commenting on the scientific studies of anatomy which were undertaken in the period 300 BC–AD 150, that we should not misunderstand the almost accidental earlier information of Egypt: 'There is so far no substantial evidence from the records of any inherent scientific interest by the Egyptians in any branch of natural knowledge'[16].

The classic text of Sir Grafton Elliot Smith (1871–1937) and Warren Royal Dawson (1888–1968), *Egyptian Mummies*[17], reproduces the Egyptian Funeral Procession from the Theban tomb of Haremhab of the Eighteenth Dynasty (Figure 6); detailed accounts of this symbolic journey across the Nile have been widely given but the work, from the tomb discovered in 1908 at Biban-el-Molûk, speaks for itself. Elliot Smith and Dawson, mainly by means of a number of woodcuts, provide illustrations which include the head of the mummy of Ramesses V, showing a dense eruption which is probably smallpox; the mummy of a very elderly woman of the Twenty-first Dynasty, where the embalmers have covered bedsores with patches of gazelle-skin; the liver, showing gallstones, from a mummy of the Twenty-first Dynasty; the mummy of a priest of Amen, of the same dynasty, but afflicted with Pott's Disease of the spine; a vertebral body showing tuberculous caries from a mummy of the Middle Kingdom; an

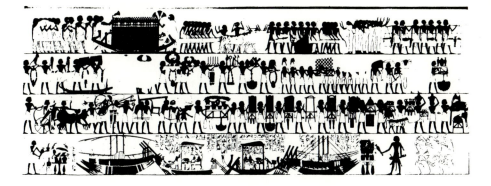

Figure 6: Egyptian funeral procession – from the Theban Tomb of Haremhab, Eighteenth Dynasty. [*From: Grafton Elliot Smith and Warren Royal Dawson, Egyptian mummies. London, Allen and Unwin, (1924).*]

osteosarcoma of the femur from a Fifth-Dynasty mummy; the talipes, or club-foot, of the Pharaoh Siptah; the gross bone changes, due to leprosy, in a mummy of the sixth century AD from Nubia; a predynastic skull with the mastoid process destroyed by disease, and the fractured forearm of a Fifth-Dynasty mummy with the bones still encased in crude wooden splints. Earlier, in 1908, Elliot Smith had provided a complete paper on *The Most Ancient Splints*[18].

The Edwardian era was bright with the results of the exploration of Egypt and Sir William Osler (1849–1919), in his *The Evolution of Modern Medicine*[19] of 1921, provided a picture of the mummy of the priest of Amen, already mentioned, marking this as showing a 'Spinal Curvature'. Osler also noted[20] that, 'One of the most prevalent . . .' of the diseases of Egypt 'appears to have been osteo-arthritis. . . . The majority of the lesions appear to have been the common osteo-arthritis, which involved not only the men, but many of the pet animals kept in the temples.' But the priest's curvature was more than just that and Elliot Smith with Sir Marc Armand Ruffer (1859–1917), in a contribution *Pott'sche Krankheit an einer ägyptischen Mumie* of 1910, showed that this was a case of Pott's spine with a massive psoas abscess – the abscess being (Figure 7) on the right side of the eviscerated abdominal cavity of the mummy and tracking down from the tuberculous spine[21].

Ruffer noted another disease present in old Egypt. Having already described a process by which mummified tissues could be prepared for histological examination, and reporting that in mummies of the Eighteenth to Twentieth Dynasties 'atheroma, pneumonia, renal abscesses, and cirrhosis of the liver are plainly recognizable', he found, in 1910, that the kidneys of two mummies of the Twentieth Dynasty exhibited the calcified eggs of *Bilharzia haematobia*[22]. Thus, the great infectious diseases mingled with the degenerative diseases in Ancient Egypt. The latter kind of illness was highlighted by Samuel George Shattock (1852–1924) who, in 1909, demonstrated to the Pathology Section of the Royal Society of Medicine, a set of microscope sections of the aorta of King Menephtah, the reputed Pharaoh of the Exodus. These sections showed[23] 'senile calcification of the aorta, the bony, parallel, elastic lamellae being perfectly

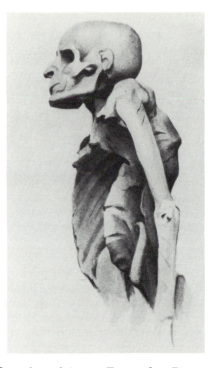

Figure 7 Mummy of a priest of Amen, Twenty-first Dynasty, afflicted with Pott's disease. [*From: Grafton Elliot Smith and Marc Armand Ruffer. Pott'sche Krankheit an einer ägyptischen Mumie. Giessen, A. Töpelmann, (1910).*]

preserved, and the interlamellar material thickly strewn with calcium phosphate.' Menephtah was an old man, but Egypt clearly knew arteriosclerosis.

Ruffer, in *Studies in the Palaeopathology of Egypt*, edited by Roy Lee Moodie (1880–1934) and published in 1921[24], brought together a collection of papers which had appeared in various journals; this work, with the later writings of its editor, forms one of the most important contributions to the subject. Among these later writings *Paleopathology: An Introduction to the Study of Ancient Evidences of Disease*[25] provided an extensive section on diseases of the Ancient Egyptians; this book provided a biographical sketch and memorial to Sir Marc Armand Ruffer.

It is clear that the prescriptions of the papyri, despite the benign climate of Egypt and the hygiene of its inhabitants, had to be used against a very wide range of the gravest human diseases.

A curiosity was the medicinal use of human mummy. The virtues of natural black bituminous material exuded from the earth in certain places, and in Latin called *mumia*, were discussed by the Greeks, later regarded as a panacea by the Persians, and described as 'mummy' until quite modern times. From late Ptolemaic times bituminous materials were used for embalming and it seems that the cures attributed to *mumia* were attributed also to the mummified. Elliot Smith and Dawson ascribe the earliest use of mummy as a drug to a Jewish physician of

Alexandria about AD 1200[26]. The practice became common and a source of both trade and fraud. Thomas Joseph Pettigrew (1791–1865), in his *History of Egyptian Mummies*[27], provides a considerable discussion of the subject in what was the first major monograph on mummies before the study of Elliot Smith and Dawson 90 years later. It is, of course, evident that the records of ancient pathology are grossly incomplete, favouring those diseases which affect bone. A reliable account of these conditions and the pathology of the Ancient Egyptians and Nubians was given by G. Elliot Smith and Frederic Wood Jones in the Annual Report for 1907–8, *The Archaeological Survey of Nubia: Report on the Human Remains*[28] – a special volume of 374 pages, with maps, the plates being separately bound.

Late in the nineteenth century it was suggested that syphilis, one of the diseases most likely to leave its marks on teeth and bones, existed in Ancient Egypt: the discussion of the turn of the century ended with Grafton Elliot Smith's paper to the *Lancet* (*The alleged discovery of syphilis in prehistoric Egyptians*) of 1908, in which he refuted earlier reports with the statement that 'syphilis did not occur in Egypt' before contact with Europe was established[29]. Elliot Smith was, in fact, demonstrating that the bony appearances previously thought to be due to syphilis were probably due to the attack of insects ages after the bones had been buried.

Even if they escaped syphilis, the Egyptians suffered not only the many illnesses already mentioned but also gout, adhesions from an appendix abscess, pleural adhesions – as shown in different mummies – and frequent arthritis, perhaps the most common disease shown in these human remains. Trauma was also frequent and the skull lesions described in the *British Medical Journal* for 1908 by F. Wood Jones (*The examination of the bodies of 100 men executed in Nubia in Roman times*)[30] remain memorable if the photographs are inspected.

The Hearst Medical Papyrus caught the interest of the pharmacologist Chauncey D. Leake (1896–1978), author of *The Old Egyptian Medical Papyri*[31] of 1952. Leake and his colleagues had been stimulated by Breasted's splendid analysis of the Edwin Smith Surgical Papyrus of 1930. Breasted's remarkable work was clearly impressive and had a lasting effect on Leake's own views. Part of the reason for this was that the main text of the Edwin Smith Papyrus shows a degree of professionalism and an absence of demonology that makes it almost unique. Even primitive and superstitious man understood that surgical conditions, such as broken bones, are not mended by spells – and the so-called Surgical Papyrus is, in its main text, consistently more rational than many of the other papyri. Leake has this to say[32]: 'There was magic endeavour in approaching disease popularly in old Egypt just as there is now in our culture. On the other hand, there is clear evidence from the surviving documents of a rational professional effort toward the systematic analyses of diseased conditions and toward the application of empirical observation in their management.'

The Hearst Papyrus, of about 1550 BC, is incomplete and exists in 18 columns, but is frayed at the beginning and end; it was first described by George Reisner (1867–1942), who received it when he led the Hearst Expedition to Egypt in 1899. It contains a greater number of invocations and recitals than the Ebers Medical Papyrus and has about 255 prescriptions intended for a great variety of medical conditions. They are poorly organized and a number of times repeated.

Some of them occur in the Ebers as well as the Berlin Medical Papyri.

Hearst is, therefore, a practitioner's recipe book and Leake, who was preoccupied with it for a number of years, wrote that[33]:

> Therapeutic principles are usually based on etiological considerations. The old Egyptians, like most primitive people, had clear and reasonably sound methods of handling direct external physical disabilities, such as fractures and injuries resulting from falls, or from such obvious causes as blows. About these matters there was apparently no uncertainty, no speculation regarding appropriate methods, no 'magic', no irrational nor superstitious procedure. Primitive surgery and obstetrics seem quite generally to be of this character. On the other hand, internal disorders, particularly what we now call infectious diseases, have no obvious etiology. Their onset is usually insidious and not readily to be correlated with any specific circumstance. Under these conditions it is not surprising that speculation and fear should inspire conviction of supernatural causes, with resulting and logical use of supernatural and magical methods of treatment. A demoniacal etiology for disease requires treatment directed toward expelling the demon or appeasing it. Thus magical procedures are a natural and logical feature of that portion of primitive medicine concerned with internal diseases.

Leake's figures show that the Ebers Papyrus quantified 72% of its prescriptions (599 of its 829). The Hearst Papyrus, of the same period, gave drug amounts in 47% of its prescriptions (121 of its 255) – most of its non-quantitative recipes being for external application.

The Hearst Papyrus is now at Berkeley and was studied by G. A. Reisner in 1905[34], by Wreszinski in 1912[35] and later, after World War II, by Leake and a number of others.

The later Egyptian papyri include that of Erman (about 1550 BC and now in Berlin); the London (of about 1350 BC); the Berlin (of roughly 1350 BC) and the Chester Beatty (of about 1200 BC) now in London. The last of these was carefully reviewed by Frans Jonckheere in a study published in 1947[36].

Each of these documents, interesting in itself, makes no fundamental difference to the conclusion. Neither do the studies of more recent years greatly modify the overall initial impression gained of the papyri. These later studies include the magnificent analyses of the seven professional Egyptian medical papyri (omitting the markedly superstitious Erman Papyrus) of the German Egyptologist, Herman Grapow. Grapow's works culminated, after a long series of publications, in the *Grundriss der Medizin der alten Ägypter*, of which the first volume appeared in 1954[37]. We have also the fine summaries of the main papyri in *A History of Medicine*[38], the study on a grand scale by Henry Ernest Sigerist (1891–1957), of which the first two volumes were of 1951 and a decade later.

These summaries and analyses with the writings of other commentators – and especially those of Steuer and Saunders (1959)[39] – make it evident that early and primitive attempts at therapy are, in internal medicine, frequently directed by aetiological concepts of the cause of disease. Edward Theodore Withington (1860–1947), in his *Medical History from the Earliest Times*[40], commenting on the Berlin Papyrus, wrote that it 'somewhat resembles that of Ebers, but is smaller and of later date. It contains 170 prescriptions, no less than 28 being enemata, a form of medication the origin of which was universally ascribed to the Egyptians.' He also noticed that 'the most remarkable thing about Egyptian medicine is its non-progressive character. More than 1000 years before Hippocrates we find a knowledge of anatomy and physiology quite equal to that of the Father of Medicine, together with a copious and varied materia medica, comprising mineral as well as vegetable remedies; yet . . . the Greek physicians of Alexandria seem to have learnt nothing from the Egyptians, and Galen mentions their medical writings with contempt. Let us try to find some causes for this remarkable failure.'[41]

These causes, the aetiological considerations, and the Egyptian professional use of enemata are, it appears, linked by a common intellectual concept. Ebbell, writing of the Ebers Papyrus, showed the use of bowel cleansing to have been entirely rational[42]:

> Among the drugs evacuative remedies were dominating. They are not only prescribed for diseases in the intestinal tract, but in many cases where it seems absurd for us to use laxantia, thus for several skin-diseases, for instance exudation, eating ulcer and spotted baldness. This was certainly due to the Egyptians, like the ancient Greeks, imagining that these and other ailments were caused by certain disease-producing humours or a *materia peccans* in the belly, and that it was thus necessary to have this unsound matter removed by means of purgation.

Robert O. Steuer and J. B. de C. M. Saunders, in the brilliant monograph already mentioned (*Ancient Egyptian and Cnidian Medicine: The Relationship of their Aetiological Concepts of Disease*) complete the explanation with their discovery of the meaning of the Egyptian technical term *whdw*[43]:

> In the transition of Ancient Egyptian medicine from magico-religious concepts to empirico-rational practice, there came into existence a technical medical term, *whdw*, which represents an idea of great significance in the preliminary and tentative gropings of the mind of man toward a scientific theory of internal disease and the development of a rational therapy. This well-known term had been interpreted variously by Egyptologists and medical historians, doubtless conditioned by contemporary views of specific nosological entities, as leprosy, smallpox, syphilis, or as a symptom, pain, or inflammation. We were able to establish in a previous study that the term actually refers to a basic aetiological principle or materia peccans adherent to the fecal content of the bowel. On absorption, this was believed to cause the coagulation and destruction of the blood, leading to the suppurative conditions with which Egypt abounds, or to the eventual putrefaction and corruption of the body.

Beginning perhaps in the Egyptian ideas of the prevention of bodily putrefaction by mummification, and transposed from religion to medicine when even professionally these subjects were close, we have a fully-grown, non-magical aetiological theory, showing a natural, physical cause for the diseases of internal medicine, and developed from the apparent putrefaction of the bowel. Cadaveric putrefaction and the suppuration of pathology were united and the concept of *wḥdw* forms the rationale of the Ancient Egyptian physician.

The idea of a putrefactive essence or principle spreading from the bowel to the bloodstream and thence to the bodily tissues, as we would call them, led the physicians to resort to emetics, purges and enemata and, once the pyogenic principle had contaminated the vascular channels, to blood-letting. Throughout the Dark Ages, almost until modern times, the sick were weakened by the venesection that was part of this kind of ritual.

These ideas add a good deal of significance to the prescriptions which, in the Ebers Papyrus, aim 'to clear out purulency in the belly' (p. 9). In the terms of Ancient Egyptian medical belief this may have seemed entirely rational.

The ideas persisted, providing the Middle Ages with a tradition of blood-letting and peculiar means of therapeutics. Another Egyptian legacy, but one which remains part of modern medicine, is the conventional symbol for a prescription or medical recipe – $\textrm{R}_x$. This sign, a direct descendant from the earliest days, is the slightly modified symbol representing the eye, the Egyptian symbol of sacrifice, which, according to the myth of Osiris, the youthful god Horus lost in his battle with the transcendent god Set.

The changing interpretations of what Ancient Egyptian medicine might have meant can be followed in the writings of authors working in successive decades in the century that has resulted in modern therapeutics. Withington (1894), writing before more than a handful of specifics were known[44], commented on the 'remarkable failure' of medicine in Egypt and its essentially 'non-progressive character'. He could find little to explain these things except the 'predominance of the priesthood' and the fact that the 'learned Egyptian was, before all things, a scribe or writer'. He considers the Greek, as a man of speech and argument, likely to do profoundly better than these generations of copyists.

Charles Singer (1876–1960), began his book, *A Short History of Medicine* (1928)[45], with the very direct statement 'Scientific Medicine began with the Greeks.' However, Singer acknowledged that the Greek debt to the civilization of Egypt was considerable. He expresses the debt in this way[46]:

> Many drugs were derived from Egypt and others were suggested by Egyptian practice. The basis of Greek medical ethics, too, can be traced to Egypt. Some of the practical devices of Greek Medicine, such as the forms of the surgical instruments, were of Egyptian origin. Nor can we neglect the statement made by the Greeks themselves, that mathematical knowledge – the test and index of all scientific growth – came to them first from Egypt. Lastly, we note that the Egyptians deified a physician, Imhotep, in exactly the way that the Greeks deified their physician, Aesculapius.

Ebbell (1937) developed much the same thought from his translation[47] of the Ebers Papyrus:

> It must then at once be pointed out that Greek medicine is by no means so original as people were formerly inclined to believe, but that a very great deal of it has been taken over from the ancient Egyptians. This is especially conspicuous in *materia medica*; an overwhelming number of remedies in the medical papyri are found in Dioskurides and are prescribed against exactly the

same diseases, so there can be no doubt that the Greeks must have borrowed them from the Egyptians.

By 1952, Leake, a pharmacologist, was impressed with the rational nature of the Egyptian achievement and the standard of practice[48]:

> From the evidence available, it would appear that (1) the ancient Egyptian physicians were relatively keen and accurate observers; (2) they possessed a systematic method of examination; (3) they were exploring the principles of diagnosis; (4) they had an idea of the significance of prognosis, and thus were aware of the natural course of untreated disease, and (5) they had accumulated a large body of tested agents and methods for the treatment and management of sickness. It is surprising that there is not more evidence of supernaturalism in the medical papyri. The various 'recitals' may reasonably be interpreted as 'prayers' for skill and guidance, not only in regard to handling the patient but also in respect to the measurement of drugs. Taken as a whole the evidence from the papyri indicates a relatively high standard of medical practice in old Egypt.

Nevertheless, he notes that 'Poppy seeds seem to have been used as carminatives. Opium, with its active alkaloids, can only be obtained by natural drying of the juice of the unripe seed capsule of the poppy. This was apparently not known to the old Egyptians.'[49] The point is of great interest – opium being perhaps the most useful drug from antiquity. The first clear account of its preparation seems to have been that of Scribonius Largus (*c.* AD 1–50)[50].

Henry Ernest Sigerist[51] continues to take his quotations of the Ebers Papyrus from the translation of Ebbell – showing the continued importance of the 1937 Englishing of the old text. However, it is in the more recent of the studies of these twentieth century authors that we find the most tentative and cautious conclusions of all: Paul Ghalioungui, writing as Senior Professor of Medicine at Ain Shams University, Cairo, and with medical qualifications from both Cairo and London, in his *Magic and Medical Science in Ancient Egypt*[52] questions 'the possibility of some day seeing our way clearly in Ancient Egyptian Medicine.' He notes the many items the Greeks inherited from Egypt and adds: 'If the Egyptian soil revealed one day all its secrets, if the Sphinx could break its silence, if the tattered, crumbling or lost papyri would re-assemble . . . we should be entitled to give a verdict on what Ancient Egyptian medicine was, and on the place it occupied in the origins of modern thought'[53].

In the present state of knowledge there is obviously something attractive about this level of reticence: any judgement we might now make rests only on the remnants of what was, for centuries, a populous civilization. But, with these limitations, what might be made of these very significant remains?

Osler, as if teaching the meaning of *wḥdw* but lecturing in 1913, concluded that the 'Egyptian civilization illustrates how crude and primitive may remain a knowledge of disease when conditioned by erroneous views of its nature'[54]. When a hypothesis becomes a belief, and the scribes or printers transmit that belief, then a high civilization can indeed contain a remarkably crude and primitive medicine.

If we think of the strange materia medica and the curious prescriptions of the Ebers and other medical papyri, the mind might recall the prophet Jeremiah who said of the virgin daughter of Egypt, 'in vain shalt thou use many medicines; for thou shalt not be cured'[55].

Mesopotamia

At much the same time as the Valley of the Nile was providing one cradle of human civilization, Mesopotamia, on the eastern side of the vast land mass of Arabia, was providing another. Mesopotamia comprised the fertile lands between the Tigris and Euphrates which, at their southern limits, join together to form the Shatt-el-Arab flowing into the Persian Gulf – the arm of the Indian Ocean lying between Persia and Arabia. Mesopotamia, roughly modern Iraq, was itself formed of the two ancient kingdoms of Babylonia, to the south, and the more northerly area of Assyria.

Babylonia corresponds to the southern plain lying between modern Baghdad and the Persian Gulf; Assyria lay to the north around present-day Mosul. Both of these great kingdoms took their names from their capital cities – Babylon, to the south, and Ashur in Assyria. West of these kingdoms were the vast areas of Syria and Arabia; to the East, lay Armenia, Media, and Persia (now Iran) – with Parthia still further to the East.

Within each of the Mesopotamian kingdoms there were great cities: Nineveh, the ancient monument of Assyria, on the left bank of the Tigris, opposite Mosul; and Babylon, capital of the Babylonian Empire, standing on both banks of the Euphrates, some 60 miles south of modern Baghdad. Babylon was of such legendary beauty that its hanging gardens were numbered among the seven wonders of the Ancient World. Older still was the Sumerian city of Ur – the biblical 'Ur of the Chaldees' is usually identified with it. Ur was located on the Euphrates, about 150 miles south-east of Babylon, and its excavations have revealed the great temple (about 2300 BC) with its *ziggurat*, or stage tower. C. Leonard Woolley, in his interestingly illustrated article *Babylonian Prophylactic Figures*[56], of 1926, showed, from the discoveries at Ur, the ancient Babylonian custom of burying beneath the floor of the house small clay models and figures which would secure the home and its occupants against sickness and evil spirits.

It is said that it was from the city of Ur that Terah and his son Abraham set out for Canaan, their long migration taking them, at first, north-west along the course of the Euphrates to Haran, in northern Syria, where – far to the north of Canaan – Abraham and his family first settled (Figure 8).

Comrie (1909) speaks[57] of Assyria as 'those lands inhabited by peoples of Semitic race who contended for many centuries with one another for the plains of the Euphrates and the Tigris, and who strove for mutual annihilation with a determined ferocity before which today we stand appalled.' In the fourth or fifth century BC the Sumerians invaded Mesopotamia, to be gradually absorbed by these resident Semitic Akkadians. Thus, the oldest real civilization was that of the Sumerians, employing a pictographic script and using a language which became the speech of the learned. Successive invasions gradually overwhelmed the Sumerian dynasties, leading, as supremacies changed, to the founding of the Old Babylonian Empire, about 2000 BC. Within the dynasties of this Empire the life of King Hammurabi (1955–1912 BC), ruler of both Northern and Southern

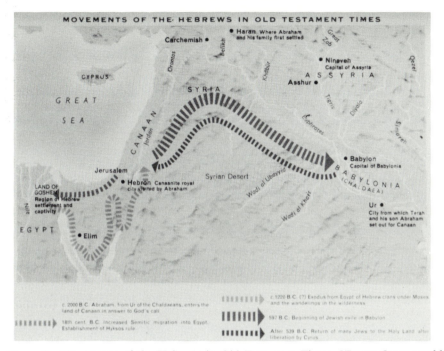

Figure 8   Movements of the Hebrews in Old Testament Times. [*From: Great world atlas. London, Reader's Digest Association (1968).*]

Babylonia, stands out as the founder of a Code of Law of great medical and cultural significance.

The Code of Hammurabi (Figure 9) is enshrined on the imposing stone monument discovered at Susa in 1901 by the French Assyriologist, Jean Vincent Scheil; it is now preserved in the Louvre in Paris. The dates of the reign of Hammurabi vary, by 90 or even more years, according to which chronological reconstruction is used but the text of the monument is in the Akkadian (Semitic) language and, although a Sumerian version has not yet been discovered, it is clear that the Code was intended to be of wide influence and to 'establish justice in Sumer and Akkad'.

A classic study of the subject is the widely-read *The Code of Hammurabi King of Babylon about 2250 BC* – a work published by Robert Harper in Chicago in 1904[58]. The Code regulated most of the activities of life and was quite specific about many aspects of medical practice. It stipulated the fees the practitioner was to receive for success, and the penalties to be exacted for failure. It provides the first known system of medical ethics and makes it clear that, even at that early date, those practising medicine received a distinct status.

Most of the provisions of the Code seem to relate to the practice of surgery – a circumstance which reminds us of the way that the medical arts tend to develop. Warren Dawson, in his book *The Beginnings, Egypt and Assyria*[59], of 1930, writes that 'the Babylonians had no physicians, according to Herodotus, and they brought their sick into the market-places in order that passers-by might confer

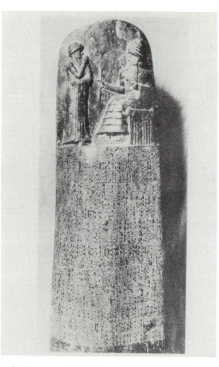

Figure 9 The Code of Hammurabi (about 2250 BC). [*From: William Osler. The evolution of modern medicine . . . New Haven, Yale Univ. Press (1921).*]

with them upon their symptoms in the hope that the patient might elicit from someone who had been similarly afflicted advice as to how to proceed to effect a cure.' Clearly, a dangerous business – indicating that, as in Egypt at a comparable time, nothing useful was known about internal medicine. Thus, for the medically sick a passer-by's guess was as good as any that could be obtained – and this at a time when the elements of simple, practical surgery were already established.

The Code of Hammurabi provides rewards and punishments for surgical acts which not only varied according to the rank of the sufferer but also seem designed to warn off the wandering charlatan – the man who might couch for cataract, producing a dramatic clearing of vision but leaving behind him, as he migrated on, an eye destroyed by infection. The Code provided for the removal of the hand of a surgeon held sufficiently guilty.

About 1758 BC the Babylonian Empire was destroyed by the Hittites – but its culture somehow survived and emerged some 600 years later. Power seems slowly to have moved to the North and, about 1140 BC, shifted to such a degree that Assyria was able to become independent of Babylonia; within less than half a century, Assyria came to rule Babylon. The expression of this great political change was that, some 1100 years before Christ, the king Tiglathpileser I rose to such power that he was able to consolidate the mighty Assyrian Empire and, about 750 BC, Nineveh became the capital of his people.

The weakened city of Babylon was finally destroyed about 700 BC, leaving the Assyrians masters of the whole of Mesopotamia. Their supremacy was marked by the reign of Ashurbanipal (668–626 BC) who, at Nineveh, promptly set about establishing a library intended to encompass the totality of available knowledge. The ruins of this library were excavated in 1849 – yielding many thousands of clay tablets with their cuneiform characters providing vast numbers of historical, literary, religious, magical, astronomical, and medical texts. It is to one man, Reginald Campbell Thompson (1876–1941), a devoted student of these tablets for much of his lifetime, that we owe most of our understanding of these ancient texts of Assyrian medicine.

Within less than a century of Ashurbanipal the might of Assyria was gone. In 612 BC the Babylonians, allied with their neighbours, the tribes of the Medes, destroyed Nineveh, bringing to an end the Empire of Assyria. Babylon came to rule once again – the zenith of the Second Babylonian Empire being marked by the reign of Nebuchadnezzar II from 604 to 561 BC. The ultimate end of both Assyria and Babylon came when in 539 BC Cyrus, the Persian king, entered Babylon. Within a few short years Babylon was destroyed and the Persians, followed by Greeks, Romans, Arabs, and Ottoman Turks became the successive conquerors of the tracts of Mesopotamia.

It is said that from the sixteenth century before Christ, from the days of the New Empire when the civilization of Egypt stood at its height, and through all this long history in Mesopotamia, routes of trade ran from Memphis, in Egypt, by way of Palestine, to Nineveh. The routes conveyed letter-posts, many of which carried messages written in cuneiform characters impressed with a three-cornered stylus upon clay.

Morris Jastrow, who was Professor of Semitic Languages in the University of Pennsylvania, devoted a fine and sizable paper, *The medicine of the Babylonians and Assyrians*, to the medicine of Mesopotamia and to its fullest expression in the cuneiform tablets of Nineveh. Jastrow's paper[60], of October 10, 1913 read before William Osler, shows that, 'the treatment of disease as revealed in the medical text of Ashurbanipal's library must revert to a period of at least 2000 BC'; it shows also that the essential features of this ancient Mesopotamian medicine were the use of incantations, the resort to vast numbers of magical rites, the persistent practice of divination (especially liver-divination), and the adjunctive and unimportant place given to drugs.

Jastrow says that, 'the belief that disease is due to demonic possession is universal at a certain stage of human culture, but in Babylonia and Assyria this belief is extended to include all the mishaps and accidents of life'[61]. Thus, over great territories and for centuries at a stretch the cause and cure of disease was bound up with demonic possession – and the treatment of disease consisted of forcing or coaxing the demon out of the patient's physical body. The incantations were to effect this. At times the attendant magic was of the simple and primitive kind in which knots were, at intervals, tied in a thread or a cord, symbolizing the imprisonment of the demon that had been driven from the body. The medicines frequently comprised foul or rotting substances (forming a *Dreckapotheke*, to use the term quoted by Jastrow[62]), so noxious that they would disgust the demon and drive it out.

R. Campbell Thompson's *Assyrian Medical Texts*, an article of 1924, provides an example[63] of the type of incantation used in this primitive type of magic:

> Incantation for a Sick Eye. Ritual for this: red wool, white wool separately thou shalt spin: seven and seven knots thou shalt tie (in each): as thou tiest, thou shalt recite the charm; the thread of red wool thou shalt tie on his eye which is sick; the thread of white wool thou shalt tie on his eye which is whole, and he shall recover.

From the same source an incantation or charm for the eye[64]:

> Incantation for a Sick Eye. Ritual for this: Charm. In Heaven the wind blew and brought blindness to the eye of the man: from the distant heavens the wind blew and brought blindness to the eye of the man. Unto the sick eye it brought blindness; of this man his eye is troubled, his eye is pained. The man weepeth grievously for himself.
>
> Of this man, his sickness Ea hath espied and (said) 'take pounded roses, perform the Charm of the Deep, and bind the eye of the man'. When Ea toucheth the eye of the man with his holy hand, let the wind which hath brought woe to the eye of the man go forth!

And a third one, this using more of the materia medica[65]:

> If a man's eyes are sick and full of blood, unguents (only) irritating (?) the blood, blood (and) tears coming forth from the eyes, a film closing over the pupils of his eyes, tears turning to film, to look oppressing him: thou shalt beat leaves of tamarisk, steep them in strong vinegar, leave them out under the stars; in the morning (i.e. on the morrow) thou shalt squeeze (them) in a helmet: white alum, storax, 'Akkadian Salt', fat, cornflour, *nigella*, 'gum of copper', separately thou shalt bray: thou shalt take equal parts (of them), put them together; pour (them) into the helmet (in) which thou hast squeezed (the tamarisk); in curd and *šuniš*-mineral thou shalt knead (it), (and) open his eyelids with a finger (and) put it in his eyes. (While) his eyes contain dimness, his eyes thou shalt smear, and for nine days thou shalt do this.

From the second part, that of 1926, of Campbell Thompson's *Assyrian Medical Texts*, both parts being in the *Proceedings of the Royal Society of Medicine*[66], an incantation for toothache – this condition being thought to be due to a worm in the tooth, identified with the maggot of figs:

> *Incantation for Toothache*. Charm. After Anu made the heavens, the heavens made the earth, the earth made the rivers, the rivers made the canals, the canals made the marsh, the marsh made the Worm. The Worm came weeping unto Samas, (came) unto Ea, her tears flowing: 'What wilt thou give me for my food, what wilt thou give me to destroy?' 'I will give thee dried figs (and) apricots.' 'Forsooth, what are these dried figs to me, or apricots? Set me amid the teeth, and let me dwell in the gums, that I may destroy the blood of the teeth, and of the gums chew their marrow. So shall I hold the latch of the door.' 'Since thou hast said this, O Worm, may Ea smite thee with his mighty fist!'

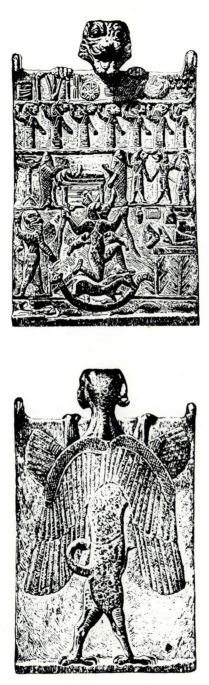

Figure 10 Assyro-Babylonian bronze amulet, Paris. [*From: Morris Jastrow. The medicine of the Babylonians and Assyrians (1913–1914).]*

Finally, and again from the second article, a charm associating liver with night-blindness[67]:

> If a man's eyes suffer from 'Sin-lurmâ' (night-blindness), thou shalt thread *makut* of the liver of an ass (and) flesh of its neck on a cord (and) put it on his neck, prepare a water-pot; on the morrow thou shalt spread a cloth in the sun, prepare a censer of pine-gum: (then) thou shalt let this man stand behind the cloth in the sun. A priest shall take seven (rounds of) bread; he whose eyes are sick shall take seven (rounds of) bread: [(then) the priest] shall say [to] the sick man, 'Receive, O clear of eye:' [the si]ck man shall say to the priest, 'Receive, O dim of eye' . . . Thou shalt chop up the *makut* of the liver . . ., assemble some children and they shall say thus: '. . .', they shall say: thou shalt mix curd and the best (?) oil together, apply to his eyes.

The demons addressed in many of these incantations and involved in these primitive rituals have been studied by numerous authors, including Warren R. Dawson, who published his *Magician and Leech, A Study in the Beginnings of Medicine with special reference to Ancient Egypt* in 1929[68]. They have also been widely illustrated, for great numbers of provocative examples remain; one such example is shown in Figure 10.

Only marginally less important than all of these charms and magic in Babylonian–Assyrian medicine was the highly-developed art of divination: as everything came from the gods, the intent of the gods could, it was thought, be foretold in the signs they obtrude in the skies, or that man could discern in the normally-hidden entrails of animals. Jastrow, in his study of this subject[69], wrote 'The first, and probably the oldest, of these methods was the endeavour to divine the future through the inspection of the liver of a sacrificed animal, based on the widespread notion among primitive people that the liver, as the bloody organ *par excellence* – blood being associated with life – was also the seat of the soul.' The clay model (Figure 11) of the liver of a sheep (the model is now in the British Museum) is a teaching aid from a Babylonian temple school; used for instruction in liver-divination, it is of about 2000 BC and has an accompanying text to allow small features of the liver and associated structures to be used in prognosis and foretelling.

There were two other main means of divination. In the first, that of birth omens, the signs noted at the time of birth were regarded as showing, for the individual, his future health, life and disease: the concept seems to have been that whatever was different or dissimilar, at the beginning of life, foretold what the pattern of growth must bring. The third system of divination was astrology, heaven and earth being thought of as two sides of the mirror of divine intent. Thus, the skies revealed all that the gods had prepared for those upon Earth. Out of these predictions, and the knowledge of the skies that they gave, there very slowly arose a real prowess in the practical science of astronomy.

Clearly, in practice, the three aspects of Assyrian and Babylonian medicine – exorcism, magic, and divination – must have merged. In just the same way the medical remedies used must have slowly provided some empirical knowledge of the value of indigenous herbs and a number of minerals.

Knowledge of these Mesopotamian remedies is, to an amazing degree, the work of one man, R. Campbell Thompson, from whom extensive quotations

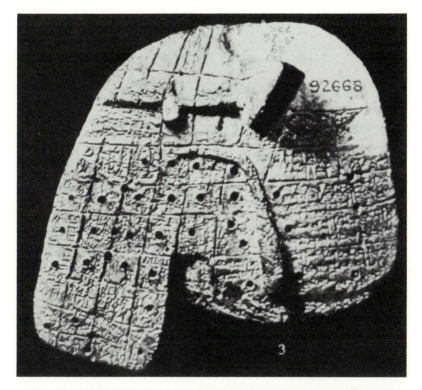

Figure 11   Clay model of the liver of a sheep. Used in a Babylonian Temple-School for instruction in liver-divination (British Museum, about 2000 BC). [*From: Morris Jastrow. The medicine of the Babylonians and Assyrians (1913–1914).*]

have already been given. Thompson published *The Devils and Evil Spirits of Babylonia* in two volumes in 1903 and the following year[70]. Interestingly, Campbell Thompson, Fellow of Merton College, Oxford, dedicated this work to his father, Reginald E. Thompson, a physician.

Beginning work on the tablets in the British Museum before 1906, Campbell Thompson published *Assyrian Medical Texts from the Originals in the British Museum* in 1923. This book contained 107 plates providing the text of 660 cuneiform medical tablets, most of them not before published. In his Preface he announced his intention[71]:

> Lest there should be any misapprehension on another point, I propose to bring out the translations very shortly. The work of editing so many texts is a long business; and it became obvious, when I set about them again after my return from the War, that the old method of leaving the vegetable drugs unidentified, or translated haphazard, would lead us nowhere. No satisfactory translation of these texts was possible until the plants had been in some measure worked out; and to this end I spent a large part of two years at work on the 250 vegetable drugs known to the Assyrian botanists. The results will appear shortly under the title of *The Assyrian Herbal*.

This devotion to working out the botanical identifications is one of the things which most distinguished Thompson's work – and which makes it almost more informative than any of the comparable studies of the medicine of Ancient Egypt. *The Assyrian Herbal*[72] followed in 1924 (after its presentation to the Royal Society on March 20th that year) and was followed by *Assyrian Prescriptions for Diseases of the Chest and Lungs* (1934)[73], and a number of specific publications of special systems.

Vegetable drugs occur most frequently in *The Assyrian Herbal*, as is shown by the following table from this handwritten text, presumably too expensive to publish in any other way due to its scripts:

Table 1   *The Assyrian Herbal, R. Campbell Thompson*[72]

Drugs∗	*Species*	*Occurrences*
Vegetable	250	4600
Mineral	120	650
Other, and unidentified	180	630
Totals	550	5880

∗ Numbers exclude the solvents, vehicles, excipients, etc.

Of the remedies for illnesses of the chest we can take two examples[74]:

> If a man is affected in the lungs, thou shalt spread powder of tar over a thorn-fire, let it (the smoke) enter his anus, . . ., his mouth and nostrils, it shall make (him) cough (?): thou shalt bathe him with water of *Vitex*; let [his tongue] take refined oil. Let him eat a mixture of fine-ground flour with fat: thou shalt bray *Ammi*, let him drink (it) in beer [and he shall recover].
>
> If ditto, thou shalt bray *Ammi*, spread it over a thorn-fire, let it (the smoke) enter his anus . . . [his mouth] and his nostrils, it shall make (him) cough (?): thou shalt bathe him with water of *Vitex*: thou shalt anoint the whole of his body with curd: thou shalt bray linseed either in milk (?) . . ., bind on him for three days, and let his tongue hold honey (and) refined oil, . . . [and he shall recover].

It is apparent that the great number of prescriptions that Campbell Thompson translated, either in whole or in part, range from the purely magical, for example[75]:

> If a man's eyes are sick . . . [thou shalt pound] the brain of an eagle in harlot's milk [and apply].

to the useful[76]:

> [If a man]'s [head] is full of scabies and itch, thou shalt bray sulphur, mix it in cedar-oil, anoint him.

The latter example reminds us that the Assyrians are usually credited with having introduced sulphur into the pharmacopoeia.

Unlike the prescriptions in the Egyptian papyri, the Assyrian remedies usually had no distinct titles – they begin with a phrase ('If a man's eyes are sick . . .' or 'If a man's head is full of scabies and itch . . .') which shows the purpose. Another difference is that, unlike the Egyptian prescriptions, the Assyrian texts very seldom give the quantities of the ingredients used. Charms, incantations, spells and the like are also more common in the Mesopotamian tablet texts than in the papyri of Egypt – though they are much more obvious in the later papyri and those of lay origin than they were in the early and professional writings. As Campbell Thompson's translations show, many of the Assyrian texts are fragmentary and, while the general sense of most of them can be understood, there are not many so undamaged that they become suitable for quotation. Despite these differences, there is a great deal of similarity between the medical texts of the Egyptian and Assyrio-Babylonian physicians.

One plant which kept its magical Assyrian significance into mediaeval times and beyond was the mandrake – famous in the Bible, and still famous in the herbals of the First Elizabethan reign. Campbell Thompson showed that the word 'mandrake' is the Assyrian word for 'plague-god plant' changed by the merchants who took it into Europe as the Greek *mandragora* – this being derived from the Assyrian *nam-ta-ira* by simple metathesis of the consonants *m,n*. Warren Dawson[77] recalls this particular point and remarks that whilst the Assyrians often used mandrake for medicinal purposes, the Egyptian pharmacopoeia does not mention it.

The herbs, weeds, thorns, woods, roots, juices, stones, minerals and accessories of the Assyrian herbal provide, as we have seen, something approaching 600 substances. Among the plants and shrubs these include anise, carraway, cassia, colewort, colocynth, coriander, cummin, cynoglosson – a name which is the equivalent of the Greek term for 'grain' or 'wheat' – jasmine, liquorice, lily, leek, mint, mushroom, mustard, nard, onion, radish, rocket, Star of Bethlehem (ornithogallum) – and many reeds and thorny plants, the seeds, juices, and leaves all being utilized. Among the trees and shrubs the authors already noted mention the use of the bark, roots, sap, seeds, twigs – and above all the fruit – of the cedar, cypress, fig, myrtle, olive, tamarisk, and willow. Of these sources several provide items which have been, or remain, part of recent therapeutics: the dried succulent fruit of *Ficus carica*, of the Moraceae, is the source of the proteolytic enzyme, ficin, and forms the basis of the Compound Figs Syrup of the *British Pharmaceutical Codex* (1973)[78]. Olive Oil (*British Pharmacopoeia*, 1980)[79] is the fixed natural oil expressed from the ripe fruits of *Olea europaea* of the Oleaceae; taken internally it has well-known culinary, nutrient, demulcent, and mildly purgative properties; externally its emollient effect is used to soften the skin and crusts in eczema and psoriasis. Sweet Birch Oil (BPC 1949)[80] – *Oleum Betulae*, Wintergreen Oil – remains in use. An important natural salicylate, it used to be obtained from *Gaultheria procumbens*, of the Ericaceae, but is now obtained almost exclusively from *Betula lenta*, one of the lovelier of the Betulaceae. It contains not less than 98% of esters, calculated as methyl salicylate, and reminds us – now that the world's vast supply of analgesic salicylates is almost all obtained by synthetic means – of the beginnings of this vital group of drugs in the oldest pharmacopoeias.

Nevertheless, these ancient compendia, and the drug lists derived from their translation, can easily be misread: because the Egyptians used parts of the poppy it does not mean they knew opium; the Assyrians knew the willow, but it does not follow that they knew it as an antirheumatic. If they did, then such a rational, empirical use was an exception – the common, characteristic use of drugs being as an adjunct to magic.

When the great schools of medicine arose in Cos and Cnidos they had little to learn, and much to discard, from Babylon. With Hippocrates (about 460–370 BC) a whole new and splendid era set in – but to the last days of Babylonian and Assyrian history, medicine, in Mesopotamia, remained attached to the demonic theory of the cause of disease. The useful parts of the Assyrian materia medica are lost in the filth to discourage the demon. The decline of the late medicine of Egypt – marked by increased, not lessened, elements of superstition – was due to the contact with Babylon. Even the name 'magic' derives from the 'magi' – the common name of the priests of Persia, late Babylon, and the home of necromancy.

The physician of Ancient Assyria and Babylonia, like that whole civilization, has his epitaph in the words in which Ezekiel[81] recalls that 'the king of Babylon stood at the parting of the way, at the head of the two ways, to use divination: he made his arrows bright, he consulted with images, he looked in the liver.'

Judea – the biblical era, about 1500–300 BC

The early history of the Jewish people has had such a direct and lasting effect upon Western medicine that it remains of relevance, even today. This history comprises both the Biblical, Old Testament period and the later period of the Talmud, roughly from the second century BC to the seventh century AD.

No medical works, as such, have come down to us from the ancient Hebrews – our only sources of knowledge being the numerous medical and hygienic references scattered throughout the sacred, historical, and legal Hebraic literature. Thus, our main source is the Old Testament, which was first written in the Hebrew language, supplemented by the archaeological findings made in Palestine.

Whilst the written record is in many ways of generous proportions, it provides its own problems: the material does not have, as its main purpose, the record of medical events; the period covered is very long, stretching back to primitive times and extending through all the stages of national development and migration. Its extension in the Talmud, which was not complete until the fifth century or a little later, reaches into the present era. Finally, we must recognize that when the record talks of medicine it does so as the medicine of the people, not of a profession, and it has been translated and transmitted by laymen. In terms of the diagnoses there are especial uncertainties – perhaps most marked with leprosy – a disease which was the subject of important and specific health measures.

The Reformation awoke interest in Biblical study, the first systematic accounts of the medicine of the Old Testament being published early in the seventeenth century. However, it was not until the nineteenth century that meaningful studies included the Talmud and other ancient Hebraic writings. Just as R. Campbell Thompson has his own unique place in opening up the early

Assyrian medical texts so, in the Jewish writings, there is one figure, Julius Preuss, who was responsible for a massive contribution to the subject.

Julius (Yitzhak) Preuss (1861–1913) was born in Gross-Schoenbeck, Germany, where his father was the only Jewish householder. He had the great good fortune to study medicine at Berlin with Rudolf Virchow (1821–1902), the founder of cellular pathology, as his teacher. Although Preuss lived at a time of intense activity in Jewish studies, and had been preceded by great writers on the historical aspects of his subject, it was left to him to undertake virtually the first major scientifically-informed critical study of the medicine of these ancient writings. His book, *Biblisch-talmudische Medizin*... [82] (Berlin, 1911) remains fundamental to the subject. It was reprinted, and provided with a distinguished introduction by Sussmann Munter, in 1971. This introduction corrects the work of Preuss where this was needed because of later additions to knowledge; it also gives a very useful outline of the many advances which have been made in Jewish studies since the establishment of the State of Israel.

Preuss – whose study was the first substantive review of Biblical and Talmudic medicine to be written by a physician – was already gravely ill when his book was published. His remarkable knowledge of Hebraic science and literature was the product of intense study during his adult years only. In some circles he was not well understood and the detached, clinical tone of his writings was widely criticized as being cold and unfeeling. His illness led to his early death in September, 1913 but his widow survived in Israel until 1960.

The great succession of historical events that were the subject of the studies of Preuss began with the migration of the Hebrews – the tribal name apparently being derived from the words '*ever ha-nahar*', meaning 'from the other side of the river', the river being the Euphrates. During this migration Abraham and his people are said to have travelled (Figure 8) from the Mesopotamian city of Ur to the area of Haran. About 2000 BC they first moved into Canaan (in modern times Palestine). Something like 250 years later they moved with their flocks into Egypt; there they spent 430 years in servitude, coming to know not only the great civilization of Egypt but also the diseases and cruelty of the Egyptians of the time.

Eventually, after their deliverance from Egypt, the Children of Israel fled, under the leadership of Moses, to spend the next 40 years, the years of the Exodus, wandering in the vastness of the Sinai peninsula. The dates are uncertain but Percival Wood, in his book *Moses, the Founder of Preventive Medicine* [83], gives the easily remembered one, 1234 BC, as the date of the Exodus.

When they reached Canaan the Israelites conquered the people already there and divided the country amongst their own 12 tribes, named after the sons or grandsons of Jacob, descendant of Abraham. The 12 tribes remained in Canaan – apart from 70 years spent in exile in Babylonia in the fifth century BC – as a free nation. They remained free until eventually dominated by the Ptolemies of Egypt. Even then their priest-kings, the Maccabees, won their freedom by revolt in 165 BC. Before long their now precarious freedom waned and, by the time of Christ, the land had become part of the growing Roman Empire. Despite this they remain recognizable as a nation until, in AD 70, the great Temple of the Jews was destroyed by Titus – and, driven from Palestine in the dispersion, the people whose lives had formed the substance of the Old Testament became scattered throughout the countries of the world until modern times.

Canaan was not just the fertile and promised land of the Jews. It lay between Africa and Asia, forming the meeting-place between the ancient civilization of Egypt, to the west, and the equally ancient culture of Mesopotamia, the land between the Tigris and Euphrates, to the east. Because of its long coastline and access to the Mediterranean Sea, Canaan was linked with the entire southern aspect of Europe. By means of these communications and their own skills and insights into the subject, the Jews later became instrumental in carrying the medical knowledge of the Greeks to the Arabs – just as they eventually conveyed much of the medical and pharmaceutical skill of the mediaeval Arab world into Europe.

The later story of the growth of medical and therapeutic knowledge is more readily told by following its migration through the different nations that became historically involved. But at each stage of its growth the peoples who carried the Old Testament and Talmudic tradition onwards through the pattern of history were important. Dispersed as they were through the nations the compilations of their works, telling the story from the Jewish point of view, show their frequent contribution to the sciences of the lands where they were admitted to the universities; the same accounts show the persistent ethical contribution which has remained a specifically Hebraic characteristic.

The people of ancient Israel, the Jews of the period long before the dispersion, cannot be viewed as if they existed in isolation uninfluenced by the geographical communications we have discussed. Much of the culture of Egypt, and a little of that of Babylon, affected the lives of the primitive Canaanitish people and influenced the Biblical Testament. Many examples of the durability of the very earliest primitive beliefs are given by Sir James George Frazer (1854–1941) in his book, *Folk-lore in the Old Testament*, which was part of the Cambridge tradition of theology and was published in 1918[84].

Breasted[85] describes a short period of monotheism during the reign of Amen-hotep IV in the First Period of the Empire in ancient Egypt – but the belief was short-lived and not in any way characteristic of old Egypt. This was in no sense true of Israel where the belief in there being only one true God characterized the entire Jewish culture. As early as in the passage given in Genesis[86], Abraham hears his god say: '. . . I am the Lord that brought thee out of Ur of the Chaldees, to give thee this land to inherit it.' And Abraham, asking how he will know that he is to inherit it, is told to make an animal sacrifice of the heifer, the she-goat and the ram and to divide them in their midst. The sign that the sacrifice had been accepted was given to him when, as the sun went down, a smoking furnace and a burning lamp passed between the pieces of the sacrifice.

This method of sealing a covenant is in the manner of ancient Hebraic law and is met with again in the passage of Jeremiah[87] where it says: '. . . the covenant which they had made before me, when they cut the calf in twain, and passed between the parts thereof . . .' Frazer says[88] that the Hebrew phrase for making a covenant means 'to cut a covenant' and he continues, citing R. A. Stewart Macalister's *Reports on the excavation of Gezer*[89] and the same author's *The excavation of Gezer*[90], with the following passage[91]:

> Perhaps this discussion of Abraham's covenant may help to throw light on a very dark spot of Canaanite history. In his excavations at Gezer, in Palestine,

Professor Stewart Macalister discovered a burial-place of a very remarkable kind. It is simply a cylindrical chamber about twenty feet deep and fifteen feet wide, which has been hewn out of the rock and is entered from the top by a circular hole cut in the roof. The chamber appears to have been originally a water-cistern and to have been used for that purpose before it was converted into a tomb. On the floor of the chamber were found fifteen skeletons of human beings, or rather fourteen and a half skeletons; for of one body only the upper part was discovered, the lower part was wanting. The half skeleton was that of a girl about fourteen years of age; she had been cut or sawn through the middle 'at the eighth thoracic vertebra, and as the front ends of the ribs had been divided at this level, it is plain that the section had been made while as yet the bones were supported by the soft parts.' The fourteen other skeletons were all males, two of them immature, aged about eighteen and nineteen years respectively; all the rest were full-grown adults, of fair stature and strongly built. The position of the bodies showed that they had not been thrown in through the hole in the roof but deposited by persons who descended with them into the cave; and a large quantity of charcoal found among the bones is thought to indicate that a funeral feast, sacrifice, or other solemn rite had been observed within the sepulchral chamber. Some fine bronze weapons – spear-heads, an axe and a knife – deposited with the bodies may be regarded as evidence that the burial took place before the advent of the Israelites, and accordingly that the men belonged to a race who preceded the Hebrews in Palestine.

Even if the findings at Gezer are from a Canaanite tribe earlier than the Hebrews, the Old Testament quotations on the solemnizing of a covenant demonstrate the great significance which the idea of sacrifice had to the early Jews. The idea persisted and the concept of atonement by sacrifice has been central to the religious environment in which much of Western medicine developed.

A second example of these long-lived beliefs relates to the mandrake plant which, for centuries, was thought to have magical and medicinal properties. The story is of Jacob who, seeking a wife, 'went towards Haran' and, in doing this, met Laban. The account is in Genesis[92], where it is shown that Laban had two daughters of whom 'Leah was tender eyed; but Rachel was beautiful and well favoured.'

Jacob, as seems to have been the practice, served seven years for Rachel – only to be given Leah, as the eldest must be given first. He then served Laban for a second seven years – and was then given Rachel. Leah proved to be fertile and soon had four sons, of whom the eldest was Reuben; Rachel proved to be barren. Then comes this account[93] beginning when the little boy, Reuben, at harvest time, follows the reapers into the fields and finds the plant that becomes such a notable sign to the two women:

And Reuben went in the days of wheat harvest, and found mandrakes in the field, and brought them unto his mother Leah. Then Rachel said to Leah, Give me, I pray thee, of thy son's mandrakes. And she said unto her, Is it a small matter that thou hast taken my husband? and wouldest thou take away my son's mandrakes also? And Rachel said, Therefore he shall lie with thee tonight for thy son's mandrakes. And Jacob came out of the field in the evening, and Leah went out to meet him, and said, Thou must come in unto me; for surely I have hired thee with my son's mandrakes. And he lay with her that night. And God hearkened unto Leah, and she conceived, and bare Jacob the fifth son.

Leah was to provide a sixth son and a daughter before the account reaches the point at which we are told[94]:

...God remembered Rachel, and God hearkened to her, and opened her womb. And she conceived, and bare a son; and said, God hath taken away my reproach...

The mandrakes were of such significance to Rachel that she was prepared to bargain Jacob's company for them. Frazer says that the Hebrew name of the plant (which, by its old botanical name, was *Mandragora officinalis*) was 'dudaim' – apparently meaning that the taste of it would cause a barren woman to conceive[95].

The origin of the myth is, of course, unknown. In folk-lore and popular fancy the shape of the root had an almost human form. This was a myth that was potent enough to lead the normally factual Dioscorides[96] to say that the male mandrake was white and the female mandrake was black. The fame of the plant lasted so long that John Parkinson, the last of the great British herbalists and Apothecary to James I and VI, in his *Theatrum botanicum: The theater of plants. Or, an herball of a large extent* (1640)[97], wrote that the two sorts of the plant were known as Mandrakes and Womandrakes respectively. Parkinson has clearly understood that the myth is not to be trusted, for he adds: 'they are foolishly so called'.

In Biblical times the mandrake clearly had undiminished and wonderful properties. These seem to provide an example of that form of magic which was propounded by the sixteenth century German physician, mystic and chemist, Paracelsus (1493–1541), and is known as the 'Doctrine of Signatures'[98]. This doctrine suggests that like cures like, or that natural cures carry a sign indicating to the seeker their divinely imposed purpose. In the case of the mandrake (a plant with potent pharmacological properties) the doctrine would suggest that the plant, by resembling the human form, can beget that form and overcome barrenness. It was for this purpose that Rachel traded for Reuben's mandrakes.

Nicolas Culpeper (1616–1654), in *Culpeper's English Physician; and complete herbal...* (Sibly's edition of 1713)[99], provides an illustration which he says is 'taken from a genuine root' but the illustrations of the 'male' and 'female' Mandragora forming Figures 12 and 13 are taken from the Matthioli commentary of 1583 on the *De materia medica* of Dioscorides[311].

The third example of the persistence of old beliefs concerns the events witnessed by Saul at Endor. It is not a story typical of the Old Testament for it is characteristically Mesopotamian: the witch of Endor is one of the few scriptural witches, for necromancy had been declared 'a lethal cunning' by Saul himself.

Exodus[100] carries the injunction, 'Thou shalt not suffer a witch to live' – an edict that produced some of the burnings and sufferings of the Middle and post-Renaissance ages. Saul[101] 'had put away those that had familiar spirits, and the wizards, out of the land.' Nevertheless, when the ultimate trial of strength was forced upon him, Saul, looking at the camps of the massive army of the Philistines, 'was afraid, and his heart greatly trembled'. Disguised, and with only

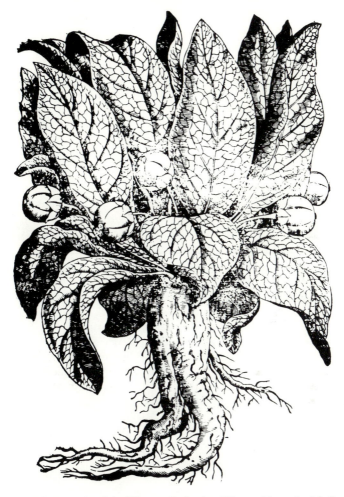

Figure 12 Mandragora 'male'. [*From: Pedanius Dioscorides. de Medica materia (edition of 1583). Royal Society of Medicine library, London.*]

two men to accompany him, he crept out at night to the witch whose home was near the field of the forthcoming battle. At his bidding she brought forth the dead Samuel. The account [102] continues:

> And he said unto her, What form is he of? And she said, An old man cometh up; and he is covered with a mantle. And Saul perceived that it was Samuel, and he stooped with his face to the ground, and bowed himself. And Samuel said to Saul, Why hast thou disquieted me, to bring me up? And Saul answered, I am sore distressed; for the Philistines make war against me, and God is departed from me, and answereth me no more, neither by prophets, nor by dreams: therefore I have called thee, that thou mayest make known unto me what I shall do.'

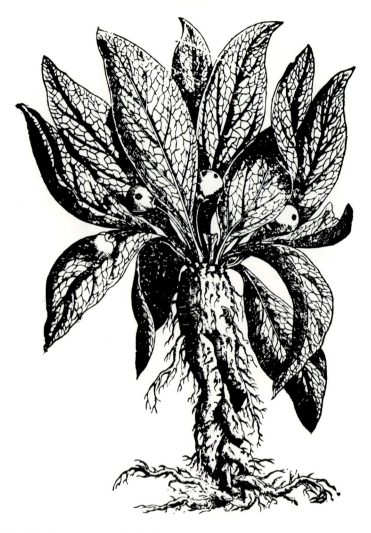

Figure 13 Mandragora 'female'. [*From: Pedanius Diocorides. de Medica materia (edition of 1583). Royal Society of Medicine library, London.*]

The result was the dreadful set of pronouncements: 'the Lord hath rent the kingdom out of thine hand' . . . 'the Lord will also deliver Israel with thee into the hand of the Philistines' and . . . 'tomorrow shalt thou and thy sons be with me.'

The passage provides one of the most obvious examples of demonology and divination in the Old Testament. Apart from this and a few similar examples the ancient scriptures are full of injunctions against such practices: the person who turned to familiar spirits was to be cut off 'from among his people'[103]; the man or woman 'that hath a familiar spirit, or that is a wizard, shall surely be put to death'[104]; 'there shall not be found among you any one that maketh his son or his daughter to pass through the fire, or that useth divination, or an observer of times, or an enchanter, or a witch, or a charmer, or a consulter with familiar spirits, or a wizard, or a necromancer. For all that do these things are an abomination. . .'[105].

Medicine was, therefore, different amongst the Hebrews than along the Nile or between the Tigris and Euphrates. The Hebraic monotheists did, however, envisage a God that could be a giver of disease, as well as healing. The followers of Moses who kept the commandments were told[106]: 'I will put none of these diseases upon thee, which I have brought upon the Egyptians: for I am the Lord that healeth thee.' The Mosaic code of mental and physical cleanliness was, in its fully developed form, of great consequence; but so was the belief that disease might be imposed by, or cured by, the divine will. The latter belief dominated the church of the Middle Ages. The code of cleanliness had, as a central aim, fitness to be in the divine presence. Thinking of this, John Young, physician and naturalist of the Glasgow, wrote[107]:

> As the Mosaic Law was not a scientific treatise, as its instructions were for the guidance of the priests, the only intermediaries between man and God, we need not complain of omissions which would have been irrelevancies had they been inserted. The general health regulations were of remarkable completeness, extending as they do to details of moral as well as of physical conduct.

Because the Mosaic code was of such profound medical and hygienic consequence it is possible to read into it purposes which may not have had any place in the minds of its originators. Thus, commenting on a book in which scientific explanations of the objects of the code had perhaps been overdrawn, Immanuel Jakobovits had this to say[108]:

> Whether the medical motive the author attributes to the laws he lists can be regarded as their rationale may be open to argument. For my part, I prefer to look upon any such medical factors in the religious legislation of Judaism as incidental rather than instrinsic in their evaluation as a discipline of life. The dietary laws in particular, I believe, primarily aimed, not at hygiene but holiness.

If the purposes of the code were purely religious, its consequences included the establishment of what we would now call preventive medicine. The people who followed these sensible and reasonable practices were promised[109] that they would be brought into a 'good land, a land of brooks of water, of fountains and depths that spring out of valleys and hills; a land of wheat, and barley, and vines, and fig trees, and pomegranates; a land of oil olive, and honey . . .' The five items that ended this list either were themselves, or were the sources of, ingredients of both the Jewish diet and pharmacopoeia.

The diseases treated with that pharmacopoeia and appearing in the Biblical accounts were discussed by Preuss (1911) along with his review of the Jewish knowledge of anatomy. Most of this knowledge came from the rituals observed in making sure that animal foodstuffs complied with the Mosaic law. Only two Hebrew terms of anatomy have clearly survived to enter the modern nomenclature and these are the corona glandis and the cauda equina. Amongst the diseases, cases of demonic possession and of the casting out of devils provide a contrast between the New Testament, in which they are frequent, and the Old Testament in which, despite its far greater length, they are infrequent.

The hygienic effects of the Jewish practices, exemplified in the *Third Book of Moses, Leviticus*, were of such value that these writings provide what appears to be the most important and beneficial document, in terms of its consequence upon medicine, before Hippocrates. The Mosaic documents provide a frank recognition of contagion and the usefulness of isolation in preventing the spread of infectious disease. The laws[110] made a difference 'between the unclean and the clean, and between the beast that may be eaten and the beast that may not be eaten'. Unclean foods include swine, rodents, and birds whose foodstuff is carrion. Among the ordinances of hygiene were the means of purification of women and the requirement of male circumcision. Amongst the decrees to prevent contagion by isolation are the remarkable rituals for both the diagnosis and management of leprosy. Almost all of Leviticus XIII and XIV is given over to this subject[111]. These texts include the idea of disfiguring disease as a divine punishment and the provisions, once the diagnosis was established, included the edict[112], 'a leprous man, he is unclean: the priest shall pronounce him utterly unclean; his plague is in his head. And the leper in whom the plague is, his clothes shall be rent, and his head bare, and he shall put a covering upon his upper lip, and shall cry, Unclean, unclean . . .' As we shall see later, these pronouncements were enshrined in the leper laws of mediaeval England.

Preuss thought that the leprosy of the Bible probably included infective eczema and older commentators have suggested that it might have included elephantiasis, smallpox, and a number of other diseases. Nevertheless, there is no doubt that the Hebrews from the days of Moses, well over 1000 years before Christ, recognized the infectious nature of some of these diseases and had laws to prevent their direct spread and transmission. The same code of hygiene provided for that benign measure, the weekly day of rest, which serves to refresh the bodily resources against disease. Considering these two measures and their effects, Karl Sudhoff (1853–1938), one of the finest of medical historians, wrote that[113], 'Two of the greatest hygienic thoughts of mankind owe their origin to Semitism . . . the weekly day of rest and the direct prophylaxis of disease.' In this level of understanding there was a great difference between the Jewish practices and those of the successors to Hippocrates – Greek medicine, throughout much of its course, remained curiously blind to the fact of contagion.

There is perhaps a darker side to the tradition. The sensible measures taken by the ancient Hebrews included the quarantining of those with infectious illnesses, the disposal or disinfection by burning or heating of contaminated clothes and furnishings, the careful disposal of excreta by soldiers, the inspection of meat, the existence of rules to prevent the adverse consequences of consanguinity, and so on. To be set against the benefits of these provisions must be placed the historical consequences of the belief that disease was caused and cured by the divine. Of the many Old Testament passages which set these two things together, that in Job[114] says 'he maketh sore, and bindeth up: he woundeth, and his hands make whole.' Many have commented on the suffering these thoughts must have brought to the afflicted; others have seen these ideas as lessening interest in the practical measures of therapeutics and have judged these ideas as having, for centuries, slowed the progress of discovering the practical means of relief.

Two things follow directly from the Hebraic expression of monotheism. One is – as pointed out by Harry Friedenwald (1864–1950) in his book *The Jews and Medicine, Essays* of 1944[115] – that the physician looked upon himself as the 'helper' or agent of divine intent. Thus, the medical person was expected to provide kind and considerate treatment and encouragement. The beginnings of proper professional relationships are to be found in the sentences such as [116], 'A good name is better than precious ointment', which became proverbs. The second consequence of monotheism and the cleanliness that became its expression was that there was no *dreckapotheke* or dung pharmacopoeia to provide the where-withal to chase off devils. In Exodus[117] we are given the formula of the precious or holy ointment: Moses, in making this material, was instructed to take 'three principal spices, of pure myrrh five hundred shekels, and of sweet cinnamon half so much, even two hundred and fifty shekels, and of sweet calamus two hundred and fifty shekels, And of cassia five hundred shekels, after the shekel of the sanctuary, and of oil olive an hin: And thou shalt make it an oil of holy ointment, an ointment compound after the art of the apothecary: it shall be an holy anointing oil.'

Myrrh (BPC, 1973)[118] is the oleo-gum-resin obtained from the stem of *Commiphora molmol* and related species of the Burseraceae. A synonym, which appears in the Old Testament, is balsamodendron. The bushes from which the resin is obtained grow mainly in Arabia and are less than 9 feet in height; they have knotted branches with twigs standing out at right-angles and ending in a protective sharp spine. The resin, obtained from natural fissures or from wounds in the bark, hardens to give reddish-brown or reddish-yellow tears with a marked aromatic odour and bitter taste. Myrrh is astringent and is used in a tincture in mouth-washes or on buccal ulcers; it is said to have a carminative action when taken by mouth. Alternative sources of the material are from Somaliland and the substance has been used from remote antiquity in incense and perfumes; it was used not only in the holy oil of the Jews but in the *Kyphi* which the Egyptians employed in embalming.

Cinnamon, both as sticks and in its powdered form, remains a common culinary spice; with the synonyms Cinnamon Bark or Ceylon Cinnamon it, like the Cinnamon Oil obtained by distillation, appears in the *British Pharmacopoeia*, 1980[119] – the monographs give the action and use of the powdered form as a flavouring agent and the oil as having a carminative action as well. The actual material is the dried bark of the shoots of the coppiced trees of *Cinnamomum zeylanicum* of the Lauraceae; it contains not less than 1% of the volatile oil, this forming the basis of the 'Concentrated Cinnamon Water' which is still recognized as an official preparation by the BP (1980).

The Calamus of the Bible is probably identical with the Calamus (BPC, 1934)[120] which is *Acorus calamus*, a member of the Arum order, Araceae. Although not botanically related to the Iris it is commonly called the Sweet Flag or Sweet Sedge. It has many other country names, including Sweet Cane, Gladdon (the 'Gladdon harvest' of the Norfolk Broads), and Cinnamon Sedge. It grows widely in Europe, Asia, Asia Minor, and America as a vigorous, reed-like, sedge beside streams, lakes, marshes and ditches. Its tall, sword-shaped leaves look very like the Yellow Flag – hence its everyday name. All parts of the plant have an unusual, pleasant fragrance which led to its feast-day use scattered on the floors of churches. The specific name, calamus, is said to be derived from the Greek word, *calamos*, meaning a reed, and the generic name, *Acorus*, from Acoron, the Greek name of the plant described by Dioscorides and used in ancient times to cure diseases of the eye. The part of the plant used in pharmacy was the dried root or rhizome which contains 1.5 3.5% of a once prized bitter aromatic volatile oil, still used in perfumery and often given, usually as an infusion, as a digestive bitter and carminative. Its place in the holy ointment was presumably due to its perfume.

Cassia (Bastard Cinnamon, Chinese Cinnamon, Cassia aromaticum, Cinnamomum) is *Cinnamomum cassia* of the Lauraceae, the pharmaceutical Cassia Bark (BPC, 1949)[121] being the dried bark containing not less than 1% of the volatile oil. It is usually used as a substitute for Ceylon Cinnamon but the oil is less fragrant and more pungent while the taste is harsher than the products of *Cinnamomum zeylanicum*. As some of its synonyms suggest, Cassia is indigenous to China; it is now cultivated in Japan, Sri Lanka, and a number of Far Eastern and South American countries. Somewhat in the manner of Cinnamon proper, the trees of Cassia are grown in coppices, the shoots springing from the roots and being harvested before they are much more than 8 or 10 feet tall. Their appearance when the delicate blossoms and flame-coloured leaves first appear is very beautiful and the dried, unripe fruits, called Chinese Cassia Buds, have been imported into Europe and used as a spice since the Middle Ages.

The second of these quite remarkable formulae, coming from Exodus and being 3000 or more years old, is given in verses 34 and 35 of Chapter XXX[122] in which Moses is told: 'Take unto thee sweet spices, stacte, and onycha, and galbanum; these sweet spices with pure frankincense: of each shall there be a like weight: And thou shalt make it a perfume, a confection after the art of the apothecary, tempered together, pure and holy...'

Stacte was certainly a fragrant spice, probably the finest kind of myrrh, the exudation of the living tree as mentioned by ancient writers, but the name was also applied to a mixture of storax and fat; it has also been thought to have been opobalsamum or tragacanth. Onycha, another word not naturalized in the English language, was the operculum of a species of *Strombus*, or other marine mollusc, which gives a penetrating aroma when burnt.

The third ingredient of this product of the art of the apothecary was Galbanum (BPC, 1934)[123] – the gum-resin obtained from *Ferula galbaniflua*, and probably other species of *Ferula*, indigenous to Persia, and members of the family Umbelliferae. It was thought that some of the drug was collected as the natural exudation of the stem of the plant but most of it was obtained by cutting the plant off at the base and allowing the exudate to harden whilst removing successive slices of the root at intervals. Apart from Persian Galbanum there is a Levant Galbanum known in commerce. The material comes in the form of small ovoid lumps, the best of which are said to be the size of a hazel nut; when broken open, these are found to be formed of clear white tears. Under dry distillation Galbanum yields a thick oil, somewhat bluish in colour, which after purification becomes a clear blue. The odour is characteristic and aromatic but the taste is bitter; both forms contain umbelliferone but Persian galbanum has the more terebinthinate odour. Galbanum used to be employed as a stimulant expectorant in bronchitis, frequently being given in a pill, generally with asafetida (the old Pilulae Galbani Compositae) – a combination which remained of value in the opinion of William Withering whose interest in it is discussed later.

Frankincense is frequently mentioned in the Pentateuch, the synonym being Olibanum. It is the gum-resin obtained from the leafy forest tree, *Boswellia Thurifera* (of the Burseraceae), a native of Arabia and Somaliland. The material contains resins, a volatile oil, gum, bassorin and plant residues. There is a magnificent description of the tree, its habitat, and the making of Frankincense, in *A Modern herbal* by Mrs M. Grieve (1931)[124].

> The trees on the Somali coast grow, without soil, out of polished marble rocks, to which they are attached by a thick oval mass of substances resembling a mixture of lime and mortar. The young trees furnish the most valuable gum, the older yielding merely a clear, glutinous fluid, resembling copal varnish.
>
> To obtain the Frankincense, a deep, longitudinal incision is made in the trunk of the tree and below it a narrow strip of bark 5 inches in length is peeled off. When the milk-like juice which exudes has hardened by exposure to the air, the incision is deepened. In about three months the resin has attained the required degree of consistency, hardening into yellowish 'tears.' The large, clear globules are scraped off into baskets and the inferior quality that has run down the tree is collected separately. The season for gathering lasts from May till the middle of September, when the first shower of rain puts a close to the gathering for that year.

The same source notes that the *kohl*, or black powder with which Egyptian women paint their eyelids, is made of charred Frankincense. The widespread use of Frankincense, sometimes mixed with benzoin and storax, as a ceremonial incense is, however, the use which has made it so well known. Mrs Grieve cites Pliny as mentioning it, as an antidote to hemlock, and Avicenna as recommending it for tumours, vomiting, dysentery and fevers. Hemlock is the product of the poisonous spotted umbelliferous plant, *Conium maculatum*, and Pliny's belief that Frankincense could be effective against such a poison suggests, not science, but magic: so great was the reputation of the incense that it could overcome even the poison with which Socrates (*c.* 470 BC–399 BC) was put to death – the story of the Athenian philosopher's last day and his drinking the hemlock being perfectly told in the *Phaedo* of Plato.

Olibanum, Frankincense (as the dried oleo-resin from the bark of *Boswellia Carterii* Birdw. and other species of *Boswellia*) remained in the BPC 1934[125] but, by then, its uses had shrunk to being 'an ingredient of incense and fumigating powders'. It was listed among the 'Deleted Monographs' of the BPC 1949[126]. It reflects the paucity of our knowledge on these subjects that T. E. Wallis, in his *Textbook of Pharmacognosy*[127] in giving the following account of the constituents of olibanum:

Olibanum consists principally of resin (60 to 70 per cent.), gum (27 to 35 per cent.), and volatile oil (5 to 7 per cent.).

Soluble in alcohol, 72 per cent.	Boswellic acid free	.	.	33·0 per cent.
	,, ,, combined	.		1·5 ,,
	Olibanoresene	.	.	33·0 ,,
	Volatile oil	.	.	7·0 ,,
	Bitter principle	.	.	0·5 ,,
Insoluble in alcohol, 28 per cent.	Gum (arabic acid with Ca and Mg)	.	.	20·0 ,,
	Bassorin	.	.	6·0 ,,
	Vegetable débris	.	.	2.0 ,,

The volatile oil is yellowish and fragrant; it contains pinene, dipentene, and phellandrene, but the aromatic constitutent is not yet known.

cites the study of Halbey from 1898. The leaflets, in their pattern of usually ten pairs with the odd one opposite, and the white or pale rose flowers of Frankincense are shown in Figure 14.

Jacob B. Glenn (1959)[128] listed a number of other drugs, including balsam, hyssop, ladanum, salt, storax gum, sulphur and tragacents, as being found in the Hebrew pharmacopoeia.

Among the many balsams or resins is Balsam of Gilead, *Commiphora Opobalsamum* of the Burseraceae, which William Woodville (1752–1805) in his *Medical Botany . . .* of 1810[129], illustrated (Figure 15) using its synonym *Amyris gileadensis*. Opobalsamum is used by Dioscorides to mean the juice which flows from the balsam tree. The balsam has been prized since antiquity, the tree growing on both sides of the Red Sea and standing 10 or 12 feet high with wand-like delicate branches. It is uncommon and so difficult to rear that it has for centuries been grown in guarded gardens the product of which is sought for its uses as a cosmetic as well as in healing. By repute, it was taken from Arabia to Judea by the Queen of Sheba as a present to Solomon – and in Judea the tree, grown particularly on Mount Gilead, acquired its popular name. The juice exudes on its own in the heat of the summer but it is helped to escape by incisions in the bark; the natural oil of the balm forms about a tenth the amount of the juice.

Its medicinal properties are shared by the Balsam of Peru (*Myroxylon Pereirae* of the Leguminosae) – a large and beautiful tree with a valuable wood like mahogany – that grows in the forests of San Salvador in Central America. Every part of the tree, including the leaves, provides an aromatic resinous juice. The beans of the tree contain Coumarin and a gum resin, distinct from the proper balsam, exudes from the trunk. Balsam of Peru – given its name from the area from which it is shipped – has been used as a stimulant, antiseptic expectorant (for it is said to be excreted by the bronchial mucous glands) and as an anti-parasitic. It has of course been used in scabies, for it destroys the itch acarus and its eggs; it has also been used to heal skin excoriations and fissures.

Balsam of Tolu, from *Myrospermum Toluiferum*, again of the Leguminosae, provides the other well-known balsam. The tree grows in many parts of South America, the balsam being gathered from angled cuts made in the bark and provided with calabash cups placed at the angle of the cut. It has a sweet,

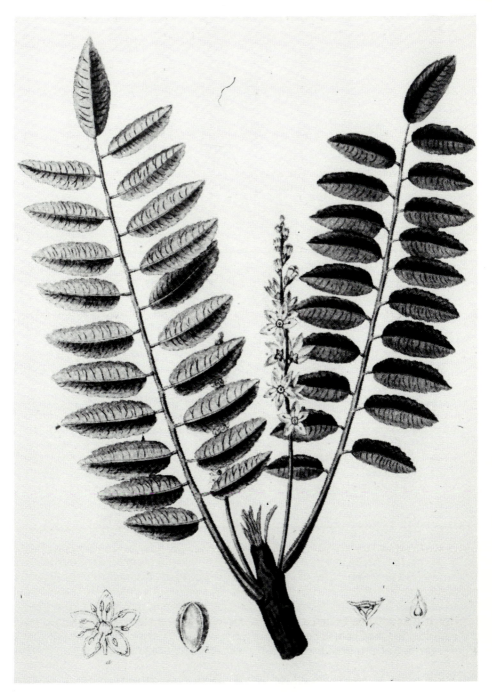

Figure 14 Boswellia Thurifera (Frankincense). [*From: Mrs M. Grieve. A modern herbal. London, Cape (1931).*]

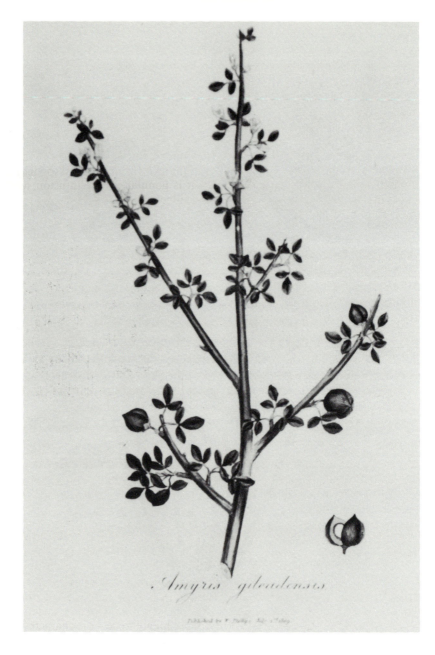

Figure 15   Commiphora opobalsamum or *Amyris Gileadensis* (The Balsam of Gilead).
[*From: William Woodville. Medical botany... London, William Phillips (1810), Vol.
III.*]

aromatic, resinous taste and is fragrant when burned. Its constituents include cinnamic acid, a volatile oil, and a little vanillin, benzyl benzoate and benzyl cinnamate. Its medical uses include its frequent inclusion in expectorant mixtures and its use as an inhalant which is reputed to clear bronchial and nasal catarrh. Tolu Balsam retains its place in the BP 1980[130] and, with Aloes, Prepared Storax, crushed Sumatra Benzoin and Ethanol, forms the basis of the Compound Benzoin Tincture BP, which is Friars' Balsam.

Hyssop (*Hyssopus officinalis* of the Labiatae) was named by the Greeks, the name recalling the use made of gatherings of the short, evergreen bushy herb in the cleaning of sacred places. It is grown, sometimes with lavender and rosemary, for use in the kitchen, in salads, and for its use (as an infusion or as hyssop tea) as a carminative and, by repute, expectorant. It is popular, as the infusion, with herbalists in the treatment of asthma and other illnesses of the chest and it forms, as the tea, one of the country remedies for rheumatism. The essential oil, obtained from the official plant by distillation, is used by perfumers.

Of the other substances listed by Glenn[131], storax gum, in the form of Prepared Storax (the purified balsam obtained from the trunk of *Liquidambar orientalis* and containing not less than 28.5% of total balsamic acids) is a BP 1980[132] item, as is Tragacanth[133] – the air-hardened gummy exudate obtained by incision or seepage from the trunk and branches of *Astragalus gummifer* and related species grown in Western Asia; the pharmacopoeial preparation is Compound Tragacanth Powder (BP). Sterculia[134] is Indian Tragacanth from *Sterculia urens* and other species of *Sterculia*. Of the inorganic materials in the list, salt[135] (Sodium Chloride as the analytical reagent grade of commerce) and Precipitated Sulphur[136], with its own monograph, are pharmacopoeial. Glenn also mentions 'ladanum' – a substance not to be confused with the opiate – and this is referred to later.

Other Biblical inorganic substances – soda and borax – were noted by Preuss[82] and these remain, as Sodium Carbonate[137] and the monographed Sodium Borate[138], part of the current pharmacopoeia. However, it is the botanical substances that provide the main puzzle for, compared with the simple and well-known inorganic salts, we know, in terms of published work, little of the activity of their active principles in pharmacological screens or their properties in organized clinical studies.

Absinthium is an example: it is also called Old Woman, or Wormwood, and is the legendary 'gall and wormwood' of Deuteronomy[139] and other Biblical references. Absinthium is the dried leaves and flowering tops of *Artemisia Absinthium* of the Compositae, a perennial undershrub. It was included in the BPC 1934[140]; this described its volatile oil, which is dark green or blue, and which contains thujone (an isomeride of camphor), thujyl alcohol, cadinene, phellandrene and pinene. The herb also contains the bitter glycoside, absinthin, and absinthic acid. Some of these substances are highly toxic – the characteristic action of absinthium being stimulation of the cerebrum, just as with camphor. The effects of chronic, as well as acute, poisoning have been carefully described. Perhaps thoroughly justifiably, the substance disappeared from the more modern pharmacopoeias but, as with many substances of this kind, we know very little, in contemporary terms, of its science.

The mandrake (Woodville's illustration forms Figure 16) has already been mentioned. As a love potion it appears in the Song of Solomon [141] where it is said: 'The mandrakes give a smell, and at our gates are all manner of pleasant fruits, new and old, which I have laid up for thee...' Culpeper (in Sibly's edition of 1713[99]) is a good deal more prosaic and says its 'fresh root is a violent purge'. He adds that '...it must be used with great caution, otherwise it will bring on convulsions'. Culpeper also notes that 'It has also a narcotic quality.' The modern name of the plant, *Atropa mandragora*, and its family, the Solanaceae, goes some way to explain the pharmacological effects noted by Culpeper. The plant is allied to Belladonna and contains the mydriatic alkaloid, mandragorine, which is probably identical with atropine or hyoscyamine.

Even the helpful plants, like the willow, have a function, in terms of their active principles, related to dose. Of this tree Leviticus [142] speaks of 'the boughs of goodly trees, branches of palm trees, and the boughs of thick trees, and willows of the brook...'

Willow Bark, the bark of *Salix alba* and other species, notably *Salix fragilis*, of the Salicaceae, was still a BPC item in 1934[143]. The same compendium[144], of a little less than 50 years ago, also described Salicin, the crystalline glycoside obtained from Willow Bark and other species of *Salix* and *Populus*. From these barks the active drug Salicin can be extracted and crystallized by very simple means. Its action is virtually that of Salicylic Acid but it is less irritant to the mucous membranes than many salicylates. It was noted (BPC, 1934)[144] 'as a specific in acute rheumatism' and was also employed in influenza. The drug was considered best administered as a mixture but, by whatever means it is given, it must provide one of the strongest links between the drugs of Biblical times and one of the most widely used remedies of today.

Salicylic acid itself (o-hydroxybenzoic acid), BP 1980[145], can be obtained either synthetically (from the sodium salt prepared from the action of carbon dioxide on sodium phenate) or naturally (by the hydrolysis of naturally occurring salicylates, such as Sweet Birch Oil)[46]. Years ago the natural product was held to be free of impurities found in the synthetic form of the acid and, for medical use, was sometimes preferred for this reason. Salicylic acid is an active antiseptic, less irritant in dilute solution than phenol; strong solutions, carefully applied, allow callosities and warts to be softened and removed from the skin. Swallowed, it is irritant to the mouth and stomach and, for internal use, has been replaced by Acetylsalicylic Acid (Aspirin). This is today's commonest drug – an antipyretic and analgesic of especial importance in treating rheumatism and acute rheumatic conditions.

Glenn[131] spoke of ladanum and Preuss[147] of laudanum, the latter being Tincture of Opium (BPC, 1968)[148]. Opium, as already mentioned, is the partly dried latex obtained from the unripe seed capsules of the Opium Poppy (Figure 17), *Papaver somniferum*, of the Papaveraceae, and Woodville[149], in his edition of 1810, provides the following anecdotal account of the history and collection of this material:

> Opium, ... is obtained from the heads or capsules of this species of Poppy, and is imported into Europe from Persia, Arabia, and other warm regions of Asia. The manner in which it is collected has been described long ago by

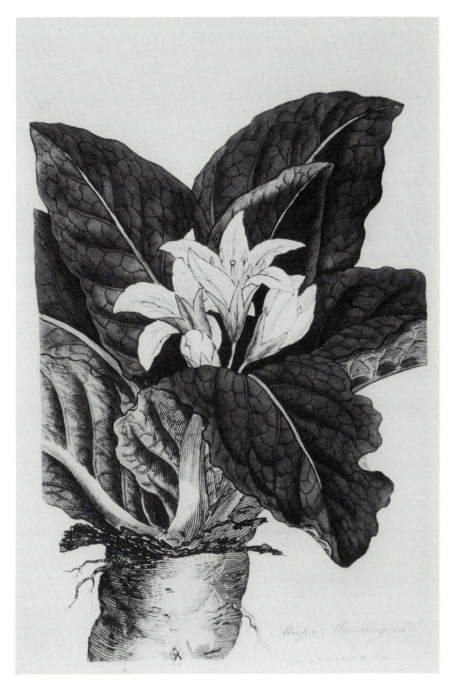

Figure 16   *Atropa mandragora* (The mandrake). [*From: William Woodville. Medical botany . . . London, William Phillips (1810), Vol. II.*]

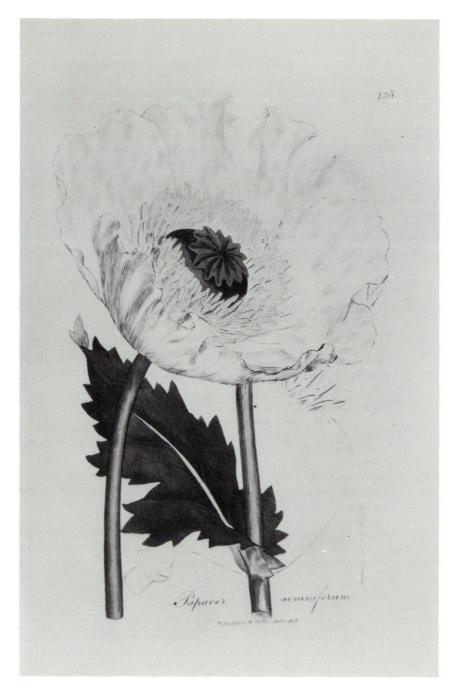

Figure 17 Papaver somniferum (The opium poppy). [*From: William Woodville. Medical botany . . . London, William Phillips (1810), Vol. II.*]

Kæmpfer and others; but the most circumstantial detail of the culture of the Poppy, and the method of procuring the opium from it, is that given by Mr. Kerr, as practised in the province of Bahar: he says, The field being well prepared by the plough and harrow, and reduced to an exact level superficies, it is then divided into quadrangular areas of seven feet long, and five feet in breadth, leaving two feet of interval, which is raised five or six inches, and excavated into an aqueduct for conveying water to every area, for which purpose they have a well in every cultivated field. The seeds are sown in October or November. The plants are allowed to grow six or eight inches distant from each other, and are plentifully supplied with water. When the young plants are six or eight inches high, they are watered more sparingly. But the cultivator strews all over the areas a nutrient compost of ashes, human excrements, cow dung, and a large portion of nitrous earth, scraped from the highways and old mud walls. When the plants are nigh flowering, they are watered profusely to increase the juice.

"When the capsules are half grown, no more water is given, and they begin to collect the opium.

"At sun-set they make two longitudinal double incisions upon each half-ripe capsule, passing from below upwards, and taking care not to penetrate the internal cavity of the capsule. The incisions are repeated every evening until each capsule has received six or eight wounds; they are then allowed to ripen their seeds. The ripe capsules afford little or no juice. If the wound was made in the heat of the day, a cicatrix would be too soon formed. The night-dews by their moisture favour the extstillation of the juice.

"Early in the morning, old women, boys and girls, collect the juice by scraping it off the wounds with a small iron scoop, and deposit the whole in an earthen pot, where it is worked by the hand in the open sunshine, until it becomes of a considerable spissitude. It is then formed into cakes of a globular shape, and about four pounds in weight, and laid into little earthen basins to be further exsiccated. These cakes are covered over with the Poppy or tobacco leaves, and dried until they are fit for sale. Opium is frequently adulterated with cow-dung, the extract of the Poppy plant procured by boiling, and various other substances, which they keep in secresy." – "Opium is here a considerable branch of commerce. There are about 600,000 pounds of it annually exported from the Ganges."

It appears to us highly probable, that the White Poppy might be cultivated for the purpose of obtaining opium to great advantage in Britain. Alston says, "the milky juice, drawn by incision from Poppy-heads, and thickened either in the sun or shade, even in this country, has all the characters of good opium; its colour, consistence, taste, smell, faculties, phœnomena, are all the same; only, if carefully collected, it is more pure and more free of feculencies."

Similar remarks have also been made by others, to which we may add those of our own; for during the last summer, we at different times made incisions in the green capsules of the White Poppy, from which we collected the juice, which soon acquired a due consistence, and was found, both by its sensible qualities and effects, to be very pure opium.

Opium, called also Opium Thebaicum, from being anciently prepared chiefly at Thebes, has been a celebrated medicine from the remotest times. It differs from the Meconium, which by the ancients was made of the expressed juice or decoction of the Poppies.

Opium is imported into Europe in flat cakes, covered with leaves to prevent their sticking together: it has a reddish brown colour, and a strong peculiar smell: its taste, at first, is nauseous and bitter, but soon becomes acrid, and produces a slight warmth in the mouth: a watery tincture of it forms an ink, with a chalybeate solution. According to the experiments of Alston, it appears to consists of about five parts in twelve of gummy matter, four of resinous matter, and three of earthy, or other indissoluble impurities.

The use of this celebrated medicine, though not known to Hippocrates, can be clearly traced back to Diagoras who was nearly his cotemporary, and its importance has ever since been gradually advanced by succeeding physicians of different nations. Its extensive practical utility however has not been long well understood; and in this country perhaps may be dated from the time of Sydenham. Opium is the chief narcotic now employed; it acts directly upon the nervous power, diminishing the sensibility, irritability, and mobility of the system; and, according to a late ingenious author, in a certain manner suspending the motion of the nervous fluid, to and from the brain, and thereby inducing sleep, one of its principal effects. From this sedative power of opium, by which it allays pain, inordinate action, and restlessness, it naturally follows, that it may be employed with advantage in a great variety of diseases. Indeed, there is scarcely any disorder in which, under some circumstances, its use is not found proper; and though in many cases it fails of producing sleep, yet if taken in a full dose, it occasions a pleasant tranquillity of mind, and a drowsiness, which approaches to sleep and which always refreshes the patient. Besides the sedative power of opium, it is known to act more or less as a stimulant, exciting the motion of the blood; but this increased action has been ingeniously, and, as we think, rationally ascribed to that general law of the animal œconomy, by which any noxious influence is resisted by a consequent re-action of the system. By a certain conjoined effort of this sedative and stimulant effect, opium has been thought to produce intoxication, a quality for which it is much used in eastern countries.

In this account Opium is differentiated from Meconium (in ancient times made of the expressed juice or decoction of the Poppy); it is also said to have been unknown to Hippocrates, although it is traced back to someone who was almost his contemporary. The date implied for the earliest knowledge of real Opium is the fourth century BC. Scribonius Largus (*De compositionibus medicamentorum liber unus*, 1528)[50], whose life spanned the period about AD 1–50, provides the first clear account of Opium. He says: 'it is made from the milk of the heads of wild poppies, not from the juice of the leaves, which the pedlars of ointments make for a profit.' He adds that, 'A little of the first is obtained with great labour, the latter is easily ground and in large amounts.' His account, and those of the great medical botanists like Woodville, suggests that the Canaanites knew Meconium, but not Opium, the source of morphine.

There have been many accounts of popular substitutes for opium – one of the more interesting appearing in Arthur Herbert Church's 1879 revision of James F. W. Johnston's *The Chemistry of Common Life*[150], first published 25 years before. At that time knowledge of chemistry and biochemistry was largely confined to what Church called 'a select class of professional persons'. Such subjects were more widely read by 1879 and such reading would have suggested a commonplace source of an alternative to the latex of the Opium Poppy. Church says that:

> In Europe, the different species of the lettuce (*Lactuca*) are capable, to a certain extent, of supplying the place of the poppy. The juice of these plants,

when collected and dried, has considerable resemblance to opium.

If the stem of the common lettuce, when it is coming into flower, be wounded with a knife, a milky juice exudes. In the open air this juice gradually assumes a brown colour, and dries into a friable mass. The smell of this dried juice is strongly narcotic, recalling that of opium. It has a slightly pungent taste, but, like opium, leaves a permanent bitter in the mouth. It acts upon the brain after the manner of opium and induces sleep.

To this crude extract the name of *Lactucarium* has been given by its discoverer, Professor Duncan of Edinburgh, who was followed by many physicians in its use as a sedative. Like opium, it dissolves in water to the extent of about one-half, and in this soluble portion the narcotic virtue resides. The principal active ingredient is supposed to be a peculiar substance named *lactucin,* of which the crude extract contains about one-fourth of its weight. It contains other active ingredients, however – the chemical nature and physiological influence of which have not as yet been rigorously investigated.

Discussion

Sir Alan Gardiner, in his *Egyptian Grammar* of 1927 and the expanded edition of 1950[151], provides a means to an increased understanding of the language of ancient Egypt. Similarly, Frans Jonckheere, in the *Autour de L' Autopsie d'une Momie, Le Scribe royal Boutehamon* (1942)[152] gives a far more detailed account of the radiological examination, unwrapping, and autopsy of a mummy than any previously mentioned.

These two works define their subjects more closely than the descriptions or records which were available – and there are constant similar additions to knowledge. In just the same way, ideas that once seemed well established undergo challenge. For example, Srboljub Živanović, in his book on *Ancient Diseases, the Elements of Palaeopathology* (1982)[153], writing of trepanning and skull injuries caused by surgery, says: 'as far as palaeopathologists are concerned, the most acceptable explanation is that pain was the primary motive for submitting to the surgical remedy of opening the skull.' This suggests that, to the contemporary specialist, the idea of letting the demons escape (as an explanation for the trephined hole in an ancient skull) is unfashionable. But primitive man would soon learn that opening the chest or abdomen to relieve pain was unsuccessful. And what causes of pain, apart perhaps from obvious local trauma, would be relieved by the size and type of hole that was trephined? While many of the challenges to old knowledge add to our understanding this particular one serves, perhaps, to make the explanation that satisfied Osler and his generation seem all the more convincing.

Discoveries also alter what was already known. Quite recently those described in *The Archives of Ebla: an Empire Inscribed in Clay*[154] – a book written by Giovanni Pettinato and translated from the Italian in 1979 – revealed evidence of a previously undescribed civilization geographically situated between the sites of the Sumerians in ancient Mesopotamia and those of the ancient Egyptians along the Nile. Pettinato and his colleagues found the remains of the palace of the ancient kings of Ebla and a royal archive of something like 10000 cuneiform tablets. From these discoveries it seems likely that in the third millenium BC Ebla must have been a great political and cultural centre trading not only with the Canaanites but also with the distant inhabitants of Egypt and Mesopotamia. The studies of the language of Ebla have begun in the fascinating work of Pettinato; these researches are complemented by the account *Ebla: an Empire Rediscovered*[155] by Paolo Matthiae, the chief excavator at Ebla, whose book appeared in 1977 after translation by Christopher Holme. So far none of the Eblaite tablets that have been translated add much to our knowledge of primitive medicine or surgery but a quite new source of information would seem to have been made available for further study.

The remnants of the civilization of ancient Egypt include the works of art depicting survival after death, the human remains of the rite of mummification, the writings of the tomb inscriptions, the account of the Book of the Dead – and so on. This great multitude of artefacts demonstrates, beyond any doubt, that a vivid belief in the supernatural played a large part in the early attempts to deal with the psychological problems of disease and death. In just the same way, the recitals contained in the Ebers Papyrus, the many strange prescriptions forming parts of Ebbell's translation of it, and the charms and incantations of the Assyrian Herbal, show the degree to which intense superstition permeated the early attempts at therapeutics. The belief in demonic possession, the practice of exorcism, and the arts of divination and astrology add to the impression. Even among the early monotheists of Canaan, the long-lasting concept of sacrifice, the mandrake fertility myth, and the story of Saul's necromancy, show how persistent other-world beliefs had become. Thus, it seems that magic is the most potent part of much of primitive religion and, perhaps to a degree which seems strange to some modern minds, magic also appears to provide the source and beginning of medicine.

Of the 829 prescriptions of the Ebers Papyrus there are very few that appear rational – and a not inconsiderable number that look positively harmful. Trauma and the obvious problems of simple surgery are more readily understood than the arcane problems of medicine. These problems are therefore tackled rationally when internal medicine remains mysterious and obscure. Early attempts at medical treatment arise from the use of magic to deal with what is totally obscure – and this produces the materia medica of the oldest civilizations. There is, in fact, little real evidence that the ancients had much by way of useful drugs – and there is a good deal to suggest that the sick would have been wise to have escaped from the primitive pharmacopoeia.

Perhaps one of the inferences that can be drawn from the remnants of the ancient civilizations is that man, faced with fears of disease and death and problems he cannot understand, develops some sort of unifying hypothesis. This produces composure and security, uniting what is known with an explanation of the unknown. Even in science a hypothesis is necessary. It is possible to look at quite sophisticated and advanced unifying hypotheses and see in them the same sort of unfounded security. Modern statistical theory, in some of its medical extensions, provides an example: the observational basis for the theory relates to simple events and their probabilities but confidence remains even when the ideas are applied to complex biological variables. We are sometimes disturbed to be reminded at the higher limits of confidence that the discussion is not of fact but of a theory.

The greatest achievement of the ancient peoples seems to have been the hygienic consequences of the Mosaic code, this being associated with the rejection of much of the gross superstition affecting the non-Judaic nations. It can be assumed that the Jews, prevented by their concept of cleanliness and its religious purpose, from developing a *dreckapotheke*, avoided a great deal of iatrogenic disease. The rejection of the grosser elements of superstition found in Egypt and Mesopotamia certainly seems to have led the Jews, in the form of the law of Moses, to the pinnacle of ancient achievement, limited though it was. Later history suggests that a similar rejection of superstition is essential if the practical arts are to develop and man is to progress with the solving of his problems by means of logic and science. As with the Jews we have had to learn that hygiene is the most potent of medicines.

Beyond the Mosaic law there is very little that can be taken for real accomplishment in the medicine of early Egypt, Mesopotamia, or Palestine. The contrast between the medicine, and the great art, architecture, and social organization of these peoples is, at first sight, startling. The people who could build the pyramids and temples of Egypt or the hanging gardens of Babylon had, it would seem, little but superstition and an evil pharmacopoeia to offer by way of internal medicine.

Thus, those who look for the beginnings of therapeutics in ancient times find little but magic. Some of it still survives: the doctor does not always demand real evidence of safety or efficacy and the patient who expects a drug at each consultation must often take it as a talisman. The conclusion cannot be evaded that a crude and primitive medicine lessened the achievement of the ancient and seemingly brilliant civilizations.

References

1. Martindale, William. The extra pharmacopoeia, incorporating Squire's Companion. Eds. Ainley Wade and James E. F. Reynolds. 27th edn., London, *Pharmaceutical Press*, 1977, p. 105
2. Morton, Leslie Thomas. A medical bibliography (Garrison and Morton), an annotated check-list of texts illustrating the history of medicine. 3rd edn., London, *André Deutsch*, 1970, p. 219
3. Lucas-Championnière, Just Marie. Trépanation néolithique, trépanation pré-Colombienne, trépanation des Kabyles, trépanation traditionnelle. Paris, *G. Steinheil*, 1912
4. Rodwell, Warwick. Wells Cathedral: excavations and discoveries. Wells, *The Friends of Wells Cathedral*, 1979 (revised 1980), pp. 16–20
5. Breasted, James Henry. A history of the Ancient Egyptians. London, *John Murray*, 1908, p. 15
6. Breasted, James H. (1908). As ref. 5 but pp. 104–105
7. Comrie, John Dixon. Medicine among the Assyrians and Egyptians in 1500 BC. *Edinburgh Med. J.,* 1909, **2** (New series), 101–129, p. 109
8. Griffith, Francis Llewellyn. The Petrie Papyri: hieratic papyri from Kahun and Gurob (principally of the Middle Kingdom). London, *B. Quaritch*, 1898
9. Comrie, John D. (1909). As ref. 7 but p. 110
10. The Edwin Smith Surgical Papyrus. Published in facsimile and hieroglyphic transliteration with translation and commentary by James Henry Breasted. 2 vols. Chicago, *Univ. Press*, 1930

11. Ebers, Georg. Papyros Ebers: Das Hermetische Buch über die Arzeneimittel der Alten Ägypter in Hieratischer Schrift. 2 vols. Leipzig, *Engelmann*, 1875
12. Comrie, John D. (1909). As ref. 7 but p. 121
13. The papyrus Ebers. The greatest Egyptian medical document. Translated by B. Ebbell. Copenhagen, *Levin & Munksgaard*, 1937
14. Wreszinski, Walter. Der Papyrus Ebers: Umschrift, Übersetzung und Kommentar. Leipzig, *J. C. Hinrichs*, 1913
15. Cave, Alexander James, Ancient Egypt and the origin of anatomical science. In: Ed. Sir Zachary Cope, Sidelights on the history of medicine. London, *Butterworth*, 1957, pp. 7–12
16. Cave, Alexander J. (1957). As ref. 15 but p. 10
17. Smith, Sir Grafton Elliot and Dawson, Warren Royal. Egyptian mummies. London, *Allen and Unwin*, 1924
18. Smith, Sir Grafton Elliot. The most ancient splints. *Br. Med. J.,* 1908, **1**, 732–734
19. Osler, Sir William, The evolution of modern medicine, a series of lectures delivered at Yale University on the Silliman Foundation in April, 1913. New Haven, *Yale Univ. Press*, 1921, p. 17
20. Osler, Sir William (1921). As ref. 19 but pp. 16–17
21. Smith, Sir Grafton Elliot and Ruffer, Sir Marc Armand. Pott'sche Krankheit an einer ägyptischen Mumie. Giessen, *A. Töpelmann*, 1910
22. Ruffer, Sir Marc Armand. Note on the presence of 'Bilharzia haematobia' in Egyptian mummies of the Twentieth Dynasty (1250–1000 BC). *Br. Med. J.,* 1910, **1**, 16
23. Shattock, Samuel George. Microscopic sections of the aorta of King Menephtah. *Vide*: Medical Societies: Royal Society of Medicine, Pathological Section. *Lancet*, 1909, **1**, 318–319
24. Ruffer, Sir Marc Armand. Studies in the palaeopathology of Egypt. Ed. R. L. Moodie. Chicago, *Univ. Press*, 1921
25. Moodie, Roy Lee. Paleopathology: an introduction to the study of ancient evidences of disease. Urbana, *Univ. Illinois Press*, 1923
26. Smith, Sir Grafton Elliot and Dawson, Warren R. (1924). As ref. 17 but p. 20
27. Pettigrew, Thomas Joseph. A history of Egyptian mummies, and an account of the worship and embalming of the sacred animals by the Egyptians . . . London, *Longman*, 1834
28. The archaeological survey of Nubia. Report for 1907–1908. Volume 2: Report on the human remains by G. Elliot Smith and F. Wood Jones. Ministry of Finance, Egypt; Survey Department. Cairo, *National Printing Dept.,* 1910. *Vide*: volume of plates accompanying Vol. 2, p. 284 ff
29. Smith, Sir Grafton Elliot. The alleged discovery of syphilis in prehistoric Egyptians. *Lancet*, 1908, **2**, 521–524
30. Wood Jones, Frederic. The examination of the bodies of 100 men executed in Nubia in Roman times. *Br. Med. J.,* 1908, **1**, 736–737
31. Leake, Chauncey Dephew. The old Egyptian medical papyri. Kansas, *University of Kansas Press*, 1952
32. Leake, Chauncey D. (1952). As ref. 31 but p. 4
33. Leake, Chauncey D. (1952). As ref. 31 but p. 34
34. Reisner, George A. The Hearst medical papyrus: hieratic text in 17 facsimile plates in collotype with introduction and vocabulary. Leipzig, *J. C. Hinrichs*, 1905
35. Wreszinski, Walter. Der Londoner Medizinische Papyrus (Brit. Museum Nr. 10059) und der Papyrus Hearst, in Transkription, Übersetzung und Kommentar. Leipzig, *J. C. Hinrichs*, 1912
36. Jonckheere, Frans. Le papyrus médical Chester Beatty. Bruxelles, *Fondation Égyptologique Reine Elisabeth,* 1947. *La Médecine Égyptienne*, No. 2
37. Grapow, Hermann. Anatomie und physiologie. In: Grundriss der medizin der alten Ägypter I. Vols. 1–9. Berlin, *Akademie-Verlag*, 1954–73
38. Sigerist, Henry Ernest. A history of medicine. Vol. 1–2. New York, *Oxford University Press,* 1951–61

39. Steuer, Robert O. and Saunders, J. B. de C. M. Ancient Egyptian & Cnidian medicine. The relationship of their aetiological concepts of disease. Berkeley, *Univ. Calif. Press,* 1959

40. Withington, Edward Theodore. Medical history from the earliest times. London, *Scientific Press,* 1894

41. Withington, Edward T. (1894). As ref. 40 but p. 22

42. Ebbell, Bendix (1937). As ref. 13 but p. 15

43. Steuer, Robert O. and Saunders, J. B. de C. M. (1959). As ref. 39 but p. 3

44. Withington, Edward T. (1894). As ref. 40 but pp. 20–23

45. Singer, Charles Joseph. A Short History of Medicine. Oxford, *Clarendon Press,* 1928

46. Singer, Charles J. (1928). As ref. 45 but p. 7

47. Ebbell, Bendix (1937). As ref. 13 but p. 25

48. Leake, Chauncey D. (1952). As ref. 31 but pp. 16–17

49. Leake, Chauncey D. (1952). As ref. 31 but p. 72

50. Scribonius Largus. De compositionibus medicamentorum liber unus. *Parisiis, ap. C. Wechel,* 1528

51. Sigerist, Henry E. (1951). As ref. 38 but Vol. 1, p. 362

52. Ghalioungui, Paul. Magic and medical science in Ancient Egypt. London, *Hodder and Stoughton,* 1963, p. 164

53. Ghalioungui, Paul (1963). As ref. 52 but pp. 170–171

54. Osler, Sir William (1921). As ref. 19 but p. 11

55. Jeremiah xlvi, 11 (AV)

56. Woolley, C. Leonard. Babylonian prophylactic figures. *J. R. Asiatic Soc.,* 1926 (Oct.), pp. 688–713

57. Comrie, John D. (1909). As ref. 7 but p. 101

58. Harper, Robert Francis. The Code of Hammurabi, King of Babylon, about 2250 BC. Autographed text, transliteration, translation, glossary, index of subjects, lists of proper names, signs, numerals, corrections and erasures, with map, frontispiece and photograph of text. Chicago, *Univ. Chicago Press* and London, *Luzac.,* 1904

59. Dawson, Warren Royal. The beginnings. Egypt and Assyria. New York, *Hoeber,* 1930, p. 59

60. Jastrow, Morris. The medicine of the Babylonians and Assyrians. *Proc. R. Soc. Med.; Sect. Hist. Med.,* 1913–14, **7,** 109–76

61. Jastrow, Morris (1913–14). As ref. 60 but p. 113

62. Jastrow, Morris (1913–14). As ref. 60 but p. 117

63. Thompson, Reginald Campbell. Assyrian medical texts. From the originals in the British Museum. London, *Oxford Univ. Press,* 1923
    Also: *Proc. R. Soc. Med.; Sect. Hist. Med.,* 1923–24, **17,** (Parts 1–2), pp. 1–34 (p. 31)

64. Thompson, Reginald C. (1923–24). As ref. 63 but p. 32

65. Thompson, Reginald C. (1923–24). As ref. 63 but pp. 28–29

66. Thompson, Reginald Campbell. Assyrian medical texts. *Proc. R. Soc. Med. Sect. Hist. Med.,* 1925–26, **19,** (Parts 1–2), pp. 29–78 (pp. 59–60)

67. Thompson, Reginald C. (1925–26). As ref. 66 but p. 8

68. Dawson, Warren Royal. Magician and leech. A study in the beginnings of medicine with special reference to Ancient Egypt. London, *Methuen,* 1929

69. Jastrow, Morris (1913–14). As ref. 60 but p. 118

70. Thompson, Reginald Campbell. The devils and evil spirits of Babylonia, being Babylonian and Assyrian incantations against the demons, ghouls, vampires, hobgoblins, ghosts, and kindred evil spirits which attack mankind, translated from the original cuneiform texts with transliterations, vocabulary, notes etc. 2 vols. London, *Luzac,* 1903–04

71. Thompson, Reginald C. (1923). As ref. 63 but p. iv

72. Thompson, Reginald Campbell. The Assyrian Herbal. London, *Luzac,* 1924

73. Thompson, Reginald Campbell. Assyrian prescriptions for diseases of the chest and lungs. *Revue d'Assyriologie et d'Archeologie Orientale.* Paris, *Leroux,* 1934, **31** (1), 1–19

74. Thompson, Reginald C. (1934). As ref. 73 but p. 18

75. Thompson, Reginald C. (1925–26). As ref. 66 but p. 44

76. Thompson, Reginald C. (1923–24). As ref. 63 but p. 2

77. Dawson, Warren R. (1930). As ref. 59 but pp. 72–73

78. The British Pharmaceutical Codex 1973. London, *Pharmaceutical Press*, 1973, p. 800
79. British Pharmacopoeia 1980. London, HMSO, 2 vols., 1980, Vol. II, Appendix IA, p. A29
80. The British Pharmaceutical Codex 1949. London, *Pharmaceutical Press*, 1949, p. 571
81. Ezekiel xxi, 21 (AV)
82. Preuss, Julius. Biblisch-talmudische Medizin Beiträge zur Geschichte der Heilkunde und der Kultur überhaupt. Berlin, *S. Karger*, 1911. Republished, with introduction by Šussman Muntner, New York, *Ktav*, 1971
83. Wood, Percival. Moses: the Founder of Preventive Medicine. New York, *Macmillan*, 1920
84. Frazer, Sir James George. Folk-lore in the Old Testament. Studies in comparative religion, legend and law. 3 vols., London, *Macmillan*, 1918
85. Breasted, James H. (1908). As ref. 5 but pp. 264–267 and 428
86. Genesis xv, 7–18 (AV)
87. Jeremiah xxxiv, 18 (AV)
88. Frazer, Sir James G. (1918). As ref. 84 but Vol. I, pp. 392–393
89. Macalister, R. A. Stewart. Reports on the excavation of Gezer. London, (ND), pp. 66–73 and 103
90. Macalister, R. A. Stewart. The excavation of Gezer 1902–1905 and 1907–1909. 3 vols., London, *John Murray*, 1912. Vol. II, pp. 429–431
91. Frazer, Sir James G. (1918). As ref. 84 but Vol. I, pp. 416–417
92. Genesis xxix, 16–17 (AV)
93. Genesis xxx, 14–17 (AV)
94. Genesis xxx, 22–23 (AV)
95. Frazer, Sir James G. (1918). As ref. 84 but Vol. II, p. 372
96. Dioscorides, Pedanius, Anazarbeus. De materia medica. Ed. Max Wellmann. 3 vols., Berolini, *Weidmann*, 1906–14, iv, p. 76
97. Parkinson, John. Theatrum botanicum: The theater of plants. Or, an herball of a large extent. London, *T. Cotes*, 1640, p. 343
98. Bombastus Ab Hohenheim, Aurelius Philippus Theophrastus [Paracelsus]. Septem libri de gradibus, de compositionibus, de dosibus receptorum ac naturalium. Basileae, *P. Perna*, 1568
99. Culpeper, Nicholas. (Ed. Sibly, E.). Culpeper's English Physician and complete herbal . . . Illustrated with notes and observations, critical and explanatory; by the late E. Sibly. 2 vols. 15th. edn., London, *W. Lewis*, 1813
100. Exodus xxii, 18 (AV)
101. 1 Samuel xxviii, 3 (AV)
102. 1 Samuel xxviii, 14–19 (AV)
103. Leviticus xx, 6 (AV)
104. Leviticus xx, 27 (AV)
105. Deuteronomy xviii, 10–12 (AV)
106. Exodus xv, 26 (AV)
107. Young, John. Essays and Addresses. Glasgow, *MacLehose*, 1904, p. 99
108. Glenn, Jacob B. The Bible and modern medicine. New York, *The Jewish Forum*, 1959, p. 47
109. Deuteronomy viii, 7–8 (AV)
110. Leviticus xi, 47 (AV)
111. Leviticus xiii and xiv (AV)
112. Leviticus xiii, 44–45 (AV)
113. Sudhoff, Karl Friedrich Jakob. Annals of medical history. 2 vols. 1917, Vol. I, pp. 113–117
114. Job v, 18 (AV)
115. Friedenwald, Harry. The Jews and medicine. Essays. 2 vols. Baltimore, *Johns Hopkins Press*, 1944–46. Vol. I, pp. 100–101
116. Ecclesiastes vii, 1 (AV)
117. Exodus xxx, 23–25 (AV)
118. BPC (1973). As ref. 78 but pp. 317 and 822
119. BP (1980). As ref. 79 but Vol. I, pp. 113–114; Vol. II, p. 839
120. The British Pharmaceutical Codex 1934, an Imperial dispensatory for the use of medical practitioners and pharmacists. London, *Pharmaceutical Press*, 1934, p. 241

121. BPC (1949). As ref. 80 but p. 223
122. Exodus xxx, 34–35 (AV)
123. BPC (1934). As ref. 120 but pp. 475–476
124. Grieve, Mrs M. A modern herbal. The medicinal, culinary, cosmetic and economic properties, cultivation and folklore of herbs, grasses, fungi, shrubs and trees with all their modern scientific uses. Ed. Mrs C. F. Leyel, London, *Cape*, 1931. Reprinted 1974, 1975. pp. 326–328
125. BPC (1934). As ref. 120 but pp. 749–750
126. BPC (1949). As ref. 80 but p. 1459
127. Wallis, T. E. Textbook of pharmacognosy. London, *Churchill*, 1946, 5th edn. 1967, p. 500
128. Glenn, Jacob B. (1959). As ref. 108 but p. 20
129. Woodville, William. Medical botany: containing systematic and general descriptions, with plates of all the medicinal plants, indigenous and exotic, comprehended in the catalogues of the materia medica, as published by the Royal Colleges of Physicians of London and Edinburgh: together with most of the principal medicinal plants not included in those pharmacopoeias. 4 vols. 2nd edn., London, *William Phillips*, 1810. Vol. III, plate 214, opp. p. 603
130. BP (1980). As ref. 79 but Vol. I, p. 459 and Vol. II, p. 833
131. Glenn, Jacob B. (1959). As ref. 108 but p. 20
132. BP (1980). As ref. 79 but Vol. II, p. 427
133. BP (1980). As ref. 79 but Vol. I, p. 460 and Vol. II, p. 711
134. BP (1980). As ref. 79 but Vol. I, p. 426
135. BP (1980). As ref. 79 but Vol. II, Append. 1A, p. A36
136. BP (1980). As ref. 79 but Vol. I, p. 440
137. BP (1980). As ref. 79 but Vol. II, Append. 1A, p. A36
138. BP (1980). As ref. 79 but Vol. I, p. 62
139. Deuteronomy xxix, 18 (AV)
140. BPC (1934). As ref. 120 but pp. 2–3
141. The Song of Solomon vii, 13 (AV)
142. Leviticus xxiii, 40 (AV)
143. BPC (1934). As ref. 120 but pp. 918–919
144. BPC (1934). As ref. 120 but pp. 917–918
145. BP (1980). As ref. 79 but Vol. I, pp. 396–397
146. BPC (1934). As ref. 120 but pp. 41–42
147. Preuss, Julius (1911 but 1971 edn.). As ref. 82 but p. xx
148. British Pharmaceutical Codex 1968. London, *Pharmaceutical Press*, 1968, p. 557
149. Woodville, William (1810). As ref. 129 but Vol. II, pp. 378–381
150. Johnston, James F. W. The chemistry of common life. Revised by Arthur Herbert Church. Edinburgh, *Blackwood*, 1879, p. v.
151. Gardiner, Sir Alan. Egyptian grammar, being an introduction to the study of hieroglyphs. 2nd. edn., Oxford, *Geoffrey Cumberlege*, 1950
152. Jonckheere, Frans. Autour de l'autopsie d'une momie, le scribe royal Boutehamon. Bruxelles, *Fondation Égyptologique Reine Elisabeth*, 1942
153. Živanović, Srboljub. Ancient diseases, the elements of palaeopathology. Translated by Lovett F. Edwards. London, *Methuen*, 1982, pp. 186–187
154. Pettinato, Giovanni. The archives of Ebla, an empire inscribed in clay. New York, *Doubleday*, 1981
155. Matthiae, Paolo. Ebla, an empire rediscovered. Translated by Christopher Holme. London, *Hodder and Stoughton*, 1977

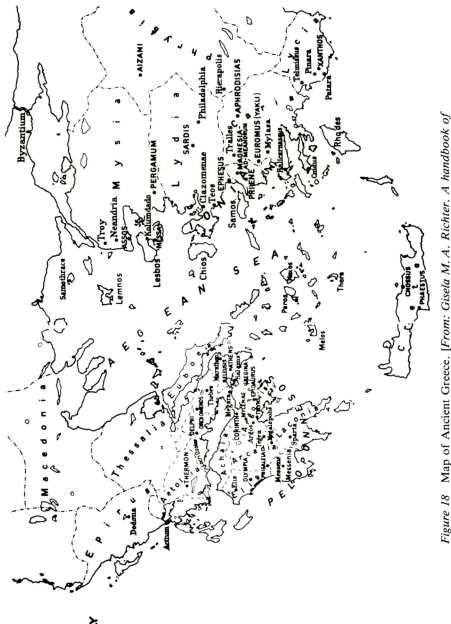

Figure 18 Map of Ancient Greece. [*From: Gisela M.A. Richter. A handbook of Greek Art, London, Phaidon Press, (1969).*]

2

The World of Greece and Rome

Ancient Greece – to about 300 BC

The Sumerian civilization of Ur was already mature when the first Neolithic waves of settlers went by sea from the mainland of Asia to the islands and coast of Greece not later than 3000 BC. They occupied Crete and the adjacent coastal regions before being reinforced by other settlers early in the Bronze Age, which began about 2600 BC in Greece. In this way, Crete became the home of another of the world's oldest civilizations – the Cretan or Minoan civilization which took its name from Minos, the legendary king, son of Zeus by Europa. It seems possible that as the source of the legend there was a historical King Minos and that the labyrinth at Knossos, the chief centre of the Minoan people, was either the royal sarcophagus or palace.

Knossos is said to have been first discovered by a Cretan merchant who, in 1878, decided to dig a well in an olive grove that had been in his family for many years. He quickly came across an ancient wall and pieces of broken pottery which a few years later were recognized by the extremely well funded archaeologist, Sir Arthur Evans (1851-1944), as being Minoan. Evans purchased the whole site (about 40 acres) in 1894 and spent the next 40 years excavating and reconstructing it. Knossos lies in the central zone of Crete, to the south of the present-day capital, Iraklion. This busy, ancient capital, situated on the northern coast of the island, possesses the second largest harbour of Crete and the world's most outstanding and interesting Minoan museum.

Sir Arthur Evans seems to have decided early in his exploration that Knossos was a Minoan Palace, but not all are agreed; today the great building is often thought of as having been principally a royal sarcophagus or burial chamber whose beginnings are obscured by the facts that it was not built to a systematic plan and what original design there was fell in ruins in an earthquake of 1730 BC. Reconstruction led to the Early Minoan (3000–2000 BC) ground strata being cut away as the foundations of the Middle Minoan (2000–1550 BC) palace were prepared. Thus, in the central court at Knossos the remains of late Neolithic buildings lie directly beneath the Middle Minoan Period paving and the whole assemblage speaks of a number of historical periods. Part of its present impressive remains are shown in Figure 19. *The Palace of Minos*[156] is the text which records the work of Sir Arthur J. Evans. The chronology of Knossos is given in R. W. Hutchinson's *Prehistoric Crete*[157] and the famous story of the unravelling of the Minoan script is told in one of the most fascinating of writings, *The Decipherment of Linear B*[158] by J. Chadwick.

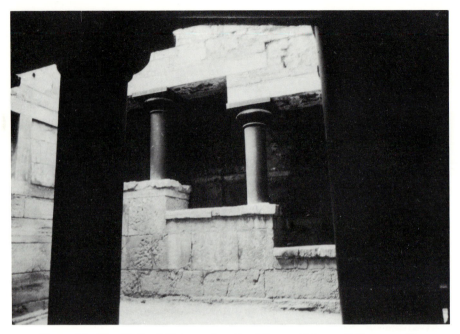

Figure 19 The Hall of Colonnades, the Minoan Palace of Knossos, Crete.

It is clear that on Crete the Minoans prospered and achieved a high degree of artistic attainment by 2000 BC or soon after. They built unfortified dwellings and palaces, as if protected from surprise attack and from enemies by the intelligence gathered by their fleets which were engaged in a widespread sea-faring trade – a perhaps unexpected situation when one remembers the bloody and appalling Mesopotamian and Syrian conflicts of the time. Nevertheless, the Minoan civilization slowly declined in importance as, one by one, the cities of Greece rose to prominence; it was followed by the Mycenaean civilization, Mycenae itself being the ancient city in the Peloponnesus some 15 miles north-east of present-day Argos.

In Mycenae the Bronze Age inhabitants and successive waves of immigrants developed their own new and remarkable culture that, after the sacking of Knossos in about 1400 BC, dominated the eastern Mediterranean. With the passage of time Mycenae was itself destroyed, probably in 468 BC.

The religion of both the Minoan and Mycenaean civilizations centred upon a female deity who, in Crete, was often represented in human form attended by cult priestesses accompanied by animal-headed humans. While this religion held sway, and between the times of the fall of Knossos and Mycenae, the people of Greece spread their settlements to Asia Minor, Italy, Sicily, the islands of the Aegean Sea, and eventually along most of the European and Asiatic coasts of the

Mediterranean. It is this which was the great and flourishing Greece depicted by Homer, the Greek epic poet whose life has usually been placed at about 1000 years before Christ in the period between 1200 and 850 BC. Whether or not Homer was a historical person, the spread of the Hellenic culture is shown by the fact that no less than seven cities: Chios, Smyrna, Rhodes, Argos, Athens, Colophon and Salamis in Cyprus, have claimed to be his birthplace. The culture of these great cities was the source of the *Iliad*, in which the poet describes the concluding weeks of the siege of Troy by the Greeks, and the *Odyssey*, in which he records the wanderings of Ulysses (Odysseus) following the fall of Troy.

By the sixth century before Christ, Greece comprised a number of city-states each of which was active in trade, most of it sea-faring, and politics. Amongst these states, Athens, Corinth, Sparta and Thebes were especially prominent and in their cities art and literature began to flourish as never before. Part of the sixth century experience comprised the lives of Thales of Miletus (639–544 BC) and Pythagoras of Samos (580–489 BC), both of whom embodied the freshness and impetus that became the chief characteristic of the civilization of Greece.

It was this classical Greek culture that, by some novel accession of thought, provided not only the beginnings of observational science but also the basis and early growth of rational and logical medicine. In biology the achievement was immense – the product of a civilization which reached its zenith in Athens in the fifth century before Christ – the Golden Age of Pericles (495–430 BC) – an Age which witnessed the life not only of Empedocles of Agrigentum (504–443 BC) but, most crucially of all, that of Hippocrates (460–370 BC), the Father of Medicine.

The individual lives of these founders of biologically-based medical thinking are represented in the chart forming Figure 20. The great epoch began as Greece won her long drawn-out struggle with the weakening, but still fearsome, Persian Empire. On land, at Marathon, a plain of Greece 25 miles north-east of Athens, the Persians invaded the mainland and camped close to the sea. There they were attacked by a Greek army, chiefly composed of Athenians, directed by Miltiades. News of the Greek victory was conveyed to Athens by Pheidippides, the Olympic champion runner who, from exhaustion, died as he entered the city. Ten years later, in 480 BC, at the Greek island of Salamis near Athens, the final massive Persian fleet was defeated by the Athenians. Each of these enormous battles, their memorials merely the record of history, took place early in the life of Pericles but the Parthenon (built between 447 and 438 in Athens) provides a monument to the fullness of the Greek Golden Age; the remains (Figure 21) of the Temple of Poseidon (430 BC), built on a promontory overlooking the sea at Sounion, provide another memorial to the years which shared the maturity of Pericles.

Even in the Golden Age the union between the Greek states remained fragile. Faced with the menace of Persia the city-states managed some kind of alliance but, with the threat for a time removed, Athens and Sparta, in 431 BC, entered upon the Peloponnesian War. In 404 BC this ended with the defeat of Athens. At first Sparta and then Thebes became the most powerful of the city-states, but each increasingly weakened the other. In 359 BC Philip of Macedon (382–336 BC), having risen to tremendous power, succeeded in making himself ruler of the whole of Greece and King of Macedonia. It was against Philip's overwhelming ambition that the Athenian orator, Demosthenes (384–322 BC) directed his famous Philippic orations, many of which have survived. Despite the protesta-

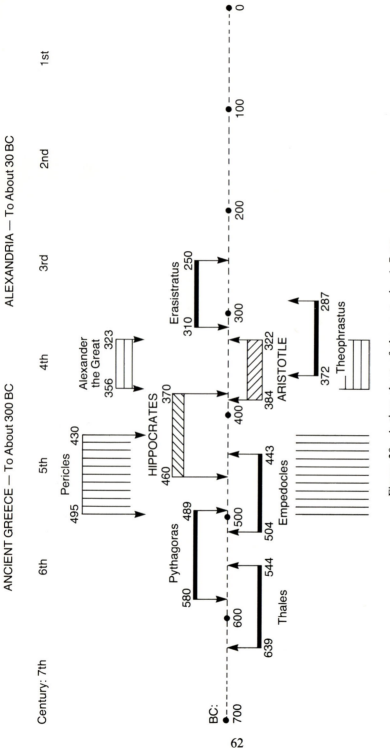

Figure 20 A time-chart of the centuries 1–7 BC.

62

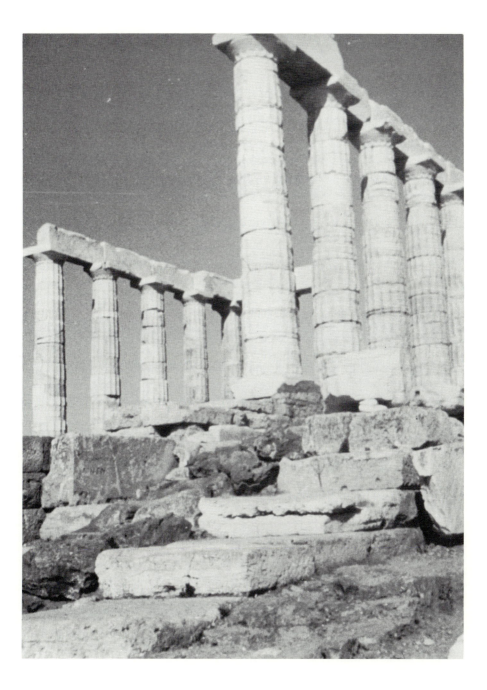

Figure 21 The Temple of Poseidon on Cape Sounion (430 BC), Greece.

tions, Philip, not only consolidated his own empire but also laid the foundations of the later conquests of his son, Alexander.

Greece is remembered for her philosophers, but the teachings and the lives of both Socrates (469–399 BC) and his pupil Plato (427–347 BC) had both already ended when, in 336 BC, Philip was succeeded by Alexander the Great and the groundwork which had been laid was used as the basis of the mightiest of all ancient military campaigns. Alexander (356–323 BC), determined to end for all time the menace of Persia, attacked the then huge Persian Empire. In 334 BC he marched his army into Asia Minor; this he conquered and, with comparative ease, overcame Phoenicia and Syria. Using his fleet, he eliminated the enemy resistance at Tyre. Egypt submitted with hardly a struggle and, having founded the city of Alexandria, he passed through Syria and on into Persia. He then traversed the historic valley of the Tigris, capturing the great Persian cities, and reached the Caspian Sea. In 326 BC, far to the east of Greece, Alexander crossed the river Indus near Attock and gained his final great victory. He returned to Persepolis, and set himself to the huge task of organizing his massive territorial gains. In the midst of this undertaking, he died.

After his death Alexander's Empire crumbled: the strength of the Greek nation had reached what can now be seen to have been its furthermost territorial limits. In the second century before Christ, the whole of Macedonia became challenged by the expanding power of Rome. Under this western assault, and with the fall of Corinth in 146 BC, the vigour of Greece faded and, before long, Greece was absorbed into the Roman Empire. By then the life of Aristotle (384–322 BC), which had overlapped that of Alexander the Great, had passed almost two centuries into the distance of history. The three centuries that remained, after Aristotle, and before the start of the Christian era, saw the intellect that characterized Greece reside for a while in Alexandria, before its great epoch, culminating in the life of Galen, began in Rome.

The roots of Greek medicine

Folk medicine, Temple medicine, and the Hippocratic tradition form the three main themes of the medicine of Ancient Greece. Emma J. and Ludwig Edelstein in their valuable *Asclepius, A Collection and Interpretation of the Testimonies*[159], provide the following quotation and translation of Isidore, Bishop of Seville (Isidorus Hispalensis; AD 570–636). Isidore's encyclopaedic work, the *Etymologiarum libri xx*[160] of 1472, presents the sum of contemporary knowledge in all branches of science. In Book IV[161] he gives a survey of the entire range of medicine, remarking that[162]:

> Prima Methodica inventa est ab Apolline, quae remedia sectatur et carmina. Secunda Enpirica, id est experientissima, inventa est ab Aesculapio, quae non indiciorum signis, sed solis constat experimentis. Tertia Logica, id est rationalis, inventa ab Hippocrate.
>
> First, methodical medicine was invented by Apollo, which pursues remedies and incantations. Second, empiric medicine was invented by

Asclepius, that is, the most tested medicine, which is founded not on indications and signs but on experience alone. Third, logical, that is, rational medicine, was invented by Hippocrates.

In this passage Isidore, one of the great educators of the Middle Ages, reviews the three great themes or varieties of the medical art and says that these are: firstly, 'remedies and incantations'; secondly, 'empiric medicine', the temple medicine invented by Asclepios and based 'on experience alone'; and thirdly, 'logical, that is, rational medicine...invented by Hippocrates'.

Isidore writing of the actual discoverers of medicine [163, 164], adds that:

Medicinae autem artis auctor ac repertor apud Graecos perhibetur Apollo. Hanc filius eius Aesculapius laude vel opere ampliavit. Sed postquam fulminis ictu Aesculapius interiit, interdicta fertur medendi cura; et ars simul cum auctore defecit, latuitque per annos pene quingentos usque ad tempus Artaxerxis regis Persarum. Tunc eam revocavit in lucem Hippocrates Asclepio patre genitus in insula Coo.

The originator and discoverer of the art of medicine is among the Greeks reputed to be Apollo. This art his son Asclepius furthered in glory and accomplishment. But after Asclepius died from the stroke of the thunderbolt, healing is said to have been forbidden. The art ceased together with its founder and remained obscured for almost 500 years until the time of Artaxerxes, the King of the Persians. Then Hippocrates, begotten of Asclepius on the island of Cos, restored it to light.

The practical roots of Greek medicine must, at the beginning, have lain in the submerged civilization of the conquered Minoan people and it may well be that the cult of the serpent – so constantly associated with Asclepius and still used as a medical emblem – was itself Minoan. Some of the hygienic ideas of the Greeks may have come from the same source for the excavations of Crete have shown that the old Minoan cities were equipped with effective sanitation and means of drainage.

There were, of course, other profound influences and the civilizations that lay along the valleys of the Tigris and Euphrates must be assumed to have provided those few demonic and superstitious beliefs that sank into Greek folk and temple medicine and affected, usually where it was most ignorant, Greek professional medical thought. There were, however, other aspects of the inheritance and it seems likely that the acquisition of Mesopotamian observational astronomy, mathematics, and numeracy by the Greeks must have been greatly to their advantage. The orderly conduct of the affairs of medicine, embodied in the Code of Hammurabi, must also have been of benefit to the Greek successors of Babylon. The Greeks derived additional mathematical knowledge and plant lore from Egypt and some of their drugs and practical means and devices of surgery seem to have had similar beginnings. Lastly, in the same way that the people of the Nile deified Imhotep, a historical figure, to provide themselves with a god of medicine, so the Greeks derived their own physician-god, Asclepius, from the same tradition.

It seems increasingly clear that the ancient civilizations influenced one another and borrowed from one another far more than used to be thought. A fairly recent example is the remarkable findings at Elba (page 52) of a very early literate civilization, geographically situated between Egypt and Mesopotamia. The existence of the people of Ebla emphasizes the close and durable communications that linked these old civilizations. By the time of the fifth century before Christ and the Greek Golden Age there must have been well-established channels of communication affecting many of the ancient means of learning. Thus all three types of medicine in Greece can be seen to have been influenced by the earlier nations – a realization which makes it surprising that Hippocrates and his followers rid themselves, to the great extent that they did, of the incubus and inheritance of the old beliefs.

But by no means all superstition died out in Greece. Of what remained, some became part of folk medicine and some sank into the substance of witchcraft. The latter vast subject has its weird pharmacological aspects and Robert Graves, in his study the *Greek Myths*[165], mentions a poisoning by a cup of wine containing wolfsbane; he tells us that 'because wolfsbane flourishes on bare rocks, the peasants call it "aconite".' He then adds: 'Aconite, a poison and paralysant, was used by the Thessalian witches in the manufacture of their flying ointment: it numbed the feet and hands and gave them a sensation of being off the ground.'[166] Assisted by a certain measure of fact, this idea was to last a long time: Margaret Murray, a distinguished Egyptologist before she started her studies on witchcraft, in her book, *The Witch-cult in Western Europe*[167], provides an Appendix in which Professor A. J. Clark discusses the formulae of the different 'flying' ointments. The first is 'Parsley, water of aconite, poplar leaves, and soot'. The second is 'Water parsnip, sweet flag, cinquefoil, bat's blood, deadly nightshade, and oil'. The third is 'Baby's fat, juice of water parsnip, aconite, cinquefoil, deadly night-shade, and soot'. All three prescriptions show a mixture of the 'dung pharma-copoeia' and pharmacologically very active plant agents. Aconite occurs in two of the formulae, and deadly nightshade (or dwale, *Atropa belladonna*, all parts of which are narcotic and poisonous from the presence of atropine) also occurs in two.

Clark[167] says that 'Aconite was one of the best known poisons in ancient times; indeed it was so extensively used by professional poisoners in Rome during the Empire that a law was passed making its cultivation a capital offence. Aconite root contains about 0.4% of alkaloid . . . the drug has little effect upon the con-sciousness, but produces slowing, irregularity, and finally arrest of the heart.' These properties would make it an effective poison but applied to the skin it had other actions – and it was these which made it so appropriate and popular in flying ointments: Martindale[168] records that 'When applied to the skin it produces tingling followed by numbness. . .'. This is, presumably, the quantum of fact behind the myth of the witches' flying.

Aconite (Aconite Root; Monkshood Root; Wolfsbane Root) is the dried root of *Aconitum napellus* agg. of the Ranunculaceae. It contains from 0.2 to 1.5% of total alkaloids, the ether-soluble alkaloids being chiefly aconitine. With large doses death is almost instantaneous. With toxic doses there is a characteristic tingling of the tongue, mouth, and skin, followed by numbness and anaesthesia; death may then occur after heart rate disturbances and muscular weakness from

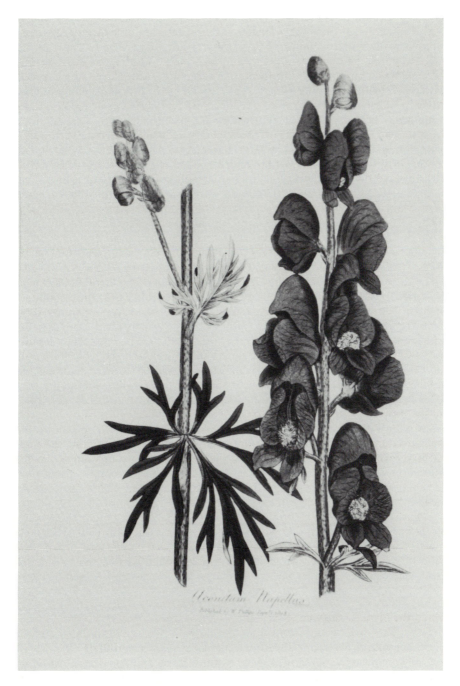

Figure 22 *Aconitum napellus* (The Monkshood or Wolfsbane). [*From: William Woodville. Medical botany . . . London, William Phillips (1810), Vol. III.*]

cardiac or respiratory paralysis. As little as 5–10 ml of tincture of aconite may be fatal. Although recognized as a dangerous therapeutic agent it was, for ages, used in very small doses to diminish the force and rate of the heart. The pharmacopoeias contain a number of preparations of modern times and these include: Aconite, Belladonna and Chloroform Liniment (BPC 1968)[169]; Aconite Liniment (also BPC 1968)[170]; Aconite Tincture (BPC 1949)[171] and Strong Aconite Tincture (the old 'Fleming's Tincture of Aconite; BPC 1949)[172]. The BPC 1934[173] contained a monograph on the active alkaloid, aconitine.

Although it is no longer part of therapeutics, Monkshood remains a common plant in England. Figure 22 shows the characteristic leaf structure, which grows brightly from the rhizome in March; it shows also the flower which, in July and August, provides tall purple spires in many of the older gardens. The original of the Figure is in *Medical Botany: Containing Systematic and General Descriptions, with Plates of all the Medicinal Plants, Indigenous and Exotic, etc.* (1810)[174]. This is the great textbook of William Woodville, not only one of the most distinguished of medical botanists but also physician to the London Smallpox and Inoculation Hospital – in which role he played an important part in the story of vaccination by Jenner.

Of the other influences on the Greeks, the thinking of the Hebrews, although dominated by supernatural concepts, is notable for its having contained singularly little witchcraft. The Witch of Endor has already been mentioned but there are few such examples; the scriptural Lilith[175] was really a lone, demonic inhabitant of the wild desert places rather than a witch. The verses that describe her say: 'And the wild beasts of the desert shall meet with the wolves, and the satyr shall cry to his fellow; yea, the night-monster shall settle there, and shall find her a place of rest.' The RV footnote is 'night-monster – Heb. Lilith'.

Babylonian belief in Lilith and such night-hags of the open spaces was strong, for the peoples of Babylon believed that such personified evil spirits came from the abode of the dead to visit pests and destruction on the living and inflict increased danger on the sick. As a result, Assyria had laws demanding the death of those who made magical potions and there were similiar sanctions at times in Ancient Egypt. It seems that where demonic forces have been most feared there has almost always arisen strong exhibitions of disapproval of non-professional meddling with them.

Thus, looking at these different influences, it seems clear that there was a whole buried or partly buried world of dark superstition clustered around the roots of Greek medicine. That the Greeks cleansed their medical art of these beliefs to the extent that was achieved forms no small part of their ultimately great achievement.

Asklepios (Asclepius; Lat. Aesculapius)

The thaumaturgical terror of Mesopotamia and the later period of Egypt, while not fully removed, was greatly lessened by the Greek Pantheon of gods with their almost human attributes. The legend was that the knowledge of medicine began with Apollo and was passed to Asklepios, son of Apollo by the beautiful nymph, Coronis. Asklepios is reputed to have become so proficient in the healing art that he was accused of diminishing the number of shadows in Hades. For this he was destroyed by the thunderbolt of Zeus. The true glory of the art then fell into decay but even in their straitened circumstances his worshippers were enabled to form a guild of physicians, the Asklepiads. The many temples of the cult comprised the famous Asklepieia, the two greatest being at Cos and Epidaurus.

Among the legendary children of Asklepios by his wife, Epione, were his daughters, Hygieia and Panacea. Their names remain alive in medicine as indicating the things which, in terms of illness, either prevent all, or heal all. In the temples they assisted in the healing rites and fed the sacred snakes which, entwined upon the staff, became the emblem of medicine.

Asklepios, then, was the god of healing, the greatness of the temple at Cos depending on its association with Hippocrates. The Hieron, 6 miles from the town of Epidaurus on the coast of Peloponnesos, opposite Sounion, was the chief centre for the worship of Asklepios; the god is shown, in a relief dated about 400–380 BC, in Figure 23. Richard Caton provides a well-illustrated account of the buildings forming the Hieron in his *Two Lectures on the Temples and Ritual of Asklepios at Epidaurus and Athens*[176].

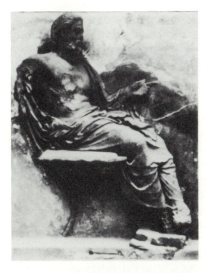

Figure 23   Asklepios. Relief from the Temple of Asklepios at Epidauros (About 400–380 BC), Athens, National Museum.

The temples were usually built on wooded hills or mountain slopes near mineral springs and the central shrine of that at Epidaurus formed a richly decorated and coloured Doric building, beautifully colonnaded and shaded, of the fourth century BC. Apart from the Temple of Asklepios, the Hieron of Epidaurus contained buildings and features which are thought to have provided a Gymnasium, a Grove, the baths of Asklepios, hostels, a Temple to Artemis and another to Aphrodite, a Stadium, long Colonnades, places for seclusion, and a number of walks and quadrangles. The Asklepieion at Athens was situated on the south side of the Acropolis, perhaps 80 feet above the mainland plain, and on a site that must have been as healthy as any that the immediate neighbourhood of Athens could provide.

The Hiereus, the priest, was the chief temple official and was appointed annually; he was not always a physician. Subordinate officials included junior priests and physicians, torch-bearers and fire-carriers (who lit the sacred flame on the altars) key-bearers, others with secular and financial duties, and priestesses (who were the ultimate carriers of the mysteries or holy things).

Probably many thousands of vigorous and fit people, as well as the sick, attended the great festivals; many of them were lodged in the nearby town, and the hamlets and villages. Patients, when they arrived, probably had an interview with the Hiereus, performed certain rites, bathed in the sacred fountain, and made offerings. An act of ceremonial purification seems to have formed an important part of the established rite. In the evening, as the practices are imagined, sacred lamps were lit and the priest recited prayers, entreating divine help and recounting divine cures. He then enjoined silence and commanded those who entered upon sleep to expect benign and healing visions from Asklepios. The sleeping chamber was a lofty and airy structure open on its south side to the colonnade. Whether, in the dim light, priests acted the part of the visiting god, or the patients responded to some anodyne or to suggestion, or the benefits depended on the regime of diet, appropriate rest, a fine climate, and the divine gift to the sick of expectation, is no longer known. The rite of the temple was called 'incubation': help was to come to the believer as in dream. After its success the patient made a votive offering – a wax, silver or gold model of the part that had been diseased – and many of these appreciative and artistic exhibits remain.

In earlier times it seems that the restoration to health achieved at such a shrine was considered purely miraculous. When the miracle failed the diseased might be led to some distant shrine, or to a hillside or hamlet to die. The impure, those about to give birth, and the moribund, were all excluded. Of the folk medicine of those in the inns and boarding-houses, and of the practices of those who cared for the mortally ill, we know little or nothing.

Thus, although today we might see the exclusion of the terminally ill and incurable as repulsive, we might also see the temple rite as providing a freedom from inappropriate drug therapy and associating this with the physical and mental means of restoration for those in whom there could be a benign outcome from their disease.

Three centuries before Christ the rulers of Rome, having failed to check a disastrous pestilence, were counselled by the Sibylline books to bring Asklepios from Epidaurus to Rome. It is said that as the galley returning from the Hieron approached Rome the sacred serpent escaped and found refuge on the island of the Tiber opposite the city – and from the city the plague then disappeared. A Temple of Aesculapius (as the Romans latinized the name of the god) was built adjacent to the island; it has been used since then, in pagan and Christian times alike, to heal the sick. It was the founding of this temple and the nature of the works wrought within it which has been said to have ensured that the staff and serpent of Aesculapius would become, and remain, the symbol of the profession of medicine.

The later literature saw Asklepios as the Antichrist and as the most significant threat to the young Christian Church. This literature is splendidly collected in the book by Emma J. and Ludwig Edelstein[159] already cited. The writings, statues and their inscriptions, coins and architectural finds, concerned with Aesculapius continue to cause interest – resulting in works like that of C. Kerényi, *Asklepios, Archetypal Image of the Physician's Existence*[177].

These studies, and others on the subject, show the healing religion of Aesculapius to have been clouded with superstition and a belief in miracles but to have presented these beliefs with elegance and mixed them with admirable practices of hygiene. In the end, however, the elegance fades in a rejection of those most grossly in need of care.

Hippocrates

The earliest of the Ionian philosophers who show the refreshment of the human spirit which began scientific biology and medicine was Thales of Miletus (639–544 BC). Thales studied under the Egyptian priests and taught that water is the primary element from which all else in nature is derived. The use of this kind of perhaps figurative language may have been of far greater antiquity; whether it was, or not, it forms a characteristic part of the sixth century intellectual process which discarded superstition and sought naturalistic explanations for natural things.

Pythagoras of Samos (580–489 BC), ultimately founder of the Italian School of Philosophers, was born on the island of Samos, a little to the north of the birth-place of Thales, and a little later. The life of Pythagoras was perhaps the hallmark of the sixth century and its new attitude to the world around it. Pythagoras probably acquired his doctrine of the mystical power of numbers when in Egypt and he carried this and the Chaldean (or neo-Babylonian) number-lore into the pattern of Greek thinking. He held number to be the first principle of the universe and taught that on the function of numbers depended the harmonies which first established, and which now maintain, the universe in its orderly motion.

In the fifth century – the century of the Golden Age of Pericles – Empedocles of Agrigentum (504–443 BC) undertook a further development of the views of Thales and his successors teaching that the four primordial elements, earth, air, fire, and water, comprised the four-fold root of all things. Empedocles, who was born at a site on the southern coast of Sicily (a fact which suggests that the intellectual awakening was quite widespread), believed that health results from the balance, and illhealth from the imbalance, of these four elements. However unlikely this theory might now seem, the idea provided the first real concept of a natural, as distinct from a supernatural, causation of disease.

This theory was of the utmost importance to the whole subsequent development of science and was not displaced until quite modern times; it is therefore worth following it a little further before returning to the great fifth century events.

Within Greek thinking particular significance was attached to the number 4 and this was used by the natural philosophers to add four qualities: dry, cold, hot, and moist, to the four elements. The characteristic qualities were related to the four elements in the following manner:

earth	=	cold	+	dry
air	=	hot	+	moist
fire	=	hot	+	dry
water	=	cold	+	moist

It was held, almost certainly before the time of Hippocrates and well before the days of Aristotle, that corresponding to the four elements and the four qualities there were four humours of the body: black bile, blood, yellow bile, and phlegm. These were thought of as being almost physiological manifestations of the four qualities, thus:

black bile	=	cold	+	dry
blood	=	hot	+	moist
yellow bile	=	hot	+	dry
phlegm	=	cold	+	moist

Frederick F. Cartwright, in his interesting recent book *A Social History of Medicine*[178], observes that 'The doctrine of humours persists in common nomenclature. We still speak of a "bilious attack" when we mean a digestive upset, still use "phlegmatic" in contradistinction to "choleric", and often speak of "good humour" and "bad humour".'

Originally, health and disease were thought to arise from either balance or imbalance of these humours and it is notable that these, seemingly strange, concepts were not only accepted by Hippocrates but were further elaborated by Galen and the Arabian physicians; in their fully developed form they were of profound influence for something like 1500 years.

The Arabian apothecaries classified their drugs and compounds according to the degrees, or relative proportions, of their different qualities. Fielding H. Garrison (1870–1935), in his substantial *An Introduction to the History of Medicine*[179], gives some examples: 'sugar is cold in the first degree, warm in the second degree, dry in the second degree, and moist in the first degree; cardamoms are warm in the first degree, cold by one-half a degree, dry in the first degree, and so forth.'

These views, resting in their early stages on the number 4, have their literal aspects – water, for example, is certainly fundamental to all forms of life – but they also have their mystical implications. That they are incorrect in a factual sense does not alter their importance: they were used in predicting the outcome of disease and, whatever the process by which the mind of man threw off some of its old terrors in the sixth and early fifth centuries, these theories represented the first determined attempts to evolve natural, as distinct from superstitious, explanations of the unknown.

To some extent these concepts were also used in the treatment of disease: lack of phlegm was treated with seafoods such as oysters which are cold and moist; but most illnesses were thought to be due to an imbalance caused by an excess of one or other of the humours – rather than by a lack of one or more humours. Thus, as time went by, too much blood (too great a moist heat, as in fever) was treated by bleeding. In the same way, an excess of phlegm was treated by purging or vomiting; an excess of yellow bile, showing in the urine, by causing sweating, and so on. The Middle Ages, and the inhabitants of Europe until the nineteenth century, were therefore bled when they least needed it and purged, vomited, and sweated in their weaknesses. These means, used sometimes with lethal enthusiasm, explain why the pharmacopoeias down the ages have been full of drugs which have these effects.

The figure '4' and the four humours were of great importance in the first great schools of medicine. Pythagoras of Samos founded what was perhaps the most famous of the early medical schools at Crotona in Italy but it is known that in certain colonial towns there were medical schools as early as the fifth century before Christ. From Crotona the views of Pythagoras, the most well known of the early philosopher-physicians, were carried throughout the then known world.

The Coan School of Hippocrates was centred on the island of Cos (Kos), one of the most eastern of the Greek islands; it lies close to the coast of what is now Turkey, midway between Samos and Rhodes. The proximity to Cnidus, on a peninsula of the mainland and the home of the Cnidian School, is remarkable: the two schools faced one another across only a small expanse of the eastern Aegean Sea – yet they contrasted fundamentally in their philosophy.

The Hippocratic or Coan School aimed at prognosis by a general study of the symptoms and signs of known diseases. It centred its attention on the patient and his individual reaction to the disease, seeing the clinical manifestations as the product of the interaction between the morbid process itself and the healing or naturally restorative powers of the body. Thus the illness was individual but often affected by very general processes, such as inflammation or cachexia. The morbid process itself was seen as causing imbalance (apepsia) of the humours, and thereby producing symptoms. The healing powers of the body brought the apeptic humours into a state of coction or balance (pepsis) and this could produce its own symptoms, such as fever or pus. Treatment aimed merely to assist the body in its work of restoration – and this resulted in rapid extrusion of the concocted humours and morbid material (crisis) or in a slower achievement (lysis) of the same process. Throughout, the patient was considered as an individual, to be understood, if he was to be understood at all, as a whole and singular being unique and peculiar to himself. It was upon this basis that the illness was to be diagnosed and the prognosis individually established.

The Cnidian School, whose greatest physician was Euryphon, reputedly author of the Cnidian Sentences, by contrast centred its attention upon the disease process itself rather than on the patient. It aimed at exact diagnosis of the morbid process and its classification and upon establishing an appropriate and specific therapy. Its actual therapy is said to have been limited to purges, milk and whey. Garrison says that 'Cnidian medicine, the medicine of library classifiers, of the pathological specimen . . . is largely the medicine of our own period of ultra-refined diagnosis and highly specialized therapy.'[180]

Of the temples of Asklepios and their part in the growth of medicine, the Asklepieion on the island of Cos is unique as having been at the birthplace of Hippocrates (460–?370 BC), himself an Asklepiad. Hippocrates, the Father of Medicine (Figure 24), is a shadowy figure and the only contemporary record of him, as a person, is said to have been written by Plato. Socrates and Plato – about both of whom we know a great deal – were contemporaries of Hippocrates. The later years of both Pericles and Empedocles overlapped the first half of his life;

the date given for his death was in the boyhood of Aristotle. These dates, perhaps as traditional as the nobility of the face of Hippocrates, would make him 90 when he died. There is no doubt that there was a historical Hippocrates, even if some of the later years ascribed to his life are those of his school or a successor.

Of the ancient biographers of Hippocrates, the most frequently quoted is Soranus of Ephesus (fl. 2nd century AD). Soranus was the chief physician of the 'methodists' and practised in Alexandria and Rome. He has two extant treatises (*On Fractures*, in J.L. Ideler *Physici et medici minores*[181], 1841, and *On Midwifery and the Diseases of Women*[182], the latter being first printed in 1838) but his most important work is *On Acute and Chronic Diseases*[183]; the latter exists only in fragments in Greek but is given in a complete fifth century Latin translation by Caelius Aurelianus. Soranus tells us that Hippocrates was born at Cos in 460 BC; that he was a member of an Asklepiad family of renown; that he travelled extensively and then returned to Cos to become the most illustrious physician of his age, and that he died in 375 BC. Other sources give a number of different dates for his death.

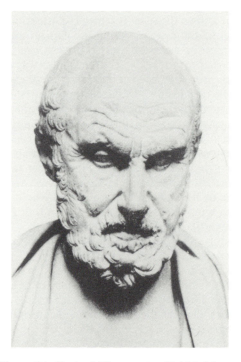

Figure 24   Bust of Hippocrates (British Museum).

In effect, he is known to us as the person whose humane presence illuminates a number of the books forming what is known as the Hippocratic Collection. His personality can be seen in these books to have been benign and his nature observant. In what are considered the authentic parts of the Collection there is an original gnomic quality of thought which suggests that the ideas have been scrutinized more than once before being given expression. The literary style has received much comment for it has a refreshing, lucid and simple quality.

Using the W. H. S. Jones translation of 1923 [184] (mentioned later) we can see the type of clinical description undertaken by Hippocrates in the book *Epidemics I*:

Case IV

In Thasos the wife of Philinus gave birth to a daughter. The lochial discharge was normal, and the mother was doing well when on the fourteenth day after delivery she was seized with fever attended with rigor. At first she suffered in the stomach and the right hypochondrium. Pains in the genital organs. The discharge ceased. By a pessary these troubles were eased, but pains persisted in the head, neck and loins. No sleep; extremities cold; thirst; bowels burnt; scanty stools; urine thin, and at first colourless.

Sixth day.   Much delirium at night, followed by recovery of reason.

Seventh day.   Thirst; stools scanty, bilious, highly coloured.

Eighth day.   Rigor; acute fever; many painful convulsions; much delirium. The application of a suppository made her keep going to stool, and there were copious motions with a bilious flux. No sleep.

Ninth day.   Convulsions.

Tenth day.   Lucid intervals.

Eleventh day.   Slept; complete recovery of her memory, followed quickly by renewed delirium.

A copious passing of urine with convulsions – her attendants seldom reminding her – which was white and thick, like urine with a sediment and then shaken; it stood for a long time without forming a sediment; colour and consistency like that of the urine of cattle. Such was the nature of the urine that I myself saw.

About the fourteenth day there were twitchings over all the body; much wandering, with lucid intervals followed quickly by renewed delirium. About the seventeenth day she became speechless.

Twentieth day.   Death.

Case V

The wife of Epicrates, who lay sick near the founder, when near her delivery was seized with severe rigor without, it was said, becoming warm, and the same symptoms occurred the following day. On the third day she gave birth to a daughter, and the delivery was in every respect normal. On the second day after the delivery she was seized with acute fever, pain at the stomach and in the genitals. A pessary relieved these symptoms, but there was pain in the head, neck and loins. No sleep. From the bowels passed scanty stools, bilious, thin and unmixed. Urine thin and blackish. Delirium on the night of the sixth day from the day the fever began.

Seventh day.   All symptoms exacerbated; sleeplessness; delirium; thirst; bilious, highly-coloured stools.

Eighth day.   Rigor; more sleep.

Ninth day.   The same symptoms.

Tenth day.   Severe pains in the legs; pain again at the stomach; heaviness in the head; no delirium; more sleep; constipation.

Eleventh day.   Urine of better colour, with a thick deposit; was easier.

Fourteenth day. Rigor; acute fever.

Fifteenth day. Vomited fairly frequently bilious, yellow vomit; sweated without fever; at night, however, acute fever; urine thick, with a white sediment.

Sixteenth day. Exacerbation; an uncomfortable night; no sleep; delirium.

Eighteenth day. Thirst; tongue parched; no sleep; much delirium; pain in the legs.

About the twentieth day. Slight rigors in the early morning; coma; quiet sleep; scanty, bilious, black vomits; deafness at night.

About the twenty-first day. Heaviness all over the left side, with pain; slight coughing; urine thick, turbid, reddish, no sediment on standing. In other respects easier; no fever. From the beginning she had pain in the throat; redness; uvula drawn back; throughout there persisted an acrid flux, smarting, and salt.

About the twenty-seventh day. No fever; sediment in urine; some pain in the side.

About the thirty-first day. Attacked by fever; bowels disordered and bilious.

Fortieth day. Scanty, bilious vomits.

Eightieth day. Complete crisis with cessation of fever.

Of the *opera omnia*, the masterwork is the *Oeuvres complètes d'Hippocrate. Traduction nouvelle avec le texte grec en regard...Par E. Littré*, published in Paris in 1839–61[185]. This monumental and scholarly Greek–French bilingual edition, one of the most important extant editions of Hippocrates, was the result of twenty-two years of diligent effort by Littré. It forms a monument to French scholarship and follows the first complete edition of Hippocrates, this having been printed in Latin and issued from Rome by Favius Calvus in 1525; there was also a Greek edition of the collected works printed by Aldus in 1526.

Perhaps one of the most useful editions of Hippocrates (it is the one from which most of the following quotations derive) is *The Genuine Works of Hippocrates. Translated from the Greek with a Preliminary Discourse and Annotations by Francis Adams* – a work published by the Sydenham Society in London in 1849[186]. This is one of the fundamental editions for the reader in English; the translation is limited to the so-called genuine works and has the advantage that it was prepared by a Greek scholar who was also a surgeon.

In those fine publications of the house of Heinemann, the *Loeb Classical Library*, there is the excellent and compact *Hippocrates. With an English Translation by W. H. S. Jones* (Vols. I, II and IV) or *E. T. Withington* (Vol. III)[184] – a set of volumes which were published in 1923–31 and which have been several times reprinted. This is the edition which, for the modern reader, sometimes replaces that of Francis Adams. It is bilingual and has a penetrating and valuable General Introduction by Jones (Vol. I). The two clinical cases previously cited (p. 75) from *Epidemics I* were taken from its translated pages. It too is limited to the works thought possibly to be genuine and its contents enable us to list the most important books of the Hippocratic collection:

Volume I contains *Ancient Medicine – Airs, Waters, Places – Epidemics I & III – The Oath – Precepts – Nutriment*.

Volume II includes *Prognostic – Regimen in Acute Diseases – The Sacred Disease – The Art – Breaths*.

Volume III has *On Wounds in the Head – In the Surgery – On Fractures – On Joints – Mochlikon*.

Volume IV provides *Nature of Man – Regimen in Health – Humours – Aphorisms – Regimen I–III – Dreams – Heracleitus – On the Universe*.

Lastly, for there are numerous editions, we have *The Medical Works of Hippocrates. A new translation from the original Greek made especially for English readers by the collaboration of John Chadwick and W. N. Mann*[187]. This work provides the results of a collaboration between Chadwick, sometime Scholar of Corpus Christi College, Cambridge, and W. N. Mann, Assistant Physician to Guy's Hospital. Thus, this edition, of modern scholarship, sees the writings of Hippocrates through contemporary medical eyes.

The Hippocratic Collection is perhaps best imagined as being the remains of the library of the school of medicine at Cos. Those particular parts of it now thought by most students to have been written by Hippocrates himself are *Airs, Waters, Places; Epidemics I & III; Regimen in Acute Diseases; On Wounds in the Head; On Fractures* and *On Joints*. Although the ethics and ideals of Hippocrates are most clearly visible in the *Oath*, it is possible that this, as a document, is an accretion or product of the leaders of the whole school; it may also contain later additions.

It would seem that the two most common complaints in ancient Greece were respiratory tract infections, especially chest troubles representing a wide range of pathologies, and malaria. With almost no knowledge of the morbid processes, as such, the diseases were described and grouped according to their symptoms. Thus, the name of a Greek disease was the name of a syndrome of symptoms and there is often no English medical term to correspond. In the *General Introduction* to the *Loeb Classical Library* edition of Hippocrates . . ., W. H. S. Jones (1923)[188] says: 'Perhaps the most remarkable point arising in a discussion of Greek diseases is the apparent absence of most infectious fevers. Plagues . . . occurred at intervals, but the medical writings in the Hippocratic collection are occupied almost entirely with endemic disease and do not describe plagues, not even the great plague at Athens. There is no mention of smallpox or measles; no certain reference occurs to diphtheria, scarlet fever, bubonic plague or syphilis.' He adds that it is doubtful if typhoid was present in Greece and implies that most cases of what read like the 'typhoid state' were really malaria. It is clear that the great problem of the Greek world, and of the ancient world generally, was malaria 'both mild and malignant, both intermittent and remittent'. 'Consumption' is frequently mentioned in the Hippocratic writings, and pneumonia, empyema, and a number of ophthalmias were well known. In addition, there was, of course, experience of a wide range of surgical conditions, some of them congenital and many of them traumatic.

Despite all this experience in the Greek world at large there is no ancient set of clinical records to compare with the succinct and realistic accounts given by Hippocrates. The 16 cases from *Epidemics III* are given in the Francis Adams, and the later, translations. It is inevitable that the reader diagnoses each case: generations of doctors have done this and it is a tribute, in its own way, to the very fine level of clinical description.

In all, Hippocrates gave clinical records of 42 cases of which 25 were fatal; these cases, recorded with typical honesty, are the only thing of their kind in the literature for what Garrison (1929)[189] estimated to be the next 1700 years. Hippocrates also described paralysis of the opposite side of the body in wounds of the head; he made the observation that epilepsy is incompatible with quartan fever and often remits after malarial infection, he showed that melancholia (mental depression) could be of exogenous or endogenous cause. Hippocrates also gave the first description of wound healing by either first or secondary intention and was the first to describe the 'succussion sound' (Hippocratic succussion) obtained when the patient, on a rigid seat, is shaken while the ear of the observer is held to the chest. He was also the first clearly to describe (in the cases of Philiscus and the wife of Dealces) the type of terminal or distressed breathing now called Cheyne–Stokes respiration. His great classic act of description, the *Facies Hippocratica*, an account of the features of a dying man, is given in the following passage from *Prognostics*[190]:

> *a sharp nose, hollow eyes, collapsed temples; the ears cold, contracted, and their lobes turned out; the skin about the forehead being rough, distended, and parched; the colour of the whole face being green, black, livid, or lead-coloured.* If the countenance be such at the commencement of the disease, and if this cannot be accounted for from the other symptoms, inquiry must be made whether the patient has long wanted sleep; whether his bowels have been very loose; and whether he has suffered from want of food; and if any of these causes be confessed to, the danger is to be reckoned so far less; and it becomes obvious, in the course of a day and a night, whether or not the appearance of the countenance proceed from these causes. But if none of these be said to exist, and if the symptoms do not subside in the aforesaid time, it is to be known for certain that death is at hand. And, also, if the disease be in a more advanced stage either on the third or fourth day, and the countenance be such, the same inquiries as formerly directed are to be made, and the other symptoms are to be noted, those in the whole countenance, those on the body, and those in the eyes; for if they shun the light, or weep involuntarily, or squint, or if the one be less than the other, or if the white of them be red, livid, or has black veins in it; if there be a gum upon the eyes, if they are restless, protruding, or are become very hollow; and if the countenance be squalid and dark, or the colour of the whole face be changed – all these are to be reckoned bad and fatal symptoms. The physician should also observe the appearance of the eyes from below the eyelids in sleep; for when a portion of the white appears, owing to the eyelids not being closed together, and when this is not connected with diarrhœa or purgation from medicine, or when the patient does not sleep thus from habit, it is to be reckoned an unfavorable and very deadly symptom; but if the eyelid be contracted, livid, or pale, or also the lip, or nose, along with some of the other symptoms, one may know for certain that death is close at hand. It is a mortal symptom, also, when the lips are relaxed, pendent, cold, and blanched.

The Hippocratic surgical writings are usually considered the only thing of value on the subject before Celsus in the time of Tiberius Caesar (42 BC–AD 37); thus, they stood for over four centuries and parts of them for far longer. The accounts given of bandaging, the treatment of congenital dislocations, and the management of fractures are particularly strong. The discussion of the nature and treatment of dislocation at the shoulder is famous and includes methods useable today; the following is from the Sydenham Society edition *On the Articulations*[191]:

> I am acquainted with one form in which the shoulder-joint is dislocated, namely, that into the armpit; I have never seen it take place upwards nor outwards; and yet I do not positively affirm whether it might be dislocated in these directions or not, although I have something which I might say on this subject. But neither have I ever seen what I considered to be a dislocation forwards. Physicians, indeed, fancy that dislocation is very apt to occur forwards, and they are more particularly deceived in those persons who have the fleshy parts about the joint and arm much emaciated; for, in all such cases, the head of the arm appears to protrude forwards. And I in one case of this kind having said that there was no dislocation, exposed myself to censure from certain physicians and common people on that account, for they fancied that I alone was ignorant of what everybody else was acquainted with, and I could not convince them but with difficulty, that the matter was so. But if one will strip the point of the shoulder of the fleshy parts, and where the muscle (*deltoid*?) extends, and also lay bare the tendon that goes from the armpit and clavicle to the breast (*pectoral muscle*?), the head of the humerus will appear to protrude strongly forwards, although not dislocated, for the head of the humerus naturally inclines forwards, but the rest of the bone is turned outwards. The humerus is connected obliquely with the cavity of the scapula, when the arm is stretched along the sides; but when the whole arm is stretched forwards, then the head of the humerus is in line with the cavity of the humerus, and no longer appears to protrude forwards. And with regard to the variety we are now treating of, I have never seen a case of dislocation forwards; and yet I do not speak decidedly respecting it, whether such a dislocation may take place or not. When, then, a dislocation into the armpit takes place, seeing it is of frequent occurrence, many persons know how to reduce it, for it is an easy thing to teach all the methods by which physicians effect the reductions, and the best manner of applying them. The strongest of those methods should be used when the difficulty of reduction is particularly great. The strongest is the method to be last described.
>
> 2. Those who are subject to frequent dislocations at the shoulder-joint, are for the most part competent to effect the reduction themselves; for, having introduced the knuckles of the other hand into the armpit, they force the joint upwards, and bring the elbow towards the breast. The physician might reduce it in the same manner, if having introduced his fingers into the armpit on the inside of the dislocated joint, he would force it from the ribs, pushing his own head against the acromion, in order to make counter-pressure, and with his knees applied to the patient's elbow pushing the arm to the sides. It will be of advantage if the operator has strong hands, or the physician may do as directed with his head and hands, while another person brings the elbow towards the breast. Reduction of the shoulder may also be effected by carrying the fore-arm backwards to the spine, and then with the one hand grasping it at the elbow, to bend the arm upwards, and with the other to support it behind at the articulation. This mode of reduction, and the one formerly described, are not natural, and yet by rotating the bone of the joint, they force it to return.
>
> 3. Those who attempt to perform reduction with the heel, operate in a manner which is an approach to the natural. The patient must lie on the ground upon his back, while the person who is to effect the reduction is seated on the ground upon the side of the dislocation; then the operator, seizing with his hand the affected arm, is to pull it, while with his heel in the armpit he pushes in

the contrary direction, the right heel being placed in the right armpit, and the left heel in the left armpit. But a round ball of a suitable size must be placed in the hollow of the armpit; the most convenient are very small and hard balls, formed from several pieces of leather sewed together. For without something of the kind the heel cannot reach to the head of the humerus, since, when the arm is stretched, the armpit becomes hollow, the tendons on both sides of the armpit making counter-contraction so as to oppose the reduction. But another person should be seated on the other side of the patient to hold the sound shoulder, so that the body may not be dragged along when the arm of the affected side is pulled; and then, when the ball is placed in the armpit, a supple piece of thong sufficiently broad is to be placed round it, and some person taking hold of its two ends is to seat himself above the patient's head to make counter-extension, while at the same time he pushes with his foot against the bone at the top of the shoulder. The ball should be placed as much on the inside as possible, upon the ribs, and not upon the head of the humerus.

4. There is another method of reduction performed by the shoulder of a person standing. The person operating in this way, who should be taller than the patient, is to take hold of his arm and place the sharp point of his own shoulder in the patient's armpit, and push it in so that it may lodge there, and having for his object that the patient may be suspended at his back by the armpit, he must raise himself higher on this shoulder than the other; and he must bring the arm of the suspended patient as quickly as possible to his own breast. In this position he should shake the patient when he raises him up, in order that the rest of the body may be a counterpoise to the arm which is thus held. But if the patient be very light, a light child should be suspended behind along with him. These methods of reduction are all of easy application in the palestra, as they can all be performed without instruments, but they may also be used elsewhere.

5. Those who accomplish the reduction by forcibly bending it round a pestle, operate in a manner which is nearly natural. But the pestle should be wrapped in a soft shawl (for thus it will be less slippery), and it should be forced between the ribs and the head of the humerus. And if the pestle be short, the patient should be seated upon something, so that his arm can with difficulty pass above the pestle. But for the most part the pestle should be longer, so that the patient when standing may be almost suspended upon the piece of wood. And then the arm and fore-arm should be stretched along the pestle, whilst some person secures the opposite side of the body by throwing his arms round the neck, near the clavicle.

6. But the method with a ladder is another of the same kind, and still better, since by it the body can be more safely counterpoised on this side; and that, while in the method with the piece of wood resembling a pestle, there is danger of the body tumbling to either side. But some round thing should be tied upon the step of the ladder which may be fitted to the armpit, whereby the head of the bone may be forced into its natural place.

7. The following, however, is the strongest of all the methods of reduction. We must get a piece of wood, five, or at least four inches broad, two inches in thickness, or still thinner, and two cubits in length, or a little less; and its extremity at one end should be rounded, and made very narrow and very slender there, and it should have a slightly projecting edge (*ambe*) on its round extremity, not on the part that is to be applied to the side, but to the head of the humerus, so that it may be adjusted in the armpit at the sides under the head of the humerus; and a piece of soft shawl or cloth should be glued to the end of the

piece of wood, so as to give the less pain upon pressure. Then having pushed the head of this piece of wood as far inwards as possible between the ribs and the head of the humerus, the whole arm is to be stretched along this piece of wood, and is to be bound round at the arm, the fore-arm, and the wrist, so that it may be particularly well secured; but great pains should be taken that the extremity of this piece of wood should be introduced as far as possible into the armpit, and that it is carried past the head of the humerus. Then a cross-beam is to be securely fastened between two pillars, and afterwards the arm with the piece of wood attached to it is to be brought over this cross-beam, so that the arm may be on the one side of it and the body on the other, and the cross-beam in the armpit; and then the arm with the piece of wood is to be forced down on the one side of the cross-beam, and the rest of the body on the other. The cross-beam is to be bound so high that the rest of the body may be raised upon tip-toes. This is by far the most powerful method of effecting reduction of the shoulder; for one thus operates with the lever upon the most correct principles, provided only the piece of wood be placed as much as possible within the head of the humerus, and thus also the counterbalancing weights will be most properly adjusted, and safely applied to the bone of the arm. Wherefore recent cases in this way may be reduced more quickly than could be believed, before even extension would appear to be applied; and this is the only mode of reduction capable of replacing old dislocations, and this it will effect, unless flesh has already filled up the (glenoid) cavity, and the head of the humerus has formed a socket for itself in the place to which it has been displaced; and even in such an old case of dislocation, it appears to me that we could effect reduction (for what object would a lever power properly applied not move?), but it would not remain in its place, but would be again displaced as formerly. The same thing may be effected by means of the ladder, by preparing it in the same manner. If the dislocation be recent, a large Thessalian chair may be sufficient to accomplish this purpose; the wood, however, should be dressed up as described before; but the patient should be seated sideways on the chair, and then the arm, with the piece of wood attached to it, is to be brought over the back of the chair, and force is to be applied to the arm, with the wood on the one side, and to the body on the other side. The same means may be applied with a double door. One should always use what happens to be at hand.

The treatise *On Fractures*[192] provides an almost equally remarkable and practical account of dealing with a fracture of the lower leg:

In such cases as do not admit of bandaging according to any of the methods which have been described, or which will be described, great pains should be taken that the fractured part of the body be laid in a right position, and attention should be paid that it may incline upwards rather than downwards. But if one would wish to do the thing well and dexterously, it is proper to have recourse to some mechanical contrivance, in order that the fractured part of the body may undergo proper and not violent extension; and this means is particularly applicable in fractures of the leg. There are certain physicians who, in all fractures of the leg, whether bandages be applied or not, fasten the sole of the foot to the couch, or to some other piece of wood which they have fixed in the ground near the couch. These persons thus do all sorts of mischief but no good; for it contributes nothing to the extension that the foot is thus bound, as the rest of the body will no less sink down to the foot, and thus the limb will no longer be stretched, neither will it do any good towards keeping the limb in a proper position, but will do harm, for when the rest of the body is turned to this side or that, the bandaging will not prevent the foot and the bones belonging to it from following the rest of the body. For if it had not been bound it would have been less distorted, as it would have been the less prevented from following the motion of the rest of the body. But one should sew two balls of Egyptian leather, such as are worn by persons confined for a length of time in large shackles, and the balls should have coats on each side, deeper towards the wound, but shorter towards the joints; and the balls should be well stuffed and soft, and fit well, the one above the ankles, and the other below the knee. Sideways it should have below two appendages, either of a single or double thong, and short, like loops, the one set being placed on either side of the ankle, and the other on the knee. And the other upper ball should have others of the same kind in the same line. Then taking four rods, made of the cornel tree, of equal length, and of the thickness of a finger, and of such length that when bent they will admit of being adjusted to the appendages, care should be taken that the extremities of the rods bear not upon the skin, but on the extremities of the balls. There should be three sets of rods, or more, one set a little longer than another, and another a little shorter and smaller, so that they may produce greater or less distension, if required. Either of these sets of rods should be placed on this side and that of the ankles. If these things be properly contrived, they should occasion a proper and equable extension in a straight line, without giving any pain to the wound; for the pressure, if there is any, should be thrown at the foot and the thigh. And the rods are commodiously arranged on either side of the ankles, so as not to interfere with the position of the limb; and the wound is easily examined and easily arranged. And, if thought proper, there is nothing to prevent the two upper rods from being fastened to one another; and if any light covering be thrown over the limb, it will thus be kept off from the wound. If, then, the balls be well made, handsome, soft, and newly stitched, and if the extension by the rods be properly managed, as has been already described, this is an excellent contrivance; but if any of them do not fit properly, it does more harm than good. And all other mechanical contrivances should either be properly done, or not be had recourse to at all, for it is a disgraceful and awkward thing to use mechanical means in an unmechanical way.

This practical procedure is made easy to understand by the diagrams[193] (Figure 25) which the Sydenham Society edition of 1849 reproduces from the splendid work of Littré, already mentioned.

Thus, Hippocrates produced fine writings not only in internal medicine but in pragmatic aspects of surgery. A man of great feeling, he was devoid of some overly simple, mechanistic explanation for things. He wrote that 'In Thasos a woman of gloomy temperament, after a grief with a reason for it, without taking to bed lost sleep and appetite and suffered thirst and nausea . . . ', showing that he was aware of the great difference between grief 'with a reason for it' and endogenous grief (Case XI, *Epidemics III*)[194]. He also ends the account of Case IX from the same book with the notes: 'Urine scanty and thin. Excreta crude, thin and scanty. It was no longer possible to do her any good, and she died'[195], showing himself concerned with much more than prognosis. Garrison (1929)[196] says that 'Behind the sensible phenomena of nature he surmised the existence of some tremendous power (*enormon*), which sets things going.'

But it is in *The Sacred Disease*, when writing of epilepsy, the disease which previous ages had seen as the hallmark of the illnesses caused by demonic

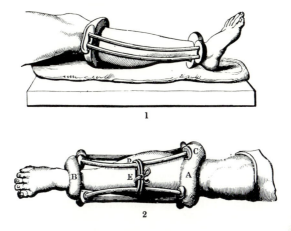

Figure 25 Hippocrates – splints in fracture by the lower leg. [*From: The genuine works of Hippocrates. Translated . . . by Francis Adams. London, Sydenham Society (1849), Vol. II.*]

possession or the direct intervention of the divine, that Hippocrates can perhaps be claimed to have achieved most. Part of the Francis Adams translation is the following[197]:

> this disease seems to me to be nowise more divine than others; but it has its nature such as other diseases have, and a cause whence it originates, and its nature and cause are divine only just as much as all others are, and it is curable no less than the others, unless when, from length of time, it is confirmed, and has become stronger than the remedies applied.

Chadwick and Mann (1950) give the following splendid version of the opening paragraph[198]:

> I do not believe that the 'Sacred Disease' is any more divine or sacred than any other disease but, on the contrary, has specific characteristics and a definite cause. Nevertheless, because it is completely different from other diseases, it has been regarded as a divine visitation by those who, being only human, view it with ignorance and astonishment.

In the translation of these authors Hippocrates adds that: 'The brain is the seat of this disease, as it is of other very violent diseases'[199], and then, still talking of the brain: 'It ought to be generally known that the source of our pleasure, merriment, laughter and amusement, as of our grief, pain, anxiety and tears, is none other than the brain. It is specially the organ which enables us to think, see and hear, and to distinguish the ugly and the beautiful, the bad and the good, pleasant and unpleasant'[200]. He sees the brain too as 'the seat of madness and delirium . . .'[201]. In this small treatise Hippocrates dismisses the old gods and superstitions and puts the mind of man in its rightful place.

The *Aphorisms* have always been famous – 'the unborn child, in the first and last stages of pregnancy, should be treated very cautiously'[202] – amongst them. They contain a number of truisms and a number of observations of great insight; the first, as given by Francis Adams in making the initial translation of its kind into English, is a gem that sparkles through the distance of time[203]:

> Life is short, and the Art long; the occasion fleeting; experience fallacious, and judgment difficult.

It is with Hippocrates and the Hippocratic Collection that medicine as we now know it can be said to have begun. It is certainly the person we know as Hippocrates who gave it its observational basis, scientific spirit and ethical ideals. Therapeutics, as we know it, began therefore at this point in time, although, largely due to lack of effective remedies, useful drug therapy is of a later date. The methods of treatment of the great Coan school centred on assisting the healing powers of nature, the *vis medicatrix naturae*, upon which the eventual outcome must still, almost always, depend. The methods aimed to provide rest, fresh air, tranquillity, a suitable diet, massage, hydrotherapy, and similar restorative measures; bleeding and purging were used when it seemed necessary but the excesses of the old pharmacopoeias were avoided – although Hippocrates was familiar with a large number of plant remedies, tisans of barley gruel, barley water, honey and water (hydromel), honey and vinegar (oxymel), and such simple things are mentioned often in the Collection and must have been frequently used. So, it would seem, was 'hellebore', often qualified as purging or black hellebore.

It is not at all certain that we know the modern equivalents of the Greek plants. Black or purging hellebore seems to have been the universal purge of the Greeks; white hellebore, the universal emetic.

Black Hellebore, the Christmas Rose, *Helleborus niger* of the buttercup family, Ranunculaceae, is a native of Europe and western Asia. It is said to have got its name (despite the fact that it has a lovely white flower) because it blossoms in midwinter – thus, the 'Christmas Rose' – but its knotty rootstock is blackish-brown externally and is markedly poisonous. The rhizome used to be used medicinally and presented in commerce as a crude drug in irregular and nodular pieces, 1–3 inches long, but white and horny within the thick blackish bark. It provides a series of glucosides and large enough doses produce cramps, vomiting and rapid purging; very large doses cause convulsions and death. It used to be especially favoured as a purge in dropsy but is now considered dangerous rather than beneficial and it has long since been dropped from the books on therapeutics. William Woodville (*Medical Botany* . . . edition of 1810)[204] says the plant 'was unknown to the gardens in this country till cultivated by Mr John Gerard in 1596'. He notes that many plants have been mistaken for this one in the confused history of the species and adds that, even in his day, the use of 'this catholicon of antiquity is now almost entirely abandoned'[205]. In a footnote Woodville remarks 'Whether our Hellebore be the same species as that said to grow in the island of Anticyra, and about Mount Olympus, so frequently alluded to by the Latin poets, is no easy matter to determine. From the accounts of Tournefort and Bellonius, who botanized these places, a species of this plant was found in great plenty, which the former supposes to be the Hellebore of Hippocrates . . .'[206]. But he then records the differences in morphology between this Hellebore of Mount

Olympus and our own Christmas Rose. For these reasons it seems an unsafe conclusion that our midwinter flower is that which Hippocrates used.

The White Hellebore is of a totally different family and has provided medicinal products of contemporary times. White Hellebore is White Veratrum (BPC 1934)[207], the dried rhizome and roots of *Veratrum album* of the Liliaceae. White veratrum is employed as a source of the alkaloids protoveratrine A and B; these alkaloids are obtained as a white crystalline powder which has a strong sternutatory action. Martindale[208] describes the ampoule dosage form of these mixed alkaloids which used to be used in the management of hypertensive toxaemias of pregnancy. Martindale[209] also lists the mixture of alkaloids obtained from the related plant, green veratrum (Green Hellebore; BPC 1954)[210], the dried roots of *Veratrum viride* (Liliaceae); these alkaloids are standardized for their total antihypertensive effect. With this substance vomiting is so prompt that death is very rare following overdosage by mouth. Woodville[211] says 'Hippocrates frequently mentions Hellebore simply, or generically, by which we are told the white is to be understood, as he adds the words black or purging when the other is meant...'

Scribonius Largus (about AD 1–50)[212] mentions the *Oath* which derives from the Hippocratic Collection and which has served as the clearest statement of the ethics of medicine until modern times. It is more than an ideal regarding the conduct of practice: it is an indenture, reminding us of the way medicine used to be taught in guilds or passed down in families, and of the way in which the initiate undertook to instruct those who would follow him and, in their turn, be bound by the oath. Parts of the Oath – and especially the parts which refer to the relationship between the physician and patient – remain the cornerstone of medicine today. There are several written forms of the Oath but in each, as in the following example, the patient and his well-being is the thing which remains sacred and inviolable[213].

THE OATH

I swear by Apollo the physician, and Æsculapius, and Health, and All-heal, and all the gods and goddesses, that, according to my ability and judgment, I will keep this Oath and this stipulation – to reckon him who taught me this Art equally dear to me as my parents, to share my substance with him, and relieve his necessities if required; to look upon his offspring in the same footing as my own brothers, and to teach them this art, if they shall wish to learn it, without fee or stipulation; and that by precept, lecture, and every other mode of instruction, I will impart a knowledge of the Art to my own sons, and those of my teachers, and to disciples bound by a stipulation and oath according to the law of medicine, but to none others. I will follow that system of regimen which, according to my ability and judgment, I consider for the benefit of my patients, and abstain from whatever is deleterious and mischievous. I will give no deadly medicine to any one if asked, nor suggest any such counsel; and in like manner I will not give to a woman a pessary to produce abortion. With purity and with holiness I will pass my life and practise my Art. I will not cut persons labouring under the stone, but will leave this to be done by men who are practitioners of this work. Into whatever houses I enter, I will go into them for the benefit of the sick, and will abstain from every voluntary act of mischief and corruption; and, further, from the seduction of females or males, of freemen and slaves.

Whatever, in connexion with my professional practice, or not in connexion with it, I see or hear, in the life of men, which ought not to be spoken of abroad, I will not divulge, as reckoning that all such should be kept secret. While I continue to keep this Oath unviolated, may it be granted to me to enjoy life and the practice of the art, respected by all men, in all times. But should I trespass and violate this Oath, may the reverse be my lot.

Aristotle

Most of the surviving early biological writings are concerned with the nature and constitution of man and it seems that this was always the centre of interest. Many of the Ionic vases, ceramics, mouldings and other art objects of the fifth and sixth centuries BC show a remarkable exactness of biological observation. They illustrate well-drawn animals, fish and birds, usually shown in relationship to man. Thus, at this early date, when it was thought that in the fetus all parts are formed simultaneously, even the embryo child was imagined as a complete, but miniature, man. It is striking that, as the Greek interest in biology awoke, the subject was explored with a spirit that was as anthropocentric as its observations were crystal clear.

The clarity of observation, and the depiction of biological things in a precise, naturalistic manner, produced works of art and science which are fresh and vivid and quite unlike the artefacts, however splendid these are, of the earlier people. But when they came to explain function the Greeks wandered at times onto far less secure ground. Thus, in the treatise *On Nourishment*, cited by Charles Singer[214] and dated about 400 BC, the pulse appears for the first time in Greek medical literature – but it appears with a physiology which was in error in a way that was to last until the days of Harvey: it saw the arteries arise from the heart and the veins from the liver. In the treatise *On Muscles*, of about 390 BC, the heart is described as sending air, fire and movement to the peripheral parts of the body, and to do this by means of arteries which were themselves moving. Despite the fact that the writer of this treatise seems to have seen arterial pulsation as movement, the beginnings of the business of science – the recording of exact observations – can be seen to begin in these early Greek texts.

Many of these first observations found their way into the early parts of the Hippocratic Collection. The finest parts of the Collection summarized the medical experience of Greece in the Age of Pericles. Many of the later observations culminated in the work of the vast and classical figure of Aristotle (384–322 BC). To the scientist it is perhaps tragic that this great progression of observation and understanding was overshadowed, and perhaps damaged, by the developments of the day in theoretical ethics and abstract philosophy. Socrates died in 399 BC shortly before the birth of Aristotle; his pupil Plato died when Aristotle was almost 40.

Greek philosophy and the rudiments of the methods of science then stood face to face – and it was soon to prove a quite unequal struggle. W. H. S. Jones, in the Introduction to his translation of *Hippocrates*... [215] says: 'The transcendant genius of Plato, strong in that very power of persuasion the use of which he so much deprecated, won the day. The philosophic fervour which longed with passionate desire for unchangeable reality, that felt a lofty contempt for the material world with its ever-shifting phenomena, that aspired to rise to a heavenly region where changeless Ideas might be apprehended by pure intelligence purged from every bodily taint, was more than a match for the humble researches of men who wished to relieve human suffering by a patient study of those very phenomena that Plato held of no account. So for centuries philosophy flourished and science languished, in spite of Aristotle, Euclid and Archimedes.'

A number of other modern writers have seen things the same way: abstract philosophy was, in its effect, as destructive to science as the most intense of the old forms of religion. The struggle was depicted in the following passage, included by Charles Singer in his brilliant, small book *Greek Biology & Greek Medicine*[216]:

> This period saw the rise of a movement that had the most profound influence on every department of thought. We see the advent into the Greek world of a great intellectual movement as a result of which the department of philosophy that dealt with nature receded before Ethics. Of that intellectual revolution – perhaps the greatest the world has seen – Athens was the site and Socrates (470–399) the protagonist. With the movement itself and its characteristic fruit we are not concerned. But the great successor and pupil of its founder gives us in the *Timaeus* a picture of the depth to which natural science can be degraded in the effort to give a specific teleological meaning to all parts of the visible Universe. The book and the picture which it draws, dark and repulsive to the mind trained in modern scientific method, enthralled the imagination of a large part of mankind for wellnigh two thousand years. Organic nature appears in this work of Plato (427–347) as the degeneration of man whom the Creator has made most perfect. The school that held this view ultimately decayed as a result of its failure to advance positive knowledge. As the centuries went by its views became further and further divorced from phenomena, and the bizarre developments of later Neoplatonism stand to this day as a warning against any system which shall neglect the investigation of nature. But in its decay Platonism dragged science down and destroyed by neglect nearly all earlier biological material. Mathematics, not being a phenomenal study, suited better the Neoplatonic mood and continued to advance, carrying astronomy with it for a while – astronomy that affected the life of man and that soon became the handmaid of astrology; medicine, too, that determined the conditions of man's life, was also cherished, though often mistakenly, but pure science was doomed.

Aristotle, the greatest of the ancient biologists, was born in 384 BC at Stagira, a Greek colony in the Chalcidice a few miles from the northern extremity of the modern monastic settlement of Mount Athos, itself a peninsula in the northern Aegean. His father, Nicomachus, was physician to the King of Macedonia and an Asklepiad of considerable standing. When he was 17 Aristotle became a pupil of Plato in Athens; after the death of Plato he crossed the Aegean to the court of the despot of Atarneus in Mysia, whose niece, Pythias, he married. It is in this region of Asia Minor that the main mass of his biological observations seem to have been made. The region is now part of north-west Turkey. It is bounded to the north by the Dardanelles and the Sea of Marmara, leading to ancient Byzantium (Istanbul). To the west it forms the Aegean coast opposite the islands of Lemnos and Lesbos (see Figure 18, p. 58). Aristotle's observations include much on the natural history of Lesbos, or Mytilene, the island lying opposite to mainland Atarneus. Ancient Troy lies a little to the north of the region Aristotle most frequently studied.

In 343 BC, at the request of Philip of Macedon, Aristotle became tutor to Philip's son, Alexander the Great. He remained in Macedonia for 7 or so years but about 335 BC, before Alexander left for the invasion of Asia, Aristotle returned to Athens; there he taught at the Lyceum before establishing his own school – the Peripatos. The bulk of his written work is thought to have been produced in the closing phase of his life between 335 and 323 BC. He died in 322 BC, at Chalcis in Euboea, a few months after his pupil Alexander.

Osler[217] applies the phrase 'the Master of those who know' to Aristotle and says: 'with justice has Aristotle been so regarded for these twenty-three centuries. No man has ever swayed such an intellectual empire – in logic, metaphysics, rhetoric, psychology, ethics, poetry, politics and natural history, in all a creator, and in all still a master. The history of the human mind offers no parallel to his career. As the creator of the sciences of comparative anatomy, systematic zoology, embryology, teratology, botany and physiology, his writings have an eternal interest. They present an extraordinary accumulation of facts relating to the structure and functions of various parts of the body. It is an unceasing wonder how one man, even with a school of devoted students, could have done so much.'

The achievement remains staggering even though it was, for centuries, eclipsed by the obsession with philosophy. In recent years it has been realized that Aristotle anticipated whole numbers of modern discoveries. How one man could have achieved so much remains a puzzle – Osler's reference to the 'school of devoted students' may be part of the answer. Some ancient writers suggest (a little improbably) that vast resources were made available to Aristotle. Others suggest that spurious works or the dissertations of students may have been mixed with his writings. These and related problems have been reviewed by Singer[218] but a greater problem is that Aristotle, like many of the ancient writers, produced fanciful and fabulous work when relying on second-hand accounts; he also slipped readily into error when conjecturing on function. What remains amazing is the number of fine and exact observations, derived from personal experience, that appear in the biological works – especially the *Historia Animalium*, *Parts of Animals* and *Generation of Animals*. The profundity of some of the psychological and philosophical books which relate to biology, including *On the Soul*, perhaps his most thoughtful book, is equally notable.

Many of the finest observations arise from what we must judge to be Aristotle's practice of animal dissection. Some of the difficulties seem to stem from extrapolating animal findings to man, human dissection being unavailable to Aristotle.

The collected works, in a Greek–Latin bilingual text, appear in *Aristotle. Opera. Edidit Academia Regia Borussica*, published in 1831–70[219]. There is also *The Works of Aristotle, Translated into English under the Editorship of J. A. Smith and W. D. Ross* of 1908–31, and this contains the important Volume IV, *Historia Animalium*, by D'Arcy Wentworth Thompson (1910)[220]. The Loeb Classical Library provides a readily available contemporary set of bilingual volumes[221].

Aristotle – the features from the Herculaneum are from a work which is probably of the fourth century BC (Figure 26) – believed that a particular principle of a non-material kind is an essential attribute of living things. He saw living forms as a progression of increased complexity, lifeless things leading, in an upward scale, to plants; and these, by means of a continuous but merging scale, to animals, molluscs, arthropods, crustaceans, cephlopods, reptiles, birds,

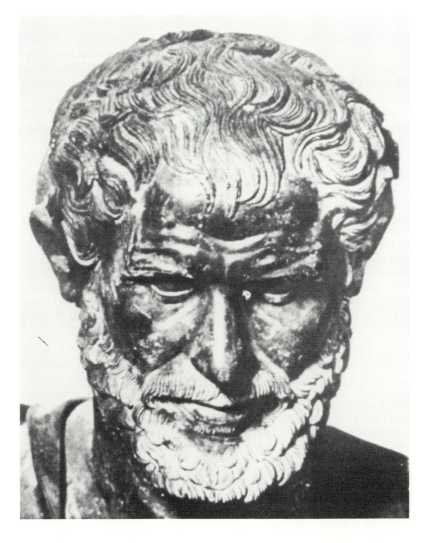

Figure 26   Aristotle. (From Herculaneum, probably 4th century BC). [*From: Charles Joseph Singer. Greek biology and Greek medicine. Oxford, Clarendon Press, (1922).*]

amphibians, fish, cetaceans, mammals, and man. In this way Aristotle seems to have envisaged an evolution – one in which the essential difference between the non-living and the living is the possession of an essential vital principle, or soul, by the latter. Many of these thoughts are seen in *On the Soul*, the more than ordinarily noble text in which he writes of a soul which is vegetative, or nutritive and reproductive; an animal, or sensitive soul; and a rational, or intellectual soul, the latter particular to man. Thus, his writings, though anthropocentric, exhibit a reverence for the simple as well as complex forms of life – an attitude which was to show in the writings of his students and especially those of his most favoured disciple, Theophrastus.

Aristotle's ideas on procreation suggested that the material substance of the embryo is derived from the female, whereas the principle of life, the soul or generative agent, was contributed by the male. Because the soul is not material it is not necessary for anything material to pass from male to female. Experiments, in later centuries, on parthenogenesis have given rise to comment on this subject – it being a fact that nothing material need pass from male to female for the stimulated ovum to replicate. But these experiments have little to do with the transmission of the male-derived and female-derived chromosomes of biology – nor do the speculations of Aristotle.

He was at his best in his account of embryology and the following is from his brilliant description of the growth of the chick embryo[222]:

> Generation from the egg proceeds in an identical manner with all birds, but the full periods from conception to birth differ, as has been said. With the common hen after three days and three nights there is the first indication of the embryo; with larger birds the interval being longer, with smaller birds shorter. Meanwhile the yolk comes into being, rising towards the sharp end, where the primal element of the egg is situated, and where the egg gets hatched; and the heart appears, like a speck of blood, in the white of the egg. This point beats and moves as though endowed with life, and from it two vein-ducts with blood in them trend in a convoluted course [as the egg-substance goes on growing, towards each of the two circumjacent integuments]; and a membrane carrying bloody fibres now envelops the yolk, leading off from the vein-ducts. A little afterwards the body is differentiated, at first very small and white. The head is clearly distinguished, and in it the eyes, swollen out to a great extent. This condition of the eyes lasts on for a good while, as it is only by degrees that they diminish in size and collapse. At the outset the under portion of the body appears insignificant in comparison with the upper portion. Of the two ducts that lead from the heart, the one proceeds towards the circumjacent integument, and the other, like a navel-string, towards the yolk. The life-element of the chick is in the white of the egg, and the nutriment comes through the navel-string out of the yolk.
>
> When the egg is now ten days old the chick and all its parts are distinctly visible. The head is still larger than the rest of its body, and the eyes larger than the head, but still devoid of vision. The eyes, if removed about this time, are found to be larger than beans, and black; if the cuticle be peeled off them there is a white and cold liquid inside, quite glittering in the sunlight, but there is no hard substance whatsoever. Such is the condition of the head and eyes. At this time also the larger internal organs are visible, as also the stomach and the arrangement of the viscera; and the veins that seem to proceed from the heart

are now close to the navel. From the navel there stretch a pair of veins; one towards the membrane that envelops the yoke (and, by the way, the yolk is now liquid, or more so than is normal), and the other towards that membrane which envelops collectively the membrane wherein the chick lies, the membrane of the yolk, and the intervening liquid. [For, as the chick grows, little by little one part of the yolk goes upward, and another part downward, and the white liquid is between them; and the white of the egg is underneath the lower part of the yolk, as it was at the outset.] On the tenth day the white is at the extreme outer surface, reduced in amount, glutinous, firm in substance, and sallow in colour.

The disposition of the several constituent parts is as follows. First and outermost comes the membrane of the egg, not that of the shell, but underneath it. Inside this membrane is a white liquid; then comes the chick, and a membrane round about it, separating it off so as to keep the chick free from the liquid; next after the chick comes the yolk, into which one of the two veins was described as leading, the other one leading into the enveloping white substance. [A membrane with a liquid resembling serum envelops the entire structure. Then comes another membrane right round the embryo, as has been described, separating it off against the liquid. Underneath this comes the yolk, enveloped in another membrane (into which yolk proceeds the navel-string that leads from the heart and the big vein), so as to keep the embryo free of both liquids.]

About the twentieth day, if you open the egg and touch the chick, it moves inside and chirps; and it is already coming to be covered with down, when, after the twentieth day is past, the chick begins to break the shell. The head is situated over the right leg close to the flank, and the wing is placed over the head; and about this time is plain to be seen the membrane resembling an afterbirth that comes next after the outermost membrane of the shell, into which membrane the one of the navel-strings was described as leading (and, by the way, the chick in its entirety is now within it), and so also is the other membrane resembling an after-birth, namely that surrounding the yolk, into which the second navel-string was described as leading; and both of them were described as being connected with the heart and the big vein. At this conjuncture the navel-string that leads to the outer after-birth collapses and becomes detached from the chick, and the membrane that leads into the yolk is fastened on to the thin gut of the creature, and by this time a considerable amount of the yolk is inside the chick and a yellow sediment is in its stomach. About this time it discharges residuum in the direction of the outer after-birth, and has residuum inside its stomach; and the outer residuum is white [and there comes a white substance inside]. By and by the yolk, diminishing gradually in size, at length becomes entirely used up and comprehended within the chick (so that, ten days after hatching, if you cut open the chick, a small remnant of the yolk is still left in connexion with the gut), but it is detached from the navel, and there is nothing in the interval between, but it has been used up entirely. During the period above referred to the chick sleeps, wakes up, makes a move and looks up and chirps; and the heart and the navel together palpitate as though the creature were respiring. So much as to generation from the egg in the case of birds.

The translation (the footnotes omitted) is by Thompson from the 1910 *Historia Animalium* in the Smith and Ross *The Works of Aristotle*[220]. A number of other examples can be given showing precise observations dating from the life of Aristotle and not improved until modern times. Charles Singer[223] has drawn attention to one such example in which, writing of the dog-fish, *Mustelus laevis*,

Aristotle talks of the young which 'develop with the navel-string attached to the womb, so that, as the egg-substance gets used up, the embryo is sustained to all appearances just as in quadrupeds'. As Singer points out such an arrangement is utterly unexpected in fishes but was surprisingly confirmed[223] when 'the whole matter was taken up by Johannes Müller about 1840'.

Against these numerous examples, and Aristotle's having named the aorta, must be set his teaching that the brain was a gland secreting cold humours to prevent overheating of the body by the fire of the heart – one of those ideas which went against the far more reasonable views of Hippocrates and which was to reappear, modified in form, in Galen. Altogether Aristotle described some 500 kinds of animals, producing original observations one after the other. The body of his descriptive work shows him to have been the master biologist not only of antiquity but also for the 2000 years that preceded Linnaeus. It is in this capacity, as a master of observational and factual biology, that Aristotle is increasingly read and remembered.

Theophrastus

Theophrastus of Eresos (372–287 BC) was the pupil to whom, on his death, Aristotle left his botanic garden and library. What we know of his personal life suggests that he was born in or about 372 at Eresos in Lesbos. As a young man he went to Athens and became a pupil of Plato and it is probably from Plato that Theophrastus first acquired the principle of classification which runs through all his later works on biological and especially botanical materials. The habit of classification held an important part in the later thinking of Plato – for it was by such groupings that he hoped to evolve those metaphysical 'ideal forms' which would provide the ideal world set apart from changing phenomena.

Aristotle had been a pupil of Plato and Theophrastus was his junior by only some 15 years. When Plato died, Theophrastus became the pupil, and probably the personal friend, of Aristotle. When in turn, aged 63, Aristotle died he left to Theophrastus the care of his son, the autograph of his own books, and the garden in the grounds of the Lyceum.

Theophrastus enjoyed not only the tuition of Plato and Aristotle but also his participation in the careers of Philip of Macedon and Alexander the Great. It was from observers taken into Asia by Alexander that Theophrastus learnt more of medicinal botany and added to his knowledge of plants and their uses. He lived to be a great age, the date of his death usually being placed in or about the year 287 BC when he was 85 years of age. In accordance with his will (preserved by Diogenes Laërtius of the 3rd century AD, author of the *Lives of the Philosophers*[224]) Theophrastus was buried, without extravagant expense, in the grounds of the garden of the Lyceum.

Like Aristotle, he was a writer of a great number of volumes. The principal extant works are the nine books of his *Enquiry into Plants* and the six books of the *Causes of Plants*. The *editio princeps* is the Aldine edition in Greek printed at Venice in 1495–8[225] but the Latin version of Theodore Gaza, the Greek refugee, was not only earlier but was based on a better manuscript – this is the Theophrastus *De historia plantarum* first printed at Treviso (*imp. B.*

Confalonerium de Salodio) in 1483[226]. The Loeb Classical Library edition is the excellent *Theophrastus, Enquiry into Plants and Minor Works on Odours and Weather Signs, with an English translation by Sir Arthur Hort*[227] – a work published in 1916. Somewhat remarkably, this represents the 'first attempt at an English translation of the "Enquiry into Plants" '.

Theophrastus begins Book 1 of his *Enquiry into Plants* with an account of the parts of plants, their composition and an attempt at classification – showing a totally methodical approach to his rambling, difficult subject. Any sort of formal classification eluded him, as it was to elude botanists for so many centuries. In his text, having thought of the manifold parts of plants and compared these with animals he realizes that the complexity of the subject puts a true classification beyond him[228].

> In fact your plant is a thing various and manifold, and so it is difficult to describe in general terms: in proof whereof we have the fact that we cannot here seize on any universal character which is common to all, as a mouth and a stomach are common to all animals; whereas in plants some characters are the same in all, merely in the sense that all have analogous characters, while others correspond otherwise. For not all plants have root, stem, branch, twig, leaf, flower or fruit, or again bark, core, fibres or veins; for instance, fungi and truffles; and yet these and such like characters belong to a plant's essential nature. However, as has been said, these characters belong especially to trees, and our classification of characters belongs more particularly to these; and it is right to make these the standard in treating of the others.

He could not approach a classification based on the way plants might reproduce themselves, for there was no real knowledge of the sexual parts of plants – but he explores this [229]:

> Taking, as was said, all trees according to their kinds, we find a number of differences. Common to them all is that by which men distinguish the 'male' and the 'female,' the latter being fruit-bearing, the former barren in some kinds. In those kinds in which both forms are fruit-bearing the 'female' has fairer and more abundant fruit. . . .

But it is with palms that Theophrastus comes closest to a real concept of fertilization[230]:

> With dates it is helpful to bring the male to the female; for it is the male which causes the fruit to persist and ripen, and this process some call, by analogy, 'the use of the wild fruit.' The process is thus performed: when the male palm is in flower, they at once cut off the spathe on which the flower is, just as it is, and shake the bloom with the flower and the dust over the fruit of the female, and, if this is done to it, it retains the fruit and does not shed it. In the case both of the fig and of the date it appears that the 'male' renders aid to the 'female' – for the fruit-bearing tree is called 'female' – but while in the latter case there is a union of the two sexes, in the former the result is brought about somewhat differently.

It is in the second volume of the 1916 translation by A. J. Hort that Theophrastus (in his Books VI-IX) achieves one of his great successes. In these books he describes under-shrubs; herbaceous plants, including wild herbs, cereals and pulses; the medicinal properties of herbs, and the juices of plants. Of the minor works, that *Concerning Odours* is really a fairly extensive study on perfumes.

Theophrastus, writing in the fourth century, gave an account of silphium – one of the great drugs of antiquity, much in use in his lifetime, but lost to us since. The silphium that he knew came from Cyrenaica and he described it as having a thick root, a stalk like a ferula, and a leaf like celery; he says that silphium was found over a wide tract of Libya and avoids cultivation[231]:

> The silphium has a great deal of thick root; its stalk is like ferula in size, and is nearly as thick; the leaf, which they call *maspeton*, is like celery: it has a broad fruit, which is leaf-like, as it were, and is called the *phyllon*. The stalk lasts only a year, like that of ferula. Now in spring it sends up this *maspeton*, which purges sheep and greatly fattens them, and makes their flesh wonderfully delicious; after that it sends up a stalk, which is eaten, it is said, in all ways, boiled and roast, and this too, they say, purges the body in forty days. It has two kinds of juice, one from the stalk and one from the root; wherefore the one is called 'stalk-juice,' the other 'root-juice.' The root has a black bark, which is stripped off. They have regulations, like those in use in mines, for cutting the root, in accordance with which they fix carefully the proper amount to be cut, having regard to previous cuttings and the supply of the plant. For it is not allowed to cut it wrong nor to cut more than the appointed amount; for, if the juice is kept and not used, it goes bad and decays. When they are conveying it to Peiraeus, they deal with it thus:– having put it in vessels and mixed meal with it, they shake it for a considerable time, and from this process it gets its colour, and this treatment makes it thenceforward keep without decaying. Such are the facts in regard to the cutting and treatment.
>
> The plant is found over a wide tract of Libya, for a distance, they say, of more than four thousand furlongs, but it is most abundant near the Syrtis, starting from the Euesperides islands. It is a peculiarity of it that it avoids cultivated ground, and, as the land is brought under cultivation and tamed, it retires, plainly shewing that it needs no tendance but is a wild thing. The people of Cyrene say that the silphium appeared seven years before they founded their city; now they had lived there for about three hundred years before the archonship at Athens of Simonides.

Silphium is an example of a drug used by countless numbers of people for long periods of time. It was frequently mentioned by Hippocrates and the great medical classicists of antiquity, and yet is a drug of which we know nothing of any active pharmacological principle that might have earned it such a singular place in history. It seems that it was discovered at the time of the colonization of Cyrene in 631 BC. The Greek colonists left Santorini (Thera) and settled on the island of Platea; they were told of an inland source of water and moved to colonize the area of this natural spring – a spring which is said to still provide part of the water for the town of Cyrene. Gradually the district they had occupied along the coast of North Africa became known as a source of supplies and a granary for Greece and Rome.

Silphium became an item of commerce to the extent that it appeared on the coins of the colony and is brilliantly shown on the Attic tetradrachm of Cyrene of about 480 BC. It was so important that the earliest coins of the new colony, minted between 570 and 525 BC, show the fruit, leaf or plant of silphium and it continued to appear on coins until the period 246–221 BC during the reign of Ptolemy III. Thus, for something like 400 years – from the beginning of the period of colonization until about 200 BC – silphium seems to have been one of the main exports of Cyrenaica.

Four hundred years later, by about AD 200, conditions in the colony seem to have become so bad, worsened by the Jewish revolt of AD 115, that the export of silphium became almost impossible. In AD 365 an earthquake practically destroyed Cyrene as a city – and it is usually assumed that by this date, if not before, silphium of Cyrene was replaced, both as an item of commerce and as a medicine, by the supplies of the pungent drug asafoetida coming from Media or Syria.

The botanical identification of the drug has been considered, and its history reviewed, by Chalmers L. Gemmill in his 1966 article *Silphium*[232]. The most likely candidate for the drug Theophrastus described is *Ferula tingitana*, or a plant very close to it. Gemmill says '*Ferula tingitana* is rare in Cyrenaica today, but it does still exist in that region'[233]. In England it is still sometimes grown as a garden plant.

The references to silphium by the ancient authors are so frequent that its uses seem to have been ubiquitous; some of them merged with those of asafoetida, its successor. Asafoetida (BPC 1949)[234] is an oleo-gum-resin obtained from the living rhizome or root of *Ferula assafoetida* and probably other species of *Ferula*, of the Umbelliferae. Its actions remained of interest to William Withering, the discoverer of digitalis, and it is in connection with his correspondence that the plant will be met with again.

The everyday example of this group of plants is, of course, fennel (*Foeniculum vulgare* of the Umbelliferae), now widely available for use in salads and an ingredient of skin cleansing lotions and gripe water in the older recipes. Fennel is also a genus (Foeniculum) of yellow-flowered umbelliferous plants, allied to dill, but distinguished by the cylindrical, strongly-ribbed, fruit. The giant fennel is *Ferula communis*.

Silphium is an example of the plant lore of Theophrastus which has been lost to modern practice. A common example of that lore which has reached from the writings of the Greeks to our own times, is the male fern. Of this plant, and its medical uses, Theophrastus says[235]:

> Of male-fern no part but the root is useful and it has a sweet astringent taste. It expels the flat worm. It has no seed nor juice: and they say it is ripe for cutting in autumn.

Clearly the Greeks not only knew the male fern as an anthelmintic but they recognized its specific activity against the tapeworm, which they had distinguished from the roundworm (*Ascaris lumbricoides*).

Male Fern (BP 1973)[236] is the rhizome, frond-bases, and apical bud of *Dryopteris filix-mas* agg. of the Polypodiaceae. It was just as in our gardens and hedgerows today, and was collected late in the autumn, cleaned of the roots and dead portions, and carefully dried so that it kept its internal green colour.

Treated like this it contains not less than 1.5% of filicin – the mixture of ether-soluble substances which can be obtained from it and of which the activity is mainly due to the flavaspidic acid content.

Male Fern Extract (BP) was an effective anthelmintic for the expulsion of tapeworms (*Taenia* species) and was sometimes used to rid the body of intestinal and liver flukes as in clinical clonorchiasis. Deservedly, it has been displaced by less toxic, more effective, more modern drugs – but it is interesting to examine a frond of the male fern, its circular, brown centres of spores on the underside, and recall the centuries down which the extract of its root was the answer to one human parasite.

Theophrastus was enough of a pharmacologist to notice that repeated use can sometimes diminish the efficacy of drugs and that they do not have the same effect on all constitutions. He brings out these observations in the following passage[237]:

> The virtues of all drugs become weaker to those who are accustomed to them, and in some cases become entirely ineffective. Thus some eat enough hellebore to consume whole bundles and yet suffer no hurt; this is what Thrasyas did, who, as it appeared, was very cunning in the use of herbs. And it appears that shepherds sometimes do the like; wherefore the shepherd who came before the vendor of drugs (at whom men marvelled because he ate one or two roots) and himself consumed the whole bundle, destroyed the vendor's reputation: it was said that both this man and others did this every day.
>
> For it seems that some poisons become poisonous because they are unfamiliar, or perhaps it is a more accurate way of putting it to say that familiarity makes poisons non-poisonous; for, when the constitution has accepted them and prevails over them, they cease to be poisons, as Thrasyas also remarked; for he said that the same thing was a poison to one and not to another; thus he distinguished between different constitutions, as he thought was right; and he was clever at observing the differences. Also, besides the constitution, it is plain that use has something to do with it.

The contribution made by Theophrastus has been summarized by Charles Singer in his *Studies in the History and Method of Science*[238] and by a number of other authors, including Henry Osborn Taylor[239]. The great contribution was to make an intellectually systematic attack on the subject and codify existing knowledge in an orderly way. Theophrastus distinguished the external organs of plants and clearly described the structure of the perianth members of flowers, but without attaining any real knowledge of their sexual nature. He closely observed the development of seeds and was fascinated by the phenomena by which plants replicate; he also studied the relationships between the structure and habits of plants and so began the later studies of plant ecology. Beyond this, he grasped that there is a relationship between the structure and function of plants and saw the need for a general classification of the many forms of plant life. Thus, by early in the third century BC, Theophrastus had laid the basis of scientific, and with it, medical botany.

There is an affinity of tone between the genuine writings of Hippocrates and those of Theophrastus. The Hippocratic writings mention some 236 plants, the *De Historia Plantarum*[227] of Theophrastus describes 455 plants and summarizes all that was known at the time of the medicinal properties of each. Theophrastus therefore provided the first work that can be considered an extensive and precise herbal.

Many writers have remarked on the tone of the writings of Theophrastus. Certainly he brought to bear upon his observance of natural things a sympathy much like that which Hippocrates had given to his clinical descriptions. It may well be this level of innate understanding which singled out Theophrastus in the mind of Aristotle.

With the death of Theophrastus, about 287 BC, real progress in the biological sciences disappeared from the ancient Greek world. There were, of course, writers of lesser ability but their works form part of a tradition which led, from the date of the founding of Alexandria in 332 BC, to Greek science and Greek culture becoming firmly implanted in Egypt. From this date Alexandria was to remain the capital of Egypt for 1000 or more years – and for the first of these centuries Alexandria flourished as a great centre of Hellenic culture and knowledge.

This Hellenistic Age – the period from 323 to 30 BC, from the date of the death of Alexander the Great to the time of the incorporation of Egypt into the Roman Empire – was the period which nurtured medicine in Alexandria. Medicine was no longer a small, useless body of knowledge. Nor was it part of magic. Working without the means of human dissection, without either experimental physiology or pathology, using just the unaided intellect and senses, it may be that it had advanced almost to its limits. Greek medical science may have advanced as far as in the circumstances it could have been taken. The point, and it is a considerable point, that Charles Singer[234] has made is that 'This was done by a process of pure scientific induction.'

In terms of science this concrete and rational system of thought was new. The inductive method of reasoning, once evolved, affected all subsequent Western schools of medicine. In its clearer form after the Renaissance it still affects the everyday practice of the art.

The Hippocratic tradition and the medicine of classical Greece contained much that was unsurpassed until the nineteenth century. Percussion, auscultation, and the modern additions to the physical senses of the physician; anaesthetics, antisepsis, blood transfusion, the cellular and microbial theories and the remaining accomplishments of the last two centuries, may have dwarfed the Greek achievement. But the heart of that accomplishment was the recognition of the *vis medicatrix naturae* and the hygiene of its means of support.

Alexandria – to about 30 BC

In Alexandria, as part of the university-like Museum with its vast library of over half a million volumes and with teachers of the calibre of Archimedes (*c.* 287–212 BC) and Euclid (fl. *c.* 300 BC), the greatest medical school of antiquity was established.

In Ptolemaic and later Roman Egypt, Alexandria was the cultural centre as well as the repository of traditional native lore. It was also the populous home of the wealthy who, even though their religious beliefs changed, maintained the time-honoured custom of mummifying the dead. The Alexandrian anatomists were therefore able to associate with the hereditary guild or caste of embalmers and add to their knowledge. The process of these additions was hastened by the debasement and degeneration of the methods of mummification which, though still traditional, were no longer the formal expression of profound religious convictions. Less and less care was given to the preservation of the remains of the dead and more to the ceremonial – the bandages and wrappings, the amulets and cartonnage coffins – that accompanied it. Many of these late mummies are nothing much more than eviscerated, resin-soaked corpses obviously in a neglected state even before the ritual began. It was now the ritual that mattered – but its neglect of the physical remains and its method of handling gave access to parts of the body previously dealt with only to preserve them. There seems little doubt that the anatomists of Alexandria carried exploration well beyond the bounds needed for ritual mummification.

Praxagoras (fl. c. 340 BC), a native of Cos, had recognized that of the blood vessels only the arteries showed pulsation. Hippocrates had given a somewhat confused account of the heart and vascular system, and this account may well have been derived from Egyptian sources. Aristotle had not really differentiated the vessels carrying blood and had written of the nutriment oozing from the blood vessels into the tissues of the body in the way in which water drains from unbaked pottery. Like Hippocrates, he used the term *arteria* for the trachea. Praxagoras, seeing that the arteries are usually empty after death, thought that they contained the *pneuma*, or vital spirit; he therefore used the term *arteria* for the arteries and called the windpipe the *arteria tracheia*, the ribbed or rough pipe of air; it is from this use that we derive the word trachea. At much the same time Diocles (fl. c. 350 BC) wrote his treatise *On the heart*[240] and in this described the cardiac valves, atria and the columnae carnae – possibly deriving part of his information from much earlier Egyptian sources and the knowledge of the embalmers.

All of these observations were made before formal dissection of the human was permitted but, after the death of Alexander the Great, when Egypt fell into the hands of his general, Ptolemy, this was allowed. Even though the books of the era are largely lost and reach us by means of inclusions in the works of much later writers, the evidence of dissection is irrefutable. By the time of the third Ptolemy, when the Museum of Alexandria had grown to greatness, dissection was by no means uncommon.

The two outstanding medical figures of Alexandria were Herophilus of Chalcedon (fl. c. 300 BC), usually looked upon as the founder of scientific anatomy, and Erasistratus of Chios (c. 310–250 BC), often regarded as the first experimental physiologist. The presence of these two teachers and their associates ensured that the museum and library of Alexandria became the means of preserving the Greek texts and, eventually, of carrying the learning of Greece into the Roman world.

Both Herophilus and Erasistratus were accused, by Celsus and Tertullian, of human vivisection in their thirst for knowledge. Perhaps, as we know of most of their work only through the writings of others, we shall never really know the truth of these accusations. Celsus, in *De Medicina*[241], is unequivocal: he says, 'They hold that Herophilus and Erasistratus . . . laid open men whilst alive –

criminals received out of prison from the kings – and whilst these were still breathing, observed parts which beforehand nature had concealed . . . ' Later on he refers more than once to the subject and, when writing that the Art of Medicine needed to draw instruction from evident causes, he qualified this by saying, 'But to lay open the bodies of men whilst still alive is as cruel as it is needless. . .' [242].

Herophilus certainly distinguished the arteries from the veins, described the meninges and the fourth ventricle, named the prostate and duodenum, placed the seat of intelligence in the brain, and made a number of other discoveries. Erasistratus described the cerebral ventricular system, traced the cranial nerves to the brain, settled the origin of the great arterial and venous cardiac vessels, named the tricuspid valve, wrote accurately upon the trachea, chordae tendineae, atria and the remaining endocardial valves, and postulated a capillary system. His knowledge could certainly have come only from dissection and he seems to have seen that the heart is a pump. Thus, he appears to have come close to an understanding of the circulation – an appreciation then lost until the vitally important seventeenth century discovery by Harvey.

Greek medicine, with all of its Alexandrian additions, was spread, in the third century before Christ, into the ancient lands of Mesopotamia. Syria, and the adjacent countries, acquired the Hippocratic medical teaching of Greece from Alexandrian Egypt. In Syrian hands the Greek teaching was mixed with the retained astrological and numerical tradition of the Assyrian and Babylonian peoples. Syria therefore becomes, for a second time, important – for Syria was soon to become the platform from which this mixed tradition of medicine, practised for over 1000 years, entered the mediaeval Western world. Great imperfections of the texts were inevitable for in the early Middle Ages the Greek manuscripts in their Syriac versions were translated into Hebrew or Arabic, and then to Latin.

These translations and the resulting imperfections of the texts were, however, later than the changes in Alexandria; in the second century before the Christian era, the Empirics arose from the declining Alexandrian school. The changes in outlook involved in this transition affected both the physicians and their rulers. Of the latter, Mithridates, King of Pontus (120–63 BC), achieved lasting medical fame by trying to design a universal antidote to poisoning. His formula was modest in its number of ingredients – but still is, in some ways, the beginning of polypharmacy. It was the basis, as more and more ingredients were added, of the 'mithridates' and 'theriacs' that form so large a part of the pharmacy of the Middle Ages and were conspicuous in the prescribing habits of physicians until the early part of the eighteenth century. The school of Empirics, in this way, left an unfortunate legacy of multiple therapy and polypharmacy. This troublesome bequest may have been counterbalanced by the practices of Erasistratus who, even though his contempories were much in favour of extensive blood-letting, used this form of therapy only seldom and favoured regulated exercise, diet, the vapour bath and restorative techniques in therapy; he favoured also the practical means of hygiene in the prevention of disease.

With the absorption of Egypt into the Roman Empire in 50 BC and the ending of the Ptolemaic dynasty by the death of Cleopatra 30 years before the beginning of the Christian era, Alexandria fell from scientific importance. The great city and Museum remained highly active in the teaching of mathematics, astronomy, and a number of subjects, including geography. But in medicine, the fame and importance of the school is synonymous with the reputation and discoveries of Herophilus and Erasistratus.

The pre-eminence of Greece ended with the destruction of Corinth in 146 BC; when Egypt became part of the strong and expanding Roman Empire roughly 100 years after the fall of Corinth, the future of medicine rested to no small extent in Rome. That it was still largely Greek medicine makes its growth in its new climate perhaps all the more singular and unexpected.

Greek Medicine in Rome – to about AD 200

While, in Egypt, the Roman span lasted from 30 BC to AD 476, throughout the whole of this period the southern half of the Italian peninsula, previously colonized by the Greeks, remained unconquered – a factor of the greatest importance in medical history. Clifford Allbutt (1836–1925), in his *Greek Medicine in Rome*[243], made the point that Southern Italy 'was not Italian even in name, but in name was Magna Graecia, and in character Greek; and this character, until blighted by malaria, it maintained.' The whole area was of Greek culture from the sixth century before until the tenth century after Christ – and from Magna Graecia there was a stream of cultural influence which later helped to found the school of Salerno.

The original medicine of Rome contained little by way of science and was interwoven with religion, superstition, and magic. The Roman religious cults contained many deities, a complex number of which were worshipped as domestic household gods. The robust attitude of the citizens seems to have resulted in disease being regarded as something of a sign of weakness, the heads of the households dealing with their own sick by invoking the domestic gods and resorting to an extensive herbal pharmacopoeia. Medicines, and the care of the infirm or ill were of less moment than the brilliant concepts of social order, organization and hygiene for which the Roman civilization is famous.

In the years in which Rome was established and expanded, medicine was practised by a lowly despised class, almost of slaves. It was not until after the fall of Corinth that increasing numbers of physicians came to Rome from the mainland of Greece and began to win some measure of respect for their skills. It was a slow process, full of complexities, many of which have been finely reviewed by W. H. S. Jones in his *Philosophy and Medicine in Ancient Greece*[244]. Jones' book is made additionally notable for its translation of *Ancient Medicine*, a work which, unlike many of the books of the Hippocratic Collection, appears as a finished, carefully constructed study containing a polemic against the intrusion of philosophic speculation into medicine. It contains also a theory of the subject with a spirited defence of the old, well-established clinical and observational method.

Long before the arrival of the Greek physicians with this tradition, both the civic and architectural means of hygiene had been established in Rome. Sanitation and bathing were main features of the life of the city – as were the *cloacae*, the subterranean sewers and drains, established from the sixth century before Christ. The Cloaca Maxima, still in use, dates from that period and serves as part of the main drainage system of Rome. In the same way, the remains of the series of great aqueducts that supplied the city with its millions of gallons of potable water a day can still be seen. Clean water, of a quality seldom reached before the present century in the towns of Europe, was a health-giving part of everyday life in the homes of ancient Rome.

Civic measures – showing how far back such ideas reach – included the law of about 450 BC which gave instructions to town officials regarding the cleanliness of the streets, the maintenance of clean water supplies and the requirement that burials were not to occur within the city walls. These laws included a requirement that the body of a woman dying in late pregnancy was to be opened in an attempt to extract a live child. In this practice lay the origin of Caesarean section, by which it is said Julius Caesar (102–44 BC) was delivered. This particular Caesar made his mark upon Roman medicine by taking steps to improve the subordinate position of physicians in Rome: perhaps to advance military surgery he conferred citizenship on the practitioners of medicine in the city. Following this improvement *valetudinaria*, or infirmaries, were provided, at first for the sick poor and servicemen; from this sort of resource a definite hospital and public health system grew and highly efficient surgical services came to be provided for the all-important army.

As these changes progressed the migrant Greek physicians came to be more and more trusted and their despised status changed. It was rather dramatically improved by Asclepiades of Bithynia (124–56 BC), who dominated the first half of the last century before the Christian era and who stood out in both tact and ability from the Empirics and their Dogmatist descendants of the earlier school of Alexandria. To Asclepiades must go the credit of having established Greek medicine in Rome on a respectable footing.

What is left of his writings is preserved in the Greek edition of the *Fragmenta. Digessit et curavit C. G. Gumpert* of 1794[245]. The very useful *Asclepiades, his Life and Writings* by R. M. Green[246] includes a translation of Gumpert's *Fragmenta*.

Asclepiades moved to Rome and practised medicine there in the great Age of Cicero, Horace, and Virgil, two centuries before Galen, and at a time when the Romans had already reached the peak of luxurious living. Tactically, he understood how to make Greek medicine acceptable to the Romans – his methods were virile and active and yet luxury-loving; he added careful dietetic care to his medicines, and his means of treatment included the fine bathing, rocking, and sea journeys so much enjoyed by the Romans even in health. Most of what is known of the techniques of Asclepiades comes from the comments of others. The *Preface* to Gumpert's *Fragmenta* cites Galen's comments that Asclepiades often employed venesection and so readily criticized the doctrines of Hippocrates and the previous centuries that he considered the ancient methods merely 'a meditation of death'[247].

In his everyday practice he seems to have been less radical than might be expected, placing great reliance on supportive, Hippocratic methods of treatment. Opposed to the idea that disease is due to an imbalance of the humours, he considered man subject to physical laws in nature; there was, therefore, now and again a mixing of theory with his practice of the art of medicine. A number of innovations are credited to him: he is said to have been the first to associate

101

hydrophobia with the bite of rabid animals; he is also said to have been the first to describe tracheotomy and to have been among the first to treat mental illness humanely. He gave specific instructions on the use of music to relieve the mentally ill and allowed the use of wine to lessen anxiety and facilitate sleep.

From the evil-averting and healing temple god, Aesculapius, there descended, as time advanced, a whole order of priests who received the name Asclepiades. Gradually this name became proper to all who were bound by oath to the schools which flourished in the name of Aesculapius, chiefly at Cos and Cnidus. Thus, various men, many of them notable, occur in the writings of the ancients and are given the name Asclepiades. It is hard not to confuse them. They included Asclepiades, known as Pharmacion, who wrote a special book describing the composition of drugs. However, none of them reach the stature of Asclepiades the Bithynian who alone, it seems, made Greek medicine accepted in Rome.

In the first century of the Christian era a wide variety of beliefs persisted – many of them dividing folk medicine from professional medicine and the lives of the privileged from the rest of the population. Beliefs regarding the underworld and its earthly manifestations proved especially durable despite considerable affluence. Superstitions then inhabited the life of the city even when it was far advanced in providing the measures of preserving the public health for which Rome is renowned.

Despite the ability to produce these measures, and the Code of law and the social order which distinguishes the Roman civilization, people still thought that eating parts of particular animals would heal illnesses and, as a healing rite, the sacrificial rituals of primitive peoples and the Romans continued up to the time of Porphyry (AD 234–305). The strength and persistence of these beliefs can now cause surprise. Some of their roots lay in the incubus of the 'foundation sacrifice' which demanded a sacrifice buried in the foundations to bring good luck and well-being upon a house. R. A. Stewart Macalister provides, in his book *The Excavation of Gezer*[248] photographs of the skeleton of an old woman buried beneath the corner foundations of an early Syrian dwelling; he also includes illustrations of a similar infant burial within a stone jar forming part of the ground structure of a house. As time passed the brutality of these beliefs was lessened by the sacrifice being replaced by a primitively-shaped human figure in precious metal which served as a talisman.

In Rome, the heart, liver, and brain – the ancient triad of life – were highly valued and blood was esteemed as the greatest of remedies. Scribonius Largus, in the first half-century after the birth of Christ, recorded the drinking of his own blood by the patient as a potent therapeutic rite. At much the same period, Celsus, describing the last resource in the treatment of epilepsy (which he calls 'comitialis' because the Romans called the disease *comitialis morbus* as a meeting of the *comitia* was adjourned if a member was attacked by it, since it was still considered a divine manifestation) says[249]:

> Some have freed themselves from such a disease by drinking the hot blood from the cut throat of a gladiator: a miserable aid made tolerable by a malady still more miserable.

While such things continued, the professionals of medicine organized themselves and the medical teachers of Rome, with their pupils and apprentices, combined to form colleges and societies; these eventually constructed for themselves a meeting place on the Esquiline Hill. These efforts were supported by the Emperors who, possibly to assist in the training of surgeons for the legions, built the *auditoria*, or teaching halls.

Celsus

The medicine of the first two centuries of the Christian era is dominated by the writings of three great figures: Celsus, Dioscorides, and Galen. Even though Rome produced no physcian of the stature of Hippocrates, the teaching of these three – one a layman, the second a medical botanist, and the third a physician and experimental physiologist – influenced medical science throughout the Middle Ages and to the beginnings of modern times.

Even though medicine in Rome was almost entirely in Greek hands the best account of it comes to us in *De Medicina* – the splendid work of Aulus Cornelius Celsus (fl. AD 10–37), a Roman of noble birth and subject of Tiberius Caesar (42 BC–AD 37). W. H. S. Jones[250] has suggested that the tradition that the first name of Celsus was Aurelius must be wrong, as Aurelius is not a *praenomen*. Almost all look upon *De Medicina* as being the surviving part of a great encylopaedia encompassing all the knowledge of the day; the lost parts are said to have dealt with agriculture, the military arts, rhetoric, philosophy and jurisprudence. Little is really known of the personal life of the author of these treatises but some say that he was born about 25 BC.

It is by no means clear that he was a professional physician. His surviving writings read as if he had an extensive personal knowledge of the materia medica and a practical familiarity with minor surgical procedures, including bleeding and cupping. His work is a compilation from the Greek authors and the writers of Alexandria and is marked by a purity of Latin and precision of literary style. Both of these assets, added to the usefulness and wide compass of *De Medicina*, must have helped to ensure its survival.

Celsus is perhaps best regarded as a man of letters experienced in the medical affairs of a large household and estate and a wider circle beyond. It is a striking fact that he is the only one of the great Greek and Roman medical writers of antiquity to use Latin – a point which demonstrates the importance of the Greek culture in the medicine of Rome. Apart from *De Medicina* there is no other source from which we can learn so much of the condition of medical science prior to the first century of the present era.

Of this work, now universally acknowledged as ·the oldest major medical document available after the Hippocratic writings, there is a fine edition, the *De Medicina* of Nicolaus (Laurentius), published in 1478 and edited by Bartholamaeus Fontius[251]. The original manuscript of the work of Celsus, written about AD 30, was lost during the Middle Ages but was rediscovered in Milan in 1443. The *editio princeps*, printed in Florence in 1478, was one of the first medical books to be printed, such was its vast importance. The work afterwards went through more editions than almost any other treatise in science – there being 49 printed editions by 1841.

The most readily accessible form of the work is the fine, bilingual, three volume edition of *De Medicina* translated by W. G. Spencer and published by Heinemann[241] between 1935 and 1938 as part of the Loeb Classical Library. In this edition, from which the following quotations and extracts are taken, the Latin and English are set opposite one another on the page.

De Medicina shows that in many departments of medicine knowledge had advanced beyond that of the days of Hippocrates; the moral tone of the book remains high, although without the noble and detached beauty of the authentic books of Hippocrates. Anatomy had improved, and with it surgery; Celsus seems to carry forward the improvements in knowledge of Alexandria. With some striking exceptions the lines of treatment are sensible and humane. The pharmacopoeia had become extensive without being burdensome and was virtually free of the 'dung pharmacopoeia' of Egypt and Assyria. It contained some topical applications which might still be considered useful and a number of items from which medicines of quite modern times were derived.

The three volumes of Spencer's edition[241] contain the eight books which comprise the work of Celsus. Book I gives an excellent summary of the Dogmatist, Methodic, and Empiric Greek Schools of medicine and contains sensible advice on dietetics and general health care. Book II deals largely with matters of diagnosis, prognosis, and symptomology. Book III deals well with internal ailments and Book IV (less satisfactorily) describes local diseases of the body. Books V and VI are the vital ones from the point of view of therapeutics. These books deal with the drug treatment of disease but their weakness is the great lack of knowledge of internal medicine of the times of Celsus. Books VII and VIII deal with surgery and show how far even operative surgery had advanced.

Acknowledging the achievement of the Father of Medicine, Celsus wrote[252] of 'Hippocrates of Cos, a man first and foremost worthy to be remembered, notable both for professional skill and for eloquence, who separated this branch of learning from the study of philosophy.' He is equally telling in his comment on the Bithynian[253]: 'Asclepiades said that it is the office of the practitioner to treat safely, speedily, and pleasantly.' The robust Roman attitude to being reluctant to consult doctors shows in the paragraph with which he opens his Book I[254]:

> A man in health, who is both vigorous and his own master, should be under no obligatory rules, and have no need, either for a medical attendant, or for a rubber and anointer. His kind of life should afford him variety; he should be now in the country, now in town, and more often about the farm; he should sail, hunt, rest sometimes, but more often take exercise; for whilst inaction weakens the body, work strengthens it; the former brings on premature old age, the latter prolongs youth.

There are famous phrases in which Celsus shows an aphoristic wisdom that is both medical and at one with that of the people. These include his comment that 'the middle-aged sustain hunger more easily, less so young people, and least of all children and old people.'[255] He recognizes the transmissibility of infectious disease in a way that goes beyond the earlier Greek understanding and says that even a healthy man should observe suitable measures during a pestilence and these should include travel abroad, taking a voyage, walking in the open, avoiding fatigue, excesses of temperatures and venery[256].

Celsus also remarks[257] that 'a practitioner should know above all which wounds are incurable, which may be cured with difficulty, and which more readily. For it is the part of a prudent man first not to touch a case he cannot save, and not to risk the appearance of having killed one whose lot is but to die . . . ' He then goes on to say which cases cannot be saved.

Even the youngest and most modern students of medicine learn one aphorism of Celsus – the famous citation from Book III[258, 259]:

> Notae vero inflammationis sunt quattuor: rubor et tumor cum calore et dolore.

> Now the signs of an inflammation are four: redness and swelling with heat and pain.

But there are fine and discerning passages and excellent segments of clinical description, perhaps at their best in the accounts of malaria[260], epilepsy[261], and phthisis[262].

Some of the attempts at treatment in difficult situations seem over-enthusiastic: 'severe fever, when the bodily surface is reddened, and the blood-vessels full and swollen, requires withdrawal of blood; so too diseases of the viscera, also paralysis and rigor . . .'[263]. Celsus talks of controlling violent forms of madness by fettering and says 'Anyone so fettered, although he talks rationally and pitifully when he wants his fetters removed, is not to be trusted, for that is a madman's trick.'[264] He says that if the madman 'says or does anything wrong, he is to be coerced by starvation, fetters and flogging.'[265] There are some rather strong treatments for the illness (hysteria) that comes 'from the womb of a woman'[266] and, recognizing that hydrophobia can be due to the bite of a dog that is mad, Celsus advises, 'In these cases there is very little hope for the sufferer. But still there is just one remedy, to throw the patient unawares into a water tank which he has not seen beforehand.'[267]

In the use of the pharmacopoeia, much of it herbal, Celsus is practical and the element of the fabulous disappears. At the beginning of his Book V he writes of medicaments and says that some practitioners would not treat disease without using drugs but others avoid them; all know they can cause harm and, of themselves, provide problems[268, 269]:

> I have spoken of those maladies of the body in which the regulation of the diet is most helpful: now I pass on to that part of medicine which combats them rather by medicaments. These were held of high value by ancient writers, both by Erasistratus and those who styled themselves Empirics, especially however by Herophilus and his school, insomuch that they treated no kind of disease without them.

> On the other hand, Asclepiades dispensed with the use of these for the most part, not without reason; and since nearly all medicaments harm the stomach and contain bad juices, he transferred all his treatment rather to the management of the actual diet. But while in most diseases that is the more useful method, yet very many illnesses attack our bodies which cannot be cured without medicaments.

In the early books of *De Medicina* Celsus mentions a number of drugs already described: these include 'black hellebore root, or polypody fern root'[270], used as a purge; 'white hellebore root'[271], used as an emetic; 'poppy, lettuce, and mostly the summer kinds in which the stalk is very milky'[272], which he employs to produce sleep. He adds that: 'If...patients are wakeful, some endeavour to induce sleep by draughts of decoction of poppy or hyoscyamus; others put mandrake apples under the pillow.'[273] Many of his plant remedies contain, it will be noticed, potent and now isolated plant principles or alkaloids.

The second volume of the W. G. Spencer translation of *De Medicina* begins with an excellent 'List of Medicamenta'[274] which is of the greatest usefulness: it does, in fact, summarize most of what is known of the pharmacopoeia at the time of Celsus.

Not all of the medicaments are herbal – copper in various forms, aluminium salts, the yellow trisulphide of arsenic (orpiment) and other forms of arsenic, bitumen, zinc ores from Cyprus, calcium salts (the oxide, silicates and sulphate), lead salts, the oxides, silicates and sulphates of iron, salt, antimony sulphide and sulphur all appear in the Roman pharmacopoeia. Of these substances the entry for copper can serve as an example of the 'List of Medicamenta' provided by Spencer[275]:

Aes Cyprium or Cuprum; copper.

Many forms of this were used in prescriptions;

(1) Aerugo; basic subacetate and carbonate of copper or verdigris. This was scraped off sheets of copper which had been steeped in vinegar and used as an astringent, repressive or caustic,

(2) Chalcitis; basic carbonate and sulphate of copper, copperas or green vitriol. This was mixed with oak bark or galls to make *atramentum sutorium*, blacking, and used as a caustic and exedent, to arrest haemorrhage, to clean wounds and form a scar,

(3) Aes combustum; calcined copper ore.

This was used as an erodent, or was fused with salt, sulphur or alum into a sulphate chloride and oxide of copper and used to make emollients and eye salves,

(4) Flos aeris or Chalcanthus; red oxide of copper.

This substance was like millet seeds and was produced by pouring cold water on molten copper and used as an exedent, or as an agglutinant for wounds,

(5) Squama aeris; black oxide of copper, copper scales.

These were chipped off molten copper, and when washed, pounded and dried acted as a mechanical aperient,

(6) Chrysocolla; borate, carbonate and silicate of copper, gold solder.

This was used as an erodent and caustic,

(7) Diphryges; sulphide and oxide of copper, mixed with iron and zinc ores.

This was used as an exedent and caustic and for cleaning ulcerations,

(8) Stomoma; red oxide of copper, copper scales hardened in the fire.

These were used to arrest haemorrhage and in making an eye salve,

(9) Psoricum; itch salve, consisted of chalcitis and cadmia boiled together in vinegar to form hydrated oxides of copper and zinc, and then buried underground till used, the preparation was also applied to the eyelids,

(In this list the cross references have been omitted.)

The first century pharmacopoeia included, amongst its botanical materials, Absinthium[276] (*Artemisia absinthium*), the twigs of which provided wormwood, the dried flowers wormseed, and from which the bitter oil, absinth, was distilled. Absinth was used as a carminative and diuretic, as a topical agent, and as a remedy for worms. Celsus advises that 'for round worms which especially trouble children, . . . a decoction of wormwood or hyssop in hydromel or cress seeds pounded up in vinegar'[277] is among the remedies that can be given.

The direct link between the Roman use of the *Artemisia* species and the remedies of the twentieth century is that Santonica (BPC 1934)[278], or Wormseed, is the dried, unexpanded flowerheads of *Artemisia cina* and other species of *Artemisia* of the Compositae; it contains not less than 2% of santonin. It used to be administered as a decoction or infusion for the expulsion of roundworms (*Ascaris lumbricoides*) or threadworms (pinworms; *Enterobius vermicularis* or *Oxyuris vermicularis*). Santonin (BP 1963)[279] was the crystalline lactone obtained from santonica; it was formerly much used as an anthelmintic in the treatment of infestation with roundworm but has now been superseded by other less toxic remedies. Poisoning with it chiefly affected vision making white objects look green, blue or yellow (xanthopsia) but large doses caused fits which could be followed by coma and death. The British Pharmaceutical Codex for 1968[280] showed it among the list of drugs deleted from that edition.

Silphium (it was probably either *Ammoniacum thymiatum, Dorema ammoniacum* or *Ferula tingitana*) was well known to Celsus, the juice of the plant being used in incense in his time and his own practice finding a place for it. The resin contained salicylic acid and a volatile oil; it was used as either a cleanser of wounds, an emollient, or an ingredient in poultices, plasters and eye salves.

We have already noticed Celsus referring to 'decoction of poppy or hyoscyamus'[273] as a hypnotic, but elsewhere, recounting treatments for spastic or soft tissue pain, as after paralysis, he says: 'It is also of service to mix fat with pounded henbane and nettle seeds, equal parts of each, and put this on, also to foment with a decoction of sulphur.'[281]. In addition to this use as a local anodyne, Celsus used the bark of the henbane as a poultice for joints, the leaves in an eye salve, the juice for earache, and the root for toothache. Purified forms of these substances remain in everyday medical and surgical use today.

Hyoscyamus, or Henbane leaves, is the dried leaves, or leaves and flowering tops, of *Hyoscyamus niger* (Figure 27) of the Solanaceae; it contains not less than 0.05% of alkaloids calculated as hyoscyamine. The calculation is made in terms of hyoscyamine as this is the chief alkaloid of hyoscyamus but there are lesser amounts of hyoscine and atropine. Thus, hyoscyamus has the central and peripheral actions of atropine and for long remained in use to counteract the griping pains produced by strong purgatives, intense intestinal hurry, or smooth muscle spasm in the urinary tract. Hyoscyamine (BPC 1934)[282] is obtained from a number of solanaceous plants and is the laevo-isomer of atropine into which it can readily be converted either by heating or the action of alkali; it is usually used as either the hydrobromide or sulphate and its anticholinergic effects are even more potent than atropine. Hyoscine (Hyoscine hydrobromide BP[283]; Scopolamine hydrobromide) is, of course, an anticholinergic agent with central and peripheral actions; the main central symptoms are drowsiness leading, as a function of dose, to coma. The central depression is sometimes preceded by stimulation but the effect is different from atropine for hyoscine acts as a powerful hypnotic. Thus, hyoscine hydrobromide has been used in acute mania and delirium, including delirium tremens, to produce calming and a rapid induction of sleep. It remains in important use as part of pre-operative medication and, in obstetrics, has been used with morphine or pethedine to produce the state of analgesia and amnesia known as 'twilight sleep'; it has had important uses in the symptomatic relief of conditions like postencephalitic parkinsonism and finds use in the eye as a mydriatic and by mouth as a means of preventing or lessening motion sickness. Certainly the Roman use of hyoscine-like substances as powerful hypnotics, and some of its uses in the eye, seem an exact predictor of current practice.

Celsus also included the juice, the fleshy red calixes, and the fresh or dried bark of *Mandragora officinarum*, the mandrake, in several prescriptions and it is interesting that this plant also yields the alkaloids hyoscine (scopolamine) and atropine.

The knowledge of the practitioners of Rome included many active pharmacological agents, although not all of their uses anticipate those of today. One such agent, 'willow leaves boiled in vinegar'[284], would provide the drug salicin, previously mentioned, and elsewhere Celsus writes of ascites advising that: 'It is good besides to measure every day with string the circumference of the abdomen, and to put a mark where it surrounds the belly, then the day following to see whether the body is fuller or thinner, for the thinning shows a yielding to the treatment. Nor is it unserviceable to take the measure of his drink, and of his urine . . . '[285] We might be surprised to find, at this date, such clinical acumen but he then goes on, mentioning the treatment Asclepiades used in a patient 'who had lapsed from a quartan into dropsy'[286], and suggests: 'It is useful also to suck a boiled squill bulb[287].' Most of the prescriptions of Celsus are for topical application but he refers again to sucking 'a boiled squill bulb'[288], to sipping 'vinegar of squills'[289, 290], and there seems no doubt that he is advising squill taken by mouth as a diuretic and treatment for dropsy.

Squill (BPC 1934)[291] is the White Squill, the dried sliced bulb of the white or Mediterranean squill *Urginea maritima* (*U. scilla*) (Figure 28) of the Liliaceae. It contains the potent glycosides scillarin A and B and has an irritant effect on the stomach, so that it has been used for its reflex expectorant action, and a digitalis-like action on the heart. From December, 1974, for a period, the British Pharmaceutical Codex allowed Indian Squill (*Urginea indica*) to be substituted for White Squill due to the shortage of the latter in the United Kingdom. The action of squill is much less certain, and it is more likely to cause vomiting than, digitalis but it is, nevertheless, remarkable that the practitioners of the days of Celsus seemingly knew of and used appropriately, an effective cardiac glycoside.

Lastly, we can notice the comment that 'if there is paralysis of the tongue . . . he should gargle a decoction of thyme, hyssop or mint . . . '[292] This is as

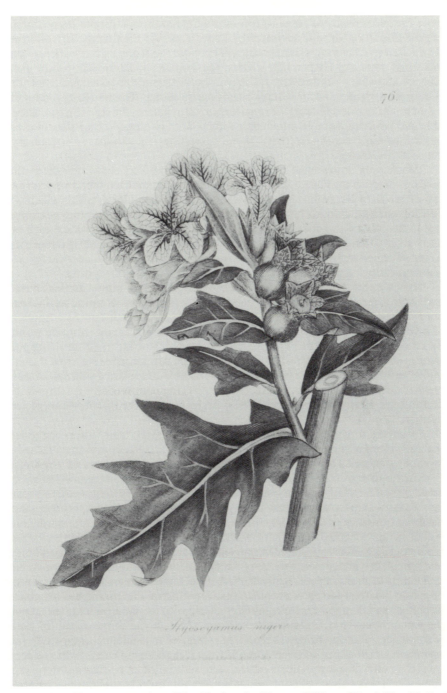

Figure 27 Hyoscyamus niger (The Henbane). [*From: William Woodville. Medical botany . . . London, William Phillips (1810), Vol. II.*]

close as Celsus seems to come to recognizing the antiseptic properties of thyme but the phenol or carbolic acid used by Lister is akin to the thymol derived from thyme flowers. Thymol is weaker than phenol but, so many centuries before the microbial theory of Pasteur, the nearest the Romans could have hoped to have come to knowing of its antiseptic properties would have been to recognize its usefulness as a gargle and in wound cleansing. Even so, Thyme (BPC, 1949)[293], Common or Garden Thyme, *Thymus vulgaris* (Labiatae), the source of an agreeable and aromatic volatile oil which contains not less than 40% of phenols and has known antimicrobial activity, is an interesting place to leave the pharmacopoeia of Celsus.

The surgical knowledge of the day had advanced to equal or exceed the progress made in medicine. Celsus was aware that traumatized blood vessels that cannot retract will continue to bleed copiously; he wrote: 'blood-vessels which are pouring out blood are to be seized, and round the wounded spot they are to be tied in two places and cut across between so that the two ends coalesce each on itself and yet have their orifices closed.'[294] Of wounds he says: 'It is dangerous when a wound swells overmuch; no swelling at all is the worst danger: the former is an indication of severe inflammation; the latter that the part is dead.'[295]

There is more difficulty when it comes to descriptions of major surgical events and the text reads as if Celsus lacks personal experience and, at times, as if he has not even seen such operations. Tonsillectomy[296] is mentioned, but the account is hardly practical. A graphic description is given of the extraction from the womb of a dead fetus[297], but it is hard to imagine the woman concerned surviving and there is no mention of a midwife or other practical woman assisting, even though midwives are mentioned in roughly contemporary accounts of normal labour. Neither does Celsus describe the technique of Caesarean section – an important and historic Roman procedure, usually performed following the death of the mother.

Traumatic surgery seems to have been another matter: later writers suggested that, advanced by gladiatorial and military experience, surgery in Rome reached a level of excellence which, once lost, was not regained until the time of Ambroise Paré in the sixteenth century. In the writings of Celsus there are passages showing great clinical acumen; to take one example: 'Therefore after a blow on the head first we must enquire whether the patient has had bilious vomiting, whether there has been obscurity of vision, whether he has become speechless, whether he has had bleeding from the nose or ears, whether he fell to the ground, whether he has lain senseless as if asleep; for such signs do not occur unless with fractured bone; and when they are present, we must recognize that treatment is necessary but difficult. If in addition there is also stupor, if the mind wanders, if either paralysis or spasm has followed, it is probable that the cerebral membrane has also been lacerated; and then there is little hope.'[298] Faced with the same patient, very much the same sequence of questions would run through the mind of the modern practitioner. Celsus also gives good accounts of couching a cataract[299] (an operation which was in use from antiquity until, in modern times, it was replaced by extraction); the plastic repair of a superficial mutilation by the raising of skin flaps which were then relieved of tension[300]; the use of a ligature to control bleeding during surgical operations[301]; the dangerous procedure of perineal lithotomy[302], and the procedure of amputation[303]. Of this Celsus says that it

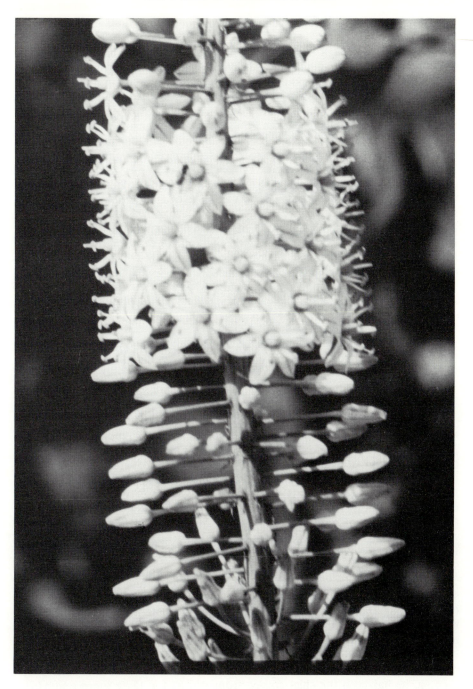

Figure 28 Urginea maritima (The White or Mediterranean Squill), Crete.

'involves very great risk; for patients often die under the operation, either from loss of blood or syncope.'[303] He adds that, 'It does not matter, however, whether the remedy is safe enough, since it is the only one'[304]; he then gives directions for a technique which was used many times in World War I to produce rounded stumps in those which had become pointed after emergency amputation.

There seems to be some recognition of the need for surgical cleanliness and Celsus, in describing the details of lithotomy, says that the surgeon must carefully pare his nails[305]; a number of times he shows a very clear understanding of the principle of surgery which demands the drainage of pus. He shows an equally clear appreciation of the need to excise dead, sequestered bone, as in the passage: 'A free flow of pus also indicates a fragment of bone; so then too it is proper to extract the fragment; sometimes also when the bone is injured a fistula is formed which has to be scraped out.'[306] In Book VIII he gives a serviceable account of the anatomy of the skeleton – reflecting the advances in knowledge made in Alexandria. In all, the eight books of *De Medicina* remain interesting and strangely akin to our modern thinking throughout. The cadence and quality of their language, and the justice done to them by their translator, can be appreciated from the passage in which he discusses the ways in which bone becomes damaged, beginning with the sentence[307,308]:

> Omne autem os, ubi iniuria accessit, aut vitiatur aut finditur aut frangitur aut foratur aut conliditur aut loco movetur.

> Now when any bone has been injured, it either becomes diseased or splits or is broken or perforated or crushed or displaced.

Dioscorides

Another Latin who owed almost everything in his great encyclopaedia, the *Natural history*[309], to Greek writings was Pliny the Elder (AD 23–79), a member of the landed class of Romans but one who, by dint of great industry and intelligence, assembled together the views and knowledge of the time on the nature, form and uses of plants and animals. This work, even though Pliny was devoid of critical or real scientific skill, became the main vehicle by which the Greek knowledge of natural history was transmitted throughout the Middle Ages. It remained important until the Renaissance brought the refreshed texts of Hippocrates and Aristotle to the readers and printers of the late fifteenth century.

A work of a quite different calibre, and one which has decided the form of every modern pharmacopoeia as well as virtually determining both popular and scientific plant nomenclature, is the *De materia medica* of Pedanius Dioscorides (fl. AD 54–68). Dioscorides was the originator of the materia medica and it is his book which is the authoritative source of information on the plant, animal, mineral and other drugs and remedies of antiquity.

Dioscorides does not provide the clinical observation and careful clinical record of Hippocrates nor does he match the creative originality of Aristotle; even so, he has been the chief source from which, for 15 or more centuries, herbalists of all nations have drawn their inspiration and physicians much of their instruction.

⊲ΠΕΔΑΚΙΟΥ

ΔΙΟΣΚΟΡΙΔΟΥ

Α Ν Α Ζ Α Ρ Β Ε Ω Σ,

ΠΕΡΙ ὕλης ἰατρικῆς.   ΒιΒλία ε′.
ΤΟΥ αὐτω̃, πἑρὶ Δηλητηρίωμ φδρμάκωμ, Ϭι φῇ αὐ ϧ̃ν προφυλακῆς.   ΒιΒλίομ Α′.
ΤΟΥ αὐτω̃, πἑρὶ ἰοβόλωμ, ϗ̀ν ὦ Ϭι πἑρὶ λυασω̃ντὸ κυνὸς.   ΒιΒλίομ Α′.
ΤΟΥ αὐτν̃, πἑρὶ σημμφώσεως ϧ̃ν ὑπἑ ἰοβόλωμ δεδηγμῴωμ.   ΒιΒλίομ Α′.
ΤΟΥ αὐτν̃, πἑρὶ θἑραπείας ϧ̃ν ὑπἑ ἰοβόλωμ δεδηγμῴωμ.   ΒιΒλίομ Α′.

⊱ PEDACII DIO

SCORIDAE ANAZARBEI,

DE MEDICA MATERIA   **LIBRI V.**

DE LETALIBVS VENENIS, EORVM΄QVE
præcautione & curatione.De cane rabido:Deq̃ notis quæ
morsus ictus΄ue animalium uenenum relinquen-
tium sequuntur:Deq̃ eorum curatione   **LIB. VNVS.**

Interprete Marcello Vergilio
Secretario Florentino.

EIVSDEM Marcelli Vergiln in hosce Dioscoridis libros commē
tarij doctissimi,in quibus præter omnigenam uariãq̃ eruditionē,col
latis aliorum Interpretum uersionibus,suæ tralationis ex utriusq̃ lin
guæ autoribus certissima adferuntur documenta.Morborum præte
rea atq̃ humani corporis uitiorum genus omne, quoq̃ subinde me-
minit Dioscorides,diligentissime explicatur.

❧COLONIAE☙

OPERA ET IMPEN-

ⓢ IOANNIS SOTERIS, AN-
NO M D XXIX.
Mense Augusto.
(٭)

Cum gratia & priuilegio Imperiali,ad Sexennium.

Figure 29 Pedanius Dioscorides. Title page from: *De medica materia . . . Interprete Marcello Virgilio (1529). [Royal Society of Medicine library, London.]*

113

☙ΠΕΔΑΚΙ PEDACII˙DI

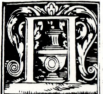

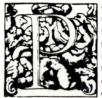

ΟΥ. ΔΙΟΣΚΟΡΙΔΟΥ ΑΝΑ-
ζαρβέως πἐ ὕλης Ἰατρικῆς,
ΒΙΒΛΙΟΝ
ΠΡΩΤΟΝ.

OSCORIDAE ANAZARBEI DE
medica materia, Liber Primus, Interprete MARCELLO VIRGI
LIO, Secretario Florentino.

OST MVLTOS NON
ueteres tātum sed iunio
res etiā, qui de medica-
mentoꝝ cōfectionibus,
uiribus & probatione
scripserunt, conabimur
& nos charissime Aree
de nobis id tibi ostende
re, nō uano nec sine ratiōe studio idem hoc ne
gotiū suscepisse: propterea ꝗ eoꝝ alꞇ rem nō
absoluerūt, alii ex historia plurima tradiderūt.
Bithynus siꝗdē Iolas & Tarētinus Heraclides,
relicta penitus herbaꝝ doctrina, tantisꝗ in hac
re metallico & odorametō
rūꝗ omnes meminerūt. Herbarius praeterea
Crateias & Andreas medicus (hi enim caeteris
omnibus diligētius hāc parte tractasse uident)
utilissimas radices multas, herbasꝗ aliquas in
descriptas reliquerūt. Veruntñ pro antiquiori
bus testandū illud est, in paucis quae tradita ab
eis fuerūt, ꝗd exactū erat, eos tradidisse. Iunio
ribus aūt nequaꝗ assentiendū, ex quoꝝ nūero
Tyleus Bassus est, Niceratus, Petronius, Nigér
ꝗ & Diodotus, Asclepiadae omnes, qui cōmu-
nē notaꝗ omnibus, & in uitae humanae usu quo
tidianā materiū exacta descriptione dignā exi
stimātes, medicas remedioꝝ uires, & probatio
nes in decursu tradiderūt: nō experiētia reꝝ ui
res, probationes & efficaciā metiētes, sed uano
de causis sermone, usꝗ ad cōtentionis tumorē
ubiꝗ; rē extollētes, & alia pro aliꞇs aliꝗ descri
bētes: Siquidē qui inter eos excellere Niger ui
def, euphorbiū ait oleastelli herbaꝫ in Italia na
scētis, liquorē: & androsemon eandē hyperico
esse: & aloēm in Iudea fossilē nasci. Pluraꝗ alia
his similia, lōge à ueritate falsoꝫ exposuit: quae
omnia eius hominis indicia sunt, qui nō prae-
senti inspectiōe & oculatus iudex, sed ex histo
ria alioruꝗ traditiōibus ea docuerit. Peccaue
rūt praeterea & in ordine, coniungētes aliꞇ quae
disconuenirēt: aliꞇ ex literaꝫ ordine deinceps
describētes, generaꝗ & potestates eoꝝ à cōge
neribus suis nō ob aliā sanè causam disiungen
tes, quàm ut facilius eoꝝ meminissēt. Nos aūt
à prima ferè iuuētute indefesso quodā cogno-
a   scendae

Figure 30 Pedanius Dioscorides. Text page from: *De medica materia ... Interprete Marcello Virgilio (1529).*

114

As with many of the figures of antiquity, the details of his life are obscure. Born in Anazarba in Cilicia he tramped much of the then civilized world as a Greek army surgeon in the service of Nero (AD 37–68). He used these opportunities to become the first to write at length on the medical applications of botany. He described some 600 plants or plant principles, about 100 more than Theophrastus. Of all of these many plants, 90 or so remained in use at the outbreak of World War I.

Some have commented unfavourably on the scientific content of *De materia medica* but it seems evident that Dioscorides set out to facilitate the use of plants in therapeutics, and describe the practices of his day, rather than attempt the work of the systematic botanist. His uncritical record of the uses of plants represents the record of their apparent success – it is not a formal attempt to evaluate their specific activities. Even today, when the means of making such evaluations are far better understood, the clinical pharmacological testing of pure herbal remedies has advanced only a little way beyond Dioscorides.

Dioscorides wrote in Greek and had some recognition of the nature of families of plants long before the first meaningful classifications of Linnaeus. In *De materia medica* he describes the various names of each drug and its sources; the means of its identification and of showing that it has not been adulterated; the method of its preparation for administration, and its actions and uses.

De materia medica was first printed in Greek by Aldus Manutius in 1499; the first translation in Latin was published in 1478. After the incunabula, there were a number of versions and commentaries but no early translation in English. Of the early editions, Figure 29 shows the title page of the 1529 translation by Marcello Virgilio[310]; Figure 30 illustrates the way in which the Greek and Latin texts are given in parallel in this lovely edition. Figures 12 and 13, the Mandragora 'male' and 'female' respectively, come from the slightly later 1583 version forming part II of the commentary by Petri Andreae Matthioli Senensis[311].

Earlier than any of these printed editions is the glorious Juliana Anicia manuscript, parts of which are thought to have been copied from originals of the first century BC. This work is one of the earliest datable Greek codices in existence and was written in capitals to form the wedding gift of Juliana Anicia, daughter of Anicius Olybrius, Emperor of the West in 472. Juliana eventually married, probably in 487, Aerobindus, a high-ranking officer in the service of the Byzantine Emperor Anastasius. The manuscript is thought to have been given her on this occasion.

This great manuscript (Med. Graec. I) – earlier in the Royal Library at Vienna – was published in facsimile, as *Dioscurides, Codex Aniciae Julianae picturis illustratus, nunc Vindobonensis Med. Gr. I*, by A. W. Sijthoff in 1906[312]. Figure 31 represents the title page and Figure 32 an illustrated text page from the copy of this huge two volume work in the care of the Librarian of the Royal Society of Medicine, London.

The first English writer fully to realize the significance of *De materia medica* was John Goodyer, the botanist of Petersfield, Sussex. Goodyer understood the importance of this first-century compilation of medical and botanical knowledge and, between 1652 and 1655, laboriously transcribed the entire Greek text with an interlinear English translation on over 4500 quarto pages. Perhaps because he failed to find a patron, Goodyer's manuscript was never printed and,

DIOSCURIDES

Codex Aniciae Iulianae picturis illustratus, nunc Vindobonensis Med. Gr. I

phototypice editus

Moderante Iosepho de Karabacek

Bibliothecae Palatinae Vindobonensis Praefecto

praefati sunt Antonius de Premerstein, Carolus Wessely, Iosephus Mantuani

Accedit tabula lithographica

PARS ALTERA

qua codicis folia 204 – 491 continentur

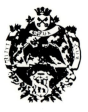

LUGDUNI BATAVORUM

A. W. SIJTHOFF

1906

' NT SEQUITUR

Figure 31 Pedanius Dioscorides. Title page from: *Dioscurides Codex Aniciae Julianae . . . moderante Josepho de Karabacek* (1906). [*Royal Society of Medicine library, London.*]

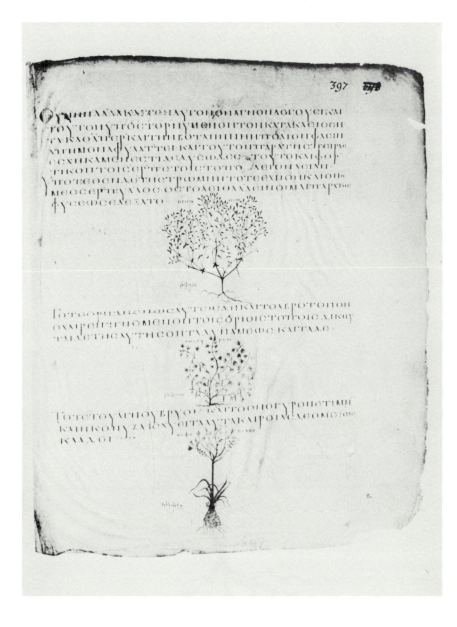

Figure 32 Pedanius Dioscorides. Text page from: *Dioscurides Codex Aniciae Julianae... moderante Josepho de Karabacek* (1906).

by 1664, was deposited, with the rest of his outstanding botanical library, in Magdalen College. From there it was published at Oxford by Robert T. Gunther, the edition – the first to give Dioscorides to Englishmen – appearing in 1934 and being illustrated from the work prepared for Juliana Anicia. This book, still widely available, is entitled *The Greek Herbal of Dioscorides, Illustrated by a Byzantine A.D. 512, Englished by John Goodyer A.D. 1655, Edited and First Printed A.D. 1933 by Robert T. Gunther*[313]. From this volume Figure 33 represents the illustration of the Horehound (*Marrubium vulgare* of the Labiatae). This plant, widely known as the White Horehound, is found all over Europe and is indigenous to Britain. It is made into Horehound Ale which is drunk in Norfolk and other country districts and has always been esteemed for its medicinal qualities. Egyptian priests are said to have called it the 'Seed of Horus' and it has been frequently used for coughs and colds and is still used, by herbalists, as an expectorant and for the relief of asthma when productive cough is a problem. Of this popular herb, John Goodyer, in his seventeenth century English, says it is[314]:

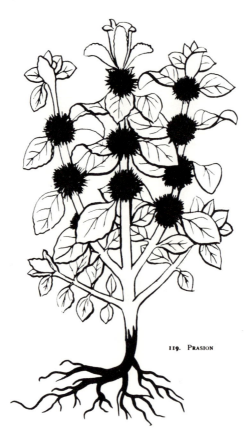

119. PRASION

Figure 33   Marrubium vulgare (The Horehound). [*From: Robert T. Gunther. The Greek herbal of Dioscorides . . . London, Oxford Univ. Press (1934).*]

a shrub of many branches from one root, somewhat rough, white, 4-cornered in ye rodds, but ye leaf is equal to ye great finger, somewhat round, thick, wrinkled, bitter to ye taste. But ye seed on ye stalks by distances, & ye flowers as ye vertebra of ye backbone, sharp. It grows in places near to houses, & rubbish of buildings. The dry leaves of this, with ye seed being sodden with water, or juiced when green is given with honey to ye phthisicall asthmaticall, & to such as cough, & if dry Iris be mixed with it it brings up thick stuff out of ye Thorax.

We have previously noticed *Artemisia absinthium* (page 107), the source of wormwood, wormseed, and absinth – and a remedy advocated by Celsus for infestation with roundworms. Gunther's *Greek Herbal* . . . provides an illustration (Figure 34) of the related *Artemisia campestris* or *Artemisia vulgaris* and John Goodyer gives this description of its characteristics and habitat [315]:

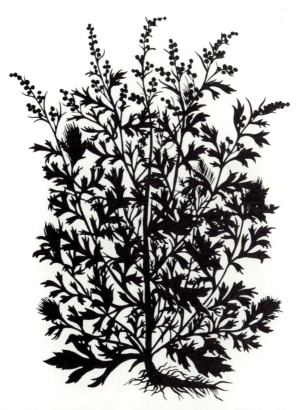

Figure 34 Artemisia (probably *A. vulgaris,* St. John's Plant). [*From: Robert T. Gunther. The Greek herbal of Dioscorides . . . London, Oxford Univ. Press (1934).*]

it grows for ye most part in places near ye Sea, a shrub-like herb, like unto wormwood but greater & hauing ye leaves grosser. There is one sort of it prosperous, having broader leaves and rods, another lesser, ye flowers little thin white, of a strong smell, it flowers in ye summer. But some do call ye slender-branched little herb in ye Mediterranean parts, single in ye stalk, extremely small, abounding with flowers, of a tawnie yellow by colour, Artemisia Monoclonos. But ye scent of this is sweeter than of that. They both do warm & extenuate.

Artemisia abrotanum (Compositae) is Southernwood, the southern or foreign Wormwood, a native of the south of Europe; it is a common garden plant in England for it was introduced into this country in 1548; it seldom flowers in our northern climate but its finely-divided, greyish-green leaves are familiar and it is called Old Man or Lad's Love. Its traditional uses are like those of Wormwood and it is employed as an emmenagogue and anthelmintic.

It is frequently difficult to be sure that the plants described by the classical writers are correctly identified in terms of modern botanical species, and this is so with the Byzantine drawing given in Figure 34. Of the possibilities, *Artemisia campestris* is the Field Southernwood, common in much of Europe but rare in Britain. *Artemisia vulgaris* is the Mugwort or St. John's Plant which grows in the hedgerows and waysides of many parts of England. It is closely allied to the Common Wormwood but lacks the essential oil of the latter. It was used to flavour beer (hence, possibly, the name 'Mugwort') before hops were introduced for this purpose; old superstitions also connect it with the name of John the

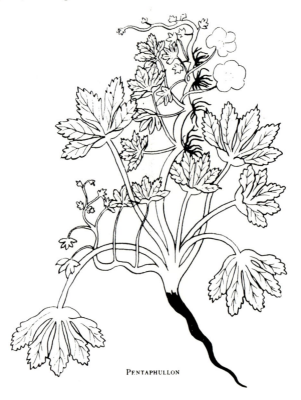

PENTAPHULLON

Figure 35   Potentilla reptans (The Cinquefoil). [*From: Robert T. Gunther. The Greek herbal of Dioscorides . . . London, Oxford Univ. Press (1934).*]

Baptist. Its traditional use is as an emmenagogue, for which purpose it is often given with Pennyroyal and Southernwood. Its constituents include a volatile oil, an acrid resin, and tannin.

Tannin has found medicinal uses since long before Dioscorides and the Cinquefoil, *Potentilla reptans*, from *The Greek Herbal...*, forms Figure 35. The Romans called this Quinquefolium and John Goodyer describes it in his enjoyable prose in the following way[316]:

> It hath leaves like unto mint, five upon every stem but rarely any where more, cut in round about like a saw: ye flower pale-white, yellowish like gold. It grows in moist places & by rivers, but it hath a reddish root somewhat long, thicker than black Ellebore, but it is of much use.

Martindale[317] notes that the related *Potentilla erecta* (Rosaceae), which is the Common Tormentil or Erect Cinquefoil, is the source of the pharmaceutical product Tormentil Rhizome. This is the dried rhizome of the Erect Cinquefoil and contains not less than 15% of tannin. It has been used both internally and on the skin and mucous membranes as an astringent, usually as a tincture.

Dioscorides describes plant after plant that achieved great medicinal importance and he seems faithfully to record the therapeutic practice of his time. From his work stems much of the medical botany and drug treatment of the intervening centuries. Thus, *De materia medica*, with its splendid editions which vie with one another for their level of interest and rich associations, forms one of the monuments of the history of medicine. Its content of observational science uncritically mixed with folklore and tradition emphasizes the state of the medical art of the time. In the form of the Robert Gunther edition, *The Greek Herbal...*, it puts the pharmacopoeia of the first century into the modern practitioner's hand.

Clinicians who followed Dioscorides included Aretaeus the Cappadocian (AD 81–c. 138), who has often been considered second only to Hippocrates in his ability to present fine descriptions of disease. The first edition of Aretaeus was a Latin translation printed in Venice in 1552; the first Greek printed edition appeared in Paris 2 years later. Aretaeus was a follower of the 'Pneumatic School' of Greek medicine and his interesting accounts of clinical illness, and its treatment with the therapeutic means of the day, can be found in *The Extant Works of Aretaeus, the Cappadocian*. This excellent version, which includes the Greek text, was edited and translated by Francis Adams for the Sydenham Society and published in London in 1856[318].

Rufus of Ephesus (c. AD 98–117) was born shortly after Aretaeus and was known to all mediaeval physicians. He enjoyed a long reputation as a surgeon and left the first formal work on human anatomy. He is said to have dissected apes and other animals and is of some importance in comparative anatomy and in understanding how this subject could advance surgery. He described the decussation of the optic nerves and the capsule of the crystalline lens and gave the first clear account that has survived of the structure of the eye. In medicine he is remembered as having given the first good account of bubonic plague and as having written on gout. He is particularly renowned for his work on haemostasis and for his descriptions of the methods of arresting haemorrhage.

Only 12 of his 36 known works survive. His first Greek edition was printed in 1554 and there is the slim, attractive volume of bilingual title (*Ruffi Ephesii, De vesicae renumque morbis. De purgantibus medicamentis. De partibus corporis humani . . .*) which was published in Paris in 1554[319]. There is also a Greek–Latin bilingual text of 1726 (Gulielmus Clinch)[320] and the first French edition, with both Greek and Latin texts, was published in Paris in 1879[321].

Soranus of Ephesus (AD *c.* 117–138), the third of this group of medical figures who flourished in the period between Dioscorides and Galen, remains famous for having left a work on gynaecology, obstetrics, and the diseases of infants, which remained important until the Middle Ages. The work was illustrated with diagrams which were not utterly unrealistic and which were copied into manuscripts of the ninth century. Soranus corrected the Hippocratic misconception that a male embryo originated in the right and a female in the left half of the uterus – a fallacy which Singer[322] points out was 'derived originally from Empedocles and Parmenides, but perpetuated by Latin translations of the Hippocratic treatises until the seventeenth century.' Soranus is of special interest to the modern physician as having been one of the first to give a clear discussion of the subject of contraception and the means employed in Roman times.

His Greek text shows Soranus to have been not only knowledgeable and critical but also singularly attached to a straightforward presentation of his material. His work reads as if he is lecturing for lay as well as professional audiences. His attitudes, presumably widely acceptable at the time, include clear statements against superstition. Discussing the qualities of a good midwife he says 'She will have a quiet disposition, for she will have to share many secrets of life. She must not be greedy for money, lest she give an abortive wickedly for payment; she will be free from superstition so as not to overlook salutary measures on account of a dream or omen or some customary rite . . .'[323] Later in his treatise he specifically says that a wet-nurse should neither be superstitious nor prone to ecstatic states[324].

Ethics in Rome had changed since the days of Hippocrates and Soranus refers to the problem of determining if a child is worth rearing in a way that suggests that weaklings might not always have been succoured. He also comes out quite clearly with recommendations for abortificants, for use when necessary, but describes contraceptives which can be used to prevent this. In the very helpful *Soranus' gynecology* translated and introduced by Owsei Temkin and published in 1956, his list of useful contraceptives is the following[325]:

Pine bark, tanning sumach, equal quantities of each, rub with wine and apply in due measure before coitus after wool has been wrapped around; and after two or three hours she may remove it and have intercourse.
Another: Of Cimolian earth, root of panax, equal quantities, rub with water separately and together, and when sticky apply in like manner.
Or: Grind the inside of fresh pomegranate peel with water, and apply.
Or: Grind two parts of pomegranate peel and one part of oak galls, form small suppositories and insert after the cessation of menstruation.
Or: Moist alum, the inside of pomegranate rind, mix with water, and apply with wool.
Or: Of unripe oak galls, of the inside of pomegranate peel, of ginger, of each 2 drachms, mould it with wine to the size of vetch peas and dry indoors

and give before coitus, to be applied as a vaginal suppository.

Or: Grind the flesh of dried figs and apply together with natron.

Or: Apply pomegranate peel with an equal amount of gum and an equal amount of oil of roses.

Then one should always follow with a drink of honey water. But one should beware of things which are very pungent, because of the ulcerations arising from them. And we use all these things after the end of menstruation.

Soranus is known to have written almost 20 works on various aspects of medicine. The *Gynaecology* is the most important of those preserved in their original Greek but short treatises *On Bandages, On Fractures*, and a *Life of Hippocrates*, are ascribed to him. One of his most interesting writings, *On Acute and Chronic Diseases*, has come down to us in the Latin paraphrase, usually regarded as being almost a translation, of the fifth or sixth century Caelius Aurelianus. Soranus was the most outstanding of protagonists of the 'Methodist School', as is shown in the title of the paraphrase just mentioned: *Caelii Aureliani, Siccensis, Medici Vetusti, Secta Methodici, De Morbis Acutis & Chronicis, Libri VIII...*, the Opera of 1722[326]. The Latin and Greek text of the work on surgical subjects, such as fractures, comprises the *Graecorum Chirurgici libri Sorani...*, published in 1754[327] and including both Soranus and Oribasius; Soranus also appears in Volume 1 of the *Physici et Medici Graeci Minores* edited by I. L. Ideler and published in 1841[328].

The fame of Soranus as an obstetrician lasted until the seventeenth century and is still remembered. St. Augustine is said to have called him 'medicinae auctor nobilissimus'[329] – he seems also to have been distinguished by both breadth of learning and pragmatism.

A treatise on medicine, written about AD 150, and which throws some added light on the period of Greek medicine in Rome in the years just before the ascendancy of Galen, is the rather remarkable *Anonymus Londinensis*, now the British Museum Papyrus 137. This was found and its importance recognized in 1891 and was deciphered by Sir Frederick Kenyon. A Greek text was published in 1893 and a German translation 3 years later. The work contains extracts from a lost collection recording the opinions of many of the early Greek physicians already mentioned. The interesting book, *The Medical Writings of Anonymus Londinensis*, by W. H. S. Jones[330], presents the Greek and English text and, in its excellent commentary, provides an insight to the 'Nature of Greek Thought' and 'The Nature of Greek Medicine'.

Galen

There remains what Singer[331] has called 'the huge overshadowing figure of Galen'. Second only to Hippocrates in importance in classical Greek medicine, Galen dominated all branches of medicine until the time of Vesalius. He was the most voluminous of the ancient medical writers and is esteemed as the virtual founder of experimental physiology.

The vast literary output of Claudius Galenus (AD 131–201) seems almost to arise from the circumstances of his life and personality. He was born at Pergamos in Asia Minor in the year AD 131 and his father, Nicon, was a well-established architect in that ancient city. Galen is said to have recorded that, unlike his amiable and benevolent father, his mother was evil-tempered and quarrelsome to the point at which she used to bite her serving-maids.

Pergamos contained not only a fine Asclepieum but also a library second only to that of Alexandria itself. In the city Galen studied Platonic, Aristotelian, Stoic and Epicurean philosophy and then, at 17, began his studies of medicine. He continued his excellent education in the great centres at Smyrna and Alexandria.

On returning to his own city he was made surgeon to the gladiators before, when he was about 31, his ambitions took him to Rome. There, within a few years spent as a demonstrator of anatomy and practitioner of medicine, he achieved so considerable a reputation that his patients came to include even the Emperor Marcus Aurelius (AD 121–180) himself. This fact has something to say of the character of Galen for Marcus Aurelius, not only emperor but also Stoic philosopher, had ameliorated the conditions of the slaves, reformed the civil laws and, although corruption was almost universal, shown himself in his *Meditations*[332] to have been self-denying, just and unaffected even by the exercise of supreme power.

Medical practice in Rome was, at this time, at as low an ebb as the morals and way of life of the community and Galen soon showed his contempt for his fellow practitioners. In AD 168, faced with frank and threatening hostility from his medical colleagues, he fled from Rome and returned to his native city of Pergamos. There he wrote at great length until, within a year, he was summoned back to Rome by imperial mandate.

Marcus Aurelius, about to undertake an expedition against the German tribes threatening the northern frontiers of the Empire, wanted Galen to travel with him. From this responsibility Galen managed, in some way, to extricate himself and remain in Italy. Having been born in one of the cities forming the seven churches of Asia listed[333] and lambasted[334] by St. John, he seems, from about the time of the expedition to Germany, to have withdrawn to study, teach and travel – and, above all, to enter upon a period of vast literary activity. He experimented, dissected animals, theorized and compounded all these activities into a life of great purpose and energy. It is probable that he died about the end of the century, but we know little of the circumstances of the closing years of Galen's personal history.

The Codices are No. 2267 of the Bibliothèque Nationale, Paris and No. 275 in the Library of St. Mark, Venice and there have been a considerable number of editions, translations and commentaries. There was a Latin translation by Linacre published in London in 1523 and this work played a notable part in the English Renaissance. The first printed edition of Galen's *Opera omnia* was the five volume Greek text of Andreas Asulanus and J. B. Opizo published in Venice in 1525[335]. Subsequent *Opera omnia* include the great 20 volume text of C. G. Kühn (Leipzig, 1821–33)[336] and the four volume work of B. G. Teubner (Leipzig, 1914–22)[337]; the former of these works provides the Greek and Latin text, the latter the Greek text only. Of all these great works there is one small volume, *Galen, On the Natural Faculties*[338], which epitomizes the whole of this writer's enormous output; this volume, which gives the Greek text of this particular book and an English translation by Arthur John Brock, was published by Heinemann and G. P. Putnam's Sons as part of the Loeb Classical Library in 1916. In his

Introduction to this valuable book Brock remarks that, 'If Galen be looked on as a crystallisation of Greek medicine, then this book may be looked on as a crystallisation of Galen.'[339] It is from the English translation of this bilingual edition that the quotations that follow are taken.

It must be observed that Galen's hectoring manner of delivery, his insensitivity to animal suffering, his theorizing, and the fact that he is, above all things, a profound teleologist, provide ceaseless difficulties for the modern reader. It was not always so, for some of these qualities seem to have been those that most helped the writings of Galen to dominate the centuries until Vesalius gathered courage enough to write of his doubts on Galen's idea that blood passed through the intraventricular septum of the heart, and Harvey dispelled Galen's physiology of the circulatory system with his own discoveries which, in the seventeenth century, revolutionized the subject.

Galen's teleology is of the kind which sees each structure that exists in the body, and each of its functions, as displaying the intent and design of an intelligent being. The concept that everything that lives and breathes represents the direct result of the Creator's plan and purpose fitted so well with the theological beliefs of the Middle Ages, whether these were Jewish, Moslem, or Christian, that Galen's widespread influence was assured. Its ultimate effect was, however, destructive: the teachings of Galen became themselves sacrosanct and served to inhibit the very kind of fresh approach and experimentalism which Galen had undertaken.

Galen's theorizing led him to convince himself that structures existed when his eyes had not seen them, but when their existence would explain what he very well knew. His description of the physiology of the circulatory system provides the most obvious example. His account of the nutrition of the tissues (as we would now call them) of the body is remarkable: 'Numerous conduits distributed through the various limbs bring them pure blood, much like the garden water-supply, and, further, the intervals between these conduits have been wonderfully arranged by Nature from the outset so that the intervening parts should be plentifully provided for when absorbing blood, and that they should never be deluged by a quantity of superfluous fluid running in at unsuitable times.'[340] He showed by experiment that the arteries contain blood and not air and studied the movements of the heart, the action of the valves, and the pulsatile forces of the great vessels; he came within a stone's throw of understanding the circulation – by conceiving the function or presence of the capillary network – when he wrote: 'If you will kill an animal by cutting through a number of its large arteries, you will find the veins becoming empty along with the arteries: now, this could never occur if there were not anastomoses between them.'[341] Then he throws it away by convincing himself of something that is not there but which would have explained so much else if it had been[342]:

> Similarly, also, in the heart itself, the thinnest portion of the blood is drawn from the right ventricle into the left, owing to there being perforations in the septum between them: these can be seen for a great part [of their length]; they are like a kind of fossae [pits] with wide mouths, and they get constantly narrower; it is not possible, however, actually to observe their extreme terminations, owing both to the smallness of these and to the fact that when the

animal is dead all the parts are chilled and shrunken. Here, too, however, our argument, starting from the principle that nothing is done by Nature in vain, discovers these anastomoses between the ventricles of the heart; for it could not be at random and by chance that there occurred fossae ending thus in narrow terminations.

Galen's physiology of the circulatory system imagined an ebb-and-flow movement of the blood arising from and falling back to the liver. Much of the subsequent history of the medicine and therapeutics of circulatory disease is bound up with this concept and those related to it. The whole scheme is beautifully shown in the diagram, from Charles Singer's *Greek Biology and Greek Medicine*[343], which forms Figure 36.

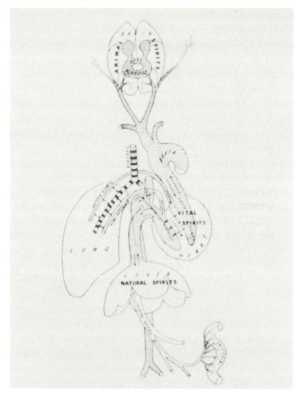

Figure 36 Galen's physiology. [*From: Charles Joseph Singer. Greek biology and Greek medicine. Oxford, Clarendon Press (1922).*]

According to Galen's final picture of the physiology the basic principle of life is a pneuma (an anima or spirit) which is drawn into the body from the overall world-soul during respiration. From the lungs the pneuma passed to the left ventricle. A further pneuma reached the left ventricle and this was the natural spirits arising from the liver (the source of innate heat to Galen) and passed, in part, through the intraventricular pores which Galen had discovered teleologically. In the left ventricle the natural spirits derived from the liver and the external pneuma arising from the lungs were elaborated to a higher form of spirit, the vital spirits, which were distributed with the blood by the arterial system, so reaching the various parts of the body. In the arteries the blood, coming from the heart, ebbed and flowed and could be felt to pulsate as it did so. In the brain the vital spirits were elaborated to an even higher kind of pneuma, the animal spirits, which were distributed to the peripheral parts of the body by the nerves which were thought to be hollow. This idea involved the discovery of structures which, in the human, do not exist, in both the brain and liver. It is a remarkable commentary on the fact that human dissection, long allowed in Alexandria, was no longer available to Galen. The net effect was that the essence of Galenic physiology – that the liver was the source of the veins and the heart of the arteries – became Galen's unfortunate bequest to the centuries.

Something of Galen's tone can be seen in the passage in which he speaks of those 'who had allowed themselves to be shown the ureters coming from the kidneys and becoming implanted in the bladder . . .' and who 'had the audacity to say that these also existed for no purpose.'[344] Both his experimental approach and his unfeelingness in vivisection are shown in his account of the means of refuting such people[345]:

> We were, therefore, further compelled to show them in a still living animal, the urine plainly running out through the ureters into the bladder; even thus we hardly hoped to check their nonsensical talk.
> Now the method of demonstration is as follows. One has to divide the peritoneum in front of the ureters, then secure these with ligatures, and next, having bandaged up the animal, let him go (for he will not continue to urinate). After this one loosens the external bandages and shows the bladder empty and the ureters quite full and distended – in fact almost on the point of rupturing; on removing the ligature from them, one then plainly sees the bladder becoming filled with urine.
> When this has been made quite clear, then, before the animal urinates, one has to tie a ligature round his penis and then to squeeze the bladder all over; still nothing goes back through the ureters to the kidneys. Here, then, it becomes obvious that not only in a dead animal, but one which is still living, the ureters are prevented from receiving back the urine from the bladder. These observations having been made, one now loosens the ligature from the animal's penis and allows him to urinate, then again ligatures one of the ureters and leaves the other to discharge into the bladder. Allowing, then, some time to elapse, one now demonstrates that the ureter which was ligatured is obviously full and distended on the side next to the kidneys, while the other one – that from which the ligature had been taken – is itself flaccid, but has filled the bladder with urine. Then, again, one must divide the full ureter, and demonstrate how the urine spurts out of it, like blood in the operation of venesection; and after this one cuts through the other also, and both being thus divided, one bandages up the animal externally. Then when enough time seems to have elapsed, one takes off the bandages; the bladder will now be found empty, and the whole region between the intestines and the peritoneum full of urine, as if the animal were suffering from dropsy.

Galen describes other vivisections and yet, even if their cruelties have to be ascribed to the manners of the times, he does establish himself as a logical and diligent experimentalist. In his clinical practice he regarded himself as a follower of Hippocrates, whom he more than once called 'most divine Hippocrates'[346], and whom he revered for his practice of observation as a means of providing a truthful and reasonable source of learning. Galen had at his disposal not only the medicine of Hippocrates, of more than 500 years earlier, but also the biological knowledge and wisdom of Aristotle, and the discoveries in anatomy made in Alexandria; to these resources he added a considerable series of researches and discoveries of his own.

The knowledge inherited by Galen was not all, and in all departments, helpful. He based his pathology, and much of the non-experimental parts of his physiology, on a combined doctrine of the bodily humours and Pythagorean number lore; within this system he introduced the doctrine of the four temperaments and a number of non-factual explanations of bodily functions which were not then understood.

In pharmacy Galen developed the practice of using herbs in complex mixtures which became known as 'galenicals'. They remained part of medical practice until the advent of specific agents which could be used as single drugs swept them away. Clifford Allbutt, in his *Greek Medicine in Rome*[243], talking of the traditional pharmacy that led up to Galen's day, wrote: 'Egypt never even turned towards experiment or scientific development . . . On the contrary, the burden of a copious but ill-assorted and altogether empirical and traditional pharmacy, treasuring prescriptions even a thousand years old, must have lain heavily upon the Greeks of Alexandria, and in after times contributed to the long oppression of Galenism.'[347] Allbutt also notes, writing of this same period, that 'About the middle of the second century the materia medica, and the shops of the public pharmacists, were subjected . . . to official inspection; first, for the Imperial household and Court, and so afterwards for the public.'[348] If this is right then the beginnings of drug regulatory control must be dated from the lifetime of Galen. Despite his polypharmacy, Galen's *De simplicibus*[349], written about AD 180, was the only Greek herbal in any way comparable to that of Dioscorides and it was later extensively copied.

The heights of Galen's achievement included his making the vital discoveries that the heart outside the body pumped for a time – showing that it not only acted as a pump but did so of its own rhythm; equally vitally, he demonstrated that the arteries contained blood. He gave the first adequate account of the mechanism of respiration and provided a set of writings which enshrined the whole of the real knowledge of the circulatory, respiratory, and nervous systems which his successors were to possess until the Renaissance was established.

The life of Galen seems to have consisted of ceaseless travels, the making of many discoveries, and the generation of a vast volume of writings, many of them of value. That his dogmatic, teleological spirit imprisoned many later generations was partly due to those generations being preoccupied with theology and to the desertion of the natural sources of Galen's own discoveries. The life of Galen coincided with the greatest period of the Roman Empire. After his time the Empire gradually fell away, and slowly the Dark Ages of Europe began.

In medicine the change was far more sudden: with the death of Galen, about AD 200, all anatomical and physiological experiment ceased. Men still suffered from illnesses and sought relief but they attempted nothing which could have used the methods of science or advanced the broad principles of knowledge. In the Western World, after the death of Galen, the science of medicine ceased to have a history and there followed 1000 years of oblivion.

Discussion

The beginnings of Greek medicine lay firstly in the folk medicine of the people, a medicine which transmitted part of the inheritance of Egypt and Mesopotamia; secondly, in temple medicine and the worship of Asklepios, the god of healing; and thirdly in Hippocratic medicine, the foundation upon which the whole edifice of modern medicine has been raised.

The very beginnings of scientific medicine must be placed in the sixth century BC. By the fifth century, during the Golden Age of Pericles, medicine almost free of superstition had become firmly established. Medical art of this rational, logical kind reached its acme in antiquity in the life of Hippocrates. We have little knowledge of the means whereby the fifth and sixth century Greeks effected the transformation which took their interest from the supernaturalism and superstition of the earlier civilizations to the enquiries which marked their growth as a people. This growth was so notable that Charles-Edward Winslow, in his study *The Conquest of Epidemic Disease . . .* , wrote: 'The Hebrews gave us a universe of moral law; but the Greeks clearly visualized for the first time in human history a universe of natural law.'[350] The means whereby the old demonic past was shaken off and Greek naturalism begun, forms one of the great puzzles of history. That the mummified dead of Egypt, in their afterlife, and the demons of Babylon, as they infested the living, found no place of abode in Minoan Crete or the islands of Greece is no surprise. But why it should be so, is without explanation.

The 42 clinical cases described by Hippocrates and his treatises *On Fractures, On Joints* and *On Wounds in the Head* are perhaps the most remarkable of all of the early Greek documents. The clinical records were the only thing of their kind for virtually 1700 years; the surgical writings were equally modern in spirit, critical, and practical to the level at which some of the techniques are usable. So fully does the thinking of Hippocrates discard the ancient superstitions that he was able to write, of epilepsy, the 'Sacred Disease', 'this disease seems to me to be nowise more divine than others; but it has its nature such as other diseases have, and a cause whence it originates, and its nature and cause are divine only just as much as all others are . . . '[197] Few of the schools of medicine that were to arise in the centuries following Hippocrates equalled the realism of the 'Father of Medicine' – and none bettered the achievement by which this directness was linked with the most sensitive principles of ethics.

Despite its points of excellence, Greek medicine was, throughout its history, unable to recognize its false beliefs – such as the doctrine of the four humours. Had it not have been for the dogmatism of Galen this system, rooted probably in Chaldean number lore, would have been less durable; as it was, the doctrine, though false, was far less damaging than dogmatically-repeated errors of observation, like Galen's channels by which part of the circulating blood volume was supposed to pass through the intraventricular septum. This latter idea inhibited the discovery of the blood circulation and even inhibited Vesalius who, though he could find no evidence for these mysterious channels could not bring himself resolutely to dismiss them. No scientist can explore new ground except by means of some sort of hypothesis: it is one thing to have an erroneous hypothesis, which time and experiment will put right; it is another to transmit errors of fact or develop hypotheses incapable of experiment or verification. Time dealt as might be hoped with the magic of the number 4, its mystical significance, and the four humours – and retained Hippocrates, his observational method, reliance on natural explanations, and his ethics.

Of the circumstances which affected the growth of medicine more than might be expected, malaria and the geographical security of Southern Italy are two of the more influential.

Many of the clinical cases described by Hippocrates seem clearly to be malaria or, as with the accounts given by Celsus and other Greek and Roman writers, the cerebral or haemolytic complications of malaria. The fever, anaemia, enlargement of the spleen, and other features of chronic forms of this infestation are conspicuous in the writings of the time. The seemingly increasing effect of the malaria parasite, as it was carried from man to man, has been explored by W. H. S. Jones in his book, *Malaria and Greek History*, of 1909; this book contains an essay on *The History of Greek Therapeutics and the Malaria Theory* by E. T. Withington[351]. The essay, along with many other writings, emphasizes the damaging part which malaria played on the later history of Rome.

The other great factor was the geography of Southern Italy. Discussing this subject, Clifford Allbutt wrote that this region 'was not Italian even in name, but in name was Magna Graecia, and in character Greek; and this character, until blighted by malaria, it maintained.'[243] It is of the greatest importance to the growth and transition of medical culture that from the sixth century before Christ to the tenth century AD Southern Italy was in language and character Greek – and from Magna Graecia there flowed a steady stream of cultural influence which later helped to found the school of Salerno.

Some of the Greek schools of medicine of classical times considered drugs important in therapeutics. Others thought them unimportant but it is at this point in history that we meet with some of the early records of effective drugs used for what would still be considered appropriate indications. Examples include the male fern used for the treatment of tapeworm infestation and opium used to promote sleep and relieve severe pain.

Most of these drugs were, of course, botanical and, in his different works, Hippocrates mentions something like 236 plants; the *De historia plantarum* of Theophrastus described about 455 plants and plant principles and summarizes all that was known at the time of the medicinal properties of each. About 300 years later, Celsus, in *De medicina*, gave an extensive account of the Greek pharmacopoeia in use in Rome and, roughly in the middle of the first century AD, Dioscorides, in *De materia medica*, not only described some 600 plants and plant principles but also provided a herbal which formed the basis of the materia medica until modern times.

The use of male fern extract to eradicate tapeworm[235] was clearly described by Theophrastus (p. 95), the gifted pupil of Aristotle. In one of the most important of the records of ancient Rome the production of real opium was first clearly described by Scribonius Largus, in *De compositionibus medicamentorum ...* [50], early in the first century AD. Thus the Romans used drugs we still use today. The writings of Celsus contain a list of the drugs and prescriptions in use in Rome at or about the time of Scribonius Largus (although they do not clearly mention opium). This fascinating pharmacopoeia of Celsus is brilliantly presented in the 'List of Medicamenta' with which W. G. Spencer begins the second volume of his text and translation of *De medicina*[241].

This List includes a number of items which, perhaps surprisingly, find a place in contemporary pharmaceutical products. Thus, it contains *Acacia Arabica*, the tannin-containing gum mucilage which was used as an astringent to arrest bleeding and agglutinate the exudate from wounds, and which appears in the BP 1980 as Acacia[352], the 'air-hardened gummy exudate flowing naturally or obtained by incision of the trunk and branches of *Acacia senegal* L. Willdenow and other species of *Acacia* of African origin.' We have powdered acacia in our Compound Tragacanth Powder.

Vinegar was used constantly by the Romans and valued as a styptic and for internal use; we still use it as a vehicle, as in Squill Vinegar BP[353]. The oxides and salts of copper were used, as caustics and exedents to cleanse wounds and promote granulations and healing. The aloes of the days of Celsus were used as aperients and, for the same purpose, remain in the current BP. Our pharmacopoeias speak of the residue obtained by evaporating the juice of the leaves of Barbados Aloes[354] or Cape Aloes[355] as providing laxatives and sources of hydroxyanthracene.

The metals in Spencer's List include several salts and earths of Aluminium and we still have Alum BP[356] (Aluminium Potassium Sulphate) as an astringent; we have also Aluminium Powder BP[357] as a topical protective, and the important Aluminium Glycinate[358], Dried Aluminium Hydroxide[359], and Dried Aluminium Phosphate[360] among the pharmacopoeial, much-used antacids. The BP 1980 preparations derived from Aluminium include Burow's Solution[361] (Aluminium Acetate Ear Drops), Compound Aluminium Paste[362], and the ubiquitous antacids – Aluminium Hydroxide Tablets[363], Aluminium Phosphate Tablets[364], Compound Magnesium Trisilicate Tablets[365], Aluminium Hydroxide Mixture[366] and Aluminium Phosphate Mixture[367].

Celsus used anise against flatulence and as a diuretic and we still have Aniseed (Anise)[368], the dried fruit of *Pimpinella anisum* L, Powdered Aniseed (as a carminative), Anise Oil[369] (obtained by distillation from the dried fruits of the star anise, *Illicium verum* Hook. f., or from the dried ripe fruits of *Pimpinella anisum* L.) and a preparation called Concentrated Anise Water[370] in the BP. Star anise, it might be noted, is a source of the rodent hepatocarcinogen, safrole, which in both the rat and mouse is metabolized to the far more potent carcinogen, 1´-hydroxysafrole (Borchert *et al.*, 1973)[371] – an example of a cancer-causing agent from plant sources. Another aromatic used by Celsus was dill and this, as Dill Oil BP[372], remains with us as a useful carminative obtained by distillation from the dried ripe fruits of *Anethum graveolens* L. It is, of course, widely used in medicines to relieve colic in babies.

Arsenic is, to us, a reagent for the laboratory but Celsus used the yellow trisulphide of arsenic, orpiment, and the golden disulphide of arsenic in prescriptions for cleaning wounds and ulcers; he does not mention the very toxic, arsenious oxide, white arsenic, which can be obtained by heating either of these substances and seems not to recognize them as poisons. He mentions zinc ores from Cyprus and these survive in our language because when they were heated in water (producing zinc carbonates and hydrosilicates) they adhered to the reed (*calamus*) with which they were stirred so that the name 'calamine' is still used for zinc lotions. Our Calamine BP[373] is a basic zinc carbonate lightly coloured with ferric oxide; we have many topical uses for zinc and the pharmacopoeial salts include Zinc Sulphate[374] (an astringent), Zinc Undecenoate[375] (an antifungal agent), and Zinc Chloride[376] and Zinc Oxide[377] (among the reagents). The preparations include Zinc Sulphate Lotion[378], Zinc Sulphate Eye Drops[379], Zinc Cream[380], Zinc and Coal Tar Paste[381], Zinc and Salicylic Acid Paste (Lassar's Paste)[382], Zinc and Castor Oil Ointment[383] and a number of everyday medical items of today, including Zinc Paste Bandage[384], Zinc Paste and Coal Tar Bandage[385] and the familiar Zinc Oxide Surgical Adhesive Tape[386]. The number of additional surgical dressings in the current pharmacopoeia shows the widespread usefulness of these zinc-based materials.

Celsus had calcium oxide, quick lime; and gypsum, sulphate of lime which, mixed with the carbonate of lime, produced Plaster of Paris, among his salts of calcium. He used ash produced by burning various substances, such as stag's horn, containing lime, to produce erodents and caustics but would not have known calcium as a mineral whose almost exact balance in the body is essential for life nor could he have suspected our multiplicity of pharmacopoeial calcium salts and derivatives – these include Calcium Carbonate[387], and the Chloride[388], Phosphate[389], Hydroxide[390], Lactate[391], Gluconate[392], Acetate[393], Hydrogen Phosphate[394], and Sodium Lactate[395] of Calcium, as well as the Dried Calcium Sulphate[396] (which is Plaster of Paris) in addition to tablets and other preparations based on these substances.

Cardamom appeared in the first century lists of drugs and was used internally as a diuretic and externally as a counter-irritant and erodent; it remains with us as Cardamom Fruit BP[397] (the dried, nearly ripe fruit of *Elettaria cardamomum* Maton var. *minuscula* Burkill) from which is obtained Cardamom Oil[398], the source of the Aromatic[399] and Compound Cardamom Tinctures[400] used as carminative and flavouring agents.

Spencer notes the mention of castor oil by Celsus who used it as an emollient but not as an aperient, although this was described by both Dioscorides and Galen; both uses – laxative and emollient – are given by the BP 1980 for Castor Oil[401], the fixed oil obtained by expression from the seeds of *Ricinus communis* L.

The 1980 BP mentions Saffron[402] in its Introduction, noting that it is the subject of a monograph in the European Pharmacopoeia but not in the British Pharmacopoeia; however, the EP standards are applicable in the United Kingdom. This does, perhaps, reflect the greater interest and more systematic study of herbal medicines in Germany and other European countries than in Britain. Saffron, a condiment and pigment, was of importance to the ancients and was obtained from the styles and stigmas of *Crocus sativus* – the low, ornamental plant with grass-like leaves and large lily-shaped flowers of the Iridaceae. It has been cultivated down the centuries for the sake of its yellow stigmas and was the *Karcom* of the Hebrews; it comes in the words of the Song of Solomon[403]: 'Thy plants are an orchard of pomegranates, with pleasant fruits; camphire, with spikenard, Spikenard and saffron; calamus and cinnamon, with all trees of frankincense; myrrh and aloes, with all the chief spices: A fountain of gardens, a well of living waters, and streams from Lebanon.'

Saffron was well known to the Greeks and Romans and was later introduced, as the Saffron Crocus, into cultivation in Spain by the Arabs who gave it its modern name *Zaffer*, or Saffron; the Greeks called it *Krokos* and the Romans *Karkom* and it is from these words that our own Crocus seems to arise. In ancient times the yellow dye of the flower was the perfection of beauty but the perfume of the water of saffron was prized as much as the colour; Celsus had a host of uses for it and it was esteemed in eye salves and used as a diuretic, emmenagogue and as an antidote.

From a quite different family, the Liliaceae, comes the Meadow Saffron, the Autumn Crocus, *Colchicum autumnale*, which grows wild in meadows especially on limestone and whose root, or corm, is the source of the poisonous alkaloid, colchicine[404], used in the treatment of gout. The flowers are light purple or white and like the crocus but for their six stamens. After the flowers form in the autumn the ovaries remain under the ground until spring when they are carried up on elongating peduncles and ripen. Colchicine retains a monograph in the BP, the preparation being Colchicine Tablets; the pure substance has uses in arresting the culture of chromosomes and the flower, growing in the Chelsea Physic Garden in London, forms Figure 37.

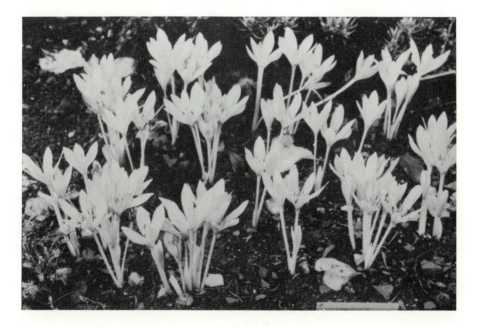

Figure 37   Colchicum autumnale (The Meadow Saffron) *at Chelsea Physic Garden, London.*

Celsus also mentions the Dittany of Crete. This is *Origanum Dictamnus* of the Labiatae family and it was famed by the people of classical times as a treatment for wounds. Spencer[405] says that it was named after Mount Dicte, in Crete, where it grew in abundance. Woodville says this of it and its oil[406]:

> The leaves of this plant are apparently very warm and aromatic; of an agreeable smell, and hot biting taste. They impart their virtues both to water and rectified spirit. Distilled with water, they give over a moderately strong impregnation to the aqueous fluid; from which, if the quantity of Dittany be large, there separates, ... a small portion of a yellowish essential oil, of a highly pungent aromatic taste and smell, and which congeals in the cold into the appearance of camphor.
>
> Both the Greek and Roman writers have fabled this plant into great celebrity; of which a single instance, related by the Latin Poet, affords a beautiful illustration.

Woodville's illustration of the plant forms Figure 38. His reference to the 'single instance, related by the Latin Poet' is to Virgil's *Aeneid*,[407] and the single prescription in which Celsus specifically mentions it is in his Book V: 'A draught for the expulsion of a dead foetus or placenta consists of ammoniac salt ... or of Cretan dittany ... in water.'[408]

Of what might seem the somewhat prosaic, oxides, silicates, and sulphates of iron, Celsus recorded the use of haematite (ferric oxide mixed with the silicates and sulphates of aluminium, and deriving its name from its colour which resembles dried blood), red ochre (the sulphates and sulphides of iron), yellow ochre (the mixed sulphates of iron with copper and lead), *Ferrugo* or *Robigo* (the rust of iron), *Squama ferri* (ferrous oxide, the scales chipped from red-hot iron rods) and a number of other iron-based substances used to stop bleeding, clean wounds, and – in the case of the yellow ochre from Attica – make new flesh grow. Only once does he mention the internal use of iron: having written that 'the spleen when affected swells, and with it simultaneously the left side; and this becomes hard and resists pressure. The abdomen is tense: there is even some swelling of the legs'[409], he goes on to describe the possible treatments and includes: 'water in which a blacksmith has from time to time dipped his red-hot irons; since this water especially reduces the spleen.'[410] This is interesting as it seems likely that the most common cause of a swollen spleen that the Romans would have seen was malaria and the swelling of the legs may have been its secondary anaemia. As Spencer[411] points out, treatment by *ferrugo*, the rust scale of iron, was mentioned by Pliny and fully described by Dioscorides. Of the medicinal uses of the rust of iron, Dioscorides, in John Goodyer's translation[412], says:

> But ye rust of iron doth bind, being put to doth stay ye womanish flux, & being drank it causeth inconception, but being anointed on with vinegar it heals Exanthemata & is of fit use for ye Paronychiae, & ye Pterygia, and scabrous eye-lids, & ye Condylomata, & it doth strengthen ye gums; & being anointed on doth help ye podagricall, & doth thicken ye Alopeciae. But iron made burning hot, quenched in water, or wine, & drank, is good for ye Coeliacall dysentericall, splenicall, cholericall & for a dissolved stomach.

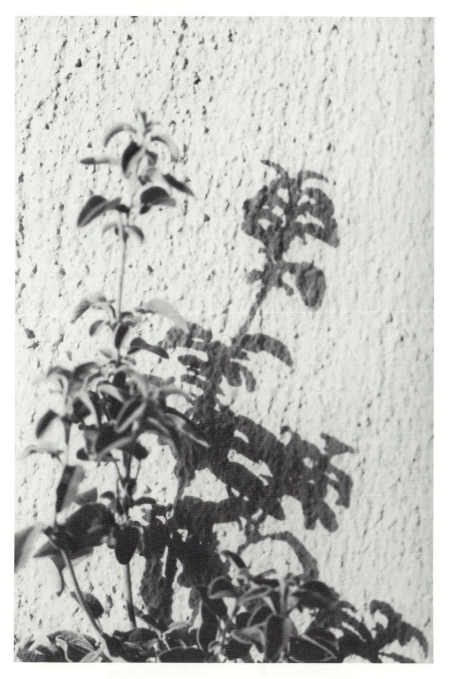

Figure 38 Origanum Dictamnus (The Dittany of Crete).

Our BP of today includes Ferrous Succinate[413], Sulphate[414], Gluconate[415], Fumerate[416] and Dried Ferrous Sulphate[417] as well as the colloidal Iron Sorbitol Injection[418] and Iron Dextran Injection[419] – the latter two giving iron in their ferric forms.

Ficus carica (Figure 39), the common fig[420] and a member of the Urticaceae, has been prized, both in its fresh and dried forms, since the earliest days. It is many times mentioned in the Scriptures and is indigenous to Persia, the whole of Asia Minor, and Syria but now grows wild in most of the Mediterranean countries and is prolific in Greece and the Greek islands. The Greeks are said to have received it from Caria in Asia Minor – hence its specific name – but it is widely cultivated and there is a fine example in the grounds of Lambeth Palace, London. Celsus used it externally to clean wounds, possibly due to its content of digestive ferments such as papain; many of the ancient authors mentioned its laxative properties and for this purpose it is retained in the contemporary pharmacopoeia, along with the Compound Fig Elixir[421].

The BP 1980 also contains Gentian[422], 'the dried underground organs of *Gentiana lutea* L.', which is used as a bitter, as is *Erythraea centaurium*, the Centaury Gentian or fever-wort. The Gentians are an extensive group of plants, amounting to almost 200 species, and deriving the name of the genus from Gentius, the King of Illyria in 180–167 BC, who is reputed to have discovered the medicinal properties of this group of plants. Most of the European gentians are blue but the Yellow Gentian, *Gentiana lutea*, an Alpine and sub-alpine plant that reaches the Balkans but not Britain or Northern Europe in its habitat, provides the root from which is extracted the bitter most frequently employed in medicine. Celsus mentions Gentian only in a prescription for an antidote but in the eighteenth century Gentian wine was drunk to stimulate the appetite before meals. Martindale[423] notes that the dried partially fermented rhizome and root of *Gentiana lutea* (Gentianaceae) contains a glycoside, sugars, and alkaloids. It is considered to be unrivalled as a tonic able to stimulate the appetite even during jaundice; it has also long been used as a febrifuge and emmenagogue and is supposed to have anthelmintic and antiseptic properties. Of the Powdered Gentian in the current pharmacopoeia, the official preparation is the Concentrated Compound Gentian Infusion[424].

Another of the vegetable bitters known to Celsus was derived from the rootstock of *Inula helenium*, the Wild Sunflower and one of the largest of our herbaceous plants, which is of the Compositae; it is also called Elecampane and the most abundant product of the root is Inulin[425]. This is in the BP as the polysaccharide granules obtained from the tubers of *Dahlia variabilis, Helianthus tuberosus*, and other genera of the family Compositae. Inulin is rapidly removed from the circulation following injection intravenously and is predominantly eliminated in the urine by glomerular filtration. Thus, Inulin Injection is still used as a diagnostic agent to measure the glomerular filtration rate and thereby provide an estimate of renal function.

Hyoscyamus niger, the Henbane, and the alkaloids hyoscyamine and hyoscine have been previously mentioned but the plant (Figure 27) was used by Celsus as a hypnotic, the seeds as a topical anodyne, the bark as a poultice for joints, the leaves in an eye salve, the juice as a remedy for earache, and the root for toothache. This potent substance – perhaps one of the most potent of the use-

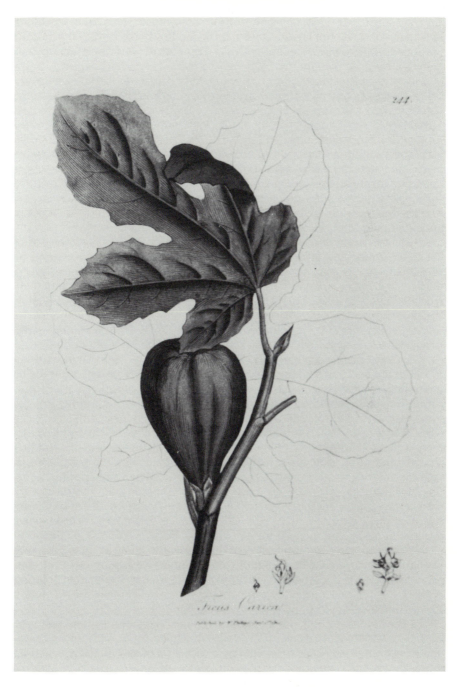

Figure 39 Ficus carica (The Common Fig). [*From: William Woodville. Medical botany . . . London, William Phillips (1810), Vol. IV.*]

ful plant medicines – remains with us as a parasympatholytic agent used as an antispasmodic and both Hyoscyamus Leaf[426] and Powdered Hyoscyamus Leaf[427] are found in the pharmacopoeia with the Dry Extract, and the Tincture being among the official preparations.

One of the medicines used by Celsus to relieve cough was lavender, his source being *Lavandula Stoechas* from the isles of Hyères (Stoechades). This is another herbal remedy still with us, even if only as a fragrance and garden flower: our Lavender Oil BP[428] is obtained by distillation from the fresh flowering tops of *Lavendula intermedia* Loisel (the English oil) or *Lavendula angustifolia* P. Miller (the foreign oil of lavender). Mint and catmint were also perfumes of supposed medicinal value and well known to Celsus who used *Mentha piperita*, peppermint, as a carminative; *Mentha viridis*, green mint, as a diuretic and a treatment for coughs; *Mentha pulegium*, pennyroyal, as a stimulant and skin cleanser; and Mentastrum (possibly wild mint) against snake bite. Celsus writes: 'At si cerastes aut dipsas aut haemorrhois percussit . . . Trifolium quoque et mentastrum et cum aceto panaces aeque proficiunt.'[429] (But when cerastes or dipsas or haemorrhois has bitten a man . . . Trefoil, and wild mint and allheal-juice, with vinegar, are equally effective.) Spencer[430] notes that *Coluber cerastes* was the horned viper of the desert, *Coluber vipera* was called dipsas as its bite produced great thirst, and *Haemorrhois* is not identified; at this point he translates mentastrum as wild mint. We have Peppermint Leaf BP[431] (the dried leaves of *Mentha x piperita* L.) and the official Peppermint Oil[432] in addition to Spearmint Oil BP[433] from *Mentha spicata* L. and *Mentha x cardiaca* (Gray) Bark.

The last of the metals that we shall note appearing amongst the prescriptions of Celsus are lead and sodium. Galena, sulphide of lead, was used, after further processing, to arrest bleeding; lead slag was used as an emollient and in a dressing for burns and ulcers; litharge, the oxide of lead separated after heating lead and silver ores, was used to clean wounds and septic skin lesions and the like; white lead, basic lead acetate, was made by pouring vinegar over shavings of lead, and then heated to produce the yellow and red oxides of lead; it was used on new wounds and ulcers and for headache and joint pain. For the latter uses the medicament was applied externally, as with most Roman prescriptions of the time. Of the salts of sodium, sodium chloride, common salt, was included in many prescriptions; rock salt was used in one of the eye salves; salt of some form was used in an enema; and various naturally occurring mixed carbonates and nitrates of soda and potash were used, usually as erodents, poultices for abscesses, or means of maturing sites of inflammation. Of all of these substances we have pharmacopoeial monographs on Sodium Chloride[434], the Carbonate Monohydrate[435] and Carbonate Decahydrate of Sodium[436], and other reagents. As with our pharmacopoeia (which contains Sulphur Ointment BP)[437], that of Rome contained sulphur.

Of *Populus alba* (see p. 46), Celsus, describing remedies for severe toothache says: 'The bark of white poplar roots boiled in diluted wine . . . '[438] may be used – and we have here the recipe for preparing a decoction of salicin, the crystalline β-glucoside obtained from the bark of young shoots of various species of *Salix* and *Populus* especially *S. fragilis* (BPC 1954)[439]. There is no evidence that Celsus or any of his successors for many centuries understood the antipyretic and analgesic actions of salicin, any more than the preparation of the pure crystalline form of the drug was imagined – but we have here one of the beginnings of the salicylates, probably best and safest of the analgesic, antirheumatoid drugs of today. Representing the very simple members of the salicylate series we have Salicylic Acid[145] itself, Methyl Salicylate[440] (which is to be dispensed when 'Oil of Wintergreen, Wintergreen or Wintergreen Oil' is prescribed or demanded) and Salicylic Acid Ointment[441] among the monographs of the BP 1980.

One plant carries the name of Rome into the modern *British Pharmacopoeia* and that is Chamomile Flowers BP[442] whose official synonyms are 'Roman Chamomile Flowers' and 'Anthemis'. Chamomile Flowers are the dried flower heads of the cultivated double variety of *Anthemis nobilis* L. (*Chamaemelum nobile* L.) and these contain not less than 0.4% of their volatile oil. Chamomile has been used as an aromatic bitter and, in large doses, as an emetic. The infusion, 'chamomile tea' is a country remedy for indigestion and a poor appetite. A poultice of the flowers is applied externally to 'draw' inflammation and cause local abscesses to point and evacuate. Chamomile Oil (BPC 1949)[443] is blue when fresh when it has a strong aromatic odour; it contains esters of angelic and tiglic acids and has been used as a potent and pleasant aromatic carminative and flavouring agent. Celsus and the Romans obtained their chamomile from Pyrethrum or *Herba salivaris; Anthemis pyrethrum* and their uses of the drug included the treatment of toothache and promotion of salivation to cleanse the mouth. It kept this use throughout the Middle Ages but its history is said to go back to the Egyptians who 'reverenced it for its virtues'[444]. The origin of the name 'chamomile' is from the Greek *kamai* (on the ground) and *melon* (an apple), the plant smelling strongly of apples, especially when crushed, and being somewhat low to the ground, and thus the chamomile, or 'ground-apple'.

The remaining plant drugs used by Celsus and still represented in our official pharmacopoeia include *Radix dulcis*, liquorice; and *Radix pontica*, which was almost certainly rhubarb. Liquorice BP[445] is the dried unpeeled root and stolons of *Glycyrrhiza glabra* so that the approved synonyms are Liquorice Root or Glycyrrhiza. Rhubarb BP[446] is the rhizome, deprived of most of its bark and dried, of *Rheum palmatum* (and possibly other species and hybrids of *Rheum*, Polygonaceae, excepting *R. rhaponticum*) cultivated in China and Tibet. It is a mild anthraquinone purgative which is unusual in that it exerts an astringent action after purgation.

Among the potent botanical drugs of Roman times we find *Scilla*, squill, already noticed on page 108, and found as Squill[447] (the bulb of *Urginea maritima*) and Indian Squill[448] or Urginea (the bulb of *Urginea indica*) – both BP preparations being the bulb, collected soon after the plant has flowered, stripped of its outer coverings, sliced and dried. Perhaps unexpectedly we still have Squill Oxymel[449] (Squill, bruised, acetic acid, purified water, and purified honey) listed among the official monographs.

We have also Thymol BP[450] and Celsus had *Thymbra capitata*, Cretan thyme, a source of the antiseptic oil of thyme. Prepared Storax BP[451] (the purified balsam from the trunk of *Liquidambar orientalis*) appears in our pharmacopoeia and Celsus had *Styrax*, or storax, and prized the perfume of this balsam which resembles the fragrance of jasmin; similarly, we have Tragacanth BP[452] (the air-hardened gummy exudate from the trunk and branches of *Astragalus gummifer* and related species) and Celsus had *Tragacantha* from *Astragalus Creticus*.

Our rubefacient Turpentine Oil BP[453] (the old Oleum Terebinthinae) – a household substance of which three teaspoonsful, 15 ml, can be fatal in children – is obtained by distillation and rectification from turpentine, the oleoresin obtained from various species of *Pinus* of the Pinaceae; the BP contains Turpentine Liniment[454] and White Liniment[455] but Celsus had *Terebinthus*, the resin from *Pistacia terebinthus*, the turpentine tree, and used it with pitch resin as an erodent or internally in patients with dyspnoea. Finally, without attempting to make this comparison complete, we still have the condiment Ginger BP[456], synonym Zingiber, the scraped or unscraped rhizome of *Zingiber officinale*, and this is a substance that Celsus included in his pharmacopoeia and used in an antidote. Just as Celsus used a pharmacopoeial wool, so we have Wool Fat BP[457] and Hydrous Wool Fat BP (Lanolin)[458].

Today's doctor, armed with his modern knowledge, would not find himself helpless with the Roman pharmacopoeia – he could do something useful for indigestion, hyperchlorhydria, costiveness, severe constipation, microcytic anaemia, scabies, photosensitivity, napkin rash, auricular fibrillation, congestive cardiac failure, otitis externa, skin excoriation round a fistula, infantile colic, sunburn, athlete's foot, chronic dermatitis, calcium deficiency, mania, sleeplessness, smooth-muscle spasm, salt deficiency, fever needing an antipyretic, rheumatoid conditions needing an analgesic, septic conditions of the skin and mucous membranes needing an antiseptic, a traumatic lesion needing adhesive strapping, and a reduced fracture needing immobilization. Some of the remedies that would need to be used would be less effective and perhaps more toxic than those available from other sources today but, by reading Scribonius Largus, opium, most potent of the anodynes, could be prepared and, by adding hyoscyamus, a reasonable premedication for pre-operative use could be derived. By extending the reading to the BPC of half a century ago, tapeworm, roundworm, and pinworm could be treated. Even by keeping to the BP 1980 items which the doctor could prepare from the constituents of the Roman pharmacopoeia, and by using salt, water, and a monosaccharide to prime and fuel the duodenal cell-wall electrolyte pump, a child gravely threatened by infantile diarrhoea could be rehydrated.

The list of remedies that could be made in this way and the conditions that, to a useful degree, could be treated, is incomplete – but it is not nothing. Even if it were made complete it would, of course, still remain a far call from what would be expected of even the most isolated doctor of today.

But, without using any drugs, today's doctor, remembering the benign outcome of much human disease, and ensuring that he avoided all harm, could take advantage of the great legacy of Greece: disease could be regarded in a way free from superstition, the most perceptive of ethics could be adopted, the necessity of clinical observation could be remembered, and the Hippocratic understanding of the *vis medicatrix naturae* could be used to illuminate contemporary practice.

References

156. Evans, Sir Arthur J. *The Palace of Minos.* 5 vols., 1921–36
157. Hutchinson, R. W. *Prehistoric Crete.* Harmondsworth, Middx. 1962. Revised 1968
158. Chadwick, J. The decipherment of Linear B. Harmondsworth, Middx. 1961
159. Edelstein, Emma J. and Edelstein, Ludwig. Asclepius, A collection and interpretation of the testimonies. 2 vols., Baltimore, *Johns Hopkins Press,* 1945
160. Isidore, Bishop of Seville [Isidorus Hispalensis]. Etymologiarum libri xx. Augsburg, *G. Zainer,* 1472

  Also Isidori Hispalensis episcopi etymologiarum sive originum libri xx. Recognovit brevique adnotatione critica instruxit W. M. Lindsay. 2 vols. Oxonii, *E. Typographeo Clarendoniano,* 1911

  Also English trans. (medical and anatomical sections) of the Etymologiae: *Trans. Am. Philos. Soc.,* 1964, **54**, pt. 2
161. Isidore, Bishop of Seville (1472). As ref. 160 but Etymologiae, IV, 4, 1
162. Isidore, Bishop of Seville (1472). Ref. 159, Vol. I, p. 186
163. Isidore, Bishop of Seville (1472). As ref. 160 but Etymologiae, IV, 3, 1–2
164. Isidore, Bishop of Seville (1472). As ref. 159, Vol. I, p. 185
165. Graves, Robert. Greek myths. London, *Cassell,* 1958, p. 333
166. Graves, Robert (1958). As ref. 165 but p. 519
167. Murray, Margaret Alice. The witch-cult in Western Europe. Oxford, *Clarendon Press,* 1921. Re-issued 1962, p. 279
168. Martindale, 27th edn. (1977). As ref. 1 but p. 1716
169. BPC (1968). As ref. 148 but p. 1138
170. BPC (1968). As ref. 148 but p. 1137
171. BPC (1949). As ref. 80 but p. 1351
172. BPC (1949). As ref. 80 but p. 1352
173. BPC (1934). As ref. 120 but pp. 53–55
174. Woodville, William (1810). As ref. 129 but plate 165
175. Isaiah xxxiv, 14 (RV margin)
176. Caton, Richard. Two lectures on the temples and ritual of Asklepios at Epidaurus and Athens. Reprinted from '*Otia Merseiana*', 1899.

  Also: The temples and ritual of Asklepios at Epidauros and Athens. Liverpool, *University Press,* 1900
177. Kerényi, C. Asklepios, Archetypal image of the physician's existence. London, *Thames and Hudson,* 1960
178. Cartwright, Frederick F. A social history of medicine. London, *Longman,* 1977, p. 3
179. Garrison, Fielding H. An introduction to the history of medicine with medical chronology, suggestions for study and bibliographic data. Philadelphia & London, *W. B. Saunders,* 1913. 4th. edn. 1929, p. 89
180. Garrison, Fielding H. (1929). As ref. 179 but p. 99
181. Soranus, of Ephesus. (On fractures) In Physici et medici graeci minores. Julius Ludovicus Ideler. 2 vols. Berolini, *G. Reimeri,* 1841. Vol. I, p. 248 et seq.
182. Soranus, of Ephesus. De arte obstetricia morbisque mulierum quae supersunt. Ex apographo F. R. Dietz. Regimontii Pr., *Graef et Unzer,* 1838
183. Soranus, of Ephesus. (On acute and chronic diseases.) *Vide*: Caelii Aureliani, siccensis, medici vetusti, secta methodici de morbis acutis & chronicis libri viii. Amstelaedami, *Ex Officina Wetsteniana,* 1722
184. (Hippocrates). Hippocrates, with an English translation by W. H. S. Jones. 4 vols., London, *Heinemann,* 1923–31. Vol. I, pp. 193, 195 and 197
185. Hippocrates. Œuvres complètes d'Hippocrate. Traduction nouvelle avec le texte grec en regard... Par E. Littré. 10 vols. Paris, *J. B. Baillière,* 1839–61
186. (Hippocrates). The genuine works of Hippocrates. Translated from the Greek, with a preliminary discourse and annotations by Francis Adams. 2 vols. London, *Sydenham Society,* 1849
187. (Hippocrates). The medical works of Hippocrates. A new translation from the original Greek made especially for English readers by the collaboration of John Chadwick and W. N. Mann. Oxford, *Blackwell,* 1950

141

188. Hippocrates (Trans. of 1923–31). As ref. 184 but p. lvi
189. Garrison, Fielding H. (1929). As ref. 179 but p. 95
190. Hippocrates (Trans. of 1849). As ref. 186 but Vol. I, pp. 236–237
191. Hippocrates (Trans. of 1849). As ref. 186 but Vol. II, pp. 568–574
192. Hippocrates (Trans. of 1849). As ref. 186 but Vol. II, pp. 538–539
193. Hippocrates (Trans. of 1849). As ref. 186 but Vol. II, plate VIII
194. Hippocrates (Trans. of 1923–31). As ref. 184 but Vol. I, p. 277
195. Hippocrates (Trans. of 1923–31). As ref. 184 but Vol. I, p. 235
196. Garrison, Fielding H. (1929). As ref. 179 but p. 99
197. Hippocrates (Trans. of 1849). As ref. 186 but Vol. II, p. 847
198. Hippocrates (Trans. of 1950). As ref. 187 but p. 179
199. Hippocrates (Trans. of 1950). As ref. 187 but p. 183
200. Hippocrates (Trans. of 1950). As ref. 187 but p. 190
201. Hippocrates (Trans. of 1950). As ref. 187 but p. 190
202. Hippocrates (Trans. of 1923–31). As ref. 184 but Vol. IV, p. 135
203. Hippocrates (Trans. of 1849). As ref. 186 but Vol. II, p. 697
204. Woodville, William (1810). As ref. 129 but Vol. III, p. 474
205. Woodville, William (1810). As ref. 129 but Vol. III, pp. 475–476
206. Woodville, William (1810). As ref. 129 but Vol. III, p. 476
207. BPC (1934). As ref. 120 but p. 1106
208. Martindale, 27th edn. (1977). As ref. 1 but p. 674
209. Martindale, 27th edn. (1977). As ref. 1 but p. 657
210. The British Pharmaceutical Codex 1954. London, *Pharmaceutical Press*, 1954, p. 338
211. Woodville, William (1810). As ref. 129 but Vol. IV, p. 755
212. Scribonius Largus (edn. of 1528). As ref. 50
213. Hippocrates (Trans. of 1849). As ref. 186 but Vol. II, pp. 779–780
214. Singer, Charles Joseph. Greek biology and Greek medicine. Oxford, *Clarendon Press*, 1922, p. 13
215. Hippocrates (Trans. of 1923–31). As ref. 184 but Vol. I, p. 8
216. Singer, Charles J. (1922). As ref. 214 but p. 17
217. Osler, Sir William (1921). As ref. 19 but p. 69
218. Singer, Charles J. (1922). As ref. 214 but pp. 22–23
219. Aristotle. Opera. Edidit Academia Regia Borussica. 5 vols. Berolini, *Reimer*, 1831–70
220. Aristotle. The works of Aristotle translated into English under the editorship of J.A. Smith and W.D. Ross. 12 vols. Vol. IV – Historia animalium by D'Arcy Wentworth Thompson. Oxford, *Clarendon Press*, 1908–52. (Vol. IV, 1910)
221. Aristotle. Aristotle. 23 vols. London, *Heinemann*, 1926–1960. These include: On the soul, Vol. VIII, Trans. W.S. Hett, 1936. Historia animalium, Vol. IX–XI, Trans. A.L. Peck, 1965–1970. Parts of animals, Vol. XII, Trans. A.L. Peck, 1947. Generation of animals, Vol. XIII, Trans. A.L. Peck, 1942
222. Aristotle (Trans. of 1910). As ref. 220 but pp. 560b, 561 a & b
223. Singer, Charles J. (1922). As ref. 214 but p. 37
224. Diogenes Laertius. Lives of eminent philosophers. Trans. R.D. Hicks. 2 vols., London, *Heinemann*, 1925
225. Theophrastus of Eresos. De historia plantarum. Venice, 1495–98
226. Theophrastus of Eresos. De historia plantarum. [Treviso], (*imp. B. Confalonerium de Salodio*, 1483)
227. Theophrastus of Eresos. Theophrastus. Enquiry into plants and minor works on odours and weather signs. Translated by Sir Arthur Hort. 2 vols. London, *Heinemann*, 1916
228. Theophrastus (edn. of 1916). As ref. 227 but Vol. I, pp. 13 and 15
229. Theophrastus (edn. of 1916). As ref. 227 but Vol. I, p. 203
230. Theophrastus (edn. of 1916). As ref. 227 but Vol. I, p. 155
231. Theophrastus (edn. of 1916). As ref. 227 but Vol II, pp. 15, 17 and 19
232. Gemmill, Chalmers L. Silphium. *Bull. Hist. Med.*, 1966, **XL** (4), 295–313
233. Gemmill, Chalmers L. (1966). As ref. 232 but p. 304
234. BPC (1949). As ref. 80 but pp. 119–121
235. Theophrastus (edn. of 1916). As ref. 227 but Vol. II, p. 319

236. British Pharmacopoeia 1973. Published on the recommendation of the Medicines Commission pursuant to the Medicines Act 1968. London, *HMSO*, 1973, p. 278
237. Theophrastus (edn. of 1916). As ref. 227 but Vol. II, pp. 305–307
238. Singer, Charles. Studies in the history and method of science. Ed. Charles Singer. 2 vols. Oxford, *Clarendon Press*, 1917–1921, Vol. II, p. 98
239. Taylor, Henry Osborn. Greek biology and medicine. London, *Harrap*, 1922
240. Diocles of Carystus. *Vide*: Oribasius. Collectionum medicarum reliquiae. 4 vols. Lipsiae, *Teubner*, 1928–31
241. Celsus. De medicina. With an English translation by W. G. Spencer. 3 vols., London, *Heinemann*, 1935–38, Vol. I, p. 15
242. Celsus (edn. of 1935–38). As ref. 241 but Vol. I, p. 41
243. Allbutt, Sir Thomas Clifford. Greek medicine in Rome. The Fitzpatrick lectures on the history of medicine delivered at the Royal College of Physicians of London in 1909–1910, with other historical essays. London, *Macmillan*, 1921, p. 11
244. Jones, W. H. S. Philosophy and medicine in Ancient Greece. Supplements to Bull. Hist. Med. No. 8. Baltimore, *Johns Hopkins Press*, 1946
245. Asclepiades of Bithynia. Fragmenta. Digessit et curavit C. G. Gumpert. Vinariae, *Industrie-Comptoir*, 1794
246. Green, Robert Montraville. Asclepiades, his life and writings. Connecticut, *Elizabeth Licht*, 1955
247. Green, Robert M. (1955). As ref. 246 but p. 110
248. Macalister, R. A. S. (1912). As ref. 90 but Vol. II, pp. 426–437
249. Celsus (edn. of 1935–38). As ref. 241 but Vol. I, p. 339
250. Celsus (edn. of 1935–38). As ref. 241 but Vol. I, p. viii
251. Celsus, Aulus Aurelius Cornelius. De medicina. Florentiae, *Nicolaus/Laurentius/*, 1478
252. Celsus (edn. of 1935–38). As ref. 241 but Vol. I, p. 5
253. Celsus (edn. of 1935–38). As ref. 241 but Vol. I, p. 231
254. Celsus (edn. of 1935–38). As ref. 241 but Vol. I, p. 43
255. Celsus (edn. of 1935–38). As ref. 241 but Vol. I, p. 65
256. Celsus (edn. of 1935–38). As ref. 241 but Vol. I, p. 79
257. Celsus (edn. of 1935–38). As ref. 241 but Vol II, p. 67
258. Celsus (edn. of 1935–38). As ref. 241 but Vol. I, p. 272
259. Celsus (edn. of 1935–38). As ref. 241 but Vol. I, p. 273
260. Celsus (edn. of 1935–38). As ref. 241 but Vol. I, pp. 279–289
261. Celsus (edn. of 1935–38). As ref. 241 but Vol. I, pp. 333–339
262. Celsus (edn. of 1935–38). As ref. 241 but Vol. I, pp. 325–327
263. Celsus (edn. of 1935–38). As ref. 241 but Vol. I, p. 159
264. Celsus (edn. of 1935–38). As ref. 241 but Vol. I, p. 291
265. Celsus (edn. of 1935–38). As ref. 241 but Vol. I, p. 303
266. Celsus (edn. of 1935–38). As ref. 241 but Vol. I, p. 447
267. Celsus (edn. of 1935–38). As ref. 241 but Vol. II, p. 113
268. Celsus (edn. of 1935–38). As ref. 241 but Vol. II, p. 3
269. Celsus (edn. of 1935–38). As ref. 241 but Vol. II, p. 3
270. Celsus (edn. of 1935–38). As ref. 241 but Vol. I, p. 169
271. Celsus (edn. of 1935–38). As ref. 241 but Vol. I, p. 175
272. Celsus (edn. of 1935–38). As ref. 241 but Vol. I, p. 211
273. Celsus (edn. of 1935–38). As ref. 241 but Vol. I, p. 297
274. Celsus (edn. of 1935–38). As ref. 241 but Vol. II, pp. xv–lxiii
275. Celsus (edn. of 1935–38). As ref. 241 but Vol. II, pp. xvi–xvii
276. Celsus (edn. of 1935–38). As ref. 241 but Vol. II, p. xv
277. Celsus (edn. of 1935–38). As ref. 241 but Vol. I, p. 439
278. BPC (1934). As ref. 120 but p. 925
279. British Pharmacopoeia 1963. Published under the direction of the General Medical Council pursuant to the Medical Act 1956. London, *Pharmaceutical Press*, 1963, p. 716
280. BPC (1968). As ref. 148 but p. xxiv
281. Celsus (edn. of 1935–38). As ref. 241 but Vol. II, p. 349
282. BPC (1934). As ref. 120 but pp. 538–539
283. BP (1980). As ref. 79 but Vol. I, p. 232

284. Celsus (edn. of 1935–38). As ref. 241 but Vol. II, p. 287
285. Celsus (edn. of 1935–38). As ref. 241 but Vol. I, p. 317
286. Celsus (edn. of 1935–38). As ref. 241 but Vol. I, p. 317
287. Celsus (edn. of 1935–38). As ref. 241 but Vol. I, p. 319
288. Celsus (edn. of 1935–38). As ref. 241 but Vol. I, p. 321
289. Celsus (edn. of 1935–38). As ref. 241 but Vol. I, p. 391
290. Celsus (edn. of 1935–38). As ref. 241 but Vol. I, p. 417
291. BPC (1934). As ref. 120 but p. 937
292. Celsus (edn. of 1935–38). As ref. 241 but Vol. I, p. 371
293. BPC (1949). As ref. 80 but pp. 913–914
294. Celsus (edn. of 1935–38). As ref. 241 but Vol. II, p. 81
295. Celsus (edn. of 1935–38). As ref. 241 but Vol. II, p. 91
296. Celsus (edn. of 1935–38). As ref. 241 but Vol. III, p. 373
297. Celsus (edn. of 1935–38). As ref. 241 but Vol. III, pp. 455–461
298. Celsus (edn. of 1935–38). As ref. 241 but Vol. III, pp. 503–505
299. Celsus (edn. of 1935–38). As ref. 241 but Vol. III, p. 351
300. Celsus (edn. of 1935–38). As ref. 241 but Vol. III, p. 363
301. Celsus (edn. of 1935–38). As ref. 241 but Vol. III, p. 401
302. Celsus (edn. of 1935–38). As ref. 241 but Vol. III, pp. 427–453
303. Celsus (edn. of 1935–38). As ref. 241 but Vol. III, p. 469
304. Celsus (edn. of 1935–38). As ref. 241 but Vol. III, pp. 469–471
305. Celsus (edn. of 1935–38). As ref. 241 but Vol. III, p. 431
306. Celsus (edn. of 1935–38). As ref. 241 but Vol. III, p. 371
307. Celsus (edn. of 1935–38). As ref. 241 but Vol. III, p. 492
308. Celsus (edn. of 1935–38). As ref. 241 but Vol. III, p. 493
309. Plinius *Secundus*, Gaius. Histoire naturelle de Pline. 20 vols. [in 10]. Paris, *C. L. F. Panckoucke*, 1829–40.
    Also: Natural history. English translations by W. H. S. Jones, H. Rackham and D. E. Eichholz. 10 vols. London, *W. Heinemann*, 1948–63
310. Dioscorides, Pedanius, *Anazarbeus*. De medica materia, Liber primus, Interprete Marcello Virgilio, Secretario Florentino. Coloniae, 1529
311. Dioscorides, Pedanius, *Anazarbeus*. Petri Andreae Matthioli Senensis,... Commentariorum in VI. libros Pedacii Dioscoridis Anazarbei, de Medica materia. Venetiis, 1583, part II, pp. 422–423
312. Dioscorides, Pedanius, *Anazarbeus*. Dioscurides Codex Aniciae Julianae picturis illustratus, nunc. Vindobonensis Med. Gr. 1. phototypice editus... moderante Josepho de Karabacek, Lugduni Batavorum, *A. W. Sijthoff* 1906
313. Gunther, Robert T. The Greek herbal of Dioscorides illustrated by a Byzantine AD 512, Englished by John Goodyer AD 1655, Edited and first printed AD 1933. Oxford, *Univ Press*, 1934
314. Gunther, Robert T. (1934). As ref. 313 but pp. 349–350
315. Gunther, Robert T. (1934). As ref. 313 but p. 357
316. Gunther, Robert T. (1934). As ref. 313 but p. 435
317. Martindale, 27th edn. (1977). As ref. 1 but p. 220
318. Aretaeus *the Cappadocian*. Τα Σωδομενα. The extant works of Aretaeus, the Cappadocian. Edited and translated by Francis Adams. London, *Sydenham Society*, 1856
319. Rufus of Ephesus. De vesicae renumque morbis. De purgantibus medicamentis. De partibus corporis humani. Sorani de utero & muliebri pudendo. Parisiis, *Turnebum*, 1554
320. Rufus of Ephesus. De vesicae renumque morbis. De purgantibus medicamentis. De partibus corporis humani... Nunc iterum typis mandavit Gulielmus Clinch. Londini, *J. Clarke*, 1726
321. Rufus of Ephesus. Œuvres, texte collationné sur les MSS., traduit pour la première fois en français avec une introduction. Publication commencée par Ch. Daremberg, continuée et terminée par Ch. Émile Ruelle. Paris, *Baillière*, 1879
322. Singer, Charles (1922). As ref. 214 but p. 121
323. Rufus of Ephesus. Soranus' gynecology. Trans. Owsei Temkin. Baltimore, *Johns Hopkins Press*, 1956, p. 7
324. Rufus of Ephesus (Temkin edn. of 1956). As ref. 323 but p. 93

325. Rufus of Ephesus (Temkin edn. of 1956). As ref. 323 but pp. 64–65
326. Soranus of Ephesus (edn. of 1722). As ref. 183
327. Soranus of Ephesus. Graecorum chirurgici libri Sorani unus de fracturarum signis Oribasii duo de fractis et de luxatis e collectione Nicetae ab antiquissimo et optimo codice Florentino . . . Florentiae, *ex typographio Imperiali*, 1754
328. Soranus of Ephesus (edn. of 1841). As ref. 181
329. Soranus of Ephesus (Temkin edn. of 1956). As ref. 323 but p. xxiv
330. The medical writings of Anonymus Londinensis. By W. H. S. Jones. Cambridge, *University Press*, 1947
331. Singer, Charles (1922). As ref. 214 but p. 122
332. Marcus Aurelius Antoninus. The Meditations of the Emperor Marcus Antoninus. Ed. A. S. L. Farquharson. 2 vols. 1944
333. Revelations i, 11 (AV)
334. Revelations ii, 12 (AV)
335. Galen. Opera omnia. Ediderunt Andreas Asulanus et J. B. Opizo. 5 vols. Venetiis, *in aedibus Aldi, et Andreae Asulani soceri*, 1525
336. Galen. Opera omnia. Editionem curavit C. G. Kühn. 20 vols. [in 22]. Lipsiae, *C. Cnobloch*, 1821–33
337. Galen. Opera omnia. 4 vols. Lipsiae, *B. G. Teubner*, 1914–22
338. Galen. On the natural faculties. With an English translation by A. J. Brock. London, New York, *Putnam*, 1916
339. Galen (edn. of 1916). As ref. 338 but p. xxv
340. Galen (edn. of 1916). As ref. 338 but pp. 325,327
341. Galen (edn. of 1916). As ref. 338 but p. 321
342. Galen (edn. of 1916). As ref. 338 but p. 321
343. Singer, Charles (1922). As ref. 214 but Fig. 11 opp. p. 66
344. Galen (edn. of 1916). As ref. 338 but p. 57
345. Galen (edn. of 1916). As ref. 338 but pp. 59, 61
346. Galen (edn. of 1916). As ref. 338 but p. 293
347. Allbutt, Sir Thomas C. (1921). As ref. 243 but p. 357
348. Allbutt, Sir Thomas C. (1921). As ref. 243 but p. 359
349. Galen. De simplicium medicamentorum facultatibus librii xi. *Vide* Ref. 336
350. Winslow, Charles-Edward Amory. The conquest of epidemic diseases. A chapter in the history of ideas. Princeton, *University Press*, 1943 p. 55
351. Jones, William Henry Samuel. Malaria and Greek history. To which is added The history of Greek therapeutics and the malaria theory, by E. T. Withington. Manchester, *Univ. Press*, 1909
352. BP (1980). As ref. 79 but Vol. I, p. 13
353. op. cit. Vol. II, p. 838
354. op. cit. Vol. I, p. 20
355. op. cit. Vol. I, p. 21
356. op. cit. Vol. I, p. 485
357. op. cit. Vol. I, p. 25
358. op. cit. Vol. I, p. 23
359. op. cit. Vol. I, p. 23
360. op. cit. Vol. I, p. 24
361. op. cit. Vol. II, p. 550
362. op. cit. Vol. II, p. 704
363. op. cit. Vol. II, p. 730
364. op. cit. Vol. II, p. 730
365. op. cit. Vol. II, p. 783
366. op. cit. Vol. II, p. 684
367. op. cit. Vol. II, p. 685
368. op. cit. Vol. I, p. 37
369. op. cit. Vol. I, p. 36
370. op. cit. Vol. II, p. 839
371. Borchert, Peter *et al.* 1′-hydroxysafrole, a proximate carcinogenic metabolite of safrole in the rat and mouse. *Cancer Res.*, 1973, **33**, 590–600

372. BP (1980). As ref. 79 but Vol. I, p. 158
373. op. cit. Vol. I, p. 68
374. op. cit. Vol. I, p. 481
375. op. cit. Vol. I, p. 481
376. op. cit. Vol. I, p. 516
377. op. cit. Vol. I, p. 480
378. op. cit. Vol. II, p. 683
379. op. cit. Vol. II, p. 570
380. op. cit. Vol. II, p. 548
381. op. cit. Vol. II, p. 706
382. op. cit. Vol. II, p. 706
383. op. cit. Vol. II, p. 702
384. op. cit. Vol. II, p. 908
385. op. cit. Vol. II, p. 909
386. op. cit. Vol. II, p. 916
387. op. cit. Vol. I, p. 490
388. op. cit. Vol. I, p. 71
389. op. cit. Vol. I, p. 74
390. op. cit. Vol. I, p. 73
391. op. cit. Vol. I, p. 73
392. op. cit. Vol. I, p. 71
393. op. cit. Vol. I, p. 70
394. op. cit. Vol. I, p. 491
395. op. cit. Vol. I, p. 74
396. op. cit. Vol. I, p. 75
397. op. cit. Vol. I, p. 82
398. op. cit. Vol. I, p. 83
399. op. cit. Vol. II, p. 833
400. op. cit. Vol. II, p. 834
401. op. cit. Vol. I, p. 84
402. op. cit. Vol. I, p. xxxi
403. The Song of Solomon iv, 13–15 (AV)
404. BP (1980). As ref. 79 but Vol. I, p. 124
405. Celsus (edn. of 1935–38). As ref. 241 but Vol. II, p. xxx
406. Woodville, William (1810). As ref. 129 but Vol. II, p. 357
407. Virgil. Aeneid. Trans. H. R. Fairclough. London, *Heinemann*, 1916–18
408. Celsus (edn. of 1935–38). As ref. 241 but Vol. II, p. 65
409. Celsus (edn. of 1935–38). As ref. 241 but Vol. I, pp. 416–417
410. Celsus (edn. of 1935–38). As ref. 241 but Vol. I, pp. 416–417
411. Celsus (edn. of 1935–38). As ref. 241 but Vol. II, p. xxxiii
412. Dioscorides (Gunther edn. of 1934). As ref. 313 but p. 631
413. BP (1980). As ref. 79 but Vol. I, p. 193
414. op. cit. Vol. I, p. 193
415. op. cit. Vol. I, p. 192
416. op. cit. Vol. I, p. 191
417. op. cit. Vol. I, p. 194
418. op. cit. Vol. II, p. 626
419. op. cit. Vol. II, p. 625
420. op. cit. Vol. I, p. 195
421. op. cit. Vol. II, p. 556
422. op. cit. Vol. I, p. 209
423. Martindale, 27th edn. (1977). As ref. 1 but p. 255
424. BP (1980). As ref. 79 but Vol. I, p. 209
425. op. cit. Vol. I, p. 240
426. op. cit. Vol. I, p. 235
427. op. cit. Vol. I, p. 235
428. op. cit. Vol. I, p. 252
429. Celsus (edn. of 1935–38). As ref. 241 but Vol. II, pp. 118–120

430. Celsus (edn. of 1935–38). As ref. 241 but Vol. II, p. 118
431. BP (1980). As ref. 79 but Vol. I, p. 333
432. op. cit. Vol. I, p. 334
433. op. cit. Vol. I, p. 423
434. op. cit. Vol. I, p. 409
435. op. cit. Vol. I, p. 408
436. op. cit. Vol. I, p. 408
437. op. cit. Vol. II, p. 701
438. Celsus (edn. of 1935–38). As ref. 241 but Vol. II, p. 247
439. BPC (1954). As ref. 210 but pp. 658–659
440. BP (1980). As ref. 79 but Vol. I, p. 287
441. op. cit. Vol. II, p. 701
442. op. cit. Vol. I, p. 92
443. BPC (1949). As ref. 80 but p. 568
444. Grieve, Mrs. M. (1931). As ref. 124 but p. 185
445. BP (1980). As ref. 79 but Vol. I, p. 258
446. op. cit. Vol. I, pp. 389–390
447. op. cit. Vol. I, p. 424
448. op. cit. Vol. I, p. 424
449. op. cit. Vol. II, p. 702
450. op. cit. Vol. I, p. 454
451. op. cit. Vol. I, p. 427
452. op. cit. Vol. I, p. 460
453. op. cit. Vol. I, p. 469
454. op. cit. Vol. II, p. 682
455. op. cit. Vol. II, p. 682
456. op. cit. Vol. I, p. 209
457. op. cit. Vol. I, p. 478
458. op. cit. Vol. I, p. 479

3

The Dark Ages and the Renaissance

The Middle Ages – to about AD 1450
The Byzantine Period

If the beginning of scientific medicine is placed at about 600 BC, during the life-time of Thales of Miletus, and it is recognized that it continued to make important advances until the death of Galen at the end of the second century AD, then it is clear that its progressive lifespan lasted for a period of 800 years. After the Dark Ages in Europe we cannot place the beginnings of modern scientific Western medicine much before the end of the fifteenth century. Thus, our own system has been evolving for barely five centuries – a little more than half the total course of Greek medicine and science.

The Mediaeval Period – from about AD 200 to AD 1450 – was the span of the Dark Ages in Europe. The end of this period was marked by the date of the capture of Constantinople by the Turks in 1453 – a date that serves to remind us that during our Dark Ages the lights of the Muslim Empire shone brightly; at this time it was within the Muslim Empire that learning was continued. In order to watch the means whereby medical culture was preserved in the 1200 years that followed the death of Galen it is, therefore, necessary to look to Byzantium where, as the influence of Rome gradually declined and Christianity strengthened and spread, power was to reside for a period (AD 395–1453) of over 1000 years.

This process began in the year 330 when Constantine the Great (AD 288–337), having become ruler of the whole Roman Empire, transferred the capital from Rome to Byzantium, the ancient city which had been built by the Greeks on the Bosphorus and which was later to become Constantinople and eventually modern Istanbul. Constantine at first tolerated the Christian sect and then, after becoming attached to the faith, made it the state religion.

In 335 Constantine elected his nephew, Julian (AD 331–363), joint ruler. Julian, once Emperor, tried but failed to restore pagan worship; he also turned to the outstanding physician of the day, Oribasius (AD 325–403), demanding that a summary should be made of all of the available medical knowledge. Thus, Oribasius became cast in the role of a compiler of existing knowledge rather than an original writer, but his output was immense: in 70 volumes he compiled an encyclopaedia embracing all of the medicine, hygiene, therapeutics and surgery from the days of Hippocrates to his own times. This was the *Synagoge* of which only 17 volumes have survived. Perhaps because of the unwieldiness of the work,

149

and for the convenience of his son, he prepared a synopsis. Both of these works remain greatly valued as Oribasius is recognized for the accurate quotation of his sources and for the fact that his writings preserve much that would have otherwise been lost.

The *Synagoge* was first printed by Aldus Manutius in Venice in 1554 or the following year. The editions of the nineteenth century include the *Oeuvres d'Oribase, texte grec, en grande partie inédit . . .* [459], printed in Paris in 1851-76. There is also the *Collectionum medicarum reliquiae* [460] of 1928-31 which contains a selection from the writings of a number of the authors of antiquity; collectively the editions are important for an understanding of the early means of therapeutics, for Oribasius assembled and analysed a vast quantity of the information then available on the remedies and medicines of the physicians of Greece and Rome.

The last sole ruler of the Empire of Rome was Theodosius I (Theodosius the Great, AD 346-395), who, on his death, divided his possessions between his sons, Arcadius (AD *c.* 377-408) and Honorius (AD 384-423). Honorius took the Western portion of the inheritance and soon became subject to the sequence of barbarian invasions that provided the final cause of the downfall of the Western Empire. To stem the threat to Rome the legions in Northern Europe were withdrawn and, in Britain, by the year 409, the great Northern Wall built by the Romans stood unguarded. Of these events, distant but to be of great effect on Byzantium, Helen Waddell [461] wrote: 'Within about a twelvemonth the barbarians had swept across France: they were in the vineyards of Bordeaux; they were encamped beneath the Pyrenees. All France "smoked like a funeral pyre". This was in 406: four years later, Alaric was in Rome . . .' In this passage and her account of these events Waddell comments on her translation of the verse of Claudian Claudianus (*c.* 370-405), the last authentic poet of the classical tradition, a Greek who rose to high office under the Emperor Theodosius and whose Latin vividly describes the ebbing of the strength of Rome. From Britain the last message asking for the means of defence provoked from Honorius the words: 'The cantons should take steps to defend themselves' [462] – a phrase which ended the rule of Rome in Britain. In 410, Alaric (AD *c.* 370-410), King of the Visigoths, led his people through Italy and, faced only with the weakness and vacillation of Honorius, pillaged the city of Rome.

Throughout the West the period after the fall of Rome was marked by the ravages of the barbarians and a series of attempts to build communities and nations out of unstable tribes. The Dark Ages were marked also by the spread of Christianity and ecclesiasticism, the rise of feudalism and the ascendancy of folk medicine. What little real medical practice survived did so in monastic hands, but for a period of 600 years – a span of time which could have almost encompassed the lives of Hippocrates and Galen and all that lay between them – Europe lay in intellectual and material waste. During this long period there occurred almost no event of importance to the progress of medicine or science.

Whilst in the West the remains of classical learning which survived did so in the hands of monks and a few scholars, none of whom excelled Isidore, Bishop of Seville whose *Etymologiarum . . .* has already been noted, events in the East were more favourable. When the great Empire of Theodosius I had been divided, Arcadius, the more fortunate of his sons, had taken the Eastern portion with his capital at Byzantium. Here the effects of the barbarian invasions were less dramatic: although the intellectual outlook of the Byzantine Empire was ultimately changed just as radically as in the West, the Byzantine change was far more gradual.

In the Empire of Arcadius the means of government survived and the Greek tradition and its manuscripts were better preserved and more widely used than in the West. Thus, in Byzantium the Greek authors could still be read in versions of the texts which were much less remote from the originals than those in use in Europe. It is of the first importance that the Christian Church generated a number of heretical sects and, for use as they migrated, these sects prepared their own translations of the Greek writers. These translations preserved the old learning and some of its attitudes and transferred it, altered only in language, to regions where it was more welcome and relevant.

Of all these heretics none are more important than the followers of Bishop Arius (d. *c.* AD 335) who believed that Christ is not divine but was a created being. Condemned at the Council of Nicaea in AD 325, Arius was driven from the Church – leaving behind him a new spirit of enquiry. Nestorius (d. *c.* AD 451), who had been nominated to the See of Constantinople by Theodosius II (AD 401–450) in 428, went a good deal further – by opposing the use of the title *Theotokos* (bearer of God), which was used for the Blessed Virgin, Nestorius insisted, in effect, that Mary was the mother of Christ, but not in the sense of the Church doctrine. Nestorius, damaged at the Council of Ephesus in 431, was deposed and exiled in 436. Against this expulsion a centre of resistance arose in the renowned school of theology at Edessa in Syria (the modern Urfa in Turkey) and it was here, where they had excellent hospital and medical facilities, that the Nestorians gathered before fleeing on to Persia in AD 489.

During their time at Edessa the Nestorians established fine facilities for teaching in the two hospitals; once in Persia they set up an even better centre of medical education at Gondisapor. This became the famous school which Garrison[463] has called 'the true starting-point of Mohammedan medicine' – and it was the medicine of Islam that, by these means, became the custodian of the medicine of Greece.

In Gondisapor the Nestorians translated the Greek medical texts into Persian and established generations of Persian-trained physicians who became the major medical teachers. Thus the Byzantines, driven by their religious beliefs from Byzantium, became the Nestorian translators who passed the medicine of Greece and Rome to the Muslim world from their home in a remote segment of Persia.

Much of their energy seems to have been occupied with their custodial function. One of the few to show any real originality was Alexander of Tralles (AD 525–605), brother of the architect of St. Sophia at Constantinople, whose *Practica* shows additions to the text of Galen. The book was printed in 1504[464] and there is the *Original-Text und Uebersetzung* published in 1878–79[465] and a French edition of 1933–37[466]. Although, in the main, Alexander Trallianus was a compiler, the work[466] contains a most original chapter on intestinal worms and vermifuges; this mentions fern-root, chenopodium, and santonin and the contribution to knowledge is extensive enough for many to prize the *Practica* and consider Alexander to have been the first parasitologist. He is also often said to have been the first to mention the use of rhubarb as a purgative and colchicum in gout.

Before considering Paul of Aegina, the final considerable medical figure of the Byzantine Period, it is important to reflect upon the intensity of beliefs which separated the multitude of religious sects in the early centuries of the Christian era. These beliefs affected medicine as all else in the history of ideas. An example comes from a recent finding. Quite by accident a group of gnostic treatises were discovered in Egypt in 1945. One of these tractates, *The Gospel of Thomas*, has aroused very great interest and it seems likely that the study of the whole of this unique collection will greatly revise our understanding of early Christianity and its mental environment. The discovery was made by two peasants digging in a cemetery near the Egyptian town of Nag Hammadi. The results are given in *The Nag Hammadi Library in English* published in Leiden[467] in 1977. The book provides a far more complex and unsorted view than has, by convention, reached us of the events of the time.

Judaic thought has had a singular and important effect of its own on the growth of medicine. The final codification of this thought spanned much of the Byzantine Period. The literature of the Talmud (from which is drawn our knowledge of the ideas that were current among the Jews during the period AD 200–600, the dates of the Talmudic Period) began when the Mishnah was edited and concludes with the Gemara. The Mishnah was compiled in Palestine and was a recording in writing of the Jewish religious and civil law, already preserved for many centuries by oral tradition. In Palestine, for some 300 years, there had existed a struggle between Hellenic culture and the Hebraic tradition. The Rabbis of the period had taken part in the struggle and had been attracted by its medical content as this related to so many of the legal, ritualistic and ecclesiastical laws and practices of the Jews. In the four centuries that followed its writing the Mishnah formed the basis of many commentaries and much of the teaching in the schools. It was used not only in Palestine but also in Babylonia where there was a large population of Jews. Gradually the commentaries overwhelmed the Mishnah in size and it is this final compilation which is termed the Gemara. The part of the Gemara that came from Palestine was edited at the beginning of the fourth century but the larger and more important portion that arose from the Babylonian colleges was completed about AD 600. The Talmud is the Palestinian and Babylonian Gemaras together with the Mishnah. To its study, and especially to the importance of its medical content, the *Biblisch-talmudische Medizin . . .* of Julius Preuss[82] makes a fundamental contribution; more recently there is the valuable *A Short History of Talmudic Medicine*[468], of J. Snowman, first published in London in 1935. This outline of the subject provides an introduction to the detailed studies of Pearlman[469] who follows all of the medical references of the Talmudic literature. The obvious direct expression of this literature on the subsequent history of medicine arises from the lives of those later medical figures, including Isaac b. Solomon Israeli, in the East, and Moses ben Maimon (Moses Maimonides), in the West, who were Jews.

The late part of the Byzantine Period is marked by the life of Paul of Aegina (AD 625–690), the author of an *Epitome*, in seven books, of medicine. He exhibits the lack of creativity of the period by explaining that all that can be known has been written by the ancients – but his writings show him to have been a skilful surgeon. They give original descriptions of lithotomy, trephination, tonsil-lectomy, and excision of the breast. The first clear description of lead poisoning also occurs in his work.

In 1528 the Aldine Press in Venice printed his first Greek edition. The first English version was *The Seven Books of Paulus Aegineta Translated from the Greek . . . by Francis Adams* – a three volume work printed for the Sydenham Society of London in 1844[470]. For those interested in drugs this is one of the treasures of the literature for, with its translation and commentaries, it sets out to provide 'a complete view of the knowledge possessed by the Greeks, Romans, and Arabians on all subjects connected with medicine and surgery'. There is a later Greek text[471], edited by Heiberg and published in 1921–24.

Paul of Aegina provides a number of vivid descriptions of surgical procedures and these make him the principal source of our knowledge of surgical practice in the early Middle Ages. In terms of drugs his work forms a basis for commentaries by Adams which take us nearer the Renaissance and can best be considered when discussing the additions to the pharmacopoeia made by the apothecaries of Arabia.

The Islamic Period

If the main contribution of the Byzantines was to preserve and transmit the ancient Greek texts, then the equivalent contribution of Talmudic medicine, like that of Biblical medicine, was not so much to list therapeutic methods as to elaborate the means of preventive medicine. These means were expressed in health rules based upon religious and ethical principles.

The Graeco-Roman world at the beginning of the seventh century is shown in Figure 40; the diagram is taken from the Silliman Foundation Lectures delivered by Sir William Osler at Yale University in April, 1913[19]. It has the practical look of Osler's teaching and shows the division of Rome into the Western and Eastern Empires, the vast regions of Christianity with the Nestorian Church spread across Mesopotamia almost to China, and the comparatively limited size of the Arabian Empire.

Confined to Arabia itself this Empire was, at first, quite small. However, Mohammed (AD 570–632) so inspired and inflamed his followers that they conquered Asia Minor, the expanse of North Africa, and the bulk of Spain, within the span of the two centuries after his death. The vigour of the effort continued in a cultural growth that established its main centres in Baghdad in the East, Kairouan in North Africa, and Cordoba in Spain.

The beginnings of this rapid growth were so vivid and unexpected that they are written of as having been incandescent: in less than 20 years the movement Mohammed had started shook the two great powers of the Byzantine Empire and the Sassanid Empire in Persia and founded a virtually new civilization. The lands occupied by the Nestorians rapidly fell to Muslim rule and the Nestorians, who had already made translations of the medical works of Greece into their own language, Syriac, adjusted to Islam.

Drawing his map (Figure 41) to show the changed events after only 100 years, Osler demonstrates the vast expanse which had come to comprise the Arabian

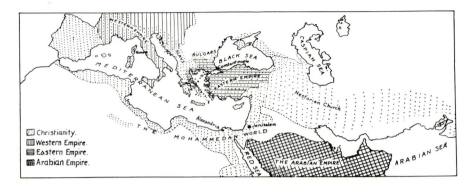

Figure 40 The distribution of the Graeco-Roman world at the beginning of the seventh century. [*From: William Osler. The evolution of modern medicine... New Haven, Yale Univ. Press (1921).*]

Empire at the beginning of the eighth century. By the ninth century a united Muslim Empire, centred on Baghdad, was firmly established. The need for the translation of the works of the peoples of Greece into Arabic, the language of Islam, was then felt everywhere. One by one, the writings that had been made into Syriac were turned into Arabic. Greek medicine, and the Greek and Roman knowledge of drugs, was by these means conveyed to the Muslim world – the Mohammedan physicians owing most of their medical learning, in the beginning, to the Nestorians.

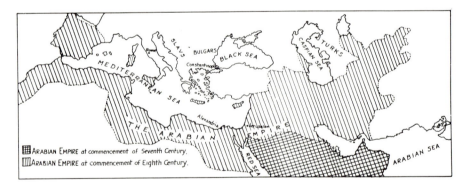

Figure 41 The Arabian Empire at the beginning of the seventh and the commencement of the eighth centuries. [*From: William Osler. The evolution of modern medicine... New Haven, Yale Univ. Press (1921).*]

The greatest of the translators who brought the Greek works into Arabic were, for geographical reasons, the medical writers of the Eastern Caliphate. During the latter part of the Mohammedan period, while medicine was being diligently studied and its texts translated, the study of anatomy was prohibited and human dissection forbidden. Thus, Arabic medicine depended for its

154

anatomy on the descriptions of Galen – a Galen whose own errors had been increased by those of the translators. Despite this, the studies of Hippocrates, Aristotle, Galen, Oribasius, and Paul of Aegina conducted by the Arabic physicians gave them, by the eighth century, considerable medical knowledge.

Amongst the earliest of those who enjoyed a level of repute of this order, and whose teachings influenced the growth of medical thought in Europe, was Mesuë the Elder (also known as Janus Damascenus; AD 777–857). Mesuë's father was a pharmacist and he grew to become head of the medical school at Baghdad and physician to the Caliph. There are a number of Latin editions of his works in the British Museum and the edition of the *Mesuë Opera* printed in Venice in 1603[472] includes a number of fine illustrations of medicinal herbs. Donald Campbell, in his book *Arabian Medicine and its Influence on the Middle Ages*[473], notes that Mesuë the Elder also wrote *Aphorisms*, a *Book of Fevers*, and *On the Pulse*, although the latter two works have not been translated.

Another whose main work lay in the translation of Greek works was Honain ben Isaac, known in the Latin West as Johannitius Onan or Humainus (AD 809–873) – a writer who, like his master Mesuë the Elder, was a Nestorian. His own books include the *Isagoge* which reviewed the Galenic system of medicine and was popular in medical studies in the later Middle Ages in Europe.

These writers and their immediate students achieve importance due to their preservation of the ancient texts, despite the limited nature of their additions to the old learning. Away from Baghdad, science and medicine were either largely lost amongst the barbarians or neglected as being of very limited interest to the Christian Church. Among the Muslims medicine continued to grow, reaching its maturity in the three great Persians known in the West as Rhazes, Haly Abbas, and Avicenna.

Rhazes, known to the mediaeval Latinists as Albubator (AD 860–932, although there is much confusion about the dates) ranks close to Hippocrates in his power to describe disease. He followed Galen in theory but Hippocrates in the simplicity of his practice and wrote an encyclopaedia of medicine which ran to 25 books and is called the *Al-Hāwī* or *Liber Continens*. In bulk it exceeds the *Canon* of Avicenna and was one of the nine volumes which composed the whole library of the medical faculty of Paris in 1395. The ninth book of the 'Continens' deals with pharmacology and formed a principal source of the knowledge of therapeutics in Europe long after the Renaissance. Although no complete manuscript exists there are a number of Latin editions; that published at Brescia in 1486[474] weighs over 17 pounds, so that the work of Rhazes provides the largest and heaviest of the incunabula.

His *Liber de variolis et morbillis*[475, 476] is the oldest and most important of the original works on smallpox and measles, the descriptions of Rhazes of these two illnesses being the most vivid and complete of antiquity. Rhazes is also said to have been the first to have introduced the orderly use of chemical preparations into the practice of medicine. He died, aged about 72, after becoming head of the hospital at Baghdad and is credited with having produced about 237 works on medicine. Most of these are now lost but he is justly remembered, not only for the duration of his influence, but for his having clearly differentiated smallpox from measles, thereby providing one of the most distinctly original contributions to medicine of the Arabians.

A near-contemporary of Rhazes was Isaac Judaeus (850–*c*. 941) who was born in Egypt, practised ophthalmology, and became famous in North Africa and his own country; he was typical of the educated Jews of his day and came to exert substantial influence on the medicine of Europe in the Middle Ages. His principal writing was a *Book of Diet* but he is a favourite subject of commentators, all of whom have remarked on the gentleness and dedication present in his writings.

The second of the great figures of Persian medicine, Haly Abbas (d. AD 994), was the author of the *Liber Regius*[477]. Haly Abbas was eminent 50 years after Rhazes. His great work, a compilation of medicine in 20 books, is also known as the *Al-Maliki*. It became the main textbook of medicine for over 100 years and, about 1070, was (in part) translated into Latin by Constantinus Africanus who gave it the title *Pantegni*. The translation is of special interest because it describes the 'Persian Fire', fulminating anthrax, and provides the Latin term for smallpox, *variola*. The section on anatomy, the *Pars practica*, is reckoned to have been the sole source of anatomical knowledge at Salerno for the century after its translation by Constantine.

The *Liber Regius*, the *Al-Maliki* or royal book, is usually regarded as having been the supreme medical work of the Arabic period. The principal Latin editions still known are those printed in Venice in 1492 and Lyons in 1523; the former was translated by Stephen of Antioch and was completed in 1127; the latter, based on the same translation, was annotated by Michael de Capella. The two versions represent one of the great works of medicine.

Mesuë the Younger (who is thought to have died about 1015) remains a vague and shadowy figure. He is probably the author of a number of books accredited to Mesuë Junior and appearing as reprints and Latin manuscripts during the Middle Ages. These include a *Simplicia*, an *Antidotarium*, and the *Grabadin medicinarum particularium* – the latter providing the *Grabadin* which became the manual of the apothecaries of the Middle Ages. The *Grabadin*, dealing mostly with the materia medica, taught Latin Europe the pharmacy and therapeutics of the Arabic-speaking peoples and was enormously important and popular. Many hundreds of editions were issued in Europe during the Middle Ages – and yet the Arabic originals have never been found and even the existence of Mesuë Junior is vouched for only by the unreliable Leo Africanus.

Europe, in the Middle Ages, learnt its medicine from Latin translations of the huge, unwieldy *Canon* of the well-authenticated Ibn Sina (AD 980–1037), the 'Prince of Physicians', known in the Latin West as Avicenna. He was born in the Persian province of Bokhara and became the most renowned of the physicians of Arabia. His writings formed the main reading of the medical scholars of Christendom and his influence was considerable throughout the whole of Islam and the West of Europe. At the age of 21 he wrote an encyclopaedia of the sciences, excepting mathematics, but is said to have become fond of pleasure and to have died, after a vast literary output, at an early age worn out by his labours and by riotous living.

The *Canon* – a massive volume of about a million words – represented the ultimate codification of the whole of Graeco-Arabic medicine. Campbell[478] says that it 'formed half the medical curriculum of European Universities in the latter part of the fifteenth century, and continued as a textbook up to about AD 1650 in the Universities of Montpellier and Louvain'. From its survival in these two centres to that late date we can estimate its effect upon the later growth of medicine. Although given to dialectical subtlety to a degree which was so marked that he is said to have stupified the physicians of Europe, his writings were ranked for centuries in the great centres of learning with those of Hippocrates and Galen.

The *Canon* was translated into Latin by both Gerard of Cremona[479] and Gerard Sabbionetta and some 30 editions founded on the Latin translations appeared in Europe. Of these, many were beautiful and Figure 42 illustrates the title page of that published in Venice in 1544; the first column of the text begins: 'Liber canonis primus, quem princeps Aboali abinsceni de medicina editit: translatus a magistro Gerardo Cremonensi in Toleto ex arabico in latinum . . .' – reminding us that the great centre of the translating movement was Toledo which, after it fell into Christian hands in 1085, provided rich and prized stores of Arabic manuscripts.

However, despite these great editions, it must be admitted that the ultimate effect of the *Canon* was to prolong and support the type of scholastic medical studies which were remote from the bedside and the direct study of disease. The effect was therefore harmful and the seventeenth century sweeping away of the great Arabian edifice of subjective and subtle reasoning was an intellectual cleansing. Even so, the beautifully wrought books of the physicians of the Eastern Caliphate had served to shelter the Greek texts and add to them their own body of clinical description. A thin but, for many, treasured work of literature also serves to remind us of Avicenna: the Persian contacts with India and places even further East had given the educated peoples of the day the game of chess, as an example of Eastern culture. No great physician frequenting the Court failed to participate, and images derived from the game resound through the poem translated by Edward Fitzgerald. The studies which resulted in parts of the book *Arabian Medicine* by E. G. Brown[480] strongly suggest that the quatrains usually ascribed to 'Umar Khayyām', and translated by Fitzgerald, originally arose long before the life of their supposed author, and from the pen of Avicenna.

The views of Avicenna, in the Eastern Caliphate, were not shared by his later Moslem colleagues of the West. The city of Toledo stands almost exactly in the centre of Spain, with Cordova to the south somewhat more than half way to the coast. In 1097, 60 years after the death of Avicenna, Toledo stood in Christian hands but surrounded on its western, southern, and eastern sides by Moslem territory. Thus, Toledo formed the meeting-place of the Latin scholars from the Christian West and the Arabic-speaking Islamic scholars of the Western Caliphate. The result was a great modification of views and the writers of the Western Caliphate – Albucasis, Avenzoar, Averroës, and Maimonides – were closer to the practical realities, and less interested in dialectic niceties and abstractions, than Avicenna.

Albucasis (b. *c.* AD 936) was born near Cordova and produced an encyclopaedia of medicine, the *Altasrif*[481] (the Collection) which has been translated a number of times. The parts on anatomy, physiology, and dietetics are derived from Rhazes; the surgical part[482], published separately, was the first independent and illustrated book on the subject. This surgical book, founded on the *Epitome* of Paulus Aegineta, was translated by Gerard of Cremona and became the standard surgical work used for centuries in Europe; it was of less influence in the

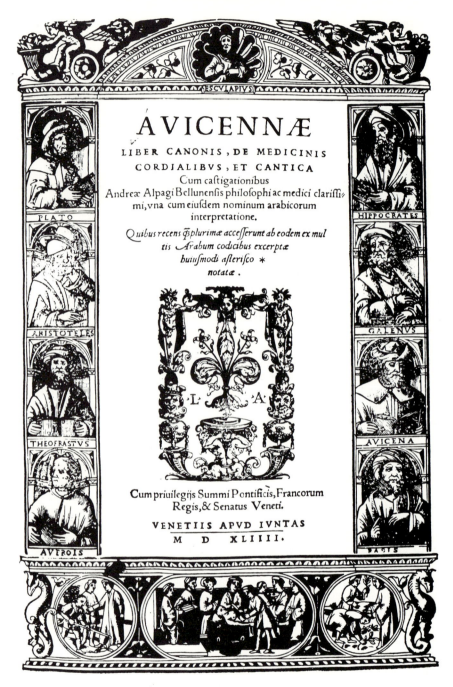

Figure 42   Avicenna. Title page from: *Avicennae Liber canonis* ... (edition of 1544).
[*Royal Society of Medicine library, London.*]

Western Caliphate itself. Albucasis has a number of other works and the *Antidotarium* by Johannes L. Tetrapharmacos is usually ascribed to him and provides a summary of the contemporary materia medica.

Avenzoar (1113–1162) was born at Seville and achieved a great reputation as a practical physician; acknowledged as one of the great thinkers of Islam, his main work is the *Altersir*, or *Teisir*[483]; in this he mentions *Acarus scabiei*, the itch-mite of scabies, the symptoms of mediastinal abscess (from which he suffered), and the procedure of tracheotomy.

Averroës (1126–1198), born in Cordova, based his final system of medicine on the philosophy of Aristotle. His views proved far more durable in the minds of those in Europe than among his own people, and Averroës, from the Western Caliphate, and Avicenna, from the Eastern, are the two principal representatives of Islamic abstract medical thought to the Christian West. His work, transliterated in the Latin West as *Colliget*[484], summarizes his knowledge of medicine from this philosophical point of view.

Maimonides, or Rabbi Moses Ben Maimon (1135–1208) is, without doubt, the best known of this group of physicians. In retrospect, he is looked upon with affection for his personal character and scholarship. Harry Friedenwald (*The Jews and Medicine, Essays* of 1944)[485] wrote that, 'Medicine was part of the discipline of Jewish scholars, and the number of those is large who followed both professions of rabbi and physician. The greatest of these was Maimonides himself.'

During the early part of the life of Maimonides Cordova was, in 1148, occupied by Almohades whose orthodox religious zeal made life for the Spanish Jews intolerable. Cordova, as a centre of learning, began to decline and Maimonides fled, passing through Palestine, to settle in Egypt. His fortune was lost in Cairo and, forced to turn to his knowledge of medicine for a living, he prospered and became physician to Saladin. He is said to have refused an equivalent appointment to Richard the Lion Heart, Richard I of England, who arrived at Acre in 1191 and was attracted by the reputation of Maimonides when he reached Palestine.

Thus, Maimonides lived during the decline of science, medicine and philosophy which formed the twilight of Arabic culture. He is regarded more as a theorist than as an active, practical physician but his meditations have served to guide many later generations of Jews and, from them, filtered into the mainstream of medicine. His chief written works include the *Book of Counsel (Tractatus de regimine sanitatis)*, a set of letters on diet and personal hygiene written for the Sultan Malek al-Afdhal ibn Saladin, and the *Aphorismen Mosis*[486], a famous collection of the aphorisms of Hippocrates and Galen. Maimonides also translated the *Canon* of Avicenna into Hebrew and produced a work, often called *Poisons and Antidotes*, which was written at the request of the Grand Vizier al-Fadil in 1198 and which was frequently quoted in the Middle Ages, even though no Latin edition was printed. There are French and German translations and a related rendering into English[487] which shows the curiously modern and scientific spirit of the work.

There is also a fine study of the writings of Maimonides by R. Levy in the first volume of *Studies in the History and Methods of Science* edited by Charles Singer in 1917[488]. Like all writings on the subject, this emphasizes the Oriental belief that it was unclean and sinful to touch the cadaver with the hands. This restriction badly affected the progress in medicine of Maimonides and his Moslem predecessors. The belief was allied to great credence in authority and permitted no real advance in anatomy and little, therefore, in physiology. Thus, Islamic medical instruction in the great hospitals of Baghdad, Cairo and Damascus was, just as with the academic studies in the principal cities of both Caliphates, limited to clinical medicine, pharmacology, and therapeutics. Chemistry was held in high regard and the Arabian interest in drugs, drug substances and ingredients and the materials of the materia medica, led to alchemy. Almost 300 years before Avicenna, and 400 years before Maimonides, alchemy had been founded, largely by Geber (AD 702–765). Geber is reputed to have discovered aqua regia and nitric acid and to have described the processes of distillation, filtration, sublimation, heating by water-baths and a number of the other basic arts of chemical science.

The tradition, in which all of this progress began, divided attempts at therapy into surgery, dietetics and pharmaceutics. The latter dominated in mediaeval times and has become of all-encompassing importance in contemporary medicine. From its early days it was split into the use of either simple or compound remedies. It remains the same today – and reaches back, as such, to the days of Galen who wrote not only *De simplicium medicamentorum temperamentis ac facultatibus*[349] but also the *De compositione medicamentorum secundum locos et secundum genera*[489]. Side by side the simple and the compound continued, over 100 Arabic authors writing about the corpus of the materia medica. Many of the works on 'simples' were written under the name of Serapion Junior (fl. *c.* 1070) but the main compilation of the materia medica of Arabia was (in its Latin translation) the *Liber magnae collectionis simplicia medicamentorum et ciborum continens*[490] of the Spaniard Ibn Baitar (d. *c.* 1248). This is the fullest work on the drugs of Islamic medicine and describes about 1400 medicaments, of which about 300 are said to have been recent introductions. The pharmaceutics of Arabia have been discussed by Manfred Ullmann in his *Islamic Medicine* of 1978[491] and provide a literature of great extent, both in the original writings and in translation. Finally, the 1847 translation by Francis Adams of *The Seven Books of Paulus Aegineta*[470] provides a fine account of the simple and compound remedies used not only by the Arabians but also by the physicians of Greece and Rome.

Of the different medicines already noticed, five prescriptions for contraceptives used by Soranus of Ephesus and containing pomegranate peel or rind are of especial interest. Pomegranate, the Grenadier, *Punica granatum* of the Lythraceae (Figure 43), provided not only the rind of the fruit but also its root, bark, and flowers to be used in remedies. Pomegranate is mentioned in the Ebers Papyrus and has formerly been much used as a symbol: it is said that the design of the fruit was used as a decoration on the pillars of King Solomon's Temple and was embroidered on the hem of the ephod of the High Priest. The stain extracted from the bark is used to give the yellow colour to Morocco leather and the root-bark was recommended as a vermifuge by both Celsus and Dioscorides. Pomegranate rind contains about 28% of gallotannic acid but no alkaloids. It has been used, in a decoction, as an astringent in the treatment of diarrhoea and dysentery but the more interesting constituents of the plant are the several forms of Pelletierine. Pomegranate Root Bark appeared in the BPC 1934[492] and

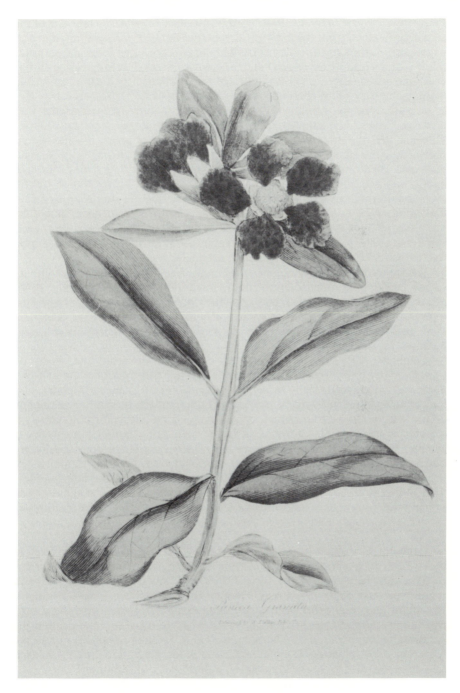

Figure 43   *Punica granatum* (The pomegranate). [*From: William Woodville. Medical botany . . . London, William Phillips (1810), Vol. III.*]

Pelletierine Tannate in the BP 1948[493] – this substance is the mixed tannates of the alkaloids obtained from the bark of the root and stems of *Punica granatum* and has a specific action on tapeworms; it is without effect on other intestinal parasites but it is now virtually never used due to its toxic effects. For long periods it has been recognized that it is contra-indicated in pregnancy. Its local effect on the motility and survival of spermatozoa seems unrecorded.

A plant drug not infrequently met with in the writings of the ancients, and used by Celsus, is Pennyroyal, *Mentha pulegium* of the Labiatae. Oil of Pulegium (Oil of Pennyroyal) BPC 1934[494] is the yellow or greenish-yellow liquid obtained by distillation from the fresh herb. Its chief constituent is the ketone, pulegone. The flower is shown in Figure 44 and the oil, with its strong mint-like odour, was used chiefly as an emmenagogue. It irritates the kidneys mildly during excretion and reflexly excites uterine contractions. The oil was also used as a flavouring agent (a use which it has officially been recommended should be prohibited)[495]. The supposed action as an emmenagogue may have been something of a euphemism: it is known that its use as an abortifacient has caused severe toxic effects, 4 ml being capable of producing convulsions[496].

We are told by Francis Adams (1847) that 'The Arabians added camphor, senna, musk, nux vomica, myrobalans, tamarinds, and a good many other articles to the Materia Medica; but, upon the whole, they transmitted the science to us in much the same shape as regards arrangement and general principles as they received it from their Grecian masters.'[497] Of this list the most useful addition was senna.

Camphor (BP 1980)[498] is obtained by distillation from the wood of *Cinnamomum camphora* of the Lauraceae and purified by sublimation. It can also be prepared synthetically from the pinene of Oil of Turpentine by conversion into camphene and subsequent oxidation. Either natural or synthetic camphor occurs as a colourless, transparent, crystalline solid and, depending on the way it has been condensed, it is known as 'bells' or 'flowers of camphor'; the blocks of camphor which are seen in commerce and widely distributed domestically are obtained by compression of the powder or sublimation. Rectified Camphor Oil (BPC 1959)[499], or Light Camphor Oil, is the lighter fractions, containing not less than 30% of cineole, of the oil obtained as a by-product during the manufacture of natural camphor; its composition varies somewhat but the heavier fractions of the crude oil, which are known as 'brown camphor oil' are used as a source of safrole.

Camphor Monobromide appeared in the BPC 1934[500] and used to be given in the treatment of headache and certain neurological conditions. Camphor Injection also appeared in the BPC 1934[501] and was used as a restorative in collapse because of its stimulating effect on the cerebral cortex and medullary vasomotor and respiratory centres. Certainly toxic doses produce epileptiform convulsions followed by paralysis and death – but the usual cause of death is the accidental administration of Camphorated Oil (Camphor Liniment) in mistake for castor oil or other domestic items that look the same. Fatalities in children have been recorded from the ingestion of as little as 1 g of camphor[502].

On the basis of the very limited evidence presently available and suggesting that camphor has a rubefacient and mild analgesic action when employed topically, a great range of preparations are used as counter-irritants in musculo-

162

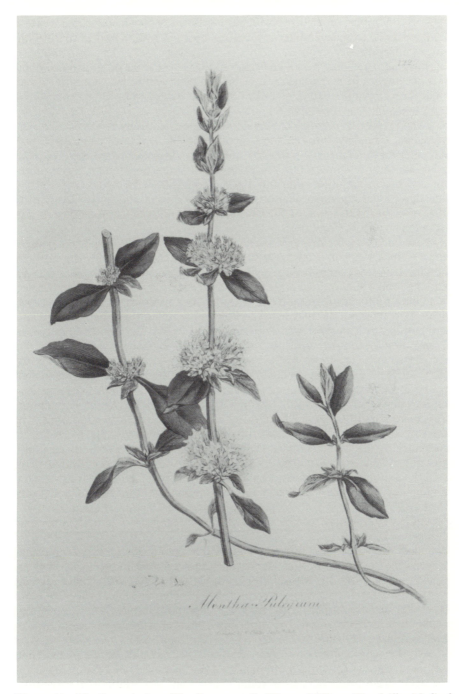

Figure 44   Mentha pulegium (The Pennyroyal). [*From: William Woodville. Medical botany . . . London, William Phillips (1810), Vol. II.*]

skeletal conditions; on evidence which is hardly more convincing it is also used, by inhalation, to relieve upper respiratory tract congestion and obstruction in simple infections.

Informed opinion moves increasingly to the view that the progressive elimination of camphor from therapeutic use, and its urgent removal in concentrated and solid forms from the environments of children, is appropriate. The subject has been fairly widely reviewed [503-507].

Senna Fruit (BP 1980)[508], or Senna Pod, is the dried fruits of *Cassia senna (C. acutifolia; C. angustifolia)* of the Leguminosae and is known commercially as Alexandrian or Tinnevelly senna; its main active ingredients are the glycosides sennoside A and sennoside B. The pods are an anthraquinone purgative useful for short-term administration but Barbara Smith[509] describes their adversely affecting rodent myenteric neurons when given chronically. Senna Leaf (BPC 1934)[510] is the dried leaflets of Alexandrian or Khartoum or Tinnevelly senna and has the same actions and uses.

Nux Vomica is the dried ripe seeds of *Strychnos nux-vomica* (Loganiaceae) and contains not less than 1.2% of strychnine. It also contains the alkaloid brucine. The seeds come from a small tree which is widely distributed over India and the Malay Archipelago and the ripe fruit, externally resembling an orange, contains a pulp and three to five of these highly poisonous seeds. In very small doses the drug was thought to act as a bitter and stimulate the appetite; it was also combined with a number of laxatives and then given to stimulate peristalsis. Preparations of this sort were listed in the BPC 1934[511] but even at that time it was recognized that the actions and uses of nux vomica were the same as strychnine (BPC 1959)[512]. Poisoning produces powerful convulsions with the body arched backwards and the teeth exposed in the 'risus sardonicus'; death from asphyxia or medullary paralysis usually follows the second to fifth such convulsion. Strychnine is a substance which is totally devoid of therapeutic justification and in the United Kingdom its use, even for the killing of animals (except moles), is forbidden by the Animals (Cruel Poisons) Regulations, 1963[513]. Perhaps a little grotesquely for such a poisonous substance the related *Strychnos Ignatii* (a woody, climbing shrub which is indigenous to Samar and other parts of the Philippine Islands) carries the name of a Saint and is known as the St. Ignatius Bean (BPC 1934)[514]; the official preparation was the Tincture of Ignatia.

Just as the greatest of the Greek drug compilations was the *De Materia Medica* of Dioscorides[313] and the main compendium of the materia medica of Arabia was assembled in the writings of Ibn Baitar, so the most important pharmacological work of Persia was the *Liber fundamentorum pharmacologiae...* of Abu Mansur Muwaffak bin Ali Harawi (fl. AD 970). This book was written about AD 970; there is an epitome by R. Seligmann dated 1830–33[515] and taken from a manuscript of about AD 1055. There is also a fine German version of 1893[516] which appeared under the direction of R. Kobert. This vast work of Abu Mansur described nearly 600 drugs.

Clearly, their contacts with new lands and new peoples led the pharmacists and apothecaries of the various parts of Arabia and the Islamic culture to exploit many old drug substances and introduce many new ones. Boric Acid was one of these remedies and was considered a valuable cleansing agent in ancient times and was used internally by Rhazes. It kept its reputation as a benign and non-toxic substance until quite modern times but R. B. Wild, in 1899[517], in an article entitled *Dermatitis and Other Toxic Effects Produced by Boric Acid and Borax*, produced one of the earlier reports showing that the substance could sometimes cause grave adverse effects. Wild mentions that Homberg, in 1702, had re-introduced the acid into medicine, after first preparing it in a crystalline form; he called his form of boric acid 'Homberg's sedative salt' and sedative, anodyne, and antispasmodic properties were claimed for it.

Boric acid is usually seen as white crystals, scales, or a white powder. It is a weak acid and its alkali salts are alkaline. The symptoms of boric acid poisoning include an almost characteristic erythematous rash with desquamation, vomiting, diarrhoea, shock, circulatory failure, coma, sometimes meningeal irritation, convulsions, and death – usually after 3–5 days and even when the source of poisoning has been removed. The difficulties are compounded by the facts that boric acid (boracic acid; borax is sodium borate) is not only absorbed from the gut but is well absorbed from abraded or damaged skin, granulating tissue, mucous membranes and serous surfaces. It does not readily penetrate intact, normal skin but, once absorbed, exhibits a prolonged half-life so that 3–7 days are necessary for full excretion of a single dose and the pharmacokinetic characteristics predispose to cumulative toxicity during repeated use.

Borax was originally imported from Persia, Japan, and China but in 1776 fairly pure supplies were detected in warm springs in Tuscany. The old form of the drug coming from the East and Far East had been called Tinical or Tankar and it is under these names that it is sometimes met with in the writings of the ancient authors. In 1856 new supplies were found in the Western parts of North America and the chief source soon became the great deposits of the salt found in Death Valley, California.

Marie Valdes-Dapena and James Arey, in 1962[518], reported three new fatal cases with pancreatic inclusions in a literature review (*Boric acid poisoning*) of 172 reported cases which, with their three additions, made the total 175; of this total 86 patients died. The fatal dose in adults of boric acid taken by mouth is thought to be 15–20 g; in infants it is 3–6 g[519]. Poisoning is almost always due either to accidental ingestion or to repeated application of pure or nearly pure boric acid to areas of denuded skin in infants. Thus, the gravest risks come from dusting babies with napkin rash with pure or nearly pure boric acid as a 'baby powder', or from feeding solutions of boric acid in mistake for other liquids, or from having concentrated forms of boric acid or borax in the home or in hospitals. Many professional bodies have drawn attention to these risks and the Pharmaceutical Society of Great Britain recommended (1956)[520] that pharmacists should not sell boric acid as a dusting powder and that such powders containing more than 5% boric acid should be labelled: 'Not to be applied to raw or weeping surfaces.' There is also a 1976 directive[521] of the Council of the European Communities relating to cosmetic products and limiting the concentration of boric acid to 5% in talcs; 0.5% in products for oral hygiene; and 3% in other products. This directive came into force in the United Kingdom in 1981[522] and, as a result, such talc has to be labelled to prevent its use on babies and boric acid is not to be present in products intended for children less than 3 years of age.

Boric acid is no longer used internally for any purpose. It is a feeble bacteriostatic and fungistatic agent which, for these uses, has been superseded by more effective disinfectants. There are monographs on both Boric Acid and Borax in the 1982 Addendum[523] to the BP of 1980 but it is doubtful if either substance has any real use (except as a buffer in pharmaceutical preparations) in contemporary therapeutics. It is another example of what used to be looked upon as a bland, natural substance now known to have been responsible for a tragic number of infant deaths and rightfully falling out of use.

The Arabians also made medicinal use of mercury – an interesting fact as, until the beginning of the present century and prior to the discoveries of Ehrlich just before the outbreak of World War I, scientific medicine recognized only three or four drugs as being truly specific (that is, able to eradicate the causative organism) and, of these, one was mercury in the treatment of syphilis.

Quicksilver (Mercury, BPC 1963)[524] was at one time given with digitalis or squill in pills or tablets because of a supposed diuretic action in cardiac oedema. Mercury with Chalk was used as a purgative in children until it was found that it could cause acrodynia (pink disease): early in the decade after 1950 it was shown that this syndrome, the cause of many fatalities, was related to the use of mercury in teething powders, dusting powders, and paediatric ointments. As mercury can be absorbed through the skin, preparations of it in a finely divided state used to be applied locally, by inunction, in the treatment of syphilis and some chronic and intractable skin diseases. Some organic compounds of mercury and ionizable mercury salts have been used as disinfectants; salts of mercury and organic mercurials are found in parasiticides and fungicides, preservatives for eye-drops and injection solutions, and a number of organic compounds of mercury were used as diuretics.

Of the latter, Mersalyl Injection (BP 1968;[525] the same compendium contained a monograph and specification for the parent Mersalyl Acid) formed an indispensable part of medical practice until the discovery of the orally-active, thiazide-type diuretics which form one of the major advances of twentieth century therapeutics. The two or three times a week routine trip round the practice to give injections of mersalyl was one of the rituals of a few decades ago that, even today, are not readily forgotten. With the thiazides available, even though Mersalyl Injection remained in the BP 1973[526], it was omitted from the BP 1980[527] – a change which recorded the fall from use of this once essential but toxic drug.

Earlier still, Mercury was very much part of the history of the treatment of syphilis. Mercurous chloride has a marked antisyphilitic action and, in ointments of 30–50% concentration, was used as a prophylactic against syphilis. In the days when syphilis was treated or prevented with mercury, bismuth and its salts were also widely used; they were given, for their treponemicidal action, in aqueous or oily suspensions, by deep intramuscular injection. In many clinics patients sat, thus protecting their sciatic nerves, for the injection to be given; X-rays which happened to include the gluteal region often showed the tell-tale radio-opaque intramuscular spots of unabsorbed bismuth. The more general antimicrobial action of mercurial salts can be represented by the Yellow Mercuric Oxide, used in eye ointments for the treatment of blepharitis and conjunctivitis, although this can lead to absorption of mercury from the eye; another such example is Mercuric Chloride which has marked antibacterial effects due to the ability of the mercuric ion to form insoluble complexes with proteins, including those of bacterial cells.

The acute and chronic toxicity of mercury and its salts are so well known, and its uses so fully superseded by safer agents, that it has become very much an item of history. Its rightful decline from therapeutic use is marked by the list of its salts that have been relegated to use as reagents only in the 1980 BP[528]. Nevertheless, mercury was one of the very few specific drugs available at the start of the twentieth century and its replacement, by the orally-active diuretics, and by penicillin in the treatment of syphilis, forms one of the highlights of the progress in therapeutics achieved during World War II and the post-war years.

The Western Middle Ages

In the East, by the end of the Byzantine and Islamic Periods, the writings of the Greeks had not only passed through a number of languages – they had also travelled through one and a half millennia. The death of Galen took place at the very beginning of the third century. Early in the fourth century, in AD 330, Constantine had transferred the capital of the Roman Empire to Byzantium; in this same century the learning of Greece was enshrined in the Byzantine *Synagoge*[459] of Oribasius. In the fifth century the medical lore of the Greeks was carried by the migrating Nestorians to Persia where it was put into their own language, Syriac. The end of the sixth and the beginning of the seventh centuries saw the rise of Mohammed, and by the early part of the eighth century the Nestorians had been absorbed into Islam. The eighth and ninth centuries formed the period in which the Greek texts, with their more recent additions, were translated from their version in Syriac into the language of Islam, Arabic. Many of these Arabic texts were then made into Latin – some of this work being undertaken by Gerard of Cremona (1114–1187), who travelled from Italy to Toledo to learn Arabic but who stayed there for the rest of his life and produced Latin versions of the works of Rhazes, Isaac Judaeus, Albucasis, and the *Canon* of Avicenna. The vigour of this school of translators was such that their texts in Latin and the volumes which they produced were soon to play a great part in the awakening of the intellect of the whole of Europe.

There is curiously little to represent the medicine of the West during that long period in which the culture of Islam flourished in the East. Of this period Clifford Allbutt wrote: 'The chief monuments of learning were stored in Byzantium until Western Europe was fit to take care of them.'[529] As Allbutt also describes, much of that return to fitness took place, by a constellation of circumstances, in the Italian city of Salerno.

The bay of Salerno, on the western coast of the parts of Italy which, in the south, formed 'Magna Graecia', lay on the great trading routes but secure from the causes of the northern disruption. From the sixth century before Christ to the tenth century AD in this southern part of Italy classical learning persisted and Greek was spoken; it continued to be one of the main languages of life in the eastern towns of the region until the thirteenth century. All of the great languages of antiquity – Greek, Arabic, and Latin – remained in constant use in the southern cities of Italy and to such an extent that the scholars of Sicily were still translating direct from the Greek in the twelfth century.

Some 300 years before this, probably in the ninth century, a medical school had been founded looking down on the bay of Salerno; there, from about AD 820, the Benedictines had a cloister and a hospital. The principal monument of the city of Salerno is the Cathedral of St. Matteo, founded in 845, and rebuilt in 1076 and the decade that followed. In the crypt is the sepulchre of St. Matthew whose body, according to legend, was carried to the cathedral in the tenth century. In the Chapel of the Crusades, founded in the thirteenth century, is the tomb of Pope Gregory VII who died at Salerno in 1085.

The life of this cathedral must have greatly affected the medical school, the earliest independent school of its kind in Europe, as it grew and attracted students from Europe, Asia, and Africa. The school of Salerno reached its zenith in the eleventh and twelfth centuries and became the most famous centre of medical studies of the Middle Ages. Throughout the whole of this period, and until the rise of the universities, Salerno became a resort for the sick and wounded, a centre of study, and a secular centre where both men and women professors could provide access to the classical tradition.

Much of that access was provided by Constantinus Africanus (c. 1020–1087) of Carthage. Constantinus was a Christian monk who had acquired his languages by travelling and who reached Salerno in the middle of the eleventh century. His translations, and he had better Arabic than Latin, included Haly Abbas, Isaac Judaeus, many Arabic versions of Hippocrates and a number of the treatises of Galen. Thus, he made into Latin a number of important Greek, Arabic, and Jewish writers – so placing the culture and experience of Islam at the disposal of the whole of Europe. The work of Constantinus lasted, in its influence, from the twelfth to the seventeenth centuries. He has a fine, two volume *Opera*[530] published by Petrus in 1536–39.

The greatest contribution of the school of medicine at Salerno was its provision of the first comprehensive textbook of medicine written by many authors. It is believed that the total output of the school numbered over 100 texts; some of this vast range of material remains available and is given in the *Collectio Salernitana*... [531] – a work published in five volumes in 1852–9. Most famous of all of these works is the *Regimen Sanitatis Salernitanum* (or *Flos Medicae*). This is a poem in leonine hexameters, first printed in Latin in 1484; it grew to some 400 verses providing dietetic and hygienic advice on the means of preserving fitness and health. The 1901 *Magistri Salernitani nondum*[532], edited by Giacosa, provides one form of this great poem; there is also *The School of Salernum. Regimen sanitatis Salernitanum, the English version by Sir John Harington*... [533] – a composite work published in 1920 and recently reprinted.

The means of therapeutics were represented by the *Antidotarium*[534] of Nicolaus Salernitanus (fl. 1140). This important book was the first formulary to be printed once the means of doing so had been discovered. The manuscript first appeared in 1140 and included a table of weights and measures which established the apothecaries' system. It provided 139 prescriptions and included the original formula of the *spongia somnifera* – the anaesthetic sponge which can be traced back to manuscripts of the eighth century. It is small wonder that the book was considered important enough to become one of those most frequently known to generations of later writers. The *spongia somnifera* was the means of lessening the pain and horror of mediaeval surgery. The recipe called for a sponge to be steeped in a water or wine mixture of opium, lettuce, hemlock, hyoscyamus, mulberry juice, mandragora and ivy. Once prepared, the sponge was dried and kept until it was needed; it was then moistened so that the juice could be drunk and the fumes inhaled. Its reputation lasted so that it was well known to a whole range of writers extending from Boccaccio to Marlow and Shakespeare. It appears in the passage from *Othello*[535] in which Iago, after Othello's entry, says:

Not poppy, nor mandragora,
Nor all the drowsy syrups of the world,
Shall ever medicine thee to that sweet sleep
Which thou ow'dst yesterday.

Another of the great works of Salerno was the *Practica chirurgiae* written by Roger of Palermo (fl. *c.* 1170–1200). This first appeared about 1180 and describes end-to-end suture, mercurial inunction in chronic skin diseases, and the use of ashes of sponge and seaweed (a source of iodine) in the treatment of goitre. This remarkable anticipation of a much later degree of understanding of thyroid disease gives great interest to the *Glossulae quatuor magistrorum super chirurgiam Rogerii et Rolandi* edited by Daremberg and published in 1854[536]. Roger's *Practica...* was edited by his pupil Roland of Parma (fl. *c.* 1230–1240) and, although not separately printed, exists on its own as a teaching manuscript.

Roger (Ruggiero Frugardi) of Palermo, despite his recognition of cancer and his innovation of suturing the divided intestines over a hollow tube, still taught that wounds should heal by secondary intention with the production of what was later called 'laudable pus'. This idea was strongly contested by Theodoric (Teodorico Borgognoni; 1210–1298), Bishop of Cervia and a successor to Roger. Theodoric was one of the first to teach that pus will merely delay the healing of wounds; this vital observation was contained in his surgical anthology and is represented in *The Surgery of Theodoric ca. 1267...* [537], a valuable translation published in 1955–60. Garrison cites Allbutt as pointing out that 'This simple statement... makes Theodoric one of the most original surgeons of all time, for only Mondeville and Paracelsus upheld these principles before Lord Lister and von Bergmann. in the long interregnum "the advocates of suppuration won all along the line".'[538]

From these heights of achievement Salerno slowly declined. The success of the school can be traced through the literature in a host of different directions – but the decline was progressive from the mid-thirteenth century when the challenge of the great new medical schools at Montpellier, Naples, and Palermo arose. In the end, Salerno was closed by Napoleon in November, 1811. However, the writings made in Salerno, and translated centuries later, form one of the windows through which the figures of antiquity can be glimpsed.

The institutions that were the successors to Salerno arose largely from monastic or collegiate schools or from student guilds. Thus, the dates of the founding of the late mediaeval universities – Paris 1110; Bologna, 1113; Oxford, 1167; Montpellier, 1181; Padua, 1222; and Naples, 1224 – provide a calendar of the most important intellectual events of the twelfth and thirteenth centuries. Of this period there are four works on the materia medica and use of drugs that are especially attractive. These are the *De simplici medicina seu Circa instans*[539] of Matthaeus Platearius (fl. *c.* 1130–1150), a study which derived from Dioscorides and appeared about 1140 and provided the original of the first French herbal; the *De virtutibus herbarum*[540], the *Macer Floridus*, a twelfth century poem giving an account of the properties of 88 simples; the *De vegetabilibus libri vii*[541] of Albertus Magnus (1193–1280), the best work on natural history with emphasis on medical botany of the Middle Ages; and the *Medicamentorum Opus*[542] of Nicolaus Myrepsus (*c.* 1280), otherwise known as the *Antidotarium magnum* as it was the biggest truly pharmaceutical work that had appeared and contained more than 2500 formulae.

Apart from these books, two of the early universities are of special medical interest: at Bologna the study of anatomy, which had been neglected apart from the dissection of animals since before Galen, was revived and an organized medical faculty arose as early as 1156. Even in Bologna human dissection remained infrequent – but it nevertheless took place and began the slow process of correcting the classical texts, read time and time again, and translated from Greek to Syriac, to Arabic, to Hebrew, and to Latin, in various sequences. Even though the need to return to dissection and correct the texts with fresh observations was compelling, it was not until the days of Mundinus of Bologna (Mondino de' Luzzi; *c.* 1275–1326) that human dissection became anything but uncommon. The bodies used were usually those of condemned felons and, possibly as a manual for the use of his students, Mundinus, in 1316, completed his *Anothomia*[543]. This was the first modern book solely devoted to anatomy; it not only forms a milestone in the development of the subject but ably puts forward the mediaeval vocabulary, mainly derived from Arabic, of the anatomist. The book was first published in Padua in 1487. In its version which appeared a little later at Leipzig (1493) it has a title page, reproduced by Osler[544] and forming Figure 45, which shows how anatomy was then taught: the incumbent of the professorial chair sits reading, possibly from Galen, while a crude assistant removes part of the contents of the abdomen; the rest of the body is untouched, the dissection beginning at the part which will deteriorate first. A small monument to this re-introduction, by Mundinus, of human dissection – a practice neglected for the preceding 1500 years – still exists in present-day Bologna where the sepulchral bas-relief of Mondino de' Luzzi can be seen on the wall of the Church of San Vitale.

Montpellier, across the Pyrenees but close to the Spanish border, was left, as the tide of Islam receded, marked by the Arabic thinking and writing which influenced the school of surgeons that arose in the region of the university. Of these surgeons, Guy de Chauliac (*c.* 1300–1368) is the most illustrious. Greatly concerned with the need of the surgeon to have a sound knowledge of anatomy, he produced his *Inventarium et Collectorium (Chirurgia magna)* in 1363. This was first published at Lyons in 1478 (*La pratique en chirurgie du maistre Guidon de Chauliac*)[545] and there is a modern French edition published in Paris in 1890. This work, the most important that Guy de Chauliac produced, passed through many editions and adaptations and established him as the greatest surgical authority of the fourteenth and fifteenth centuries. In it he distinguished varicocele, hydrocele, sarcocele, and the like from the various kinds of hernia; he also described a radical operation for the cure of rupture. In the book, Guy also gave a good account of fractures and of their management in his day, and provided an outstanding description of the dentistry of the period. Rightfully the

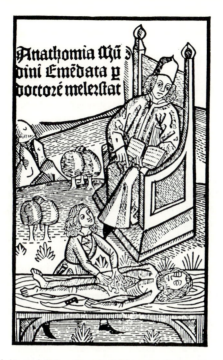

Figure 45 Mondino de'Luzzi (Mundinus). Title page from: *Anothomia* (about 1493).
[*From: William Osler. The evolution of modern medicine... New Haven, Yale Univ.
Press (1921).*]

book, the greatest text on surgery of the time, established his reputation and
allowed this to stand almost unchallenged for almost 200 years. Part of this
reputation must have rested on the work of those a generation or so older than
Guy de Chauliac who taught at Montpellier. Of these, Henri de Mondeville (*c.*
1260–1320) became the first who is known to have lectured with the aid of illustrations; he used 13 charts illustrating human anatomy and is the subject of a study
(*Die Anatomie des Heinrich von Mondeville...*)[546] published in Berlin in 1889.
An almost exact contemporary of this lecturer, whose presentations must have
refreshed those used to endless readings from the ancient authorities, was the
producer of one of the earliest important treatises on toxicology, Petrus de
Abano (1250–1315). This writer's *Tractatus de venenis...* [547] was published in
1472 and provides one of the finest, typographically, of the medicinal incunabula;
it is to this beautiful volume, and its translation into English of 1924, that those
concerned with therapeutics turn in order to see their subject represented among
the earliest volumes to be printed.

The first English medical writings of any real significance date from roughly
this period late in the Dark Ages. Before the Norman Conquest of 1066 medicine,
in England, was in the hands of the Saxon leeches, the 'wise women' of the towns
and villages, and the totally ignorant. All were using a mixture of herbal potions,
charms, spells, and gross superstitions. A scholarly study of the period is the
famous *Leechdoms, Wortcunning, and Starcraft of Early England*[548] by Thomas

171

Cockayne – a three volume work of 1864–66 which was written by a clergyman and collects together much detail of the Anglo-Saxon language and the practice of barbarian folk medicine; in Anglo-Saxon English it records the Herbal of Apuleius, it has also the Leech Book of Bald. Probably the other best-known work on the subject is the *Early English Magic and Medicine*[549] brought out by Charles Singer in 1920; this fine pamphlet is a reprint from the Proceedings of the British Academy, 1919–20. The history of medicine in Scotland from the earliest times was written by John Comrie[550] (1875–1939) who lectured at Edinburgh from 1913 – a period when Charles Singer (1876–1960) was at the forefront of the professional teaching of the history of medicine in London. The medicine of Anglo-Saxon times has also been the chosen subject of both Joseph Payne's FitzPatrick Lectures of 1903[551] and Wilfred Bonser's study[552] published in 1963.

The span of the Dark Ages in Britain is far longer than the dates usually given by general historians and Singer remarks that 'some of its documents undoubtedly date from as late as the thirteenth century.'[553] During this long period it would seem that demonology was not a particularly English characteristic. Instead there was a belief which the English shared with the continental Teutons and with the Celts. Singer[554] describes the doctrine in the following paragraph:

> It would appear that the Teutonic peoples had not the belief in possession by demons which was so characteristic of the near East where Christianity took its rise. Nevertheless a large amount of disease was attributed not to occupation by, but to the action of supernatural beings, elves, Æsir, smiths or witches whose shafts fired at the sufferer produced his torments. Anglo-Saxon and even Middle English literature is replete with the notion of disease caused by the arrows of mischievous supernatural beings. This theory of disease we shall, for brevity, speak of as the *doctrine of the elf-shot*.
>
> The Anglo-Saxon tribes placed these malicious elves everywhere, but especially in the wild uncultivated wastes where they loved to shoot at the passer-by. There were water-elves, too, perhaps identical with the Nixies of whom we learn so much from Celtic sources. Such creatures were perhaps personations of the deadly powers of marshes and waterlogged land.

A modern study of the subject is the *Anglo-Saxon Magic and Medicine*[555] of 1952 in which John Gratton became co-author with Charles Singer. This provides a full account of the beliefs and practices with which the people of the Dark Ages attempted to combat leprosy, plague and the great host of mediaeval diseases.

Many of these diseases affected the population of the times of the Norman invasion and the detailed recording of the properties of England given in the *Domesday Book* – the statistical survey of AD 1086. Even if the medicine of the time was primitive, the administration of the day was much less so and in compiling this book full advantage was taken of the experienced English administration, enlivening this with the great energy and possessiveness of the Conqueror. As an example, and because of its relevance to the important disease of leprosy, we can take the following paragraph from the *Domesday Book* volume devoted to Sussex and included in the 1976 edition edited by John Morris[556]:

In DUMPFORD Hundred
The Bishop holds ELSTED himself. He held it from King Edward.
Then it answered for 13 hides; now for 5½ hides. Land for . . .
In lordship 2 ploughs.
7 villagers with 23 smallholders have 2 ploughs.
2 slaves; a mill at 4s; a church; woodland, 10 pigs; grazing, 1 pig in 7.
Richard holds 1 hide of this manor; Osbern the cleric, ½ hide; Ralph the
    priest 1 hide, which belongs to the church.
Value of the whole manor before 1066, later and now £15.

The unit of measurement used, the hide, in the seventh and eighth centuries had meant 'land for one family'; by the time of the survey it usually, but not always, meant a number of acres, most frequently 120, and it was regularly divided into four virgates. The acre varied regionally but, in general, was as much land as could be ploughed in a long day. Some neat-minded eleventh century administrators tried to organize things so that each Hundred contained 100 hides and each hide a 100 acres – but in practice these measurements varied and there remained regional differences.

The natural science of the people 200 years or so after the *Domesday Book* is contained in the *De proprietatibus rerum*[557] of Bartholomew Anglicus (fl. 1250); this work was published in Bazel about 1470 but was written about the middle of the thirteenth century. If formed a compact encyclopaedia of what was then thought of as natural science and became the most widely read book on its subject of the Middle Ages. Caxton is reputed to have learnt to print by studying this book. There is an English translation by John of Trevisa made in 1398[558].

The medicine of the period is that of the *Rosa anglica practica medicinae a capite ad pedes*[559] written by John of Gaddesden (Johannes Anglicus; *c.* 1280–1361). John was a prebendary of St. Paul's and physician to Edward II; the work was compiled about 1314 but was printed in 1492, achieving its own place in history by becoming the first printed medical book of an Englishman. The work is characterized by its many rural simplicities and superstitions.

English surgery of just a little later was, at its best, that of John of Arderne (1307–1370), the first real surgeon of England and an exact contemporary of Guy de Chauliac. John of Arderne practised at Newark-on-Trent but moved to London in 1370. His *Treatises of fistula in ano, haemorrhoids, and clysters*[560] edited by Sir D'Arcy Power was published in 1910 but was originally compiled about 1376. Power also, at the request it seems of Henry Wellcome, translated the *De Arte Phisicali et de Cirurgia of Master John Arderne, Surgeon of Newark, dated 1412*[561]; this publication of 1922 derives from the original manuscript forming part of the Royal Library at Stockholm.

This book was the first published by the Wellcome Historical Medical Museum following its foundation in 1913; it forms a fitting beginning to the later achievements of the present-day Wellcome Institute Library, London.

From biographical details in his treatises it is assumed that John Arderne was a surgeon in the service of Henry Plantagenet and afterwards with the first Duke of Lancaster for whom he visited Antwerp in 1338, Algeçiras in Spain in 1343 and Bergerac in Aquitaine in 1347. The Duke died of plague in 1361 and Arderne may then have attached himself to the Duke's son-in-law, John of Gaunt. Philippa, the granddaughter of John of Gaunt, in 1406 married Eric, King of Norway and

Sweden, and went to live in Stockholm with what Power (in advancing this alternative explanation for the presence of the manuscript in that city) calls 'a considerable retinue of English men and women'[562]. The manuscript shows the medicine of John of Arderne to be 'essentially that of the Saxon leeches, treatment by spells, herbs and nasty or innocuous substances'[563]. His surgery, by contrast, was far ahead of his time and his fame rests upon his invention of the successful treatment for anal fistula by laying open each ramification; this technique then fell into disuse for almost 500 years before it was rediscovered to form the basis of the modern operation.

Arderne's medicine can be judged from a prescription for deafness: 'Eggs of ants and earthworms beaten up with white wine and distilled in an alembic and, after cleansing the body, injected into the ear makes the deaf hear and stops tinnitus.'[564] Or from 'the following charm (which) has been found most satisfactory in cases of cramp by many who have used it both in foreign countries and at home'[565]:

> Take a sheet of parchment and write on it the first sign ⊞ Thebal ⊞ Suthe ⊞ Gnthenay ⊞ . In the name of the Father ⊞ and of the Son ⊞ and of the Holy Ghost ⊞ Amen ⊞ . Jesus of Nazareth ⊞ Mary ⊞ John ⊞ Michael ⊞ Gabriel ⊞ Raphael ⊞ The Word was made Flesh ⊞ .
>
> The sheet is afterwards closed like a letter so that it cannot be readily opened. And he who carries that charm upon him in good faith and in the name of the Omnipotent God and firmly believes in it will without doubt never be troubled with the cramp.

The original manuscript contains anatomical drawings (Figure 46) in the centre column and quaint illustrations of some of the conditions described in its margins. Figure 46, only one portion of the complete roll of the manuscript, forms Plate II of D'Arcy Power's text – but it gives a good idea of the paucity of anatomical knowledge of the best English surgeon of the time. The original text is damaged where it would explain the treatment being given to figure 1 of the right column of the manuscript. The second figure in the right column is suffering from chaudepisse (gonorrhoea) for which the treatment is 'Parsley and boil it in water until it is turned into a mucilage let it be well shaken with oil of roses or violets and then add to it the milk of a nursing woman āā, in which liquor camphor is dissolved and inject with a syringe.'[566] (Power's marks showing uncertainties in the translation or on the manuscript are omitted.) The fourth figure, right column shows prolapse of the rectum, a condition from which Henry IV suffered so it caused a good deal of interest at the time when the document was written. The figure in the centre of the left column is using a gargle for headache due to phlegm.

John Arderne lived until the fourteenth century was well advanced and the Stockholm manuscript is dated 1412. At this date Canterbury cathedral, built chiefly in the twelfth and fourteenth centuries, already stood; the oldest college of Oxford University, founded 1249, was over one and a half centuries old. Roger Bacon (1214–1292), founder of English experimental science, had been dead for more than a century and Chaucer (c. 1340–1400) for a decade, when an unknown scholar gathered together the materials. Arderne had written and produced this

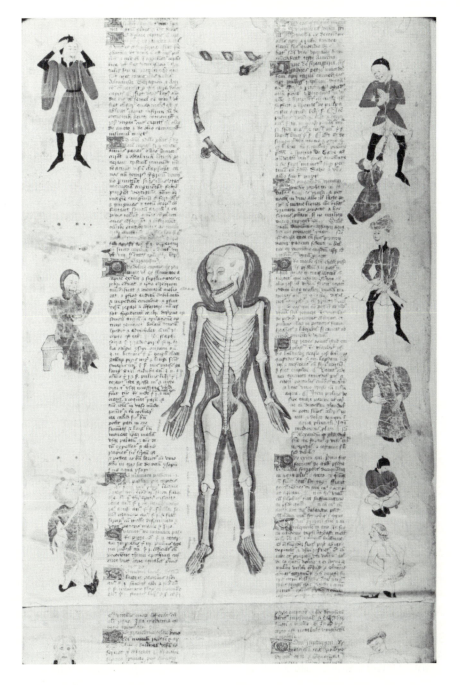

Figure 46 John of Arderne. From: *De arte phisicale et de cirurgia* (1412). [*From the* original ms., Kungliga biblioteket (the Royal Library), Stockholm.]

singular manuscript. Few things convey quite so vividly the state of the art of surgery and the practice of medicine in pre-Renaissance England as the thirteen plates, together making up the whole of the manuscript, with which Power illustrated his translation of 'Master John Arderne, Surgeon of Newark'.

The Church of the Middle Ages saw the need for faith rather than science but its teachings produced compassion and a willingness to undertake individual patient care in a way that had never before been seen. This led to the growth and foundation of hospitals which were, in themselves, one of the finest achievements of the twelfth and thirteenth centuries. The spirit of this great movement has been described by Rotha Mary Clay in her study *The Mediaeval Hospitals of England*[567]; one of the best histories of the period is *The Story of Medicine in the Middle Ages*[568] by David Riesman. There is also a fascinating collection, gathered from a number of sources, some of which are difficult to reach in themselves, in the 1965 publication of *Medical Illustrations in Medieval Manuscripts*[569] by Loren MacKinney.

It is likely that most of the early infirmaries and hospices grew alongside the cloisters but St. Bartholomew's was an exception for it was founded in 1137, by Rahere, a jester who took Holy Orders and obtained a grant of land from Henry I. Other early hospitals included the Holy Cross Hospital which was founded at Winchester in 1132 and, almost a century before John Arderne was born, St. Thomas's Hospital, founded by Peter, Bishop of Winchester, in 1215.

These were the great city hospitals but The Hospital of St. Mary, situated in St. Martin's Square, Chichester, dates from 1269 and has provided continuous care of one sort or another since then. The main infirmary and chapel block (Figure 47) was completed about 1290 and provides a unique example of the minor Mediaeval hospitals that were once common in England. Most of these hospitals had a long single roof covering both the infirmary and chapel; these buildings were quite different from the almshouses of ancient foundation, mostly of the collegiate type with small houses ranged round a quadrangle and with a separate chapel. Of these establishments fine examples remain in St. Cross at Winchester and Archbishop Abbott's Hospital at Guildford. Both types of building serve, however, to remind us of the extreme squalor of the poor people of the Middle Ages. Hygiene, as it is now known, and had been known in classic times, was non-existent; the elementary medical care given in these establishments concentrated on the Offices and Intercessions.

The thirteenth century date of the founding of St. Mary's, Chichester, coincided with the peak in the spread of leprosy that characterized the Middle Ages. A small area of the country will serve to illustrate what happened widely – for there are everywhere records, and some remains, of the mediaeval response to the threat of leprosy. Compassion, in dealing with this disease, seems to have been lessened by ancient religious prejudice and anxious attempts to limit the spread of the disfiguring infection.

One of the architectural remnants of the time is the 'Leper's window' (Figure 48) in the West wall of the little Anglo-Saxon Church of St. Paul at Elsted, Sussex. This window is possibly unique – preserved by the strength of the Anglo-Saxon stonework with its characteristic 'herring-bone' pattern. Perhaps sheltered by some outside wooden covering, the leper passed his arm through the wall to receive the sacrament. The window serves as a reminder that the leper was an

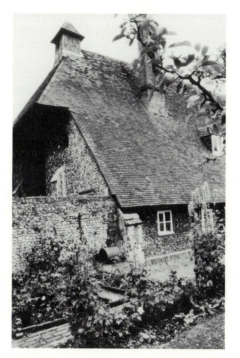

Figure 47 St. Mary's Hospital, Chichester, Sussex. The main infirmary and chapel block, completed about 1290.

outcast, often forced to live in a hut in the fields or in a separate dwelling and compelled to ring the 'Lazarus-bell' at his approach.

Many writers have studied the separate dwellings put apart for lepers; these include Charles Mercier who gave the FitzPatrick Lectures of 1914 on *Leper Houses and Mediaeval Hospitals*[570] (published 1915). To come closer to the Hundred mentioned in referring to the *Domesday Book* (p. 173), Walter H. Godfrey (*Mediaeval Hospitals in Sussex*, 1959)[571] has shown that there are records of 28 mediaeval hospitals in Sussex; nine of these were exclusively for lepers and one general hospital (Rye) made provision for leprous persons. This author says that 'These "lazar-houses" were usually built as a group of cottages within a close that also contained the chapel and buildings for the staff, but with the disappearance of the disease they became neglected and were ultimately demolished.'[572] One of these 28 Sussex lazar-houses was in the parish of Harting in Dumpford Hundred, adjacent to the parish of Elsted which has the Anglo-Saxon Church with the 'Leper's window'. The *Victoria History of the Counties of England*[573] gives the following account of the hospital at Harting:

Henry Hoese, or Hussey, founded a hospital for lepers, under the patronage of St. John the Baptist at Harting, early in the reign of Henry II. Agnes, wife of Hugh de Gundevile, gave 4 acres in Upton in East Harting to these lepers, and Henry II, some time before 1162, granted them a fair on St. John's Day, and its eve and morrow. Nothing more appears to be known of

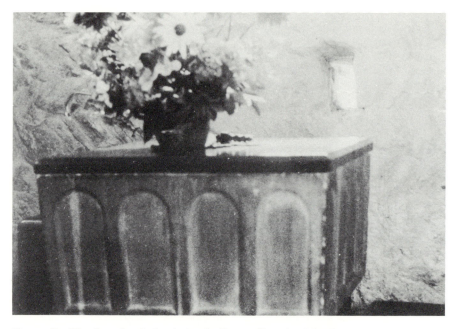

Figure 48 The 'leper's window', Anglo-Saxon Church of St. Paul at Elsted, Sussex.

this lazar-house until about 1248, when it was bought from the master of the
order of St. Lazarus by the abbot of Dureford, and absorbed into the estate of
that abbey.

Thomas Horsfield, in his book on *The History, Antiquities, and Topography of
the County of Sussex*[574] summarizes the same information with a footnote:
'Henry de Husee founded in this parish a small hospital for leprous persons, in
the reign of Henry II, afterwards subject to the abbey of Durford.' The record
can continue to be followed, like that of countless parish places in England.

At its most rigorous the exclusion of the leper involved his civil death and
subjection to ecclesiastical rites adapted from the taking of the veil. This dreadful
ceremony, a consequence of the diagnosis of leprosy, is described in the following
passage from Charles Mercier[575]:

> Wrapped in a shroud, and placed on a bier, he was carried into the church,
> his family and friends following as in funeral procession. Arrived in the
> church, which was hung with black as for a funeral, the leper was laid upon the
> ground, covered with a pall, and a requiem mass was said. He was then carried
> to the churchyard and laid beside an open grave, where the priest scattered dust
> three times upon his head, saying, ''Die to the world, be born again to God.''
> Then, while the *Libera me*, the psalm for the dead, was chanted, the leper was
> conducted to his cabin, at the door of which the priest gave him his scrip for
> alms, his stoup for water, his wallet for scraps of food, his gloves, his cloak,
> and his clapper, and addressed him in these terms: – ''While you are diseased
> you will enter no house, no inn, no forge, no mill, nor in the common well or

178

fountain will you drink or wash your clothes. You will not eat except by yourself or with other lepers. You will enter no church during service; you will mingle with no crowd. When you speak to any you will stand to leeward; when you beg for alms you will sound your clapper as a sign that you are forbidden to address anyone. You will not go out without your cloak; you will not drink but from your own fountain, nor will you draw water from any well or fountain but that which is before your door. You will always wear your gloves, and will touch no well-rope without them. You will touch no child, not even your own; and you will return to your cabin every night." In handing him the scrip the priest said: – "In this you will put the alms of the charitable, and you will remember to pray to God for your benefactors." The priest then planted a wooden cross before the door, fixed it to an alms box, and himself placed the first donation therein. The people followed his example, and then, after a prayer, the priest addressed the leper thus: – "My brother, through suffering much tribulation may you come to Paradise, where there is no sickness nor suffering, but all are pure and clean, resplendent like the sun. There you will go, if it please God. *Pax vobiscum*."

The ceremony was no idle form. The unhappy leper upon whom it was pronounced was civilly dead. His will took effect at once. His property was divided amongst his legatees and heirs.

If the leper were removed by law then he was subject to the writ known as *De leproso amovendo* which *Notes and Queries* of 1877[576], citing Judge Fitzherbert, says 'lieth where a man is a lazar or leper, and is dwelling in any town, and he will come into the church, or amongst his neighbours where they are assembled to talk with them, to their annoyance and disturbance – then he or they may sue forth that writ to remove him from their company . . .' In its Latin the writ is given in *Registrum Brevium . . .*, 1687[577].

The mediaeval medical information on leprosy came from the *Compendium medicinae*[578] published in London in 1510 of Gilbertus Anglicus (d. 1250). Gilbertus was the leading exponent of Anglo-Norman medicine at a time when the Normans improved the intellectual apparatus of the Anglo-Saxon physicians by sending them to continental Europe to be educated as clerics. Gilbertus favoured simple, Hippocratic methods of treatment but hesitated to implement these ideas; the most important aspect of his writing is that he provided an original account of leprosy and referred to smallpox as a contagious disease.

Leprosy was the most feared disease in the three centuries which followed the Norman conquest. The fear was clearly disproportionate to the incidence of the disease for, in England, it has been estimated that it is unlikely to have exceeded 4 or 5 per 1000 of the population. What is clear is that the experience of the disease in the thirteenth century led to the recognition that many fevers associated with obvious rashes, phthisis with its cough, and erysipelas with its fulminating signs, were all infectious and, like leprosy, could sometimes be spread by contact.

It is known that, at one time, there were over 200 lazar houses in England and some housed more than 100 patients; most probably held 20–30. The burden of diagnosis fell mostly on the clerics but the disease was common enough for them to be likely to know it on sight – so lessening the likelihood that they would make a mistake and pronounce (from the old Use of Sarum) 'The Office at the Seclusion of a Leper' in error. In a very literal sense the leper died before his time – once condemned to what was seen as divine punishment he could neither inherit nor bequeath property. Amongst this civic and clerical barbarism some kindliness seems, in some hands, to have prevailed, and E. B. Poland's account of *The Friars in Sussex 1228-1928*[579], a book published in the latter year but interesting for its study of mediaeval times, makes it evident that the friars not only cared for but, if need be, lived with the lepers.

The disease started to decline about the year 1315 and Cartwright[580] suggests that this 'may be connected with the widespread famine which occurred at the same time'. He concludes that 'The great mortality during the last half of the fourteenth century virtually ended leprosy in Britain.' If the measures taken to exclude the leper from the community played some part in controlling the disease, they might be thought to have had some usefulness. However, the rate at which leprosy disappeared, once the process had really begun, has suggested to many observers the occurrence of some natural calamity which decimated those already weakened by the disease.

Apart from famine, the main natural force which destroyed the lepers must be assumed to have been plague. From 1066-1300 the growth of the population seems to have been fairly progressive, suggesting that live births steadily exceeded deaths, even though the expectation of life was short. Local epidemics, most of them probably typhus associated with famine and malnutrition, are likely to have been the most obvious health problem.

Even so, only one famine of truly national proportions can be clearly identified – this was the disaster of 1257–1259. The size of the population in 1086, at the time of the Domesday survey, was about 1.25 million; by the year 1300 it had grown to about 4.25 million. These are, inevitably, only the most approximate of figures: although a good deal is known about the kings and nobles, the serfs and common people of those years were not important enough to be carefully counted.

Bubonic plague (the term 'the Black Death' to describe it was not invented until about 1820) is the virulent infection of rodents which is transmitted by fleas which are parasitic on both rats and man. The causative organism is *Pasteurella pestis* and by far the most lethal vector is the old English or Black rat (*Rattus rattus*) which readily associates with man and infests dwellings and warehouses and cities. The glandular, or bubonic, form of the disease does not usually cause grave pandemics; the fulminating, pneumonic form is a different story: being droplet-spread, so that the flea is no longer needed for its transmission, it is responsible for the rapid spread, high incidence, and massive mortality of the plague pandemics which have swept the world from time to time.

Between these outbreaks the dormant locations of the disease used to lie in the wastelands of Manchuria and the Far East. In 540-590 it broke out from these locations to sweep across Europe; waves of the disease, or some other infection similar in its mortality, remained in Europe for a time. Bede (*Opera Historica*)[581], in J. E. King's translation of 1930, describes the most noted visitation of the plague of the seventh century. The text of the Venerable Bede has the words 'subita pestilentiae lues...'[582] which the translator includes in the following passage[583]:

Now in the same 664th year of the Lord's incarnation an eclipse of the sun happened on the third day of the month of May about the tenth hour of the day: in the which year a sudden destructive plague, consuming first the southern regions of Britain, took hold also of the province of the Northumbrians; and raging far and wide with much continuance brought low in grievous ruin an infinite number of men. In the which affliction the foresaid priest of the Lord, Tuda, was carried off from the world and honourably buried in the monastery called Paegnalaech. Moreover, this affliction pressed sore on the island of Ireland with a like destruction.

The great illness seems to have been known as the 'Yellow Pest' and Bede elsewhere, writing of the same plague of 664, says of Bishop Cedd that, visiting a certain 'monastery in the time of a mortal sickness, being taken with illness of body in the same place he died'[584]; hearing of his death about 30 brethren of Cedd's old monastery journeyed to that which he had founded at Lastingham (near Whitby) but 'all died in that spot with the coming upon them of the destruction of the foresaid plague, except one little boy, who (as is well known), was saved . . .'[585].

Plague then retreated for something like eight centuries before being reactivated, probably by the opening of the trade routes to the East. Carried by migrant Tartar tribesmen, it reached the Balkan and adjacent countries, spread along the trade routes into Europe, and in 1348 was landed on the Dorset Coast at Weymouth. It remained, probably in its bubonic form, localized for a time but, within two months, erupted in its pneumonic phase and swept westwards to Devon, north into Bristol, and eastwards to London and Oxford. Held by the winter, it broke out the following spring and reached Ireland, carried there by shipping, in 1349; it was found in Scotland and Wales by 1350.

It is hardly possible to give even an approximate figure for the number who died – but the population fell, from that already given of about 4.25 million in 1300, to less than 2.5 million calculated on the basis of the Poll Tax returns of 1377. Thus, of the fairly small population of those times, it would seem that plague killed about two million.

From place to place the incidence of the disease varied. Charles Creighton, in his outstanding *A History of Epidemics in Britain* (1891)[586], taking an example of a badly affected town for which reasonable figures can be given, says of Yarmouth that 'in 1377, by the poll-tax reckoning, its population was about 3639. It may be assumed to have lost more than half its people . . .'[587].

The most reliable records were probably those kept by the monastic communities and, of these, Creighton gives some examples[588]:

At St Albans, the abbot Michael died of the common plague at Easter, 1349, one of the first victims in the monastery. The mortality in the house increased daily, until forty-seven monks, "eminent for religion," and including the prior and sub-prior, were dead, besides those who died in large numbers in the various cells or dependencies of the great religious house. At the Yorkshire abbey of Meaux, in Holdernesse, the visitation was in August, although the epidemic in the city of York was already over by the end of July. The abbot Hugh died at Meaux on the 12th of August, and five other monks were lying unburied the same day. Before the end of August twenty-two monks

181

and six lay-brethren had died, and when the epidemic was over there were only
ten monks and lay-brethren left alive out of a total of forty-three monks
(including the abbot) and seven lay-brethren.

Everywhere the grievous figure varied: 'At Ely 28 monks survived out of 43'[589]; at
Canterbury, which seems to have been specially favoured, 'In a community of
some eighty monks only four died of the plague in 1349.'[590].

This pandemic produced some of the more famous books of medicine. One of
the earliest printed medical books was the *Tractatus de epidemia et peste*[591];
published about 1470 by Valescus de Taranta (1382–1417). Some 3 years later
(1473) the *Buchlein der Ordnung der Pestilenz*[592] of Heinrich Steinhöwel
(1420–1482) appeared; this work became so well-known that it was often
reprinted and it was reproduced in facsimile in 1936. The plague also produced
the first medical book to be printed in England: this, *A litil boke the whiche
traytied and reherced many gode thinges necessaries for the . . . Pestilence*[593], was
written about 1357 by Johannes Jocobi (d. 1384), a friend of Guy de Chauliac; it
was printed in London about 1485 and became the most popular plague tract in
the England of the fifteenth century. There is a copy in the John Rylands Library,
Manchester and, from this, a facsimile reproduction was published in 1910.

The decimating plague epidemic of 1348–49 clearly changed the social
structure of mediaeval England, shaking the basis of feudalism and making the
common people, who had not previously been worth counting, a good deal more
important. After the great pandemic there was a pause. Then, in 1361, another
pandemic broke out. This is thought by most authorities to have been plague but
it produced its greatest mortality amongst children. Today such an effect, on
those born since the initial outbreak or not previously exposed, would not be
unexpected.

Gradually, plague became endemic in Europe. Eruptions of the disease, soon
to become the most feared of all illnesses, covered the long period from 1361 to
1665. The change in the natural history of this disease provides one of the more
significant lessons of therapeutics. In the mid-fourteenth century other, new
forces were having their impact on the mind of man: amongst these new
influences were the New Testament teachings, made into English by John Wycliffe
(*c*. 1324–1384) and his successors, which were bringing forward thoughts of the
care of the individual man. Everywhere enquiring minds turned from the realms
of belief to consider the practical means whereby this might be accomplished.

The Renaissance – to about AD 1600
The revival of learning

Throughout the length of the Middle Ages learning in Europe acknowledged
Theology as its master, leaving little opportunity for either creative thought or
discovery. The late fourteenth century saw some restlessness in the face of the
authoritative way in which organized religious belief was imposed – and from
about 1450 a series of important events conspired to break the old mould. This

remarkable cluster of events included the invention of printing, the fall of Byzantium, the final proof to the world of heliocentric astronomy, the great voyages of discovery like those of Christopher Columbus (1451–1506), the discovery of gunpowder and the development of the first guns able to use it to shatter the structure of feudalism.

The gathering pace of the search for learning led to a demand for manuscripts and the means of study. The possession of a store of such manuscripts was important and Montpellier is thought to have had an advantage over Paris in this respect. In the twelfth century the shortage of manuscripts had led the Universities of Paris and Bologna to organize effective means of preparing manuscript books – and when the invention of printing did come it caused great anxiety to these organizations.

The credit for the discovery, in the West, of the means of printing in a useful form is usually given to Johann Gutenberg (c. 1397–1468) of Mainz, Germany. The magnificent Gutenberg Bible was of about 1456 and the great Psalter of 1457 became the first book to use more than one printed colour; it was also the first to carry a colophon naming its printer and the date and place of publication. Printing spread with extraordinary rapidity, due to the great demand for books from the students of the growing universities, and from Mainz it spread, in the decade after 1460, throughout Germany. Presses soon appeared in Italy, France and other European countries, and these frequently were operated by itinerant German printers. Most of the early works were liturgical, theological and legal but almost 40 000 editions are thought to have been published during the fifteenth century and these included an increasing number of medical works, herbals, and associated pieces of literature. Thus, by the year 1500 many of the great texts of the Greek and Latin classics had appeared in print and become available not only in universities but also to the increasing numbers of literate people who were found among the middle class that was beginning to arise. The first English printer was William Caxton (c. 1422–1491) who returned from Bruges to London in 1476 and set up a press in Westminster where he printed about 80 books including *The Canterbury Tales* and *Mort d'Arthur*.

Some of these presses were fed, before the incunabula had been much more than begun, by the fall of Constantinople to the Turks in 1453. This ended, after over 1000 years, the long span of the Byzantine Empire – and the flight of the Byzantine scholars equipped with their precious manuscripts to Italy and the other centres of learning in Europe was one of the chief means of the Renaissance. These manuscripts brought the Greek writers of antiquity to Europe in fresh, uncorrupted texts that were rapidly carried into print, often in volumes of great excellence and beauty. Once printed, these texts were, in themselves, responsible for much of the revival of learning.

Some of the scholars stirred by the new texts were the medical humanists already well versed in Greek and Latin and equipped with a lively interest in the natural sciences and medicine. Amongst these was Leonicenus (Niccolò Leoniceno; 1428–1524), professor of medicine at Padua and Bologna and an excellent Latinist, who translated the *Aphorisms* of Hippocrates and corrected the botanical errors of Pliny in a work called *De Plinii et plurium aliorum in medicina erroribus*[594] of 1492. The texts of Pliny, despite their original errors and those of the copyists down the centuries, were considered inviolable and the work of Leonicenus was of great courage. It was greeted with a storm of opposition and it is a comment on the intellectual climate of the Renaissance that both the work and its instigator survived. The book was itself remembered by later generations of botanists and made possible the orderly and scientific description of the materia medica.

The man who did more than anyone else to restore medical learning to England was Thomas Linacre (Figure 49; 1460–1524); Linacre, a graduate in medicine at both Padua and Oxford, was a friend of Leonicenus and became physician to both Henry VII and Henry VIII. He is revered for his Latin scholarship, his grammatical works, and his foundation of lectures on medicine at both Oxford and Cambridge. Linacre travelled to Italy and seems to have been the first Englishman to have fully understood Aristotle and Galen in Greek. However, it was his unique and accurate translations of the treatises of Galen that brought the vitality of the classical writings to much of the Continent and England: these provided the works of Galen on hygiene (*De sanitate tuenda*[595], Paris, 1517), therapeutics (*Methodus medendi*[596], Paris, 1519), and psychological medicine (*De temperamentis*[597], Cambridge, 1521); these translations were followed by Galen's works on the natural faculties (*De naturalibus facultatibus*[598], London, 1523), the pulse (*De pulsuum usu*[599], London, 1523), and semeiology (*De symptomatum differentiis*[600], London, 1524). These versions made physicians and students realize how distorted the previous texts had become; they were also the means of restoring the anatomy and medicine of Galen to their rightful place in the thinking of the day. Experimental and exploratory medicine had ended with the death of Galen in 201 AD; it was Linacre's contribution to revive Galen's approach to the subject after a lapse of more than 13 centuries.

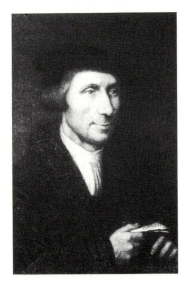

Figure 49 The portrait of Linacre at Windsor. [*From: William Osler. Thomas Linacre. Cambridge, Univ. Press (1908).*]

The practice of medicine in Britain had fallen to a parlous state by Linacre's day. Only a very small number of physicians were university graduates and only an equally small, or smaller, proportion of surgeons had been licensed by a university. All orthodox practitioners were clerks and the bishops therefore controlled the better forms of medical practice. By conferring on those clerks who had served as an acolyte the higher clerical grade of exorcist, which carried with it the power to cast out unclean spirits, the bishops could allow anyone they chose to practise medicine. Most of those who, early in the sixteenth century, practised with a bishop's licence were illiterate; apart from them, most of the practitioners of the day were illiterate barber-surgeons belonging to guilds whose guild-laws allowed them to practise only locally. Outside these two groups, licensed by either bishop or guild, a vast range of quacks, imposters, charlatans, and 'wise women' provided what little medical care the ordinary people were able to obtain.

At about this time a beginning was made on what gradually became the main source of care for the everyday people: grocer-apothecaries, often called 'pepperers', arose from the grocers and their guild and began to specialize in herbs and the drug trade. Frequently, whilst dispensing and selling their remedies, they provided elementary medical advice and decided what form the treatment should take.

Henry VIII (1491–1547), who was keenly interested in his own health as well as in public causes, brought some order into this muddled situation. In 1511–12 the monarch instigated the first Medical Act. This made it an offence to practise medicine or surgery without being either a university graduate or having a bishop's licence granted after the candidate had satisfied a panel of experts. Graduate physicians and the members of the guilds of barber-surgeons were excluded from the restrictions of the Act.

Due to the shortage of trained, even literate, people, Henry VIII's first Medical Act could do little more than limit the spread of quackery. The real need was for a body that could be involved in worthwhile medical qualifications – and this was achieved when Linacre obtained, by petition to his sovereign, Henry the Eighth's Charter establishing, in 1518, the Company of Physicians. In 1551 this body became the Royal College of Physicians of London. The Company was allowed to examine and license physicians throughout the realm and control practice within 7 miles of London; importantly, it was also allowed to ensure the purity of drugs sold in that area by the apothecaries.

There is a fine portrait of Linacre at Windsor and William Osler, in the Linacre Lecture of 1908, produced a finely turned tribute, published as *Thomas Linacre*[601].

The Renaissance artist and scientist, scholar and physician, were often one, and in Florence there was a Guild of Physicians and Apothecaries whose members shared the interest in anatomy of the artists who, from time to time, bought pigments and spices from the apothecary. It is from this type of background that Leonardo da Vinci (1452–1519) seems to have arisen. He was not only the finest draughtsman but also the greatest anatomist of Renaissance Italy.

The scientific study of the mechanics of flight began with Leonardo's research on birds. This was undertaken while he made attempts to build a flying machine and produce the work which formed the *Codice sul volo degli uccelli*[602], first printed in 1492 and republished in 1893; the same studies influence the fascinating

The Notebooks of Leonardo da Vinci[603] of which there is a fine edition of 1938.

Leonardo's chalk drawings, of the period about 1512, lay unnoticed until they caught the attention of William Hunter in the eighteenth century. They show Leonardo to have been a painstaking and skilled anatomist, well versed in the technique of dissection and able to display the relationships shown in deep dissection of the viscera. His drawings of the bones are systematic, like those of the great vessels of the heart and the brain in cross-section. He was also able to depict realistically the fetus within the uterus (Figure 71) – possibly this is what caught the eye of William Hunter who was later to produce the best atlas of its kind on the subject (Figure 101). His notes on the drawings are often in mirror-writing – a feature compatible with the cautious, secretive spirit of the age. His typically expressive drawings of the fetus at term form Figure 50.

Leonardo made something like 750 drawings of the main organs of the body and many of these show a markedly physiological approach to anatomy. The great collection of these works in the Royal Library at Windsor led to publication in a two volume edition of 1898–1901[604] and a six volume work of 1911–16[605]. However, many of the drawings were not adequately reproduced until recent years and the publications in New York of *Leonardo da Vinci on the Human Body . . .* [606] (which has an extensive apparatus by O'Malley and Saunders), dated 1952, and the *Corpus of the Anatomical Studies in the Collection . . . at Windsor Castle*[607] (edited by Keele and Pedretti) of 1980 are both instructive and exquisite.

Leonardo was a great traveller much involved in the affairs of his time. In 1470 he is known to have been working in a studio in Florence; later he was in Egypt as an engineer; in 1500 he was back in Florence as architect and engineer to Cesare Borgia. In 1506 he was in France, and he died near Amboise.

The engravings on copper and, almost to the same extent, those on wood, show the remarkable power of expression and detail of his close contemporary, Albrecht Dürer (1471–1528). Dürer's anatomical studies demonstrate his profound knowledge of the dissected body, and his great treatise on human proportion, *De simmetria . . .* (Nuremberg, 1532), is a work of fundamental importance to both anatomy and art.

These great artists of the Renaissance, Leonardo in particular, soon became the first people to seriously challenge the anatomy of Galen. The challenge continued in the work of Michelangelo (Michelangelo Buonarotti; 1475–1564), who was, by common consent, the finest monumental painter of the Renaissance. Michelangelo's knowledge of human functional anatomy and perspective fore-shortening permitted the glories of the ceiling frescoes of the Sistine Chapel (1508–12). In this work the knowledge of anatomy is so sure that Michelangelo is able to distort the normal and express the gestures, movements, and meanings of the Renaissance. He was also the architect of the profoundly moving Pietà in the Church of St. Peter, Rome, and one of the great writers of the time. The sensitive recent translation of *The Sonnets of Michelangelo*[608] by Elizabeth Jennings captures much of this expression. The promise of the new knowledge of the Renaissance and the stresses of the loss of the old mould of authority show in the passages in which Michelangelo speaks of 'Fruit from a tree too dry to bear or break'. The language is as compressed as the gestures of the frescoes.

In other hands the breaking of the old mould was forceful. Few show this more clearly than Aureolius Philippus Theophrastus Bombastus ab Hohenheim

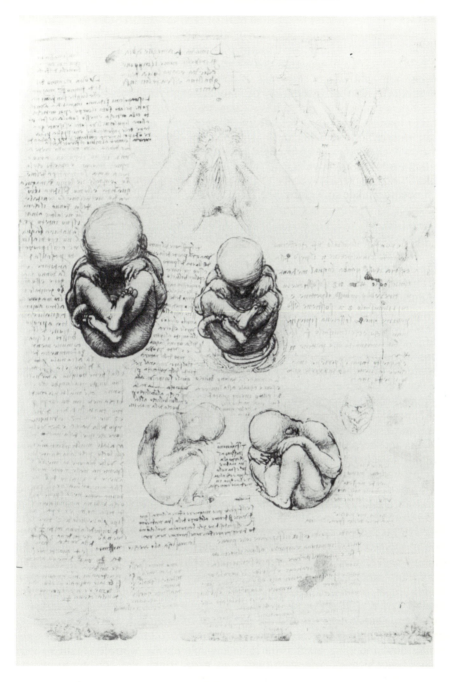

Figure 50   Leonardo da Vinci. From: *Quaderni d'anatomia...* (1911–16).

(1493–1541) who, in later life, called himself 'Paracelsus'. To shatter, in medical circles, the old grip of authority and mediaevalism, Paracelsus publically burnt the works of Galen and the *Canon* of Avicenna, then virtually the bible of medicine. It has been suggested that he adopted the titular name by which he has always been known to show his superiority to Celsus; others believe that 'Paracelsus' is a free translation of 'Hohenheim'. In either event his robust, mixed personality and contradictory but original writings provide a wealth of strange interest. Garrison[609] calls him the 'precursor of chemical pharmacology and therapeutics, and the most original thinker of the sixteenth century...' Morton[610] cites others who thought him 'uncouth, boorish, vain, ignorant and pretentious'. Osler[611] says that:

> Paracelsus is the Luther of medicine, the very incarnation of the spirit of revolt. At a period when authority was paramount, and men blindly followed old leaders, when to stray from the beaten track in any field of knowledge was a damnable heresy, he stood out boldly for independent study and the right of private judgment.

Paracelsus was born near Zürich in 1493 and his father, who was a physician, taught him both medicine and chemistry. Occultism, chemistry, and alchemy were mixed together in his early studies and he added to his knowledge of these subjects during his wide travels in the countries of Europe. When he returned to Germany he practised with great success in a number of cities and, almost always opposed by the local faculty of medicine, acquired a commanding reputation as a healer. In 1527 this reputation led to his being called to take up the chair of medicine in Basel but, as was inevitable, he quarrelled with the more timid spirits there and returned to his wanderings. In 1541 he died in Salzburg.

The paradoxes presented by Paracelsus are such that, while some of his beliefs were pure, individualized astrologic magic, others represented totally new insights and began interest in novel areas of therapeutics. In clinical practice he seems to have been a fine practitioner and surgeon who, unlike most physicians of his day, cared equally well for the noble and lowly. He was sympathetic to the therapeutic restraint of Hippocrates and yet interested in new sources of remedies. This interest led to his introducing a number of chemicals into practical therapeutics, and it is on these significant and often original introductions that much of his fame now rests. He was a sufficiently keen observer to have been the first to show a relationship between cretinism and endemic goitre; he was also among the first to understand the geographic differences in diseases. His important medical works, in their modern versions, include the *Sämtliche Werke...* [612], published in Berlin in 1922–33, and the *Theophrastus Paracelsus Werke*[613] of W. E. Peuckert of 1965–69.

The surgical works showed the same level of originality. Paracelsus was one of the few to believe in clean, near-aseptic surgical techniques and he disbelieved in the use of boiling oil for the cleansing of gunshot wounds. His *Chirurgia magna* went through many editions and translations and his famous *Grosse Wund Artzney von allen Wunden, Stich, Schüssz, Bränd, Bissz, Beyn-brüch...* [614], of 1536, became one of the leading texts of its kind.

A great deal, both for and against Paracelsus, has been written since the sixteenth century – but there is no doubt, in his favour, that he shattered much scholastic dogma, lifted a weight of authority from the shoulders of Renaissance medicine, and provoked intense interest in the medical applications of chemistry. Among his more quaint beliefs, he recognized three substances – sulphur, mercury, and salt – as being basic ingredients of all organic and inorganic bodies. In pursuit of these and related ideas he made important discoveries regarding zinc, mercury and its compounds, sulphur and its derivatives and a number of other substances. He was a strong advocate of the medicinal use of iron and antimony, producing a vogue for the latter troublesome substance which has not totally left us even today. In terms of the useful, durable things of therapeutics his reputation rests most firmly on his introduction of laudanum, tincture of opium. This introduction led to experiment with, and a better understanding of the parent drug, opium. It was therefore among the more valuable of the accomplishments of Paracelsus.

Both the name and reputation of Paracelsus were well known to Shakespeare whose *All's Well That Ends Well* (Act II, Scene iii), talking of the case of the King which must be relinquished as being incurable, has the passage:

> *Lafeu*:   Both of Galen and Paracelsus.
> *Parolles*:   So I say.
> *Lafeu*:   Of all the learned and authentic fellows...

Shakespeare was making a valid comparison for, by and large, the drugs with which the King or anyone else might have been cured were either the vegetable remedies of Galen or the chemicals typical of Paracelsus. After Paracelsus, the galenicals remained contrasted with the chemical or spagyric medicines, and the Paracelsian physicians regarded chemistry as the fundamental basis of the knowledge of medicine.

The treatise usually known as *De gradibus (Septem libri de gradibus, de compositionibus, de dosibus receptorum ac naturalium)*[98], published by Paracelsus in 1568, contains most of his practical innovations in the use of chemicals in therapeutics. Of his several contributions to the knowledge of individual diseases, his writings on syphilis were amonst the most important. The *Von der frantzösischen kranckheit drey Bücher*[615] appeared in Frankfurt in 1553; Paracelsus termed the disease 'French gonorrhoea', so beginning a confusion which lasted until the nineteenth century. He also suggested the hereditary method of the transmission of syphilis and advocated mercury, taken internally, as a remedy for the disease.

There are a number of modern commentaries on Paracelsus and the collected works include the fine, two volume, *Opera omnia Medico-chemico-chirurgica*...[616] published in Geneva in 1662; in the first of these volumes the portrait of Paracelsus forming Figure 51 appears opposite the fine title page, here shown as Figure 52.

The Herbals

The first German pharmacopoeia (*Artzneibuch*)[617] was produced by Ortolff von Bayrlant (fl. *c*. 1400), a physician in Würzburg, in 1477. The oldest printed herbal

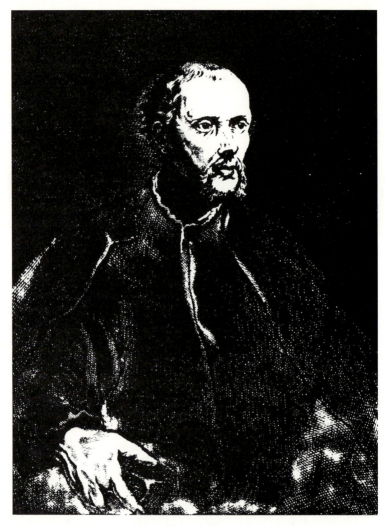

Figure 51 Paracelsus (1493–1541). Portrait from the *Opera omnia medico-chemico-chirurgica* . . . (1662), Vol. I. [*Royal Society of Medicine library, London.*]

with illustrations was the *Herbarius Moguntie impressus*[618] (1484). It is usually called the *Herbarius Moguntinus* and derives this name from the fact that it was printed in Mainz. The printer of this historic volume was Peter Schoeffer (1425–1502) who later the same year issued the *Herbarius*[619]; this was an entirely different compilation derived from much earlier material and containing some 500 crude conventional plant pictures and some fanciful pictures of animals. This fundamental work of botany (there are modern facsimile editions of 1924 and 1968) was followed by the *Ortus sanitatis*[620] (1491), one of the most important of the early herbals. There is an English translation of 1521, reprinted in 1954, and demonstrating the way that these books were beginning to assemble knowledge of

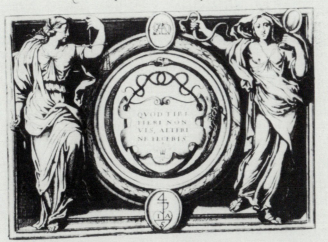

AVR. PHILIP. THEOPH.

PARACELSI

BOMBAST AB HOHENHEIM,

MEDICI ET PHILOSOPHI CELEBERRIMI,
Chemicorùmque PRINCIPIS,

OPERA OMNIA

MEDICO ~ CHEMICO ~ CHIRVRGICA,

TRIBVS VOLVMINIBVS COMPREHENSA.

EDITIO NOVISSIMA ET EMENDATISSIMA, AD GERMANICA
& Latina exemplaria accuratiſſimè collata: Variis tractatibus & opuſculis ſummâ
hinc inde diligentiâ conquiſitis, vt in Voluminis Primi Præfatione
indicatur, locupletata: Indicibusq; exactiſſimis inſtructa.

VOLVMEN PRIMVM,

Opera Medica complectens.

QVOD TIBI
FIERI NON
VIS, ALTERI
NE FECERIS

Sumptibus Ioan. Antonij, & Samuelis De Tournes.

M. DC. LIIX.

Figure 52 Paracelsus. Title page from: *Opera omnia medico-chemico-chirurgica* (1662), Vol. I.

the subject upon which most of the remedies of the day were based. Together these very early books formed the basis for the French *Le Grant Herbier*[621] or *Arbolayre (Le grant herbier en francoys, contenant les qualitez, vertus et proprietez des herbes, arbres, gommes & semences...)* published in Paris about 1520 and representing a considerable degree of accomplishment.

Genuine botanical science, replacing the more fanciful and inaccurate herbals, began with the work of the 'German Fathers' of the sixteenth century. The earliest of this group of writers was Otto Brunfels (1488–1534) of Mainz. Brunfels, a medical graduate of Basel, in producing his *Herbarum vivae eicones*[622] of 1530–36, went back to nature instead of copying the earlier writers. The result was a book based on personal observation which set a new standard; it was illustrated by 135 careful drawings by Hans Weiditz, the best wood-engraver of the day. In this book the original observations by Brunfels and the drawings seemed to go hand-in-hand, the illustrations far excelling the rest of the Latin text which drew heavily on Theophrastus, Dioscorides and Pliny.

The actual description of plants took its first fresh start since the Greeks in the *New Kreütter Buch*[623] (1539) of Brunfel's younger contemporary Hieronymus Tragus (Jerome Bock; 1498–1554), a schoolmaster born near Heidelberg, whose book was followed by a later work showing the same love of plants. Bock escaped some of the errors of Brunfels and his books were popular as the texts were lively and written in his native German.

The most beautiful of these early German herbals was the *De historia stirpium commentarii*[624] (1542) of Leonhart Fuchs (1501–1566). Fuchs was professor of medicine at Tübingen and his book,. which was published in Basel, was a deliberate attempt to advance knowledge of the materia medica. It became the most famous herbal of the sixteenth century and is a treasured volume providing an accurate and detailed account of the medicinal plants and something over 500 excellent woodcuts. Of these, Figure 53 shows the illustration of *Papaver sativum* and Figure 54 (beautifully coloured in the original) the engraving which depicts the artists of the book. It was so popular that a new edition was soon published and there is a Flemish version, of 1543, which contains woodcuts of such excellence that it is perhaps to be preferred to the original edition. The name of Fuchs is preserved in the designation of the fuchsias. Fuchs, who produced a number of smaller reprints of his book, intending these for general use, was well known as a medical figure of his time and was the author of an important work on the plague.

The most gifted but tragic of these figures was Valerius Cordus (1515–1544), a Prussian who was the son of a physician and a devoted medical botanist. He was the discoverer of ethyl (sulphuric) ether (1540); he also undertook probably the most brilliant of the early exercises in plant discovery and original description. After his death his commentary on Dioscorides was edited with exquisite care by the humanistic bibliographer, Conrad Gesner (1516–1565) of Zürich. This totally unselfish work yielded the *Annotationes in Pedacii Dioscoridis Anazarbei de medica materia*[625], published in Strasbourg in 1561. The book included the description of the preparation and properties of ether and showed that Cordus had not only modernized the plant descriptions of Dioscorides but had listed roughly 500 new species of plants. It established Cordus as the originator of phytography.

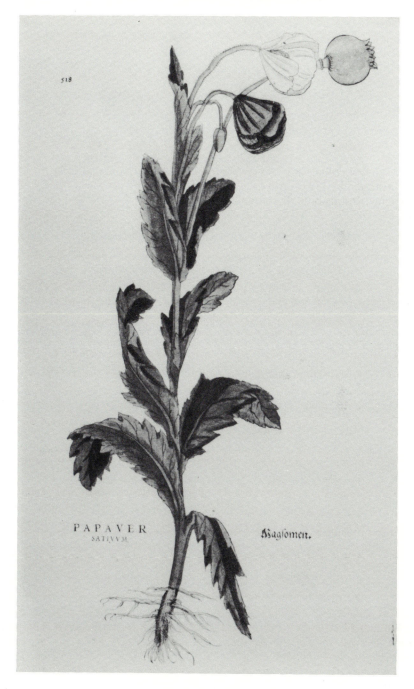

Figure 53 *Papaver sativum.* From: Leonhart Fuchs, *De historia stirpium commentarii* (1542). [*Wellcome Institute library, London.*]

193

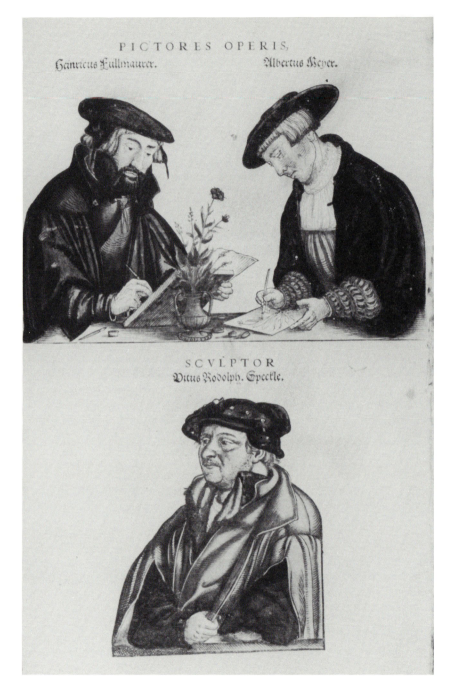

Figure 54   Pictores Operis. From: Leonhart Fuchs, *De historia stirpium commentarii* (1542). [*Wellcome Institute library, London.*]

In a curious way he also became the first to produce a real pharmacopoeia which achieved legal recognition. Holmstedt and Liljestrand[626] describe how this came about:

> In 1542 Valerius Cordus went to Italy studying at Padua, Ferrara and Bologna and continuing his work in botany. His botanical activities in the malarial regions cost him his life. In the summer of 1544 he went through Florence and Pisa towards Rome. Badly hit by a horse and suffering he died shortly after his arrival in the Eternal City in September 1544, when only 29 years old *"febri ardente extinctum"*.
>
> While on his way to Italy Valerius Cordus stopped at Nuremberg, where he remained for some time talking to the learned men and physicians of the free city. Upon hearing that he had compiled a work containing all old and new medical preparations, with many improvements of his own, the physicians of Nuremberg requested him to furnish a copy for the use of the apothecaries of that city. Valerius gave his manuscript to the Senate of that city for examination. A special committee reported that the book was the best and most complete possible, whereupon the Senate forthwith ordered that it be printed, and directed the apothecaries to prepare their medicines in accordance with its directions. The author died before the book was printed but it was issued by the Senate of Nuremberg in 1546 as a lasting memorial to that "learned and brilliant youth, Valerius Cordus".

There had been earlier town pharmacopoeias (the Venetian *Luminare majus* of 1496 and the Florentine *Nuovo receptario* of 1498) but the 1546 version of Cordus was the first to receive authorized publication and to be given official status. It is entitled *Pharmacorum omnium, quae quidem in usu sunt, conficiendorum ratio, vulgo vocant dispensatorium pharmacopolarum*[627] and the apothecaries of Nuremberg were directed to make their preparations in accordance with its directions. There is an important facsimile edition[628] published under the direction of L. Winkler in 1934 and, from this, the title page is reproduced to form Figure 55. In the process of time Cordus's *Dispensatorium* was followed by many town and regional pharmacopoeias, including the famed *Pharmacopoeia Londinensis*[629] – the first London pharmacopoeia, issued by the College of Physicians. Of this book the first edition was published on 7th May, 1618 but it was full of typographical errors and the name of the publisher was printed as 'Marriot'; a second, corrected edition appeared on 7th December, 1618 with the colophon showing 'E. Griffin for J. Marriott'. A facsimile reprint of both versions was published in 1944.

The English herbals seem to have begun with the anonymous *Here begynnyth a new mater, the whiche sheweth and treateth of ye vertues & proprytes of herbes, the whiche is called an Herball*[630], printed by Rycharde Banckes in London in 1525. Usually called 'Banckes' Herbal' it exists in only two known copies, one of which is in the British Library, London. It was reproduced, with a modern transcription, in New York in 1941. The first illustrated English herbal was the 'Great Herbal' (*The grete herball whiche geveth parfyt knowlege and understandyng of all maner of herbes and there gracyous vertues*)[631] published by Peter Treveris in 1526. This was mainly a translation of the French 'Grant Herbier'[621] which had appeared in Paris about 1520. Its woodcuts have considerable simplicity and

PHARMACORVM

OMNIVM, QVÆ QVIDEM IN

ufu funt, conficiendorum ratio.

Vulgo uocant

DISPENSATO-

RIVM PHARMACOPOLARVM,

Ex omni genere bonorum authorum, cum ueterum tum
recentium collectum, & fcholijs utilifsimis illuftra-
tum, in quibus obiter, plurium fimpliciũ, hacte
nus non cognitorũ, uera noticia traditur.

Authore

VALERIO CORDO.

ITEM

De collectione, repofitione, & duratione fimplicium.
De adulterationibus quorundam fimplicium.
Simplici aliquo abfolute fcripto, quid fit accipiendum.
Ἀντιβαλλόμενα, id eft, Succec anea, fiue Quid pro Quo.
Qualem uirum Pharmacopolam effe conueniat.

Cum Indice copiofo.

Confit at : ₴ ₤ ¡ ⁶ ₣

Norimbergæ apud
Ioh. Petreium.

Figure 55   Valerius Cordus. Title page of the 'Dispensatorium' (1546). [*From: Ludwig Winkler. Das Dispensatorium des Valerius Cordus faksimile...Mittenwald, Arthur Nemayer (1934).*]

196

Olúba is a byɔde dwellyng amõg mankynde but the turtyll doue deliteth lyuet in ꝑ feldes and dɔye trees onely The flesshe of turtyll doues is yll meate foɔ a man / bycause they haue often the fallynge sekenesse named eppilencia / wherby a persone might gette any dyseale causing grete harme to hymselfe. But the other doues ben not all holsome nouther. And a seke persone shall not eate of them. The blode vnder his ryght wynge / is good in medycynes.

☙ Foɔ the eyes. ꝛ

The same bloode dɔopped warme in the eyen wasseth the webbe therin.

☙ Foɔ impostumes. B

The blode put in open blaynes oɔ impostumes heleth thein.

☙ Caseus. Chese. Ca. CCCC. lxxviii.

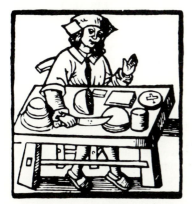

Chese is a meate not well dygestyfe and doth grete harme to them that hath a harde lyuer and mylte. Chese moch eaten dooth encrease the stone in the bladder / therfoɔe sayth the excellent mayster Constantyne. The chese is not good eaten foɔ telygrous persones dwellynge in monasteryes / but the chese which is fresshe & mylky is better to eate.

☙ Foɔ purgacyon.

The wey of chese is good foɔ seke persones it confoɔteth & lareth without harme and causeth temperatly purgacyon. The wey shall be made of the best Chepe chese ꝑ may be. Chese moche salted causeth many sekenesse & yll accydentes in a man. Fyrst it engendɔeth the stone in the bladder & letteth to pysse / & causeth ꝑ stomake slymy and without appetyte and soupleth ꝑ heed with yll humours and accydentes. Therfoɔe euery persone shall take hede foɔ to moche blyng of chese / foɔ to restrayne sekenes and pɔeserue hym selfe in helth.

☙ De Siligo. Rye.

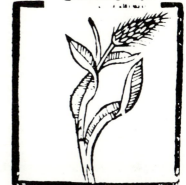

Siligo Rye nouryssheth moɔe thã barly. And the bɔede of rye nourysheth lesse thã wheate bɔede. ꝑ bɔede of rye is better foɔ thẽ ꝑ be in good helth thã foɔ seke folke / foɔ it causeth strength in a holsame body / & dyseaseth in a seke body. The wheat bɔede is onely good foɔ seke bodyes Bɔede of rye is not good foɔ them ꝑ hath a colde stomake foɔ they mare not dygest it. Take hede of eatyng all maner of bɔede ꝑ is not baken well foɔ it causeth many dyseases in the body.

Figure 56 Text page from: *The grete herball whiche geveth parfyt knowlege and understandyng of all maner of herbes and there gracyous vertues.* Southwarke, P. Treveris (1526). Edition of 1529, fol. Bb 5 verso. [*Wellcome Institute library, London.*]

charm and Figure 56 shows a typical page, in this instance illustrating the cheeses and rye.

The wine-loving churchman, scholar and doctor, William Turner (1510–1568), often called 'The Father of English Botany', produced a number of works including the very well known *A New Herball*[632]. The very fine paper, *Old English Herbals, 1525–1640*[633], given to the Royal Society of Medicine (*Proceedings*, 1912–13) by H. M. Barlow, gives the following account of Turner and the production of the three parts of his herbal:

> The first original English botanist of the sixteenth century was William Turner, Dean of Wells, Protestant divine, controversialist, and physician. He was born about 1510–15, and in 1531 was a Fellow of Pembroke Hall, Cambridge. Like his German contemporary botanists, Turner was a pronounced Lutheran, who threw himself heart and soul into the work of the reformers. He was, therefore, in constant trouble, and for preaching without a license was imprisoned and afterwards banished. Crossing to the Continent, he travelled extensively, studying botany under Luca Ghina at Bologna, and taking a medical degree either there or at Ferrara. On the accession of Edward VI, he returned to England, was appointed physician to the Duke of Somerset, became Dean of Wells in 1550, but was deprived of his office by Mary in 1553. He again crossed to the Continent and renewed his botanical studies, having a garden at Weissenberg and another at Cologne. When Elizabeth came to the throne in 1558, Turner returned, and was reinstated in his deanery, but four years later was again in trouble, being suspended for nonconformity. He died in 1568.
>
> He was the first English botanist who studied plants scientifically, and his work marks a new era in the history of the science in England. The superiority of his herbal over any of the earlier English publications is recognized immediately the comparison is made. This was published in three parts, the first in 1551.
>
> The second part was not published till eleven years later (1562) at Cologne by another printer, Arnold Birckman. The third part was printed in 1568, together with new editions of the first and second parts. This was the complete edition, published also at Cologne by the same printer, Birckman.

Of Turner's complete 1568 edition, Figure 57 shows the title page of the first and second parts, to which the third part had recently been added, and in which the names of the herbs were given in Latin, English, German, French, and Apothecaries' Latin. The first part of the complete edition was dedicated to Queen Elizabeth (Figure 58) and the third part to the 'right worshipfull Felowship and Companye of Surgiones'. Of the text pages of the volume, Figure 59 represents that giving part of the account of the 'herbe called Foxe glove, Digitalis'.

Each of these herbals made a significant contribution to the science of sixteenth century England. Turner also made a somewhat more specifically medical contribution with the *Libellus de re herbaria novus*[634], in which he treated plants as medicinal 'simples', without attempting to show their botanical relationship. But perhaps the best remembered of all the English herbalists was John Gerarde (1545–1612) whose *The Herball or Generall Historie of Plantes*[635], first published in London in 1597, became very well known. The original edition has 1392 numbered text pages (excluding the index and apparatus) and gives a

198

The first and seconde partes

of the Herbal of William Turner Doctor in Phisick/late=
ly ouersene/corrected and enlarged with the Thirde parte/ lately ga-
thered/ and nowe set oute with the names of the herbes/in Greke
Latin/English/ Duche/ Frenche/ and in the Apothecaries and Herbaries Latin/with the properties/
degrees/and naturall places of the same.

Here vnto is ioyned also a Booke of the bath of Baeth in England/
and of the vertues of the same with diuerse other bathes / moste
holsom and effectuall/both in Almanye and England/
set furth by William Turner Doctor
in Phisick.

God saue the Quene.

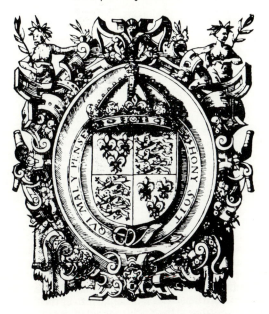

Imprinted at Collen by Arnold Birckman/In the yeare
of our Lorde   M. D. LXVIII.

Cum Gratia & Priuilegio Reg.Maiest.

Figure 57   William Turner. Title page from: *A new herball* (1568 edition). [*Royal
Society of Medicine library, London.*]

199

To the moſt noble and lear-

ned Princeſſe in all kindes of good lerninge, Quene Eliza-
beth/by the grace of God Quene of England/ France and Ireland/
Defender of the Fayth/rc. William Turner Doctor of Phyſicke/
wiſheth continual helth of both bodye and ſoule/ and daylye
encreaſe of the knowledge of Goddes holy worde/
with grace to lyue and rule Goddes
people accordyng to the ſame.

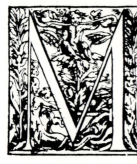

Oſt mightye and renoumed Prin-
ceſſe/after that I had made an end of þ third
parte of my Herbal/which intreateth of theſe
herbes/whereof is no mention made nether
of þ old Grecianes nor Latines/ I had ouer-
ſene agayne my firſt parte / and both corrected it and encreaſed it bery muche/ and had
alſo corrected the ſeconde parte: and the Prin
ter had geuen me warninge/ there wanted
nothinge to the ſettinge oute of my hole Her-
bal/ſauing only a Preface/wherein I might
require ſome both mighty and learned Pa-
tron to defend my laboures againſt ſpitefull & enuious enemies to al men-
nis doynges ſauing their owne/and declare my good minde to him that I
am moſt bound vnto by dedicating and geuing theſe my poore labours vn
to him. I did ſeke out euerye where in my mind/howe that I coulde come
by ſuche a Patron as had both learning & ſufficient autoritie/ioyned therewith to defend my poore labours againſt their aduerſaries/and in the ſame
perſon ſuche frendſhippe and good will towardes me / by reaſon whereof
I were moſt bound vnto aboue all other. After longe turninge this matter
ouer in my mind/it came to my memorye that in all the hole realme of En-
gland/ that there were none more fit to be Patroneſſe of my Booke / and
none had deſerued ſo muche / to whom I ſhould dedicate & geue the ſame
as your moſt excellent ſublimitie hath done : I haue dedicated it therefore
vnto your moſt excellent ſublimitie/and do geue it for the auoydinge of all
ſuſpicion of ingratitude or vnkindnes vnto you as a token and a witnes
of the acknowledginge of the great benefites that I haue recepued of your
Princelye liberalitie of late yeares. As for the ſupremitie of your power/
might and autoritie in this realme/there are none that will denye it/ſauing
onlye the bewitched hypocrites and bound men of the ſpiritual Babylon.
As for your knowledge in the Latin tonge xviij. yeares ago or more/I had
in the Duke of Somerſettes houſe (beynge his Phyſition at that tyme) a
good tryal thereof/when as it pleaſed your grace to ſpeake Latin vnto me:
for although I haue both in England/lowe and highe Germanye / and o-
ther places of my longe trauell and pelgrimage/neuer ſpake with any noble or gentle woman/ that ſpake ſo wel and ſo much congrue fyne & pure

       * ij   Latin

Figure 58   William Turner. Dedicatory page from: *A new herball* (1568 edition).

Of the herbe called Foxe gloue.
Digitalis.

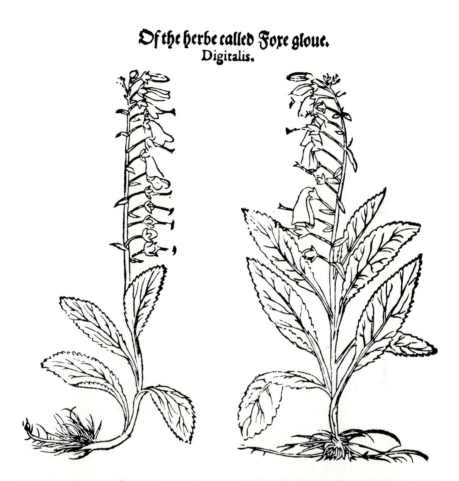

It hath a longe ftalke and in the toppe manye floures hanginge doune like belles or thumbles of diuerfe coloures / fometyme they are blewe / fometyme white / fometyme yelowifh.

The properties of Foxe gloue.

I Haue heard one that fayd / that he proued that the hole herbe / ftalkes / leues / and floures / bruifed a litle / and put betwene the horfe fadle and his back / is an excellent remedye againft the fatcye or fattones.

Figure 59 William Turner. Text page from: *A new herball (1958 edition).*

201

long list of maladies and their appropriate remedies at the back. The book was not without fault and is said to have been based upon earlier work which Gerarde failed to acknowledge; its many errors also needed correction in a second edition. This edition, of 1633, 'Very much Enlarged and Amended by Thomas Johnson, Citizen and Apothecarye of London', printed by Adam Islip and others, provides 1631 numbered text pages and brings the total number of plants described to about 2850. It has one of the finest title pages (Figure 60) of all the herbals.

The last of the great English herbalists was John Parkinson (1567–1650), a gardener's and countryman's book; the title is a pun on the syllables of the two principal books and, of these, *Paradisi in sole paradisus terrestris or a garden of flowers with a kitchen garden and an orchard*[636] is a work of leisure; it is a gardener's and countrymans book; the title is a pun on the syllables of the author's name. The second work is the *Theatrum botanicum: The theater of plants. Or, an herball of a large extent*[637], which was published in 1640. The herbals, as such, had now reached the limit of their development; some new, systematic method of dealing with their contents and material was becoming urgent. At their zenith they were, in England, represented by the Thomas Johnson edition of Gerarde's 'Herball' and John Parkinson's 'Theatrum botanicum...'. The latter, massive and splendid volume of 1755 pages describes almost 3800 plants and has been well described as 'one of the pillars of English botany'.

Interest in plant remedies was further stimulated by the success of the great Renaissance voyages of discovery and their provision of valuable drugs from far-off and exotic places. Christopher Columbus (1451–1506), born in Genoa but financed by Spain, led an expedition to find a westward route to India – and so reached the West Indies in 1492. He was reputed to be the discoverer of America and made three other voyages to the Americas. The second of these adventurers was Vasco da Gama (*c*. 1460–1524), the Portuguese navigator, who rounded the Cape of Good Hope, discovered and named Natal, and crossed the Indian Ocean to Calicut. The return journey was beset by unfavourable winds and the expedition took close on 3 months to cross the Arabian Sea. Many of his crew died of scurvy, but on his return to Lisbon Vasco da Gama became the first European to have rounded the Cape and reached India by sea. These voyages took place during the reign, in England, of Henry VII but some 20 or so years later, in the reign of Henry VIII, Ferdinand Magellan (*c*. 1480–1421) discovered (1520) the Magellan Straits, linking the Atlantic and Pacific Oceans at the extremity of South America, and now named after him. He was killed in the Philippines but one of his ships sailed on – to complete the first voyage around the world.

After these voyages the drug and spice trade became increasingly competitive in Europe. On the founding of colonies in the New World many new plants were brought back, and these included ipecacuanha, cinchona, other useful new drugs, and tobacco. The first to describe the medicinal plants of the New World was Oviedo y Valdés (1478–1557), Viceroy of Mexico, who published his *Sumaria de la historia natural de las Indias*[638] in Toledo in 1525. The first full treatise on these drugs, and for many years the most important study of the medicinal plants of Central America, was the *Dos libros. El uno trata de todas las cosas que traen nuestras Indias Occidentales...* [639] published in 1565 by Nicolás Monardes (1493–1588) of Seville. A second part of this work came out in 1571; the third

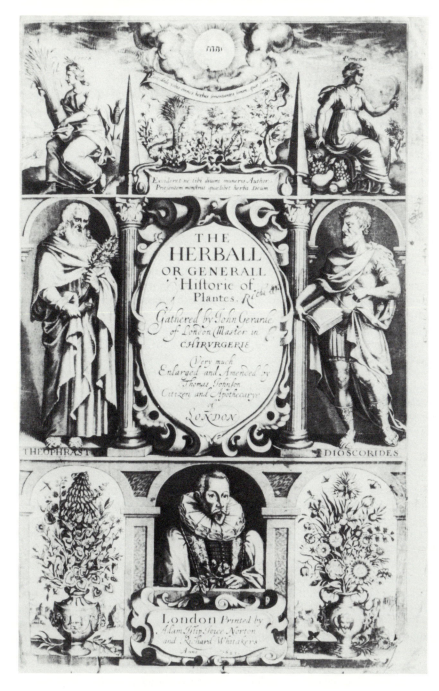

Figure 60 John Gerard. Title page from: *The herball or generall historie of plantes.*
Thomas Johnson edition of 1633. [*Wellcome Institute library, London.*]

part, together with the first two sections, appeared in 1574. Such was the longing for new remedies that when this work was translated into English, by John Frampton (fl. 1577–1596), it carried the title *Joyfull newes out of the newe found world*[640]; this appeared in 1577 and was reprinted in 1925.

The first European to attempt to describe the rich indigenous plant drugs of India was Garcia d'Orta (1501–1568) who published his *Coloquios dos simples, e drogas he cousas mediçinais da India*[641] in Goa in 1563. This was the first account of the Indian materia medica and the first European attempt at a treatise on the relevant areas of tropical medicine. It contains a classical account of cholera and was published, in an English translation by Sir Clements Markham, in 1913. The same study formed the basis for the *Tractado delas drogas, y medicinas de las Indias Orientales...*[642] produced by Cristobal Acosta (*c.* 1540–1599) in 1578; Acosta's work was little more than a translation of Garcia d'Orta but some important illustrations were added.

These few books, providing the first real studies of the plants and plant drugs of the New World, added to the contents of the great herbals of Europe; together they provide a great insight into a vast part of the therapeutics of the Renaissance. Of the whole field of study involved, a useful summary is provided by the privately-printed paper *Some Early Herbals and Pharmacopoeias*[643] produced by Douglas Guthrie in 1950 to accompany the exhibition, of the May and June of that year, in the University Library, Edinburgh. An excellent, full study, *Herbals, their origin and evolution*[644], was published by Agnes Arber in 1938.

The story of the growth of the herbals ended with the need to systematize botanical knowledge – the turning point being reflected in the magnificent '*De Plantis*'[645] (Florence, 1583) of Andrea Cesalpino (1524–1603). Cesalpino was professor of medicine at Pisa but he also taught botany and was in charge of the Botanic Garden founded in 1543. He classified plants by their fruits and was considered by Linnaeus to have been the first true systematic botanist.

Anatomy and Vesalius

The Renaissance saw not only the beginnings of chemical pharmacology, in the hands of Paracelsus, but also the addition of many vegetable substances to the herbals. These additions represented an expansion of the study of the plants and chemicals from which the new drugs were derived, and the results of these studies were entered into the first pharmacopoeias.

Part of the intellectual ferment of the Renaissance came to a head when, in 1517, Martin Luther (1483–1546), an almost exact contemporary of Paracelsus, challenged John Tetzel, a friar and seller of indulgences, to a debate. On October 31st, 1517, he fixed to the door of a church at Wittenberg a list of the 95 theses which were to form the subject of the historic discussion. It is this event which is usually taken as marking the beginning of the Reformation: the ultimate breaking of the old mould of revered authority. In 1520 the Pope issued a bull condemning the views of Luther – but the reformer publically burnt this at Wittenberg, making his breach with the established Church complete.

England also soon broke with Rome. Henry VIII had become King in 1509 and promptly married Catherine, daughter of Ferdinand and Isabella of Spain.

By about 1526 he had become enamoured of Anne Boleyn, but could marry her only upon the divorce of Catherine. The required break with the Church of Rome came in 1529 when Parliament decreed Henry supreme head of the Church in England. The work of reform was finished by the dissolution of the monasteries, with enormous cultural losses; medicine in England, at its best usually an aspect of clerical life, then began to adjust to the post-reformation years.

Its anatomy was still that of Galen, where the work of Galen was remembered and the available texts allowed it to be read. John of Arderne's anatomy, in the fourteenth century, was nothing like as good as Galen if the Stockholm manuscript (Figure 46) and his own writings are anything to go by. However, the demarcation between primitive, ancient anatomy and factual, modern anatomy was very soon to be drawn: historically, it can be placed at the date when, in 1543, the magnificent *De humani corporis fabrica libri septem*[646] of Andreas Vesalius (1514–1564) was published in Basel.

The 50 year period prior to the publication of the epoch-making masterpiece of Vesalius had opened with the appearance of the *Fasciculus medicinae*[647] of Johannes de Ketham (d. *c.* 1490) in Venice in 1491. The whole work was a collection of Renaissance medical treatises but its great importance is that it includes the first anatomical illustrations of any kind. There was a second edition (Venice, 1493) which includes four new woodcuts, each of them filling a folio page. These are, in each case, singular and very beautiful works, drawn only in outline, and full of expression.

The first (Figure 61) shows the physician, Petrus de Montagnana, lecturing from his rostrum; beneath him an old man and a woman with a child represent the patients. The second shows a pillared hall and a group of physicians in consultation. The third shows the actual process of dissection and the professor still lectures while an assistant dissects and the students listen and look on (Figure 62). The fourth engraving shows (Figure 63) a man sick with plague lying in his bed, attended by women and with two assistants carrying censers for fumigation. These remarkable woodcuts, from the Italian version of 1493 of Ketham, show the gravity which Venetian art could infuse into such subjects; they also demonstrate early Renaissance anatomizing. Not a lot had changed in the teaching of anatomy since the methods of Mundinus (Figure 45), whose *Anothomia*[543] was dated 1478.

Some of the errors of Mundinus were corrected by Berengario da Carpi (1470–1550), who provided the first mention of the vermiform appendix and gave the first account of the greater pelvic capacity of the female; he also described the thymus[648] and, a year after his first work, in 1522[649], published an improved book which included a description of the valves of the heart.

The descriptions of the next decade included the first account of the ileocaecal valve by the Spanish anatomist, Andrés Laguna (1499–1560)[650] and the appearance, in 1532, of the *De indiciis et praecognitionibus, opus apprime utile medicis...* [651], the first anatomical text by an Englishman, David Edwardes (1502–1542). Edwardes seems to have been the first to make a human dissection in England and his book, although published in facsimile in 1961, is now of such rarity that the only known copy is in the British Museum.

The idea of preparing good drawings, realistic in nature, gained ground and the best of the anatomical atlases before Vesalius was produced by Johann

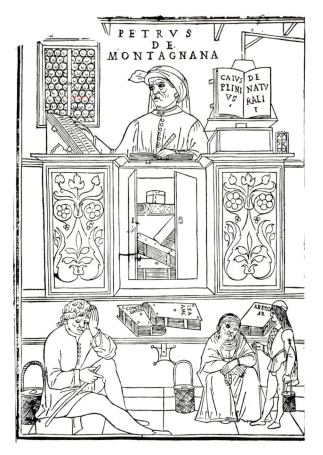

Figure 61   Petrus de Montagnana. From: Johannes de Ketham, *Fasciculus medicinae.*
Venice (1491). Edition of 1493. [*Royal Society of Medicine library, London.*]

Dryander (1500–1560), whose publications are of 1536[652] and 1537[653]. The first
book in which each muscle was shown separately was the *Musculorum humani
corporis picturata dissectio*[654] (?1541) of Giovanni Canano (1515–1579) who
suppressed his own book, with its fine copper-plates, after seeing the staggering
woodcuts of Vesalius's '*Fabrica*'.

There was, therefore, a rich but scholastic background to the studies in
anatomy of Vesalius. He was born in Belgium, of Flemish stock but German
extraction, and was a pupil of Sylvius (Jacques Dubois; 1478–1555), a committed
follower of Galen. Sylvius[655] had named the jugular, subclavian, and popliteal
blood vessels and a number of muscles with the terms we use today. Vesalius,
against the background of this traditional training, seems to have been
determined to move to where he could find the greatest opportunity to dissect. As
a result he became public prosector at Padua – and in five brisk and busy years
virtually completed his life's work, making anatomical discoveries one after the

206

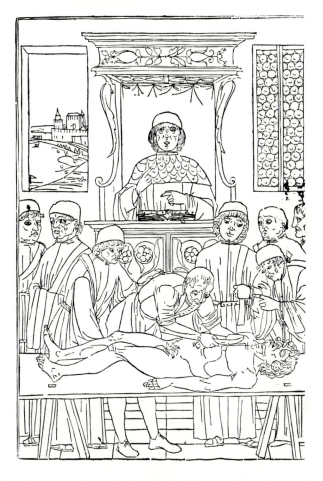

Figure 62 The dissection. From: Johannes de Ketham, *Fasciculus medicinae,* Venice (1491). Edition of 1493.

other. It is with Vesalius that a thoroughly practical basis for modern anatomy arose.

His challenge to parts of the tradition surrounded him with controversy and his old teacher, Sylvius, broke with him for opposing the views of Galen. Although at 21 he was elected to the chair of anatomy and surgery at Padua, he suffered greatly from the surrounding hostility and, in the end, not only burnt many of his manuscripts but also rejected his career in anatomy. He then, still a young man, began a long period in Madrid as court physician to Charles V (1500–1558), Holy Roman Emperor and King of Spain. He made no further really important contribution, and it is with the '*Fabrica*' that the real work of Vesalius was done.

The masterpiece had been preceded by the *Tabulae anatomicae sex*[656] of 1538. Only two copies of the original edition of this, one of the rarest of major anato-

207

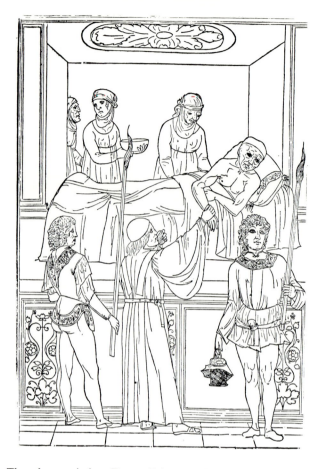

Figure 63 The plague victim. From: Johannes de Ketham, *Fasciculus medicinae,*
Venice (1491). Edition of 1493.

mical works, are known to exist. There was, however, a private reprinting for Sir
William Stirling-Maxwell in 1874 and there are modern impressions reduced in
size. Uniformly, these drawings show a radical departure from the mediaeval and
early Renaissance work that preceded them.

When, in 1543, Vesalius came to produce the magnificent *De humani corporis
fabrica libri septem* [646] he used a title page (Figure 64) which suggests one reason at
least why knowledge had advanced so far since the anatomizing (Figure 62)
shown in the Johannes de Ketham Venetian edition of the *Fasciculus medicinae* [647]
of 1493 – only some 50 years before.

The great title page, countless times reproduced, shows Vesalius himself
dissecting and demonstrating with students and a group of visitors watching.
There is a skeleton hung nearby for reference when needed, and this time it is a
student who is reading. Animals are available for a purpose which is not disclosed, and a group of what seem to be distinguished guests watch from the

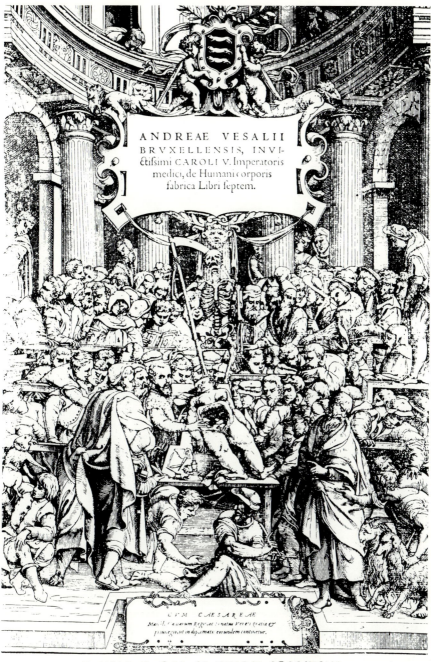

Figure 64   Andreas Vesalius. Title page from *De humani corporis fabrica* ... Basileae
(1543). [*Royal Society of Medicine library, London.*]

gallery. This point is, that the tissues and parts of the body and the instruments of dissection are in the hands of Vesalius – and the times had gone when the professor sat and read from Galen.

Vesalius provides a fine portrait of himself (Figure 65) in the woodcut that stands opposite page one of the '*Fabrica*'. The features are quite striking and are those of the man who worked at a time when knowledge was still so limited that, amongst the whole list of his innovations, he was able to draw and describe the thyroid gland for the first time.

ANDREAE VESALII.

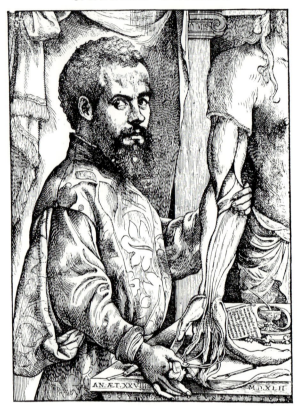

Figure 65 Andreas Vesalius. Portrait from: *De humani corporis fabrica*... Basileae (1543).

When the dissections and drawings were finished, Vesalius took enormous pains over the actual production of the work. Everywhere he had corrected and enlarged the work of Galen and he quite clearly set out to convey a detailed and accurate record of his discoveries, and of the whole of human anatomy, to the generations of anatomists who would follow him. He spent a year in Basel supervising the making of the great book – and it became fundamental to all departments of modern medical science; it is also one of the chief glories of the High Renaissance. The excellence of the illustrations can be shown in the drawings of the musculature, represented in Figures 66 and 67, taken from the library copy of the Royal Society of Medicine.

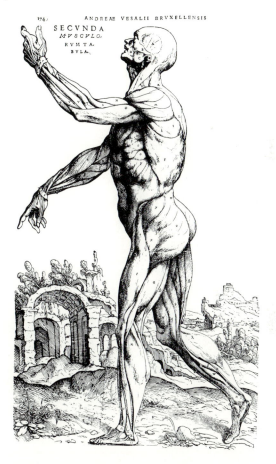

Figure 66 Andreas Vesalius. Secunda musculorum tabula. From: *De humani corporis fabrica*. Basileae (1543).

Although the volume marked the divide between mediaeval and modern anatomy, and Vesalius poured scorn on Galen's idea that the blood passed through the intraventricular septum by means of perforations that the eye could not see, he failed to understand the circulation of the blood, and this remained to be discovered by Harvey.

There is a very rare 'Epitome' (*Suorum de humani corporis fabrica librorum epitome*)[657] which was published by Vesalius in June, 1543, the same month as the '*Fabrica*'. This has (1949) been reproduced in a modern facsimile and translation; it preceded the 1555, even better, edition[658] of the '*Fabrica*'.

211

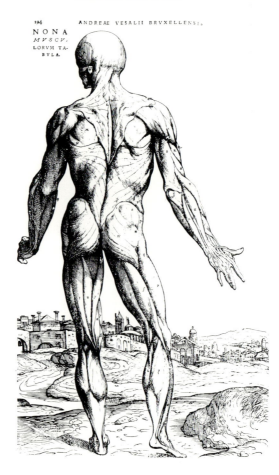

Figure 67   Andreas Vesalius. Nona musculorum tabula. From: *De humani corporis fabrica*. Basileae (1543).

These works have to be judged as being the most significant in the history of medicine since Galen. They established Vesalius as 'the Father of Modern Anatomy' and prepared for the birth of modern physiology which dates from the discoveries of Harvey. Most importantly of all, Vesalius, by the publication of the '*Fabrica*', finally ended the reverence for authority, even in science, which had constrained the centuries since Galen; the work began a new epoch of independent observation in anatomy and of discovery in clinical medicine.

The factual descriptions of Vesalius were supported by his pupil Fallopius (Gabriele Falloppio; 1523–1562) who became professor of anatomy at Ferrara, Pisa, and Padua. Fallopius was a careful and detailed dissector and became the first to discover and describe the chorda tympani and the semicircular canals. He gave a good account of the course of the cerebral blood vessels and enumerated all of the nerves of the eye. He is remembered in the names of the Fallopian tubes and the aqueduct of Fallopius which he described. His principal, and quite out-standing, work is the *Observationes anatomicae*[659], published in 1561.

However, the new teaching and spirit of Vesalius was not everywhere accepted and he was opposed not only by his old teacher, Sylvius, but also by Eustachius (Bartolommeo Eustachi; 1520–1574), who became professor in Rome. Eustachius was himself a fine anatomist and the author of the excellent *Tabulae anatomicae*[660], the publication of which was curiously delayed. The plates for this work were drawn by Eustachius and completed in 1552. For some reason, now not known, they remained unprinted and lay in the library of the Vatican until they were re-discovered early in the eighteenth century and, at that time, given by Pope Clement XI to Lancisi, his personal physician. Lancisi, realizing that the plates were even more accurate than those of Vesalius, published them, with a commentary, in 1714. It has been acknowledged that if they had appeared in 1552 Eustachius would have ranked with Vesalius as almost a co-founder of modern anatomy. As it was, in his lifetime, Eustachius produced the 1564 first edition of his *Opuscula anatomica*[661]; in this he provided observations which are funda-mental to many branches of medical science. A number of the plates in the work illustrate the structure of the kidney. Eustachius also discovered the thoracic duct, and the adrenal glands, and gave the first really accurate description of the uterus. He gave many original descriptions, including that of the cochlea and the origin of the optic nerves; he is eponymously remembered in the designation of the Eustachian tube.

Syphilis and Fracastorius

Vesalius is important in the history of pharmacology not only for his massive effect on freeing the Renaissance from the doctrines of authority but also for his pioneering effort in drug standardization. In this he was extending the concept first developed by Valerius Cordus in his 'Dispensatorium' (p. 195; Figure 55) of 1546. The pharmacological work, an epistle on the China-root, of Vesalius was of the same year (*Epistola . . . radicis Chynae decocti*[662], and is contained in a letter to his friend, Joachim Roelants (1496–1558); it was printed by Oporinus of Basel, who had printed the great '*Fabrica*'. The letter describes how Vesalius had used the China-root to treat the Hapsburg Emperor Charles V; it also shows the care and deliberation with which Vesalius used this drug and guaiacum or sarsaparilla to treat the royal patient. It makes his interest in exactly identifying the drugs and using them in meticulously measured amounts quite clear, and shows him to be observant regarding dose–response relationships. Vesalius is to be regarded as one of the earliest to have been critically interested in rational drug use and this aspect of his practice is well described in the biography *Andreas Vesalius of Brussels*[663], published in 1964 by Charles D. O'Malley.

Syphilis is significant in the history of drug use in the Renaissance. The illness was noted in Italy around 1493, soon after the return of Columbus and his crews from their second voyage to the New World. The disease spread rapidly and late in the fifteenth century became malignant in character.

Medical knowledge soon began to accumulate, Joseph Grünpeck (1473–1532) being the first, in 1496, to record[664] mixed and multiple primary lesions and to note the second incubation period of the disease. These primary lesions suggest the florid nature of the infection at that time and, in one of the earliest full treatises[665] on the subject, Niccolò Leoniceno (1428–1524) gave what is now considered a classic description of syphilitic hemiplegia. One of the best accounts of syphilis in the fifteenth and sixteenth centuries is given in the 1498 publication[666] of Francisco Lopcz dc Villalobos (1473 1549) and the full neurological manifestations of syphilis were well described by Niccolò Massa (1489–1569) in a book[667] dated 1507. Thus, a good deal was known about the rather fulminating form of syphilis affecting the European population in the years before Vesalius wrote his 'Epistle' to his friend.

The disease took its name from the most famous of all medical poems – *Syphilis sive morbus gallicus*[668] – published in Venice in 1530 by Fracastorius (Girolamo Fracastoro; 1478–1553). This poem, at one time extraordinarily well known and, from the first, a great literary success, became one of the monuments of Renaissance Latin. It is in three books and shows that Fracastorius not only recognized the venereal cause of the disease but also knew that it was specific and, despite its multitudinous features, comprised a distinct clinical entity. In the third book the poet sings the praises, as a remedy, of guaiac and introduces the shepherd, Syphilus, whose name, once accepted into common use, became that of the disease. The first complete English translation of the poem, which mentions mercury as a treatment for syphilis, was produced by Nahum Tate, later Poet Laureate, in 1686.

The success of the poem, great as it was and notable as it made the name of Fracastorius, may have served to eclipse his *De sympathia et antipathia rerum liber unus. De contagione et contagiosis morbis et curatione*[669], published in 1546, and representing a far important asset to science. It is this book which has led, of recent years, to a progressive revision of the reputation of Fracastorius, who was the first to put forward what can be recognized as a germ theory of infection. An account is given of typhus and the contagiousness of tuberculosis is suggested in the writings of Fracastorius, but the great interest of what he wrote, without the benefits of either microscopy or the techniques for culturing organisms, lies in the way in which he anticipated essential parts of modern germ theory. He described seeds or germs (*seminaria contagionum*) and seems to have thought of these, not so much as if they were living organisms but as if they were physical or chemical entities which could reproduce themselves in the right circumstances. He sees the illnesses caused by these organisms as being transmissible and specific to their individual cause. The whole account approaches a foretelling of modern knowledge and reads particularly vividly now that our understanding of the replication of viruses has blurred what once seemed a quite clear distinction between the reproductive capability of living cells and the far lesser attributes of things which are merely chemical. The '*De contagione . . .*' is available in an excellent translation by Wilmer C. Wright (1930), and the poem's modern versions in English include *Syphilis; or, the French Disease* by H. Wynne-Finch, 1935.

A great deal was added to the knowledge of syphilis in the newborn by Pietro Mattioli (1500–1577), who recognized[670] mercury as being specific in action in syphilis. Those who believe that the dreaded infection was brought to Europe from the New World rely heavily on the important *Tractado cótra el mal serpentino*[671] published in Seville, in 1539, by Rodrigo Diaz de Isla (1462–1542). This book gives an account of a new disease, obviously syphilis, which appeared in Barcelona in 1493. The account is of the early, readily contagious form of the disease affecting what is possibly a previously unexposed population.

Fracastorius discussed the aetiology of the disease in his poem. He suggests that it might have been infecting the community for a long time, gradually losing virulence, until something altered its history. He dismissed the astrological and magical explanations which were current at the time but admitted that the disease might well have been an import from the New World. The contagion was called the French Disease and, remarkably, mercury was used as a specific treatment almost from the beginning: possibly because it had long before been introduced by the Arabian apothecaries for the treatment of skin conditions. For this reason its use may have appeared appropriate to the skin lesions of syphilis.

It was also thought – as an aspect of the mystical concepts forming part of the Doctrine of Signatures of Paracelsus – that where peculiar diseases arise, there must also exist natural remedies of divine origin. These remedies, readily imported into Europe from the New World, included guaiacum, the core wood of *Guaiacum officinale*, a small resinous tree indigenous to the West Indies. The material was made into a decoction and used to treat syphilis and as a means of avoiding the salivation, dental loss, and dreadful systemic toxicity of mercury. The substance has no spirochaeticidal action but, nevertheless, remained popular. Although devoid of any satisfactorily demonstrated useful property it remained in the modern pharmacopoeias: Guaiacum Wood (BPC 1949)[672] had pharmacopoeial monographs after the last World War. The heartwood of *Guaiacum officinale* and *G. sanctum*, of the Zygophyllaceae, it is the source of guaiacum resin and an ingredient of compound sarsaparilla decoction. The only sensible use of the resin is the traditional test for occult blood in the faeces.

Other substances appeared and may have seemed effective, as the symptoms and signs of both the primary and secondary stages of the disease disappear as part of its natural history. Again, some of these came from the New World. They included sarsaparilla – the roots of various species of *Smilax* of the Liliaceae. The principal dried roots that were used were those of *Smilax medica* from Mexico, *S. ornata* from Jamaica, and *S. officinalis*, usually from Honduras. These *Smilax* species are woody vines and they kept their places in the pharmacopoeias until modern times: Sarsaparilla Liquid Extract was in the BP 1898[673]; Concentrated Compound Sarsaparilla Decoction remained in the BPC of 1949[674].

An additional remedy was sassafras, from a South American small deciduous tree, now known to be a carcinogen. The three antisyphilitic drugs, mercury, sarsaparilla and sassafras, in fact included a toxic but specifically-active metal and two ineffective plant remedies. In sixteenth century Europe the latter were (perhaps euphemistically) known as 'blood purifiers'. The name of sarsaparilla (it ended its medicinal life as a vehicle and flavouring agent for medicaments) persisted in music hall humour long after its use in the treatment of syphilis had been forgotten. There are also herbal and other 'blood purifiers' that, without any semblance of efficacy, trade upon memories of what they might purify.

Even in the sixteenth century there were some who worried about the gross toxicity of mercury and Fallopius, the anatomist, wrote an account (*De morbo gallico*)[675] opposing the use of quicksilver in the disease. The condition spread widely, and its first clear mention in the English medical literature occurs in the *Certaine works of chirurgerie*[676] published by Thomas Gale (1507–1587) in London in 1563. The whole span of the disease which could, in its manifestations, teach all aspects of clinical medicine, was covered for the sixteenth century in the *De morbo gallico omnia quae extant*[677] of Luigi Luigini (b. 1526); of this superb collection of literature Boerhaave himself published a revised and supplemented version in 1728.

Surgery and Ambroise Paré

Fracastorius, when studying at Padua, was a contemporary of both Desiderius Erasmus (1466–1536), the Dutch humanist who so greatly influenced the Reformation, and Nicolaus Copernicus (1473–1543), the Polish astronomer. Copernicus is attested to have left Padua in possession of all of the knowledge of the day in mathematics, astronomy, medicine and theology. He soon became disenchanted with the geocentric astronomy of Ptolemy, the Egyptian astronomer and geographer who had represented the earth as the fixed centre of the universe with the sun, moon, and other planets revolving around it from east to west in separate zones. Copernicus dismissed this belief and, in his *De revolutionibus orbium coelestium*[678] of 1543, showed that the earth is spherical and moves in orbit round the sun. Once established, the heliocentric astronomy of Copernicus caused a radical change in the mind of the Renaissance, compelling a previously anthropocentric world to acknowledge that the earth was by no means the centre of the universe.

The year 1543 was, therefore, auspicious: it saw not only the publication of the '*Fabrica*' of Vesalius but also the disturbing publication of the work by which, at the very end of his life, Copernicus was to transform astronomy and, by implication, challenge the account of the creation in Genesis. Whatever the impact of this challenge upon medicine it is clear that the man who, more than any other, brought the full strength of the '*Fabrica*' to bear on the surgery of the Renaissance was the Frenchman, Ambroise Paré (1510–1590).

The first work of the early German surgeons referring to the extraction of bullets and to rhinoplasty was written about 1460 by Heinrich von Pfolspeundt[679] (fl. 1460). The first proper account of gunshot wounds appeared about 1497 in a work[680] notable for its woodcuts, which are one of the earliest examples of medical illustration, written by Hieronymus Brunschwig (1450–c. 1512). A contemporary, Giovanni de Vigo (1450–1525) produced the first complete system of surgery since Guy de Chauliac, and this work[681] had a section on syphilis. The first printed picture of an amputation appeared in the *Feldtbuch der wundartzney* (1517)[682] of Hans von Gersdorff (fl. 1500) – a surgeon who performed many of these operations and came to oppose Paré's great step forwards, Paré having ended the horrendous practice of cauterizing gunshot wounds with boiling oil.

Paré abridged the '*Fabrica*' in the vernacular and used its knowledge and approach with great practicality. Born in poor circumstances and beginning as nothing more than a rural barber-surgeon's apprentice, Paré became a surgical dresser at the Hôtel Dieu in Paris and then a military surgeon; he used his experiences to become the finest surgeon of his time and to make a series of innovations of great importance to surgery. His fairly early treatise[683] on gunshot wounds, by then becoming common, was amongst his most important and was published in Paris in 1545. In this fundamental work he finally abandoned the practice of cauterizing gunshot wounds with boiling oil. In a brilliant study[684] of 1549 he revived the podalic version, previously described by Soranus of Ephesus, and made the procedure both popular and practical. He continued to make innovations and, in *Dix livres de la chirurgie, avec le magasin des instrumens necessaires à icelle*[685], provided his first description of the use of the ligature in amputation. He also introduced the use of artificial limbs, described fracture of the neck of the femur; prevented the almost inevitable castration which had previously accompanied herniotomy, and proposed syphilis as a cause of aneurysm. In 1575, in his first full-scale surgical work, collecting together many of his previous materials, he produced the splendid *Les oeuvres de M. Ambroise Paré*[686] (translated into English by Thomas Johnson in 1634). This precedes the J. F. Malgaigne editing of the *Oeuvres complètes d'Ambroise Paré* (1840–41)[687], widely considered to provide the best edition of the collected works and the great overview of the surgery of Paré.

Based on the anatomy of Vesalius, the progress made by Paré is remarkable. He stands out of an era of the crudest, most superstitious surgery as one able to illuminate the subject with good sense and enlarge it with important innovations.

His skill became a legend, and others discarded the old ideas of wound cauterization. Bartolomeo Maggi (1477–1552), professor of surgery at Bologna, in a work[688] of 1552, showed that not all gunshot suppurated; he therefore treated sound gunshot wounds with applications of saline and egg white. Thomas Gale (1507–1587), an English contemporary of Paré and surgeon to the army of Henry VIII at Montreuil, supported[689] Paré's views and disbelieved the superstition that bullets were always able to cause poisoned wounds; however, his therapy included thick ointments which must have produced a good deal of festering.

The 'weapon-salve' also received the faith of Wilhelm Fabry (1560–1634) – Fabricius, the 'Father of German Surgery' – whose *De gangraena et sphacelo*[690] was published in 1593 and who was the first to advocate amputation above the gangrenous or destroyed part. The establishment of such sound principles of surgery raised the subject in the hands of its Renaissance leaders so that the status of the surgeon changed and Peter Lowe (1560–1610), born the same year as Fabricius, became the founder of the Faculty of Physicians and Surgeons of Glasgow, after practising for many years in France. Lowe also produced *A discourse on the whole art of chyrurgerie*[691] which was published in London in 1596 and gives insight into the early years of operative surgery based on sound anatomy and accompanied by Hippocratic ethics.

The same approach began to change obstetrics. The earliest printed textbook for midwives was the *Der swangern frawen und hebammen roszgarten* (1513)[692] of Eucharius Rösslin (d. 1526) which was translated into English in 1540 by Richard Jonas and printed by Thomas Raynalde as the fascinating *The byrth of mankynde*[693]. The informed anatomical approach also showed in the splendid *La commare o riccoglitrice* (1596)[694], the first Italian obstetric textbook, in which Geronimo Mercurio (1550–1616) proposed Caesarean section in cases of contracted pelvis. It showed again in the 1609 *Observations diverses sur la sterilite, perte de fruict, feocondite, accouchements, et maladies des femmes, et enfants nouveaus naiz*[695] in which Louise Bourgeois (1563–1636), accoucheuse to the French Court, advocated the induction of premature labour in patients with contracted pelvis; it seems likely that her very sensible idea derived from Paré.

Medicine and Jean Fernel

In medicine there could be no advance to compare with the surgical progress of Paré. The doctrine of the four humours and temperaments was retained until late in the sixteenth century and, with no understanding of the general circulation of the blood, there could be no scientific physiology. The basis for rational and informed surgery provided by Vesalius was, therefore, missing in the case of the physicians – and had to await the discoveries of Harvey.

Limited progress in the descriptive elements of medicine could be made. Euricius Cordus (1486–1535), the father of the brilliant and better-known Valerius Cordus, wrote an important account[696] of the condition known as the sweating sickness. More accounts of the epidemics of this disease followed and included Joachim Schyller's (fl. 1529) description[697] of the German epidemic of 1528–30. The first English book on the sweating sickness was *A boke, or conseill against the disease commonly called the sweate, or sweatyng sickness*[698] – an account written by John Caius (1510–1573) and published in London in 1552. It came out a year after the last epidemic of the disease and describes a febrile illness with sweating accompanying fever and with pain in the limbs, nausea and vomiting, and sometimes delirium. The real nature of the disease is still uncertain. Whooping cough and hay fever were also amongst the conditions first described during the Renaissance – the former by Guillaume de Baillou (1538–1616)[699], one of the founders of modern epidemiology, and summer catarrh by Leonardo Botallo (b. 1500)[700].

With the span of life short the diseases of children attracted much attention, the first book on the subject by an Englishman being the work of Thomas Phaer (1510–1560); his *The regiment of life, whereunto is added a treatise of the pestilence, with the boke of children*[701] appeared in London in 1545. Other works described the beginnings of psychiatry. Johann Weyer (1515–1588), by means of his book *De praestigiis daemonum*[702] of 1563, is usually accounted the founder of medical psychiatry; mental illness first began to be separated from concepts of witchcraft by Reginald Scot (*c.* 1538–1599) whose book was called *The discoverie of witchcraft*[703] (1584). One of the first accounts of one particular mental illness studied systematically was the notable *A treatise of melancholie, containing the causes thereof*[704] which appeared in 1586 from the pen of Timothy Bright (*c.* 1551–1616).

Perhaps one of the greatest achievements in the medicine of the day was the publication, 11 years after the '*Fabrica*', of the *Medicina*[705] (1554) of Jean François Fernel (1497–1558) who Garrison considers 'the greatest French physician of the Renaissance'[706]. Garrison adds that: 'Having relieved the sterility of Catherine de Medici and the ill health of Diane de Poitiers, he feigned a pleurisy and other excuses to sidestep the dubious responsibility of royal physician, which was later forced upon him by Henri II.'[707]

The first part of *Medicina* was concerned with physiology and Fernel corrected a number of the errors of Galen. The second part was concerned with pathology and introduces the term for the first time in the modern sense. It is the first major treatise in which the signs and symptoms of each illness were considered in relationship to the development of the disease. Fernel became the first to describe appendicitis, endocarditis, and to differentiate true from false aneurysms. The third part of the great book dealt with treatment. It is one of the very first, perhaps the first, textbook of medicine that, in its approach, reads as a modern book. Apart from anatomy, the handling of the subject is physiological, then pathological, and then clinical – like a textbook of today. At the time the idea of devoting part or the whole of such a work to the structure of the organs in the diseased state was new. The intellectual approach of Fernel was probably as close as the Renaissance came to a comprehensive, functional view of medicine.

The *Medicina*, of 1554 – a tribute to French medicine if ever there was one, and to its humanism – contained a section (*De naturali parte medicinae libri septem*)[708] which had been issued before (1542). This part was the earliest work devoted solely to physiology and it was the first work to call the subject by its name. Fernel, for a long time, was directing physicians to study the normal body, then the changes of illness within it, and to reject tradition.

There was another remarkable book, the *Christianismi restitutio* (1553)[709], of the same period. This work was by Michael Servetus (1511–1553) and it appeared the year before *Medicina*. In this book the great physiological secret was almost unlocked: Servetus provides the first printed description of the lesser circulation. For his heresies, Servetus, by the order of Calvin, was burnt at the stake at Champel, Geneva. Most copies of the book were burnt with him. There is an imperfect copy in Edinburgh, a copy in Vienna and another in Paris. There is a modern translation of *Christianismi restitutio* by C. D. O'Malley (1953) and a later (1966) translation of the part which describes the pulmonary circulation (J. F. Fulton, *Selected Readings in the History of Physiology*).

There is a possibly even nearer grasp at the truth: in *Peripateticarum quaestionum libri quinque*, 1571[710], Andrea Cesalpino (1525–1603) comes near to the discovery of Harvey. He seems to envisage the idea of the general circulation of the blood and, in his *Quaestionum peripateticum, libri V* (1593)[711], records observations on the centripetal flow of the blood in veins. Lacking any sustained attempt at experimental proof, these ideas had no effect on Harvey or any of his contemporaries, but Cesalpino had come very close to the great understanding.

In England the Reformation quest for religious belief was represented by Cranmer's Prayer Book of 1549. This was 6 years after the '*Fabrica*' of Vesalius and 5 years before Fernel's *Medicina*. In 1533 Thomas Cranmer (1489–1556) had been made Archbishop of Canterbury. He pleased Henry VIII and proved instrumental in bringing into England the ideas of the church reformers; his affairs flourished with the establishment of the Protestant Church but, in 1553, with the accession of Mary (1516–1558), daughter of Henry VIII and Catherine of Aragon, the power of Cranmer ended. In the face of the restoration of the Catholic Church under Mary, accused of treason, he was sentenced to death and burned for heresy.

Against this background of the Reformation and Counter-reformation considerable institutions were established in England. In 1540, Thomas Vicary (*c.*

1548-1577) – who produced *The Englishman's Treasure*[712], the first English anatomy printed in the vernacular – secured the assent of Henry VIII to the formation of a United Company of Barber-Surgeons. Vicary was, in this way, following the example of Linacre of hardly 20 years before and, with royal protection, establishing a Company which could epitomize and protect proper practice over wide regions of the country. However, the Company, which had the right to anatomize the bodies of four executed criminals each year, could fine unlicensed surgeons only in London. An aspect of the Charter of 1540 which was of importance was that it relieved the surgeon of the requirement to act as barber; it also restricted the surgical efforts of the barbers to dentistry. In essence, the Charter began the separation of the surgeons from the barbers even though this long and difficult process was to take another 200 years to complete.

The progress made was very soon lost due to the lack of an adequate number of skilled practitioners. The cause was also damaged by the greed of established surgeons who were unwilling to help the poor. For these reasons further Acts of Henry VIII were passed in 1542-3 and these permitted those with a knowledge of herbal and folk medicine to administer to the indigent. Importantly, these provisions exempted those who took advantage of them from the penalties of the Charter of 1540, provided fees were charged only for the provision of the remedy itself. These exemptions not only permitted unqualified people to practise but, in a manner which affects the conduct of medicine today, materially influenced the later evolution and habits of the apothecaries.

The first part of the long reign of Elizabeth (1533–1603), daughter of Henry VIII and Anne Boleyn, was occupied with the establishment of the Church of England. During her reign the execution of Mary Queen of Scots (1542–1587) put an end to Roman Catholic plots and the defeat of the Spanish Armada in 1588 eliminated the second great threat to the throne. As the horizons of a strong settled England expanded Francis Drake (*c.* 1540–1596) became, between 1577 and 1580, the first of his countrymen to circumnavigate the globe.

One of those who in these adventurous years became widely experienced in military and naval practice was William Clowes (1540-1604). Clowes was probably the finest of the English surgeons of Elizabeth's reign; he became surgeon to St. Bartholomew's Hospital in 1581, was a fleet surgeon against the Armada in 1588, and was later made the Queen's physician. His *A prooved practise for all young chirurgians, concerning burnings with gunpowder, and woundes made with gunshot*[713], published in London in 1588, is usually reckoned to have been the finest surgical writing of the Elizabethan age. In amputating he covered the bone with integument, so providing a much improved result and a move towards the closure by a flap and the production of a rounded stump. A little earlier, Clowes had published the first original treatise on syphilis. This was *A short and profitable treatise touching the cure of the morbus gallicus by unctions* (1579)[714]. There is a facsimile reprint of 1972 and Clowes shows that something like three-quarters of the patients admitted to St. Bartholomew's were suffering from one form or another of syphilis.

The founding of the great institutions continued and in 1582 the University of Edinburgh was chartered by James VI (1566-1625), the son of Mary Queen of Scots and Lord Darnley; in 1603 he became also James I of England.

Thus, by the end of the Renaissance, medical institutions of great calibre and potential existed in both England and Scotland. Even so these great events may have changed the life of the common man surprisingly little: the everyday person probably believed what he was compelled to believe and, outside the great hospitals, was unlikely to come into contact with the limited improvements which had been made in medicine. Of the epidemics, leprosy, sweating disease, and epidemic chorea – so characteristic of the Middle Ages – had waned by the middle of sixteenth century; the most feared epidemic diseases were then plague and syphilis. The standards of medical care of the average person seem to have been those of folk medicine, the untutored herbalist, the imposter and quack: there were no drugs that had more than symptomatic efficacy and can be thought of as having been curative, apart from the very toxic forms of mercury and its derivatives used in syphilis.

Rising above this was the promise of the great hospitals, the mediaeval and Renaissance universities, and the new professional institutions. The Hospital of St. Mary of Bethlehem was converted from a monastery to a mental asylum ('Bedlam') in 1547. Bridewell was changed from being a palace to becoming a place of refuge in 1553. In the same year Christ's Hospital, once the Grey Friars' Monastery, became a charity for orphans. Thus, in a multitude of ways, the Renaissance was not only a time of re-birth but was also a time in which the new understanding found its rapid expression.

Discussion

The Dark Ages of Europe, reaching in the terms of the history of medicine from the death of Galen to the fall of Constantinople, were by no means the dark ages of Islam. In the East a great culture flourished while that of the West faded and survived in few but monastic hands. The period was that of the production of the most beautiful of manuscripts – an example (Figure 68), from the Wellcome Institute library, London, is provided by part of the first text page of the *Canon* of Avicenna translated into Latin by Gerardus Cremonensis and illuminated in Padua (J. Herbort), the work being dated 19 August, 1479.

Avicenna's work, in its several translations, is perennially interesting, and the fine study, *A Treatise on the Canon of Medicine of Avicenna...* [715] by O. Cameron Gruner (1930), is one of the several modern books which provide the interest and insight of these magnificent Islamic writings. In ending his treatise this author says: '... the time has come to close the ancient book. As we do so, we are conscious that our range of vision is widened, and our sense of responsibility deepened.' He speaks also of the fact that by the reading of Avicenna and the Persian experience, 'We face more confidently the exceptions to academic lore which are so much commoner than the rule.' Almost at the close of the book he concludes that a 'Deeper insight into the nature of man, and the wider outlook of a true philosophy does away with notions of the superiority of new over old, making clear, as it does, the necessity for combining and welding the two into a corporate whole.' These passages, written just before the great spate of modern drugs, which may not have advanced our holistic understanding in proportion to their obvious benefits, seem still worth reading. It is certainly hard to read the Islamic writers, even in translation, without developing a respect for the centuries

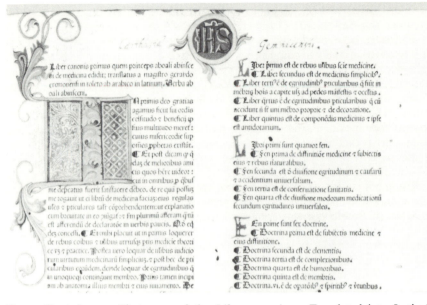

Figure 68 Avicenna. First page of the *Liber canonis*... Translated into Latin by Gerardus Cremonensis. Padua (J. Herbort). (1479). [*Wellcome Institute library, London.*]

of their tuition and the growth of their understanding.

The old remedies were relatively seldom given internally – perhaps wisely, for there were so few effective medicaments and only imprecise measurements of toxic effects. Nevertheless, medicines were not glibly given in ways that readily overcome the body's defences and it is worth recalling what Galen and his successors meant by an 'antidote'. Francis Adams (1847), in his commentary on *The Seven Books of Paulus Aegineta*[716], gives this definition:

> Those compositions which cure affections not when they are applied externally, but when taken internally, are named antidotes by the ancients. There are three different kinds of them. The first are those which are administered for deleterious substances; the second, for those animals called venomous; and the third are the remedies for affections occasioned by bad articles of food. Some antidotes profess to fulfil all these three purposes....

We would now use the word specifically, to indicate something that counteracts a poison. We would no longer use it, in a general sense, to suggest an antagonist against evil or something that acts against an attack of disease. We have certainly gone beyond using the term, as the ancients did, to signify a remedy taken internally.

But if the Islamic and Byzantine Periods have riches which outshine those of the Western Middle Ages, even ten such periods could not offer the significance of the Renaissance. Its music and art may, as the spirit of man re-awoke, remain unsurpassed. In its shedding of the ages of authority, the brightness of the Greek rediscovery and its willingness to present facts, simply as facts, it has been neither surpassed nor forgotten.

The change can be seen in the mind of one man. Leonardo, one of the greatest of artists, was a brilliant and experienced anatomist. The range of his talents can be seen, as nowhere else, in the drawings – about 600 in all – which are preserved in the Royal Library at Windsor. His work in anatomy occupied him for almost 30 years – from about 1485 to 1510–15. His interest is in the body in action, as a means to art, but it extends to a reverence to what he studies. His endowments were derived from a peasant girl, Caterina, and a Florentine notary, Ser Piero da Vinci.

Late in his life he said that he had dissected more than 30 bodies. He was born in 1452 and his first dated drawing dates from 1473. The metalpoint drawings of the 1480 decade include the early anatomical studies; his early discoveries include the maxillary antrum. In the 1490s he continued metalpoint drawing and there is a sheet (c. 1492–4) in which to 'display to men the origin of the second – first or perhaps second – cause of their existence'; he shows (Figure 69) a hemisected man and woman in coition. The drawing shows traditional ideas of the generative act:

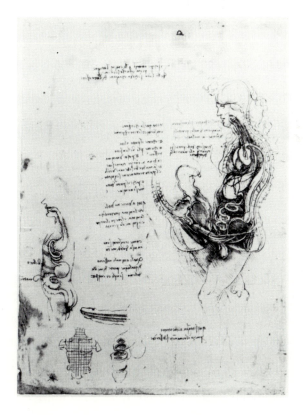

Figure 69 Leonardo da Vinci. Plate from *Quaderni d'anatomia...* Version of 1911–1916. Vol. III, Folio 3 verso.

Avicenna followed Hippocrates in believing that the thickest part of the seminal fluid, the part which carried the spirit or soul to the future embryo, came from the male spinal cord. Leonardo's drawing shows the mythical tube which carries the precious fluid from the lumbar region of the cord to the upper two passages of the penis. It shows also the way that the lower mythical tube of the male organ carries the lesser fluid from the testis to the female, just as it can carry urine. The corrugated appearance of the uterus derived from mediaeval ideas that this organ was divided into the celestial number of seven sectors; the epigastric veins are structures which Leonardo shows as leaving the upper side of the uterus with the blood of the retained menses of pregnancy; these later form milk from the breasts.

In the second part of the decade which began with the year 1500 Leonardo underwent a spate of renewed anatomical activity. This work was based on dissection and was concerned with the abdominal organs, the skeleton and musculature. In these works the artist passes beyond what might seem necessary for one concerned only with art. His drawing (Figure 70) of the male genitalia is,

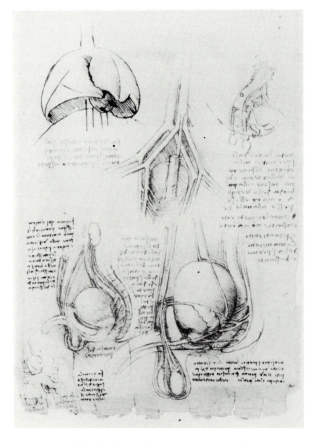

Figure 70 Leonardo da Vinci. Plate from *Quaderni d'anatomia*... Version of 1911–1916. Vol. III, Folio 4 verso.

in anatomical terms, masterly: it shows the vas deferens arising from the testis and passing to the seminal vesicles at the underside of the bladder; it shows also the ejaculatory duct entering the urethra just beyond the internal sphincter of the bladder. In each of these ways it demonstrates Leonardo's understanding of the anatomy of the region.

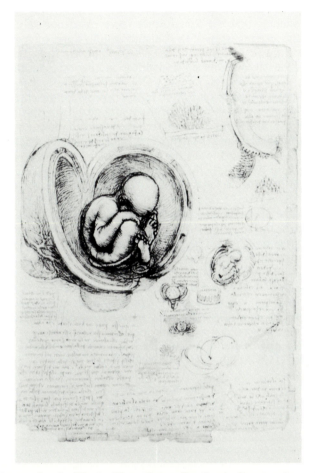

Figure 71 Leonardo da Vinci. Plate from *Quaderni d'anatomia...* Version of 1911–1916. Vol. III, Folio 8 recto.

He travelled between Milan, Florence and Rome in the years soon after 1510, settling in Rome in 1513. At this period his anatomical studies were almost continuous. Figure 71, in which he explores 'the great mystery' of the growing child in the uterus, is of this time. The particular fetus depicted shows the tucked-in heel and the winding umbilical cord, disturbingly close to the cervix, of other drawings of exactly the same period. Quite mistakenly, Leonardo shows, in the walls of the human uterus, the several interdigitating cotyledons which he had observed in a cow he had dissected a few years before. Apart from this, in the manner of the Renaissance, he has remained factual. It seems possible that the situation of the placenta below the presenting breech had brought this specimen, at or about term, to Leonardo. This is conjecture, but what is certain is that the spatial relationship of the fetus to the volume of the uterus has seldom been expressed with the same eloquence.

We can conclude that the Renaissance represented not only the revival of learning and the levering open of the old and crippling grip of authority but also the beginnings of a new attitude. This was a willingness to establish and enjoy facts for what they are without precipitately expecting explanation. Some of the records of the seeking for facts remain irreplaceable: Dürer's greatest work, *Vier Bücher von menschlicher Proportion* (1528)[717], provides an example. The first two books deal with the proportions of the anatomical form, the third represents fat and thin figures and seeks mathematical rules for the variations of the human form; the last book examines the figure in motion and studies the effects of fore-shortening. The whole work was not only new in its level of objectivity but was something done so beautifully that it lasted from the Renaissance.

The same attitude led to the founding of fact-based forms of modern science. The *Historia animalium*[718], 1551–87, of Conrad Gesner (1516–1565) is of this type: this was one of the starting points of modern zoology – a science which has its foundation in the work of Edward Wotton (1492–1555), author of the *De differentiis animalium*[719] published in 1552, and which recovered much of the spirit of Aristotle and swept away the grotesque accretions of the Middle Ages.

The respect for facts led to the beginnings of their organization. An example, of direct revelance to the development of modern therapeutics, was the 1564 *Enchiridion, sive ut vulgo vocant dispensatorium, compositorum medicamentorum, pro Reipub. Augstburgensis pharmacopoeia*[720], of which the 1613 edition became the official pharmacopoeia of Augsburg. This was the *Pharmacopoeia Augustana*, deriving directly from the 1564 work which was by Adolph Occo (1524–1606) and formed one of the very earliest of the pharmacopoeias.

The medical sciences of the Renaissance saw the surgical progress of Ambroise Paré and the physiological approach to clinical medicine of Jean François Fernel – but the greatest Renaissance achievement was the epoch-making *De humani corporis fabrica libri septem*[646] (1543) of Andreas Vesalius. The year of the publication of this book is one of the greatest dates in the history of medicine. It is also one of the landmarks along the difficult route by which the mind of man has travelled towards rationality.

The light of the Renaissance, brilliant as it was, shone against a background of wars, famines, epidemics, poor hygiene, squalid towns, the effects of a paucity of medical care, and the ravages caused by the absence of effective remedies for either the deprivations or diseases of the time. Together these factors produced a high infant mortality rate, a short expectation of life, and a slow growth of the population. To be set against all of this is the fact that where learning did exist it was refreshed by the revised, clean texts of the classics carried to the universities and the alert minds of the new middle class by the splendid, informative works of the printer.

Even if the darkness was slow to fade from the mind of everyman, the world had been set to think by Copernicus and Luther. The outline of the modern world had been sketched by Leonardo and the anatomist-artists. The beginnings of the concepts of modern science and medicine had been established by Vesalius and the great Renaissance humanists.

Those who seek to understand the process by which the mind of man obtained a finger-hold upon rational thought find it as hard to leave the study of the Renaissance as to leave the artefacts and evidences of the sixth and fifth century Greek experience.

References

459. Oribasius. Oeuvres d'Oribase, texte grec, en grande partie inédit collationné sur les manuscrits, traduit pour la première fois en français; par les Drs. Bussemaker et Daremberg. 6 vols. Paris, *Imp. nationale*, 1851–76

460. Oribasius (Oribasii). Collectionum medicarum reliquiae. In Corpus medicorum Graecorum. Ed. Ioannes Raeder. 4 vols. Lipsiae, *Teubner*, 1928–33

461. Waddell, Helen. More Latin lyrics from Virgil to Milton translated by Helen Waddell, Ed. Dame Felicitas Corrigan. London, *Gollancz*, 1976, p. 72

462. Barnett, Lincoln. History of the English language. London, *Sphere*, 1970, p. 80

463. Garrison, Fielding H. (1929). As ref. 179 but p. 127

464. Alexander of Tralles. Practica. (Lugduni, *per F. Fradin*, 1504). Vide edn. of 1522

465. Alexander of Tralles. Alexander von Tralles. Original-Text und Uebersetzung ein beitrag zur geschichte der medicin von Theodor Puschmann. 2 vols. Wien, *W. Braumüller*, 1878–79. Reprinted Amsterdam, 1963

466. Alexander of Tralles. Oeuvres médicales d'Alexandre de Tralles, le dernier auteur classique des grands médecins grecs de l'antiquité. Ed. F. Brunet. In Médecine et Thérapeutique Byzantines. 4 vols. Paris, *Geuthner*, 1933–37, Vol. 2, pp. 103–113

467. The Nag Hammadi Library in English, translated by members of the Coptic Gnostic Library Project of the Institute for Antiquity and Christianity, Ed. James M. Robinson. Leiden, *E. J. Brill*, 1977

468. Snowman, J. A short history of Talmudic medicine. New York, *Hermon*, 1935. Reprint, 1974

469. Pearlman, M. Midrash-Ha-Refuah. Tel-Aviv, 1929

470. Paul of Aegina. The seven books of Paulus Aegineta. Translated from the Greek by Francis Adams. 3 vols. London, *Sydenham Society*, 1844–47

471. Paul of Aegina. Paulus Aegineta. Ed. J. L. Heiberg. In Corpus medicorum Graecorum. Ed. Ioannes Raeder. 2 vols. Lipsiae, *Teubner*, 1921–24

472. Yuhannā Ibn Māsawayh (Mesuë Senior or Janus Damascenus). Mesuë opera. Venice, *R. de Nouimagio*, 1479. Vide edn. of Venice, 1603 pp. 41, 48, 53, and 76

473. Campbell, Donald. Arabian medicine and its influence on the Middle Ages. 2 vols. London, *Kegan Paul*, 1926, Vol. I, p. 61

474. Rhazes, Abū Bakr Muhammad Ibn Zakarīya Al-RazLiber Elhavi seu totum continentis Bubikir Zacharie Errasis filii, traducti ex arabice in latinum per Mag. Ferragium. [Brescia, *J. Britannicus*], 1486. The *Al-Hawi. or Continens*

475. Rhazes (Abū Bakr Muhammad Ibn Zakarīya Al-Rāzī). Rhazes de variolis et morbillis, Arabice et Latine. Ed. Iohannis Channing. Londini, *G. Bowyer*, 1766

476. Rhazes, Abū Bakr Muhammad Ibn Zakarīya Al-Razī). A treatise on the smallpox and measles. Translated from Arabic by William Alexander Greenhill, London, *Sydenham Society*, 1848

477. Haly Abbas ('Ali ibn-Al-'Abbās Al Majūsi). Liber artis medicine, qui dicitur regalis. Venetiis, *B. Ricius*, 1492. *The Almaleki*, or *Liber regius*

478. Campbell, Donald (1926). As ref. 473 but Vol. I, p. 79

479. Avicenna (Abu-'Ali Al-Husayn Ibn-Sina). Liber canonis. Mediolani, *P. de Lavagna*, 1473
    Vide: Avicennae Liber canonis, de medicinis cordialibus, et cantica cum castigationibus
    Andreae Alpagi Bellunensis... *Venetiis*, 1544
480. Browne, Edward Granville. Arabian medicine. The FitzPatrick Lectures delivered at the
    College of Physicians in November 1919 and November 1920. Cambridge, *Univ. Press*,
    1921. Reprint 1962
481. Albucasis (Abul-Qasim). Liber theoricae. Augustae Vindelicorum, *imp. S. Grimm & M.
    Vuirsung*, 1519. The *Altsrif* of Albucasis, the medical part
482. Albucasis (Abul-Qasim). De chirurgia. Arabice et Latine cura Johannis Channing. 3 vols.
    Oxonii, *e typ. Clarendoniano*. 1778 Albucasis' *Altsarif*, the surgical section
483. Avenzoar (Abumeron). Liber Teisir, sive rectificatio medicationis et regiminis. Venetiis, *J.
    & G. de Gregoriis*, 1490. Latin translation from the Hebrew version of 1280
484. Averroes (Abu'l Welid Muhammad ibn Ahmed ibn Rushad al Maliki). Colliget. Ferrarae,
    L. de Valentia de Rubeis, 1482. The *Kitab-al-Kullyat* or *Colliget* (Book of Universals)
485. Friedenwald, Harry (1944). As ref. 115 but Vol. I, p. 194
486. In hoc volumine hec continentur. Aphorismi Rabi Moysi. Aphorismi Jo. Dasmasceni.
    Liber secretorum Hypocratis, *etc.* (Venetiis, *J. Pencium de Leucho*, 1508). Contains the
    aphorisms of Maimonides and the writings of Mesuë the Elder
487. Bragman, Louis J. Maimonides' treatise on poisons. *Med. J. Rec.*, 1926 (July 21 and Aug.
    4), pp. 103–107, 169–171
488. Levy, R. (1917). In Singer, Charles. As ref. 238
489. Galen. De compositione medicamentorum secundum locos et secundum genera. In Opera
    omnia (edn. of 1821–1833). As ref. 336 but Vols. 12 and 13
490. Abn Bitar or Ibn-Beitar. Unprinted. *Vide* Pereira, Jonathan (1840) Part II: Tabular view
    of the history and literature of the materia medica, p. 6
491. Ullmann, Manfred. Islamic medicine. Edinburgh, *Univ. Press*, 1978
492. BPC (1934). As ref. 120 but pp. 490–491
493. The British Pharmacopoeia 1948 published under the direction of the General Council of
    Medical Education and Registration of the United Kingdom. London, *GMC*, 1948, pp.
    400–401
494. BPC (1934). As ref. 120 but pp. 731–732
495. Food Standards Committee report on flavouring agents. London, *HMSO*, 1965
496. Martindale, 27th edn. (1977). As ref. 1 but p. 1025
497. Paul of Aegina (Francis Adams edn. of 1847). As ref. 470 but Vol. III, p. 4
498. BP (1980). As ref. 79 but Vol. I, p. 75
499. British Pharmaceutical Codex 1959. London, *Pharmaceutical Press*, 1959, pp. 131–132
500. BPC (1934). As ref. 120 but pp. 267–268
501. BPC (1934). As ref. 120 but p. 266
502. Martindale, 27th edn. (1977). As ref. 1 but p. 294
503. Smith, Albert G. and Margolis, George. Camphor poisoning, anatomical and pharma-
    cologic study; report of a fatal case; experimental investigation of protective action of
    barbiturate. *Am. J. Pathol.*, **30**, 857–869
504. Aronow, Regine. Camphor poisoning. *J. Am. Med. Assoc.*, 1976, **235** (12), 1260
505. Sibert, J.R. Poisoning in children. *Br. Med. J.*, 1973, **1**, 803
506. Bellman, M.H. Camphor poisoning in children. *Br. Med. J.*, 1973, **2**, 177
507. Camphorated oil and camphor-containing drug products for over-the-counter human use;
    notice of proposed rulemaking. *Fed. Register*, 1980, **45** (189), 63869–63874
508. BP (1980). As ref. 79 but Vol. I, pp. 398–399
509. Smith, Barbara. Effect of irritant purgatives on the myenteric plexus in man and the
    mouse. *Gut*, 1968, **9**, 139–143
510. BPC (1934). As ref. 120 but pp. 944–945
511. BPC (1934). As ref. 120 but pp. 675–676
512. BPC (1959). As ref. 499 but pp. 731–732
513. The Animals (Cruel Poisons) Regulations 1963, S.I. 1963, No. 1278
514. BPC (1934). As ref. 120 but p. 545
515. Abu Mansur Muwaffak Bin Ali Harawi. Liber fundamentorum pharmacolo-
    giae... Primus Latio donavit R. Seligmann, 2 pts. Vindobonae, *Antonius Nob. de
    Schmid*, 1830–1833. Epitome from ms. of 1055

516. (Abu Mansur). *Vide* Rudolf Kobert, Historische studien aus dem Pharmakologischen Institute der Kaiserlichen Universität Dorpat. Halle a. S. *Tausch & Grosse*, 1893, **III**, 139–414

517. Wild, R. B. Dermatitis and other toxic effects produced by boric acid and borax. *Lancet*, 1899, **1**, 23–25

518. Valdes-Dapena, Marie A. and Arey, James B. Boric acid poisoning, three fatal cases with pancreatic inclusions and a review of the literature. *J. Pediatrics*, 1962, **61**, 531–544

519. Martindale, 27th edn. (1977). As ref. 1 but p. 272

520. Borax and boric acid. Pharmaceutical Society of Great Britain, meeting of Council. *Pharm. J.*, 1956 (April 21), 189–190

521. Council Directive of 27 July 1976 on the approximation of the laws of the Member States relating to cosmetic products (76/768/EEC). *Official Journal of the European Communities*, No. L 262/169–199

522. The Cosmetic Products Regulations 1978 (S.I. 1978 No. 1354), p. 35

523. British Pharmacopoeia 1980, Addendum 1982, published on the recommendation of the Medicines Commission pursuant to the Medicines Act 1968. London, *HMSO*, p. 14

524. British Pharmaceutical Codex 1963. London, *Pharmaceutical Press*, 1963, pp. 474–475

525. British Pharmacopoeia 1968, published under the direction of the General Medical Council pursuant to the Medical Act 1956. London, *GMC*, 1968, pp. 592–594

526. BP (1973). As ref. 236 but p. 290

527. BP (1980). As ref. 79 but Vol. I, p. xxvii

528. BP (1980). As ref. 79 but Vol. II, p. A235

529. Allbutt, Sir Thomas Clifford. Science and medieval thought, the Harveian Oration delivered before the Royal College of Physicians, October 18, 1900. London, *C. J. Clay*, 1901, p. 65

530. Constantine of Africa. Opera. 2 vols. Basileae, *H. Petrus*. 1536–39

531. Collectio Salernitana . . . raccolti ed illustrati da G.E.T. [*i.e.,* A.W.E.T. Henschel, C. Daremberg ed E. S. de Renzi]. 5 vols. Napoli, *Filiatre-Sebezio*, 1852–9

532. Magistri Salernitani nondum editi. Ed. Piero Giacosa. 1 vol. and atlas. Torino, *frat. Bocca*, 1901

533. The school of Salernum. Regimen sanitatis Salernitanum, the English version by Sir John Harington. History of the School of Salernum by Francis R. Packard, and a note on the prehistory of the Regimen Sanitatis by Fielding H. Garrison. New York, *Hoeber*, 1920

534. Nicolaus (Salernitanus). Antidotarium. Venetiis, *N. Jensen*, 1471

535. Shakespeare, William. Othello, III, iii

536. Daremberg, Charles Victor. Glossulae quatuor magistrorum super chirurgiam Rogerii et Rolandi. Ed. C. Daremberg. Neopoli et Parisiis, *J. B. Baillière*, 1854

537. Theodoric, Bishop of Cervia. The surgery of Theodoric ca. 1267. Translated from the Latin by Eldridge Campbell and James Colton. 2 vols. New York, *Appleton-Century-Crofts*, 1955–60

538. Garrison, Fielding H. (1929). As ref. 179 but p. 153

539. Platearius, Matthaeus. De simplici medicina seu Circa instans. *In* Nicolaus Praepositus, *Dispensarium*, Lugduni, 1537, ff. 70–96.

    Vide Dorveaux, Paul: Le livre des simples medecines traduction française du Liber de simplici medicina dictus Circa instans de Platearius . . . Paris, 1913

540. De virtutibus herbarum. Neapoli, *imp. per Arnoldum de Bruxella*, 1477

541. Albertus Magnus (Albert von Bollstädt). De vegetabilibus libri vii. Berolini, *G. Reimeri*, 1867

542. Nicolaus *Myrepsus*. Medicamentorum opus. Basileae, *per Jo. Oporinum*, 1549

543. Mondino De'Luzzi (Mundinus). Anothomia. Papiae, *Antonio de Carcano*, 1478

544. Osler, Sir William (1921). As ref. 19 but p. 105

545. Guy de Chauliac. La pratique en chirurgie du maistre Guidon de Chauliac. Lyon, *Barthelemy Buyer*, 1478

546. Mondeville, Henri De. Die Anatomie des Heinrich von Mondeville. Nach einer Handschrift der Königlichen Bibliothek zu Berlin von Jahre 1304 zum ersten Male herausgegeben von J. Pagel. Berlin, *G. Reimer*, 1889

547. Petrus *de Abano*. Tractatus de venenis. Mantua. (*Thomas of Hermannstadt*), 1472. English trans. *Ann. Med. Hist.*, 1924, **6**, 26–53

548. Cockayne, Thomas Oswald. Leechdoms, wortcunning, and starcraft of early England. 3 vols. London, *Longman*, 1864–66. Reprinted, 1961

549. Singer, Charles Joseph. Early English magic and medicine. London, *H. Milford*, 1920

550. Comrie, John Dixon. History of Scottish medicine. 2nd edn. 2 vols. London, *Baillière, Tindall & Cox*, 1932

551. Payne, Joseph Frank. English medicine in the Anglo-Saxon times. Oxford, *Clarendon Press*, 1904

552. Bonser, Wilfrid. The medical background of Anglo-Saxon England; a study in history, psychology, and folklore. London, *Wellcome Historical Medical Library*, 1963

553. Singer, Charles (1920). As ref. 549 but p. 1

554. Singer, Charles (1920). As ref. 549 but p. 17

555. Grattan, John Henry Grafton and Singer, Charles Joseph. Anglo-Saxon magic and medicine. London, *Oxford University Press*, 1952

556. Domesday Book, text and translation edited by John Morris. 2, Sussex, edited from a draft translation prepared by Janet Mothersill. Chichester, *Phillimore*, 1976, p. 17b, c

557. Bartholomew, Anglicus [de Glanvilla (Bartholomaeus)] De proprietatibus rerum. (Bazel, *B. Ruppel, circa* 1470)

558. Bartholomew, Anglicus. De proprietatibus rerum. (London, *Wynkyn de Worde*, 1495)

559. John of Gaddesden (Johannes Anglicus). Rosa anglica practica medicinae a capite ad pedes. (Papie, *J. A. Birreta*, 1492)

560. John of Arderne. Treatises of fistula in ano, haemorrhoids, and clysters. Edited by Sir D'Arcy Power, London, *Kegan Paul,* 1910

561. John of Arderne. De arte phisicale et de cirurgia. Translated by D'Arcy Power from a transcript made by Eric Millar from the replica of the Stockholm manuscript in the Wellcome Historical Medical Museum. London, *John Bale*, 1922

562. John of Arderne (edn. of 1922). As ref. 561 but p. xi

563. John of Arderne (edn. of 1922). As ref. 561 but p. viii

564. John of Arderne (edn. of 1922). As ref. 561 but p. 6

565. John of Arderne (edn. of 1922). As ref. 561 but p. 32

566. John of Arderne (edn. of 1922). As ref. 561 but p. 28

567. Clay, Rotha Mary. The mediaeval hospitals of England. London, *Methuen*, 1909

568. Riesman, David. The story of medicine in the Middle Ages. New York, *P. B. Hoeber*, 1935

569. MacKinney, Loren Cary. Medical illustrations in medieval manuscripts. London, *Wellcome Historical Medical Library*, 1965

570. Mercier, Charles Arthur. Leper houses and mediaeval hospitals. London, *H. K. Lewis*, 1915

571. Godfrey, Walter H. Mediaeval hospitals in Sussex. In Sussex Archaeological Collections relating to the history and antiquities of the County, published by The Sussex Archaeological Society. Haywards Heath, *Charles Clarke*, 1959, Vol. XCVII, pp. 130–136

572. Godfrey, Walter H. (1959). As ref. 571 but p. 131

573. The Victoria History of the Counties of England, Sussex. London, *Constable*, 1907, *II*, p. 103

574. Horsfield, Thomas Walker. The history, antiquities, and topography of the County of Sussex. Lewes, *Baxter*, 1835, Vol. II, p. 87

575. Mercier, Charles A. (1915). As ref. 570 but pp. 13–14

576. Ward, W. G. Leprosy. In Notes and queries: a medium of intercommunication for literary men, general readers, etc. London, *John Francis*, 1877 (5th series), Vol. 8, pp. 401–402

577. De Leproso amovendo. In Registrum Brevium tam originalium, quam judicialium...London, *Atkins*, 1687, pp. 267–268

578. Gilbertus Anglicus. Compendium medicinae Gilberti Anglici tam morborum universalium quam particularum nondum medicis sed et chyrurgicis utilissimum. Lugduni, 1510

579. Poland E. B. The friars in Sussex 1228-1928. Hove, *Combridges*, 1928

580. Cartwright, Frederick F. (1977). As ref. 178 but p. 29

581. Baedae (The Venerable Bede). Opera historica. With an English translation by J. E. King. I: Ecclesiastical history of the English Nation. 2 vols. London, *Heinemann*, 1930

582. Baedae (1930 but 1979 edn.). As ref. 581 but Vol. I, p. 484

583. Baedae (1930 but 1979 edn.). As ref. 581 but Vol. I, p. 485

584. Baedae (1930 but 1979 edn.). As ref. 581 but Vol. I, p. 447

585. Baedae (1930 but 1979 edn.). As ref. 581 but Vol. I, p. 447
586. Creighton, Charles. A history of epidemics in Britain. 2 vols. Cambridge, *Univ. Press*, 1891–94. Reprinted, London, *Frank Cass*, 1965
587. Creighton, Charles (1891 but 1965 edn.). As ref. 586 but Vol. I, p. 131
588. Creighton, Charles (1891 but 1965 edn.). As ref. 586 but Vol. I, p. 131
589. Creighton, Charles (1891 but 1965 edn.). As ref. 586 but Vol. I, p. 132
590. Creighton, Charles (1891 but 1965 edn.). As ref. 586 but Vol. I, p. 132
591. Valescus de Taranta. Tractatus de epidemia et peste. (Argentorati, *M. Flack*, c. 1470)
592. Steinhöwel, Heinrich. Buchlein der Ordnung der Pestilenz. Ulm, *Johann Zainer*, 1473
593. Jacobi, Johannes (Jacques; Jasme). A litil boke the whiche traytied and reherced many gode thinges necessaries for the . . . Pestilence. (London, *Willelmus de Machlinia*, 1485?) Facsimile of copy from John Rylands Library 1910
594. Leoniceno, Niccolo. De Plinii et plurium aliorum in medicina erroribus. (Ferrara, *L. de Valentia et A. de Castronovo*, 1492)
595. Galen. De sanitate tuenda, libri vi. Thoma Linacro Anglo interprete. Paris, *G. Rubeum*, 1517. *See also*: De sanitate tuenda. In his Opera. ed. C. G. Kühn, Lipsiae, 1823, **6**, 1–748. English trans. R. M. Green, 1951
596. Galen. Methodus medendi vel de morbis curandis: Thomas Linacro Anglo interprete. Lib. 40. Paris, 1519. *See also*: De methodo medendi. In his Opera. ed. C. G. Kühn, Lipsiae, 1825, **10**, 1–1021
597. Galen. De temperamentis. Cambridge, *Siberch*, 1521, *and* Galeni Pergamensis de temperamentis et de inaequali intemperie, libri tres: Thoma Linacro Anglo interprete. Facsimile, J. F. Payne, Cambridge, 1881. *See also*: De temperamentis. In his Opera. ed. C. G. Kühn, Lipsiae, 1821, **I**, 509–694
598. Galen. De naturalibus facultatibus. London, *Pynson*, 1523. *See also*: ref. 338
599. Galen. De pulsuum usu. London, *Pynson*, 1523. *See also*: De pulsuum usu. In his Opera. ed. C. G. Kühn, Lipsiae, 1823, **5**, 149–210
600. Galen. De symptomatum differentiis. London, *Pynson*, 1524. *See also*: De symptomatum differentiis. In his Opera. ed. C. G. Kühn, Lipsiae, 1823, **7**, 42–84
601. Osler, Sir William. Thomas Linacre. (The Linacre Lecture, 1908, St. John's College, Cambridge), Cambridge, *Univ. Press*, 1908
602. Vinci, Leonardo da. Codice sul volo degli uccelli. Pubblicato da T. Sabachnikoff; transcrizione e note di G. Piumati, con traduzione francese di C. Ravaisson-Mollien. Paris, *E. Rouveyre*, 1893
603. Vinci, Leonardo da. The notebooks of Leonardo da Vinci. Arranged, rendered into English and introduced by Edward MacCurdy. 2 vols. London, *Cape,* 1938
604. Vinci, Leonardo da. I manoscritti de Leonardo da Vinci della Reale Biblioteca di Windsor. Pubblicata da Teodoro Sabachnikoff. Transcritti e annotati da Giovanni Piumati. 2 vols. Parigi, *E. Rouveyre*, 1898–1901
605. Vinci, Leonardo da. Quaderni d'anatomia. I–VI. Fogli della Royal Library di Windsor, pubblicati da C. L. Vangensten, A. Fonahn, H. Hopstock. 6 vols. Christiania, *J. Dybwad*, 1911–16
606. Vinci, Leonardo da. Leonardo da Vinci on the human body. The anatomical, physiological, and embryological drawings of Leonardo da Vinci. With translations, emendations, and biographical introduction by Charles D. O'Malley and J. B. de C. M. Saunders. New York, *Henry Schuman*, 1952
607. Vinci, Leonardo da. Corpus of the anatomical studies in the collection . . . at Windsor Castle. Eds. K. D. Keele and C. Pedretti. 3 vols. New York, *Johnson Reprint Corporation*, 1980
608. (Michelangelo). The sonnets of Michelangelo translated by Elizabeth Jennings with a selection of Michelangelo drawings and an introduction by Michael Ayrton. London, *Folio Society*, 1961
609. Garrison, Fielding H. (1929). As ref. 179 but p. 204
610. Morton, Leslie T. A medical bibliography (Garrison and Morton) an annotated check-list of texts illustrating the history of medicine. 3rd edn., London, *Andre Deutsch*, 1970, p. 218
611. Osler, Sir William (1921). As ref. 19 but p. 135

612. Paracelsus (Bombastus ab Hohenheim (Aureolus Philippus Theophrastus). Sämtliche Werke... Herausg. von K. Sudhoff und W. Mathiessen. 14 vols. München, Berlin, *O. W. Barth, R. Oldenbourg*, 1922–33

613. Paracelsus, Bombastus ab Hohenheim (Aureolus Philippus Theophrastus). Theophrastus Paracelsus Werke. Besorgt von W. E. Peuckert. Bd. 1–5, Basel, *Schwabe*, 1965–69

614. Paracelsus (Bombastus ab Hohenheim (Aureolus Philippus Theophrastus). Grosse Wund Artzney von allen Wunden, Stich, Schüssz, Bränd, Bissz, Beynbrüch, und alles was die Wundartzney begreifft. Ulm, *Hans Varnier*, 1536

615. Paracelsus, Bombastus ab Hohenheim (Aureolus Philippus Theophrastus). Von der frantzösischen kranckheit drey Bücher. Franckfurt am Mayn, *H. Gülfferichen*, 1553

616. Paracelsus (Bombastus ab Hohenheim (Aureolius Philippus Theophrastus). Opera omnia medico-chemico-chirurgica, tribus voluminibus comprehensa. 2 vols. Genevae, *Sumptibus Ioan. Antonij, & Samuelis De Tournes*, 1662

617. Ortolff von Bayrlant. Artzneibuch. (Augsburg, ?*G. Zainer*), 1477

618. Herbarius Moguntie impressus. Mainz, *P. Schoeffer*, 1484

619. Herbarius. (Mainz, *P. Schoeffer*, 1484)

620. Ortus sanitatis. Moguntiae, *J. Meydenbach*, 1491

621. Le grant herbier en francoys, contenant les qualitez, vertus et proprietez des herbes, arbres, gommes & semences, *etc.* (Paris, *par Guillaume Nyverd pour Jehan Petit, et pour Michel le Noir*, ca. 1520)

622. Brunfels, Otto. Herbarum vivae eicones. 3 vols. Argentorati, *apud. I. Schottum*, 1530–36

623. Tragus, Hieronymus (Bock (Jerome)). New Kreütter Buch. Strassburg, *W. Rihel*, 1539

624. Fuchs, Leonhart. De historia stirpium commentarii. Basileae, *in off. Isingriniana*, 1542

625. Cordus, Valerius. Annotationes in Pedacii Dioscoridis Anazarbei de medica materia. Argentorati, *excud. I. Rihelius*, 1561

626. Holmstedt, Bo, and Liljestrand, Goran. Readings in pharmacology. Selected and edited by B. Holmstedt and G. Liljestrand. Oxford, *Pergamon Press*, 1963

627. Cordus, Valerius. Pharmacorum omnium, quae quidem in usu sunt, conficiendorum ratio, vulgo vocant dispensatorium pharmacopolarum. Norimbergae, *apud J. Petreium*, 1546

628. Winkler, Ludwig. Das Dispensatorium des Valerius Cordus faksimile des im Jahre 1546 erschienenen ersten Druckes durch Joh. Petreium in Nürnberg. Mittenwald (Bayern), *Arthur Nemayer*, 1934

629. Pharmacopoeia Londinensis. London, *E. Griffin for J. Marriott*, 1618

630. Here begynnyth a new mater, the whiche sheweth and treateth of ye vertues & proprytes of herbes, the whiche is called an Herball. London, *Rycharde Banckes*, 1525

631. The grete herball whiche geveth parfyt knowledge and understanding of all maner of herbes and there gracyous vertues. Southwarke, *P. Treveris*, 1526

632. Turner, William, A new herball. 3 pts. London, *S. Mierdman*; Collen, *A. Birckman*, 1551–68

633. Barlow, H. M. Old English herbals, 1525–1640. *Proc. R. Soc. Med., Sect. Hist. Med.*, 1912–13, **6,** 108–149

634. Turner, William. Libellus de re herbaria novus. Londini, *apud Ioannem Byddellum*, 1538

635. Gerard, John. The herball or generall historie of plantes. London, (*E. Bollifant for B.* and *J. Norton*), 1597

636. Parkinson, John. Paradisi in sole paradisus terrestris or a garden of flowers with a kitchen garden and an orchard. London, *H. Lownes and R. Young*, 1629

637. Parkinson, John. (1640). As ref. 97 but p. 82

638. Oviedo Y Valdés, *Don* Gonçalo Fernández de. Sumaria de la historia natural de las Indias. Toledo, *R. de Petras*, 1525

639. Monardes, Nicolás. Dos libros. El uno trata de todas las cocas que traen nuestras Indias Occidentales, *etc.* Sevilla, *S. Trugillo*, 1565

640. Monardes, Nicolás (1565). As ref. 639 but as an English translation by John Frampton: *Joyfull newes out of the newe found world*, 1577 (reprinted 1925)

641. Garcia d'Orta. Coloquios dos simples, e drogas he cousas mediçinais da India. Goa, *Joannes*, 1563

642. Acosta, Cristobal. (Costa, (Christovam da)). Tractado delas drogas, y medicinas de las Indias Orientales, con sus plantas debuxadas al bivo. Burgos, *Martin de Victoria*, 1578

643. Guthrie, Douglas. Some early herbals and pharmacopoeias. Edinburgh (*privately printed*), 1950

644. Arber, Agnes Robertson. Herbals: their origin and evolution. A chapter in the history of botany, 1470–1670. 2nd edn. Cambridge, *University Press*, 1938

645. Cesalpino, Andrea (Caesalpinus). De plantis. Florence, 1583

646. Vesalius, Andreas. De humani corporis fabrica libri septem. Basileae (*ex off. Ioannis Oporini*, 1543)

647. Ketham, Johannes de. Fasciculus medicinae. Venetiis, *per Johannem & Gregorius fratres de Forlivio*, 1491

648. Berengario da Capri, Giacomo. Commentaria cum amplissimis additionibus super anatomia Mundini una cum textu ejusdem in pristinum et verum nitorem redacto. Bononiae, *imp. per H. de Benedictis*, 1521

649. Berengario da Carpi, Giacomo. Isagogae breves perlucide ac uberime in anatomiam humani corporis a communi medicorum academia usitatam. Bononiae, *per B. Hectoris*, 1522

650. Laguna, Andrés (Lacuna). Anatomica methodus, seu de sectione humani corporis contemplatio. Parisiis, *apud J. Kerver*, 1535

651. Edwardes, David. De indiciis et praecognitionibus, opus apprime utile medicis. Eiusdem in anatomicen introductio luculenta et brevis. Londini, *R. Redmanus*, 1532. English trans., 1961

652. Dryander, Johann (Eichmann). Anatomia capitis humani. Marpurgi, *E. Cervicorni*, 1536

653. Dryander, Johann (Eichmann). Anatomiae, hoc est, corporis humani dissectionis pars prior. Marpurgi, *apud E. Cervicornum*, 1537

654. Canano, Giovanni Battista. Musculorum humani corporis picturata dissectio. (Ferrara, 1541?)

655. Dubois, Jacques (Sylvius). Isagoge. Venice, 1556

656. Vesalius, Andreas. Tabulae anatomicae sex. Venetiis, *sumpt. J. S. Calcarensis*, 1538

657. Vesalius, Andreas. Suorum de humani corporis fabrica librorum epitome. Basileae (*ex off. J. Oporini,* 1543)

658. Vesalius, Andreas. De humani corporis fabrica libri septem. Basileae, *J. Oporinus*, 1555

659. Falloppio, Gabriele (Fallopius). Observationes anatomicae. Venetiis, *apud M. A. Ulmum*, 1561

660. Eustachi, Bartolommeo (Eustachius). Tabulae anatomicae. Romae, *ex off. F. Gonzagae*, 1714

661. Eustachi, Bartolommeo (Eustachius). Opuscula anatomica. Venetiis, *V. Luchinus*, 1564

662. Vesalius, Andreas. Epistola . . . radicis Chynae decocti. Basel, Operinus, 1546. Cited by Leake, Chauncey (1975), ref. 1461, p. 95

663. O'Malley, Charles, D. Andreas Vesalius of Brussels. California, *Univ. of California*, 1964

664. Grünpeck, Joseph. Tractatus de pestilentia scorra. (?Leipzig, *Boettiger,* 1496). English trans., 1930

665. Leoniceno, Niccolò. Libellus de epidemia, quam volgo morbum Gallicum vocant. Venetiis, *in domo Aldi Manutii*, 1497. English trans., 1945

666. Lopez De Villalobos, Francisco. El sumario de la medicina, con un tratado sobre las pestiferas buuas. Salamanca, *Antonio de Barreda*, 1498. English trans., 1870 and 1939

667. Massa, Niccolò. Liber de morbo gallico. Venetiis, *in aedibus F. Bindoni ac M. Pasini*, 1507 (1527)

668. Fracastoro, Girolamo (Fracastorius). Syphilis sive morbus gallicus. Veronae, (*S. Nicolini da Sabbio*), 1530

669. Fracastoro, Girolamo (Fracastorius). De sympathia et antipathia rerum liber unus. De contagione et contagiosis morbis et curatione. Venetiis, *apud heredes L. Iuntae*, 1546. English trans., 1930

670. Mattioli, Pietro Andrea. Morbi gallici novum ac utilissimum opusculum quo vera et omnimoda ejus cura percipi potest. (Bononiae, *imp. haered. Hieronymi de Benedictis,* 1533)

671. Diaz De Isla, Rodrigo Ruiz. Tractado cótra el mal serpentino. (Sevilla, *D. de Robertis*, 1539)

672. BPC (1949). As ref. 80 but pp. 381–382

673. BP (1898). As ref. 1672 but edn. of 1898

674. BPC (1949). As ref. 80 but p. 1093

675. Falloppio, Gabriele (Fallopius). De morbo gallico. Patavii, *apud C. Gryphium*, 1563

676. Gale, Thomas. Certaine works of chirurgerie. London, *R. Hall*, 1563
677. Luigini, Luigi (Luisinus, Aloysius). De morbo gallico omnia quae extant. 3 vols. Venetiis, *apud J. Zilettum*, 1566–67
678. Copernicus, Nicolaus. De revolutionibus orbium coelestium, 1543
679. Pfolspeundt, Heinrich von. Buch der Bündth-Ertznei. Hrsg. von H. Haeser und A. Middeldorpf. Berlin, *G. Reimer*, 1868
680. Brunschwig, Hieronymus (Braunschweig). Dis ist das buch der Cirurgia Hantwirckung der wundartzny von Hyeronimo brunschwig. Strassburg, (*J. Grüninger*), 1497
681. Vigo, Giovanni De. Practica in arte chirurgica copiosa . . . continens novem libros. (Rome, *per S. Guillireti et H. Bononiensem*), 1514. English trans., 1543
682. Gersdorff, Hans von (Gerssdorff; Schylhans). Feldtbuch der wundartzney. Strassburg, *J. Schott* (1517)
683. Paré, Ambroise. La méthode de traicter les playes faictes par hacquebutes et aultres bastons à feu: et de celles qui sont faictes par flèches, dardz et semblables. Paris, *Chés viuant Gaulterot*, 1545
684. Paré, Ambroise. Briefve collection de ladministration anatomique: avec la maniere de conjoindre les os: et d'extraire les enfans tant mors que vivans du ventre de la mere, lors que nature de soy ne peult venir a son effect. Paris, *G. Cavellat*, 1549
685. Paré, Ambroise. Dix livres de la chirurgie, avec le magasin des instrumens necessaires à icelle. Paris, *imp. Jean Le Royer*, 1564. English trans., 1969
686. Paré, Ambroise. Les oeuvres de M. Ambroise Paré. Paris, *G. Buon*, 1575. English trans., 1634
687. Paré, Ambroise. Œuvres complètes d'Ambroise Paré. 3 vols. Paris, *Baillière*, 1840–41
688. Maggi, Bartolomeo. De vulnerum sclopetorum et bombardarum curatione tractatus Bononiae, *per B. Bonardum*, 1552
689. Gale, Thomas. An excellent treatise of wounds made with gonneshot. London, *R. Hall*, 1563
690. Fabry, Wilhelm (Fabricius *Hildanus*). De gangraena et sphacelo. Cölln, *P. Keschedt*, 1593
691. Lowe, Peter. A discourse on the whole art of chyrurgerie. London, *T. Purfoot*, 1596
692. Rösslin, Eucharius (Rhodion; Röslin). Der swangern frawen und hebammen roszgarten. (Hagenau, *H. Gran*), 1513
693. Rösslin, Eucharius (Rhodion; Röslin). The byrth of mankynde. London, *T. R.*, 1540
694. Mercurio, Geronimo Scipione. La commare o riccoglitrice. Ventia, *G. B. Ciotti*, 1596
695. Bourgeois, Louise (dite *Boursier*). Observations diverses sur la sterilite, perte de fruict, foecondite, accouchements, et maladies des femmes, et enfants nouveaux naiz. Paris, *A. Saugrain*, 1609
696. Cordus, Euricius. Ein Regiment: wie man sich vor der newen Plage der Englische Schwaisz genannt, bewaren, unnd so mann damit ergryffen wirt, darinn halten soll. Marpurg, 1529
697. Schyller, Joachim (Schiller). De peste Brittanica commentarioius vere aureus. Basileae, *H. Petrus*, 1531
698. Caius, John (Kaye). A boke, or conseill against the disease commonly called the sweate, or sweatyng sicknesse. London, *Richard Grafton*, 1552
699. Baillou, Guillaume de (Ballonius). Opera medica omnia. 4 vols. Venetiis, *apud A. Jeremiam*, 1734–36
700. Botallo, Leonardo. De catarrho commentarius. Parisiis, *apud B. Turrisanum*, 1564
701. Phaer, Thomas (Phayer; Phayr). The regiment of life, whereunto is added a treatise of the pestilence, with the boke of children. London, 1545
702. Weyer, Johann (Wierus). De praestigiis daemonum. Basileae, *per J. Oporinum*, 1563
703. Scot, Reginald (Scott). The discoverie of witchcraft. (London, *W. Brome*), 1584
704. Bright, Timothy. A treatise of melancholie, containing the causes thereof. London, *T. Vautrollier*, 1586
705. Fernel, Jean François. Medicina. 3 pts. (in 1). Lutetiae Parisiorum, *apud A. Wechelum*, 1554
706. Garrison, Fielding H. (1929). As ref. 179 but p. 196
707. Garrison, Fielding H. (1929). As ref. 179 but pp. 196–197
708. Fernel, Jean François. De naturali parte medicinae libri septem. Parisiis, *apud Simonem Colinaeum*, 1542
709. Servetus, Michael. Christianismi restitutio. (Vienne, *Balthasar Arnollet*), 1553. English trans., 1953 and 1966

710. Cesalpino, Andrea (Caesalpinus). Peripateticarum quaestionum libri quinque. Venetiis, *apud Iuntas*, 1571

711. Cesalpino, Andrea (Caesalpinus). Quaestionum peripateticum, libri V. Venetiis, *apud Juntas*, 1593

712. Vicary, Thomas. The Englishman's treasure. London, *J. Windet for J. Perin*, 1586. (Later editions, 1587, 1633, 1641)

713. Clowes, William. A prooved practise for all young chirurgians, concerning burnings with gunpowder, and woundes made with gunshot. London, *T. Orwyn for T. Cadman*, 1588

714. Clowes, William. A short and profitable treatise touching the cure of the morbus gallicus by unctions. London, *J. Daye*, 1579

715. Gruner, O. Cameron. A treatise on the Canon of Medicine of Avicenna incorporating a translation of the first book. London, *Luzac*, 1930, p. 567

716. Paul of Aegina (Francis Adams edn., 1844–47). As ref. 470 but Vol. III, p. 510

717. Dürer, Albrecht. Vier Bücher von menschlicher Proportion. (Nürnberg, *J. Formschneyder*), 1528

718. Gesner, Conrad. Historia animalium. 5 vols. Tiguri, *apud C. Froschouerum*, 1551–1587

719. Wotton, Edward. De differentiis animalium. Lutetiae Parisiorum, *M. Vascosanus*, 1552

720. Occo, Adolph. Enchiridion, sive ut vulgo vocant dispensatorium, compositorum medicamentorum, pro Reipub. Augstburgensis pharmacopoeia. (Augsburg, 1564)

4

The Seventeenth Century

The Age of Experiment – to about AD 1700
Locke, Galileo and Newton

The seventeenth century became a kind of post-Renaissance marked by great individualism, invention, and discovery; in science its most obvious characteristic is that it was the age of the deliberate, planned experiment. In the world at large it was an era of individual genius – the time of major parts of the lives of Shakespeare, Milton, Pepys and Wren; Rembrandt, Bach and Purcell; and, in philosophy, Descartes, Spinoza, Bacon and Locke. In the mathematical and physical sciences this was the era of Galileo, Newton and Boyle; in biology it saw the quite fundamental contributions of Leeuwenhoek and Hooke, and in medicine the seventeenth century saw the achievements of both Harvey and Sydenham.

The experimental approach showed in the works of its philosophers. Of these, the writings of Francis Bacon (1561–1626), educated at Trinity College, Cambridge, and later Lord Chancellor, made a great impact due to their vivid and lively style, their great power of reasoning, and their emphasis on the experimental method.

The process of discarding the old authoritarian system continued in the work of René Descartes (1596–1650), a student of the Jesuit College of La Flèche and the University of Poitiers. Famous for basing his philosophy on universal doubt, but recognizing that doubt cannot itself be doubted, he produced the postulate *Cogito, ergo sum* – 'I think, therefore, I am' – which epitomized the ultimate challenge to the transmission of wisdom by authority. These ideas were developed in the thinking of the Dutch philosopher, Benedict Spinoza (1632–1677), a Jew who later left that faith and whose later philosophy is really pantheistic.

But without much doubt the core of this practical type of philosophy becomes most readily available to the biological scientist of today in the splendid *An Essay Concerning Human Understanding*[721] (1689, but all copies dated 1690) of the English philosopher, John Locke (1632–1704). Locke was educated at Christ Church, Oxford, became physician and secretary to Anthony Ashley Cooper

237

(later Earl of Shaftesbury) and was ultimately Commissioner on the Board of Trade (1696–1700). The Essay, and his later writings on government, toleration, education and religion were of such important effect that Locke has often been described as the initiator of the Age of Enlightenment and the inspirer of the American constitution. He was an associate of Robert Boyle and his medical studies brought him into contact with Thomas Sydenham – whose rejection of traditional views and reliance on the powers of observation may have had a good deal to do with the eventual formation of Locke's own philosophical system.

Locke's belief that there are such things as laws of Nature became of profound significance, and the plain language which he used and the care which he devoted to the long generation of his *Essay Concerning Human Understanding* ensured that the book made its mark from the first. There were something like 30 editions in English by 1850; modern editions include the fine, two volume version edited by John W. Yolton (1961).

Locke rejected the speculative element in Descartes and thought that knowledge was to be gained by experience and reflection upon experience, in the manner in which he could see it being gained by Boyle and Sydenham. In the following passage he bases himself firmly on experience [721]:

> Let us then suppose the mind to be, as we say, white paper void of all characters, without any *ideas*. How comes it to be furnished? Whence comes it by that vast store which the busy and boundless fancy of man has painted on it with an almost endless variety? Whence has it all the materials of reason and knowledge? To this I answer, in one word, from *experience*; in that all our knowledge is founded, and from that it ultimately derives itself. Our observation, employed either about *external sensible objects, or about the internal operations of our minds perceived and reflected on by ourselves, is that which supplies our understandings with all the materials of thinking.* These two are the fountains of knowledge, from whence all the *ideas* we have, or can naturally have, do spring.

In attempting to understand how human knowledge was attained Locke looks at the beginning of knowledge in sense-perception and our awareness of it by introspection and intuition. He sees that sense-experience is not direct knowledge of the world as it is but that the senses provide the mind with material, we might call it 'ideas', which is that which seems real. Locke thus accepts that while some of the representations in the mind are exact copies of the physical world, many are not. He continues, leading away from anything which resembles supernaturalism to an empiricism which holds that knowledge of the physical world is the reality of ideas derived from sense-perceptions.

Some of his thoughts on the relationship between the senses, especially vision and touch, have greatly affected later philosophers of science. He shows great interest in the association of ideas, and in language and the function of language in knowing. His writings compel a recognition that what is real to our minds is a perception, arising from a sense impression, which needs care in its demonstration. He argues that knowledge is the result of experience and many of our beliefs derive from the association of ideas. His writings suggest prudence in the design of the experiments which will demonstrate the physical world to the senses and in the use of the means of reasoning by which we must examine experience.

The seventeenth century was marked not only by the works of the natural philosophers of science but also, even from its beginning, by a great wealth of scientific discovery. Galileo Galilei (1564–1642) began to doubt his scholastic training early in life. By 1591 he had reached the conclusions for which his name is famous that the rate of fall of a body is a function of the period of its fall and not of its weight. These conclusions were opposed to the Aristotelian view that bodies of different weights must fall at different speeds. At Padua, Galileo proved theoretically that falling bodies obey what has come to be known as the law of uniformly accelerated motion. Because of his work on gravitation, and because of his combining mathematical analysis with the experimental method, Galileo is often considered to have been the founder of modern experimental physics.

When he was in Venice in 1609 he heard of the recent invention of very simple telescopes. On his return to Padua he quickly built an instrument with a three-fold magnifying power, and he soon improved this ten-fold. Before long he produced the first instruments which could usefully be used to make astronomical observations. Because his instruments were very quickly in demand throughout Europe, Galileo is usually considered to have been the inventor of the telescope.

His observations proved that the Earth revolves around the Sun – thus finally establishing the truth of the teaching of Copernicus. Galileo, tried by the Inquisition in Rome, and ordered to recant, was forced to spend the last 8 years of his life under house arrest. His eventual legacy to science went beyond the usefulness of his discoveries – it is his belief in the expression of observational results in numbers and their subjection to mathematical analysis which represents his greatest contribution to the modern methods of experiment.

The additional work of Galileo included the novel development of the thermometer, the discovery of the law governing the vibrations of a pendulum, the making of the first attempts to measure the speed of light and weigh air, and the design of the first experiments to produce a vacuum. Despite all of these things the residual darkness of the times is shown not only by the handling of Galileo by the Inquisition but also by the publication, in 1597, of a treatise on the need for use of severe measures to combat the grave threat of witchcraft. This particular book, demonstrating a complete belief in the reality of demons and witches, was called *Daemonology*[722] – and it came from the pen of James VI, King of Scotland, soon to become also James I, King of England.

This irrational book was published just before the beginning of the seventeenth century. That century was marked by the dates of the deaths of Francis Bacon (1626), René Descartes (1650), Benedict Spinoza (1677) and John Locke (1704); one of its late and most notable achievements was the 1690 dating of the *An Essay Concerning Human Understanding* by John Locke. During this century the year 1642 saw not only the death of Galileo but also the birth of Newton.

In Isaac Newton (1642–1727) the numeracy of the seventeenth century reached its full maturity. He graduated at Trinity College, Cambridge in 1665 – just before the great pandemic of the Black Death of that year caused the University to be closed until the Spring of 1667. During these 18 months of reflection when Cambridge was in recess, Newton developed what is now known as the binomial theorem and an early form of the differential calculus, probably the most singular mathematical invention since the Greeks. Newton also analysed, by experiment, the composition of white light and explored the nature of colours, before discovering the gravitational force holding the moon in orbit.

Back at Cambridge, as professor of mathematics, he produced the reflecting telescope (as distinct from the refracting instrument) and then went on, building on the three laws of planetary motion already advanced by Johann Kepler (1571–1630), to postulate that a universal force of gravitation causes the planets to orbit the sun with a force that decreses in intensity with the square of the distance. Newton's *Philosophiae Naturalis Principia Mathematica*[723], published in 1687, embodied these and his other observations showing, for the first time, that a single Law of Nature, capable of mathematical expression, accounted for the observed phenomena of not only the Earth and skies, but also the movements of objects on Earth, its tides, and such sequences of its natural events.

Newton was 85 years old at the time of his death in 1727; he was buried in Westminster Abbey. The man then laid to rest had, for the first time, shown that the earthly and heavenly bodies are directed by the same physical laws. Newton had swept the cosmology of Aristotle, Galen, and the long tract of the Middle Ages into the errors of history. More than just a great deal of modern physical science begins with the great work of Newton; our expectation that new knowledge will be contiguous with what is already known, and the rational views by which we see the laws of nature unite the cosmos around us, stem from the '*Principia*'.

Those prepared to follow the views of Galileo and Newton included the Paduan professor, Sanctorius (Santorio Santorio; 1561–1636) who was the founder of the study of physiology in numerical terms. He introduced into medicine the idea of reducing the events of physiology to mathematical terms and began the practice of counting the pulse, measuring the body temperature, and recording the weight of the body in varying circumstances. He is always shown in the famous frontispiece plate from the later editions of his *De statica medicina* (1614)[724] in which he sits in a chair suspended from a steelyard conducting, upon himself, one of the first orderly experiments in metabolism. It is said that while Galileo was in Pisa cathedral during his first year at the university in the town, he observed a lamp swinging and found that it always needed the same amount of time to complete an oscillation, regardless of the range of the swing. Later in life he demonstrated this experimentally and went on to suggest that a pendulum might be used to regulate clocks. Using his pulse to test the synchronous character of the vibrations of a pendulum led him to the converse proposition of measuring the rate of the pulse by a pendulum. Sanctorius utilized these ideas and, in his *Commentaria in primam fen primi libri canonis Avicennae*[725] of 1625, provided the first record of the use of a pulsilogium, or pulse-clock, and a thermometer to study disease. Early in the following century Sir John Floyer (1649–1734) published *The Physician's Pulse-watch*[726] (1707–10) in which, before watches had hands to measure the seconds, he described a watch which divided the minute and allowed him to record careful observations on the rate of the pulse. A little later the first important work which advanced the ideas of Sanctorius on the clinical use of the thermometer was provided by George Martine (1702–1741) in his *Essays Medical and Philosophical*[727] of 1740.

Another of the early workers who applied the principles of Galileo to the measurement of biological events was John Graunt (1620–1674) whose *Natural and Political Observations mentioned in a following index, and made upon the Bills of Mortality*[728] represented the first book on vital statistics. Graunt, apprenticed to his father, a London haberdasher of fairly considerable substance, came to exert substantial influence in his own right. His book was based on a study of the weekly bills, or lists, of deaths and their causes which were compiled by parish clerks in the London area and extended back to 1603. His study established the mathematical approach to the understanding of the causes of mortality and the effect of these causes on the public health. Graunt was the first to notice that more boys are born than girls and he showed that the population can be estimated from an accurate death rate. The Bills of Mortality gained greatly in importance following their study by Graunt and, in 1838, merged into the returns of the Registrar-General. The achievement, considering the faulty nature of the original Bills of Mortality, was remarkable. It was followed by the *Several Essays in Political Arithmetic* (1699)[729] of Sir William Petty (1623–1687), professor of anatomy at Oxford, later professor of music, who took the first census of Ireland. Some authorities have suggested that the erudite and educated Petty may have been the real author of the study attributed to Graunt. At all events, at much the same time, the astronomer, Edmund Halley (1656–1742), produced *An Estimate of the Degrees of Mortality of Mankind, drawn from curious tables of the births and funerals at the City of Breslaw, with an attempt to ascertain the price of annuities upon lives*[730]; this work, beginning the data upon which the world of insurance is based, is a fundamental text of the science of vital statistics – a singularly English contribution to medicine. The data used by Halley were provided for him by Caspar Neumann, a pastor of Breslau.

A beginning in the development of carefully measured and recorded experiments with new chemical substances examined pharmacologically was made by Christopher Wren (1632–1723), the great architect, who collaborated with Robert Boyle (1627–1691), the pioneer chemist. Wren showed an enormous aptitude for the mathematical methods of science as well as for the demands of architecture and he rebuilt much of London after the fire of 1665.

In Oxford, Boyle undertook experiments on the properties of air. He examined the elasticity, compressibility and weight of air and discovered the inverse relationship between the volume and pressure of gases – so forming the celebrated law that goes by his name. This, Boyle's Law, appeared in a pamphlet, *A Defence of the Doctrine Touching the Spring and Weight of the Air*[731] which Morton[732] notes as having been attached to the second edition of Boyle's *The Spring and Weight of the Air* of 1662. Boyle also invented suction pumps with which air could be withdrawn from a bell jar and, experimenting with flames and small animals in the vacuum he had produced, he proved air to be essential for both combustion and life – so beginning the search for oxygen and, in his *New Experiments Physico-mechanicall Touching the Spring of the Air* (1660)[733], providing a main starting-point of modern respiratory physiology. He was the first to recognize the true nature of an element and, in 1663, formed one of the small group of natural philosophers who became known as the Royal Society.

Boyle's most important medical work, *Memoirs for the Natural History of Humane Blood, especially the Spirit of that Liquor* (1683)[734], provides one of the fundamental treatises of the biochemistry of blood. Wren and Boyle collaborated in a study in which, in 1656, they became the first to inject solutions of opium and of crocus metallorum into the veins of dogs. These studies were designed to measure the effects of the injection, the crocus metallorum being prepared by igniting antimony metal with potassium nitrate to yield liver of antimony which, when treated with water, produced the desired mixture of antimony oxides. Pharmacology thus owes to Wren and Boyle the first experiments on the intravenous injection of drugs – but these studies formed only a small part of the great contributions to chemistry that were achieved by Boyle who, assiduous enough to learn Hebrew, Greek and Syriac so that he could pursue his critical biblical studies, became known as 'The Father of Chemistry'.

William Harvey

It is no coincidence that many of these events in the philosophy of science took place either in Italy, Holland or England – for throughout much of the first half of the seventeenth century great areas of central Europe were decimated by the Thirty Years' War, fought mainly in Germany (1618–48).

In one of the places where this war was not of destructive effect, at Padua, in the chair of anatomy in which Fallopius had succeeded Vesalius, a further worthy successor had been found in the person of Girolamo Fabrizzi (Fabricius ab Aquapendente; 1533–1619). Fabricius built an anatomical theatre of great fame and distinction and in *De formato foetu* (1600)[735] and *De formatione ovi et pulli* (1621)[736] wrote at great length on embryology. He also made what can be seen, in retrospect, to have been important observations on the valves in veins.

Osler reproduces a plate (Figure 72) from the *De venarum ostiolis* (1603)[737] of Fabricius, who became the teacher of Harvey in Padua. The drawing of the valves is clear – but it seems fairly certain that Fabricius failed to understand their function. The effects of tying a vein and the centripetal nature of the flow of blood in veins had already been recorded in print by Cesalpino in works of 1571[738] and 1593[739]; however, these observations, unsupported by convincing experimental studies, had no effect on contempories at Padua, or upon Harvey. The precise drawing of the valves in veins by Fabricius hints at their function: Fabricius calls them *ostiola* (little doors), and most doors open only one way. Despite the approximation to a real understanding, Fabricius failed to grasp their importance – he probably looked on the valves as simple structures which delayed the flow of blood. At all events, this work must have had great influence on the design of Harvey's later experiments.

William Harvey (1578–1657), born in Folkestone in Kent, was a student at Padua from 1599 to 1603. He would probably have already been familiar with the very rational and interesting *De magnete*[740] of William Gilbert (1540-1603) – a work which not only showed that the Earth is a massive spherical magnet, but which also did a great deal to explain a number of phenomena previously the subject of much superstition. Gilbert's book, like the works of Newton, contributed to the growing rationalism of the times: even today it forms one of the milestones in the history of science.

Harvey returned to London, became physician to St. Bartholomew's Hospital, and in 1615 was made anatomical lecturer to the College of Physicians.

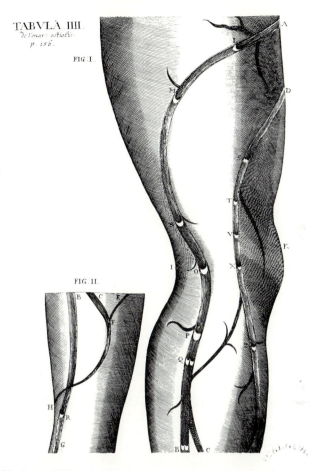

Figure 72   Girolamo Fabrizzi (Fabricius ab Aquapendente). *De venarum ostiolis.* Patavii (1603). Tabula IIII. [*Royal Society of Medicine library, London.*]

By some curious chance his lectures of the year 1616 have survived and his notes were published by the College in facsimile in 1886 (*Praelectiones anatomiae universalis*)[741]. The lecture of April 17, 1616, shows a clear appreciation of the fact that the blood must *circulate*: Osler[742], in Figure 73, shows 'the extraordinarily crabbed hand' in which these notes were written; he also gives a transscript of the original.

Although the lectures were repeated year after year they excited little comment until, 12 years later, in 1628, Harvey published a quarto volume of 74 pages entitled *Exercitatio anatomica de motu cordis et sanguinis in animalibus*[743]; this, somewhat poorly printed item, seen through the press in Frankfurt, is the most important book in the history of medicine. It came to do, for physiology, and therefore for the whole of medicine, what the '*Fabrica*' of Vesalius had done for anatomy and, thereby, for surgery. Having waited so long

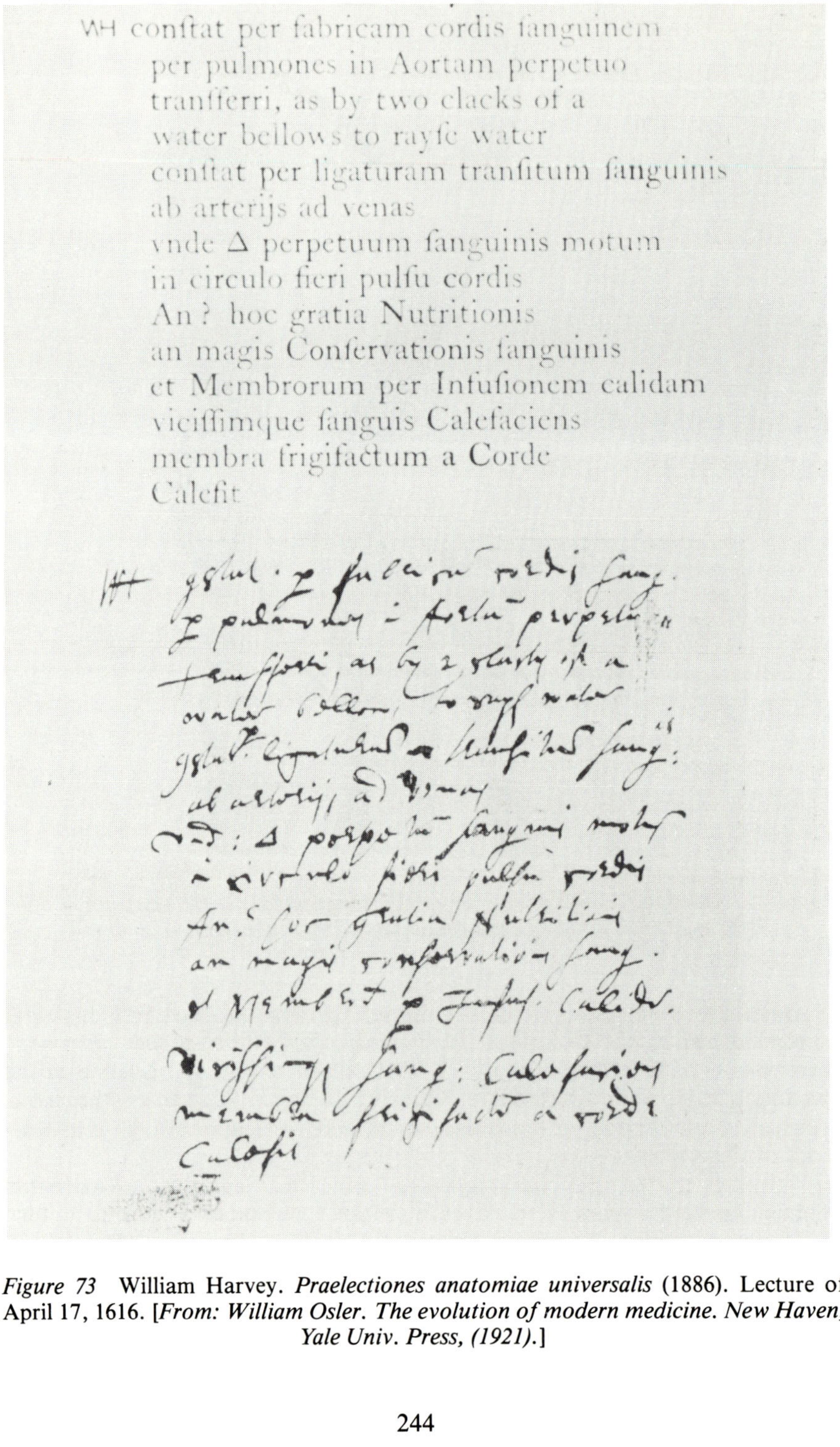

WH conftat per fabricam cordis fanguinem
per pulmones in Aortam perpetuo
tranfferri, as by two clacks of a
water bellows to rayfe water
conftat per ligaturam tranfitum fanguinis
ab arterijs ad venas
vnde Δ perpetuum fanguinis motum
in circulo fieri pulfu cordis
An? hoc gratia Nutritionis
an magis Confervationis fanguinis
et Membrorum per Infufionem calidam
viciffimque fanguis Calefaciens
membra frigifactum a Corde
Calefit

Figure 73 William Harvey. *Praelectiones anatomiae universalis* (1886). Lecture of April 17, 1616. [*From: William Osler. The evolution of modern medicine. New Haven, Yale Univ. Press, (1921).*]

244

before finally allowing publication, Harvey may have chosen to print in Frankfurt because of the famous book fair held in the city. The Latin text, with an English translation by K. J. Franklin, was published in Oxford in 1957 and there is a fine Sydenham Society edition – *The works of William Harvey. Translated from the Latin, with a life of the author, by Robert Willis*[744] – dated 1847.

'*De Motu Cordis*' shows the deliberate way in which Harvey gradually rejected the ideas of the ebb-and-flow movement of the blood passed to him since Galen. In the following passage from the translation by Willis[745], he shows his appreciation of the fact that the heart contracts and, to the hand, feels harder when it does so; he concludes, in this and related passages, that the heart expels blood by the force of its active contraction, and receives it only in relaxation. These observations dispelled the converse belief:

> We are therefore authorized to conclude that the heart, at the moment of its action, is at once constricted on all sides, rendered thicker in its parietes and smaller in its ventricles, and so made apt to project or expel its charge of blood. This, indeed, is made sufficiently manifest by the fourth observation preceding, in which we have seen that the heart, by squeezing out the blood it contains becomes paler, and then when it sinks into repose and the ventricle is filled anew with blood, that the deeper crimson colour returns. But no one need remain in doubt of the fact, for if the ventricle be pierced the blood will be seen to be forcibly projected outwards upon each motion or pulsation when the heart is tense.
>
> These things, therefore, happen together or at the same instant: the tension of the heart, the pulse of its apex, which is felt externally by its striking against the chest, the thickening of its parietes, and the forcible expulsion of the blood it contains by the constriction of its ventricles.
>
> Hence the very opposite of the opinions commonly received, appears to be true; inasmuch as it is generally believed that when the heart strikes the breast and the pulse is felt without, the heart is dilated in its ventricles and is filled with blood; but the contrary of this is the fact, and the heart, when it contracts [and the shock is given], is emptied. Whence the motion which is generally regarded as the diastole of the heart, is in truth its systole. And in like manner the intrinsic motion of the heart is not the diastole but the systole; neither is it in the diastole that the heart grows firm and tense, but in the systole, for then only, when tense, is it moved and made vigorous.

Galen knew that enough blood went from the right ventricle to the lungs to permit their nutrition but Harvey, having seen the heart as a pump, deduced, from the position and direction of the valves of the great vessels, that the contraction of the right ventricle must force all of its contained blood to the lungs, and from the lungs it must pass to the left side of the heart. The crux of the work is to dismiss the idea – held over the vast period of time since Galen – that the massive circulating blood volume could pass through the intraventricular septum. The actual quantity, and the velocity, of the blood must, as he computes, make this impossible. The same factors must, as he realizes, make it inevitable that the blood, forced from the left ventricle into the arteries, must return to it by the venous route. It must, therefore, circulate.

The passage in which, to his students, he gave this conclusion in 1616 was shown in Figure 73. The passage, from the Willis translation, in which, with some trepidation, he announced this conclusion to the world at large is contained in the following[746]:

> Thus far I have spoken of the passage of the blood from the veins into the arteries, and of the manner in which it is transmitted and distributed by the action of the heart; points to which some, moved either by the authority of Galen or Columbus, or the reasonings of others, will give in their adhesion. But what remains to be said upon the quantity and source of the blood which thus passes, is of so novel and unheard-of character, that I not only fear injury to myself from the envy of a few, but I tremble lest I have mankind at large for my enemies, so much doth wont and custom, that become as another nature, and doctrine once sown and that hath struck deep root, and respect for antiquity influence all men: Still the die is cast, and my trust is in my love of truth, and the candour that inheres in cultivated minds. And sooth to say, when I surveyed my mass of evidence, whether derived from vivisections, and my various reflections on them, or from the ventricles of the heart and the vessels that enter into and issue from them, the symmetry and size of these conduits, – for nature doing nothing in vain, would never have given them so large a relative size without a purpose, – or from the arrangement and intimate structure of the valves in particular, and of the other parts of the heart in general, with many things besides, I frequently and seriously bethought me, and long revolved in my mind, what might be the quantity of blood which was transmitted, in how short a time its passage might be effected, and the like; and not finding it possible that this could be supplied by the juices of the ingested aliment without the veins on the one hand becoming drained, and the arteries on the other getting ruptured through the excessive charge of blood, unless the blood should somehow find its way from the arteries into the veins, and so return to the right side of the heart; I began to think whether there might not be A MOTION, AS IT WERE, IN A CIRCLE. Now this I afterwards found to be true; and I finally saw that the blood, forced by the action of the left ventricle into the arteries, was distributed to the body at large, and its several parts, in the same manner as it is sent through the lungs, impelled by the right ventricle into the pulmonary artery, and that it then passed through the veins and along the vena cava, and so round to the left ventricle in the manner already indicated. Which motion we may be allowed to call circular, in the same way as Aristotle says that the air and the rain emulate the circular motion of the superior bodies; for the moist earth, warmed by the sun, evaporates; the vapours drawn upwards are condensed, and descending in the form of rain, moisten the earth again; and by this arrangement are generations of living things produced; and in like manner too are tempests and meteors engendered by the circular motion, and by the approach and recession of the sun.

In looking at the peripheral pathways by which the blood might circulate, Harvey notes that, 'The celebrated Hieronymus Fabricius of Aquapendente, a most skilful anatomist, and venerable old man, or . . . Jacobus Silvius, first gave representations of the valves in the veins . . .'[747] he then adds that the discoverer of these valves did not rightly understand their use; he follows this with these paragraphs, illustrating them with the famous four diagrams reproduced in Figure 74[748].

> But the valves are solely made and instituted lest the blood should pass from the greater into the lesser veins, and either rupture them or cause them to

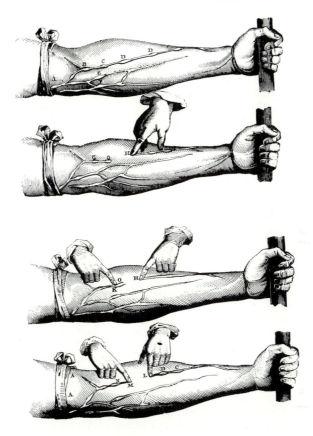

Figure 74 William Harvey. Circulation of the forearm veins. [From: *The works of William Harvey. Translated from the Latin... by Robert Willis,* London, *Sydenham Society* (1847).]

become varicose; lest, instead of advancing from the extreme to the central parts of the body, the blood should rather proceed along the veins from the centre to the extremities; but the delicate valves, while they readily open in the right direction, entirely prevent all such contrary motion, being so situated and arranged, that if anything escapes, or is less perfectly obstructed by the cornua of the one above, the fluid passing, as it were, by the chinks between the cornua, it is immediately received on the convexity of the one beneath, which is placed transversely with reference to the former, and so is effectually hindered from getting any farther.

And this I have frequently experienced in my dissections of the veins: if I attempted to pass a probe from the trunk of the veins into one of the smaller branches, whatever care I took I found it impossible to introduce it far any way, by reason of the valves; whilst, on the contrary, it was most easy to push it along in the opposite direction, from without inwards, or from the branches towards the trunks and roots. In many places two valves are so placed and fitted, that when raised they come exactly together in the middle of the vein, and are there united by the contact of their margins; and so accurate is the adaptation, that neither by the eye nor by any other means of examination can the slightest chink along the line of contact be perceived. But if the probe be now introduced from the extreme towards the more central parts, the valves, like the floodgates of a river, give way, and are most readily pushed aside. The effect of this arrangement plainly is to prevent all motion of the blood from the heart and vena cava, whether it be upwards towards the head, or downwards towards the feet, or to either side towards the arms, not a drop can pass; all motion of the blood, beginning in the larger and tending towards the smaller veins, is opposed and resisted by them; whilst the motion that proceeds from the lesser to end in the larger branches is favoured, or, at all events, a free and open passage is left for it.

But that this truth may be made the more apparent, let an arm be tied up above the elbow as if for phlebotomy (A, A, fig. 1). At intervals in the course of the veins, especially in labouring people and those whose veins are large, certain knots or elevations (B, C, D, E, F,) will be perceived, and this not only at the places where a branch is received (E, F), but also where none enters (C, D): these knots or risings are all formed by valves, which thus show themselves externally. And now if you press the blood from the space above one of the valves, from H to O, (fig. 2,) and keep the point of a finger upon the vein inferiorly, you will see no influx of blood from above; the portion of the vein between the point of the finger and the valve O will be obliterated; yet will the vessel continue sufficiently distended above that valve (O, G). The blood being thus pressed out, and the vein emptied, if you now apply a finger of the other hand upon the distended part of the vein above the valve O, (fig. 3,) and press downwards, you will find that you cannot force the blood through or beyond the valve; but the greater effort you use, you will only see the portion of vein that is between the finger and the valve become more distended, that portion of the vein which is below the valve remaining all the while empty (H, O, fig. 3).

It would therefore appear that the function of the valves in the veins is the same as that of the three sigmoid valves which we find at the commencement of the aorta and pulmonary artery, viz., to prevent all reflux of the blood that is passing over them.

Farther, the arm being bound as before, and the veins looking full and distended, if you press at one part in the course of a vein with the point of a finger (L, fig. 4), and then with another finger streak the blood upwards beyond the next valve (N), you will perceive that this portion of the vein continues empty (L N), and that the blood cannot retrograde, precisely as we have already seen the case to be in fig. 2; but the finger first applied (H, fig. 2, L, fig. 4), being removed, immediately the vein is filled from below, and the arm becomes as it appears at D C, fig. 1. That the blood in the veins therefore proceeds from inferior or more remote to superior parts, and towards the heart, moving in these vessels in this and not in the contrary direction, appears most obviously. And although in some places the valves, by not acting with such perfect accuracy, or where there is but a single valve, do not seem totally to prevent the passage of the blood from the centre, still the greater number of them plainly do so; and then, where things appear contrived more negligently, this is compensated either by the more frequent occurrence or more perfect action of the succeeding valves or in some other way: the veins, in short, as they are the free and open conduits of the blood returning *to* the heart, so are they effectually prevented from serving as its channels of distribution *from* the heart.

But this other circumstance has to be noted: The arm being bound, and the veins made turgid, and the valves prominent, as before, apply the thumb or finger over a vein in the situation of one of the valves in such a way as to compress it, and prevent any blood from passing upwards from the hand; then, with a finger of the other hand, streak the blood in the vein upwards till it has passed the next valve above, (N, fig. 4,) the vessel now remains empty; but the finger at L being removed for an instant, the vein is immediately filled from below; apply the finger again, and having in the same manner streaked the blood upwards, again remove the finger below, and again the vessel becomes distended as before; and this repeat, say a thousand times, in a short space of time. And now compute the quantity of blood which you have thus pressed up beyond the valve, and then multiplying the assumed quantity by one thousand, you will find that so much blood has passed through a certain portion of the vessel; and I do now believe that you will find yourself convinced of the circulation of the blood, and of its rapid motion. But if in this experiment you say that a violence is done to nature, I do not doubt but that, if you proceed in the same way, only taking as great a length of vein as possible, and merely remark with what rapidity the blood flows upwards, and fills the vessel from below, you will come to the same conclusion.

Harvey had used the valves to show that in the veins of the peripheral circulation the blood flows towards the heart but he had no means of seeing how the blood passed from the smallest arterial branches visible to the eye to the smallest tributaries of the veins: the demonstration of the capillaries had to await the early developments in microscopy. However, he had correctly deduced the function of the capillaries and had discovered the circulation of the blood. This vital understanding provided the foundation upon which was built much of the later knowledge of physiology. Of perhaps even greater importance was Harvey's quantitative, mathematical, and experimental approach: the ultimate contribution of 'De Motu Cordis' was to make physiology a vital, exact science from which could be developed major parts of the framework of modern medicine.

The lack of microscopy which denied Harvey sight of the capillary network more seriously limited his otherwise substantial studies of embryology. These studies were recorded in his *Exercitationes de generatione animalium*[749] of 1651. His ideas on the method by which the ovum is fertilized were wrong but he became one of the first to dispute the erroneous belief that the embryo is a preformed being. Harvey taught that the embryo was derived from the ovum by the gradual generation and aggregation of its parts. This view, rejecting the old belief that the fetus was preformed in miniature in the ovum, was elaborated well before the means existed by which the final demonstration of its truth could be effected. The book is also notable as providing, in its chapter on midwifery, the first written work on that subject by an Englishman.

Leeuwenhoek and microscopy

The facility that Harvey most greatly lacked was microscopy. Francesco Stelluti (1577–1653), in his *Persio tradotto*[750] published in Rome in 1630, provided the first book which contained illustrations of natural objects seen through a microscope. The first to apply microscopy to medicine was Pierre Borel (Borellus; 1620-1689) who is thought to have seen *Sarcoptes scabiei* and the red blood corpuscles (1653)[751]; in a slightly later work, of 1655[752], Borel collected together a mass of evidence suggesting that Zacharias (Zacharias Janssen, a Dutch spectacle-maker) invented the compound microscope in or about the year 1590. But it is to Athanasius Kircher (1602-1680), of Fulda, Germany, that the credit must be given for having been the first to employ the microscope in investigating the cause of disease: in his *Scrutinium physico-medicum contagiosae luis, quae pestis dicitur*[753], published in Rome in 1658, a year after the death of Harvey, he wrote that the blood of patients with plague was filled with 'a countless brood of worms' which were invisible to the naked eye. He could not have seen the plague bacillus with such a low power microscope and was probably describing rouleaux of red blood cells or clumps of pus cells but, even so, he was describing an appearance of disease visible only by microscopy. Kircher was also the first to make an explicit statement proposing that living animalculae, or micro-organisms, might be responsible for contagion and some infectious diseases. An account of this work was given by Marchmont Needham (1620-1678), one of the first, if not actually the earliest, Englishman to write (*Medela medicinae*, 1665[754]) on the germ theory.

Perhaps the most brilliant and extraordinary of these early microscopists was Antonj van Leeuwenhoek (1632-1723), a draper in the city of Delft and spare-time naturalist. Without any formal scientific training Leeuwenhoek showed a quite amazing level of originality and made a number of discoveries which, in their interest and importance, were surpassed by no other early microscopist. Many of these findings were communicated by their discoverer in papers transmitted to the Royal Society in London.

The work occasions modern interest and a photograph of an original Leeuwenhoek microscope (Figure 75), now in the collection of the Deutsches Museum at Munich, is provided by the courtesy of Brian J. Ford, author of the recent paper *Revelation and the single lens*[755] and of a later study. The instrument illustrated is less than 45 mm long and comprises two thin rectangular metal plates riveted together and pierced by a small aperture which is common to them both and houses a minute biconvex lens of short focal length; opposite the lens there is a needle point on which the object to be examined can be impaled and kept in exact focus by the use of rigidly mounted adjusting screws. The great virtue of the instrument was that the object being examined could not only be got into exact focus, but could then be kept there.

Leeuwenhoek is said to have made about 250 microscopes of this basic design and to have had 419 lenses, many of which he ground himself. The observations were made by holding the microscope close to the eye and illuminating it with a restricted cone of light derived from a candle or lamp-flame or a distant window; the instrument described by Ford[755] has the surprising magnification of × 266 and a resolution approaching 1 μm.

A collection in Dutch of many of the contributions which Leeuwenhoek sent to the Royal Society in London was published under the title *Ontledingen en ontdekkingen*[756] at Leiden in 1693-1718; the other great collection of his writings is the *Arcana naturae*[757] of 1695-1719. The first accurate description of the red blood corpuscles (first noted by Swammerdam in 1658) was contained in his

Microscopical observations concerning blood, milk, bones, the brain, spittle, and cuticula . . . [758] published in the *Philosophical Transactions* of 1674 and the presentations of his works in English include the fascinating translations from the Dutch and Latin editions published by Samuel Hoole in 1798–1807 [759].

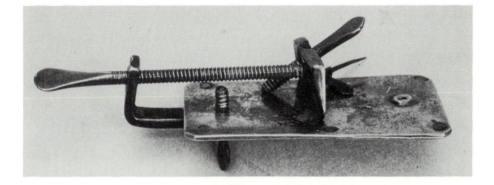

Figure 75   The original microscope of silver made by Antony van Leeuwenhoek, now in the collection of the Deutsches Museum at Munich. [*Photograph by Brian J. Ford, 1983.*]

From this translation part of Plate IV from Volume 1 is reproduced in Figure 76. Relating to the little diagram which he marks 'Fig. 1.' in this plate, Leeuwenhoek gives this account of the capillary circulation in the tadpole [760]:

> When thefe tadpoles were about eight or ten days old, I could perceive a fmall particle moving within their bodies, which I concluded to be the heart; and the fluid which was protruded from it began to affume a red colour.

Upon examining the tail of this creature, a fight prefented itfelf, more delightful than any that my eyes had ever beheld; for here I difcovered more than fifty circulations of the blood, in different places, while the animal lay quiet in the water, and I could bring it before the microfcope to my wifh. For I faw, not only that the blood in many places was conveyed through exceedingly minute veffels, from the middle of the tail towards the edges, but that each of thefe veffels had a curve, or turning, and carried the blood back towards the middle of the tail, in order to be again conveyed to the heart. Hereby it plainly appeared to me, that the blood-veffels I now faw in this animal, and which bear the names of arteries and veins, are, in fact, one and the fame, that is to fay, that they are properly termed arteries fo long as they convey the blood to the fartheft extremities of its veffels, and veins when they bring it back towards the heart. For example, I fee many blood-veffels in the tail of a tadpole taking their courfe, as reprefented in Plate IV, *fig*. 1. A B C, where the profition of the parts A and C is towards the fpine or middle of the tail, and the part B towards the edge of it. In A B, the blood is driven from the heart, and in B C, it is brought back again, and thus may we fay, that the veffel A B C, is both an artery and a vein, for it cannot be denominated an artery, farther than where the blood is driven in it to its fartheft extent, that is, from A to B; and we muft name B C, a vein becaufe, in it, the blood is returing back to the heart. And this it appears an artery and a vein are one and the fame veffel prolonged or extended.

In explaining the features of the remaining drawings in Plate IV and others of his plates, Leeuwenhoek provides equally unique accounts of many other features of the microcirculation. He discovered protozoa, bacteria and spermatozoa and was the first to give a description of the striped nature of the fibre of voluntary muscle. Amongst his innovations can be ranked the fact that, in 1719, Leeuwenhoek became the first – by using saffron to stain muscle fibres – to introduce the practice of staining into histology.

The founder of the science of histology and the greatest of the early exponents of descriptive embryology was the distinguished Marcello Malpighi (1628–1694), professor of anatomy at Bologna and Pisa. Malpighi (Figure 77) is the actual discoverer of the capillary circulation which we have noticed Leeuwenhoek describe: the *De pulmonibus observationes anatomicae*[761] of Malpighi was published in 1661; it is now very rare and comprises two letters to Borelli, the second letter containing the great discovery which completed the understanding of the general circulation and the work of Harvey. There is an English translation of this, one of the most important books in the history of medicine, in the *Proceedings of the Royal Society of Medicine*[762] for 1929–30. This same work – which shows the capillary anastomosis between the arteries and veins and thereby demonstrates the peripheral circulatory link which Harvey had deduced must exist – demonstrates also Malpighi's understanding of the fact that the trachea ends in minute bronchial filaments which reach the pulmonary tissues, themselves vesicular in nature.

Malpighi is remembered for a great deal more: his *De viscerum structura exercitatio anatomica*[763] of 1666 includes his classical account of the structure of the kidney – and this organ, in its 'Malpighian bodies', provides one element which perpetuates his name. The book also gives the first account of what we now call 'Hodgkin's disease'. It preceded the *De ovo incubato observationes*[764] of

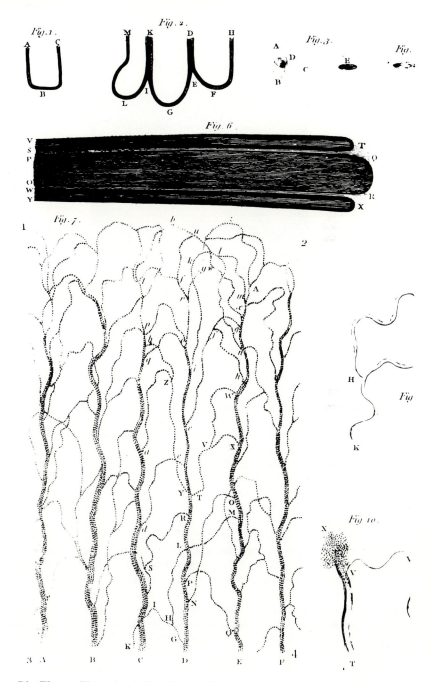

Figure 76 The capillary circulation. From: *The select works of Antony van Leeuwen-hoek ... Translated ... by Samuel Hoole.* London, *Henry Fry,* (1798–1807). Vol. I., Plate IV.

253

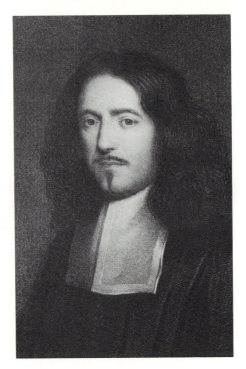

Figure 77   Marcello Malpighi (1628–1694). [*From: Thomas Joseph Pettigrew. Medical portrait gallery. London, Fisher, (1838–1840)*.]

1673, and a later work[765] of the same year, in which Malpighi gave the first description of the chick embryo examined microscopically – this account placing the whole science of embryology on the sound anatomical basis from which it has grown. In the same way that he sought to understand the unfolding of zoological anatomy, Malpighi examined the plant kingdom, approaching the subject through the microscopical study of the tissues of plants and the growth and development of plants – and these studies were recorded in the *Anatome plantarum*[766] which he published in 1675–79. His name is commemorated in the Malpighian layer of the skin and the Malpighian bodies of the spleen as well as of the kidney; one by one these memorials demonstrate not only the achievements of a great scientist but also the enrichment of knowledge which frequently follows the discovery of an invention, such as microscopy, which adds a new dimension to the unaided senses. Malpighi began the modern study of organogenesis, now so important in drug development, and one can retrace the foundations of this part of contemporary studies in his splendid *Opera omnia*[767] published by Robert Scott in London in 1686.

Those others whose imagination was captured by the microscope included Robert Hooke (1635–1703), at one time research assistant to Robert Boyle at Oxford. Hooke, Malpighi, Leeuwenhoek, and Swammerdam were all born within a decade of one another and represented the generation for which microscopy opened a new world. Hooke became the first Curator of Experiments to the newly-formed Royal Society and, in 1665, published his famous *Micrographia, or some physiological descriptions of minute bodies made by magnifying glasses; with observations and inquiries thereupon*[768]. This was the first work totally given over to microscopy and is the earliest book devoted to that subject in English. Many of its plates, almost all of them excellent and many engraved by Hooke himself, give an accurate account of much of the realm of plant histology. The historic hallmark of the book is its drawing of the microscopical structure of a piece of cork: this and the accompanying text provide the first use in the literature of science of the word 'cell' employed to describe a unit of histological structure.

Hooke's interests were wide ranging and he provides (1677) the first note on the microscopical appearance of the fungal diseases of plants – the most notorious of which is *Claviceps purpurea* or ergot, the cause, from eating bread made with ergot-infected grain, of the St. Anthony's Fire (epidemic ergotism) which swept Europe in the Middle Ages. The interest of Hooke and his friends in the physiology of respiration led him to undertake an experiment, reported as *An account of an experiment of preserving animals alive by blowing through their lungs with bellows*[769] in 1667, which showed that life could be preserved by such means without the respiratory apparatus being in motion. From such experiments began part of the search to understand the nature and mechanisms of respiratory gaseous interchange.

Sydenham and the clinicians

The first half of the seventeenth century enriched clinical medicine with names still often in use. The sciences related to medicine were astir and the turn of the century saw the work of Jean van Helmont (1577–1644), one of the principal founders of biochemistry; van Helmont invented the word 'gas', began the gravimetric analysis of urine, and wrote of the importance of ferments and gases in the *Ortus medicinae*[770] published for him by his son in 1648.

Those working in the clinical field included Francis Glisson (1597–1677) who was born in Dorset and became Regius Professor of Physic at Cambridge; in his *De rachitide sive morbo puerili, qui vulgo The Rickets dicitur* (1650)[771] Glisson provided the first reasonably full account of infantile rickets and became the first to describe infantile scurvy. In his slightly later *Anatomia hepatis*[772] of 1654 he gave the first accurate account of the integument of the liver (Glisson's capsule), by which his name is remembered. Much in advance of his time, in a publication of 1677[773], he wrote of the idea of irritability as a inherent property of all human tissue – an idea which doctors of his own day ignored but which was later shown experimentally by the great physiologist Albrecht von Haller.

Thomas Willis (1621–1675), born in Wiltshire and an astute clinician who became Sedleian Professor of Natural Philosophy at Oxford, provided the most clear and complete account of the nervous system that had been published. This formed the substance of his *Cerebri anatome: cui accessit nervorum descriptio et usus*[774] published in London in 1664. In preparing the work Willis was assisted by Richard Lower and provided with illustrations by Sir Christopher Wren. The book includes the description of the vitally important ring of arteries at the base of the brain (the Circle of Willis) and the eleventh cranial nerve (the nerve of Willis) – the former of these two structures still making Willis' name frequently heard, even though others (including Wepfer) had given earlier complete descriptions of the arterial ring. Willis is really more important as a careful and original observer of disease; he has an outstanding *Opera omnia*[775] published in Geneva in 1676–80 and is accounted second only to Sydenham amongst the clinical men of his day.

Willis' other contributions to anatomy and physiology included his account of the spinal nerves and the dorsal chain of ganglia which he called the 'intercostal nerve'; he wrote also on the process of fermentation in digestion and drew an analogy between putrefaction and fermentation. He wrote a chapter of one work on the sense of hearing and noted the sweetness of the urine in diabetes mellitus – so differentiating this condition from diabetes insipidus. His excellent accounts of clinical illnesses include what is probably the first record of an epidemic of cerebrospinal fever, a description of what is almost certainly myasthenia gravis, and a fine description recognizing general paralysis of the insane for the first time. He also gave a classic description of hysteria, an account of whooping cough ('puerorum tussis convulsiva, chincough dicta'), named puerperal fever, and wrote the first description of epidemic typhoid. Willis, in his discussion *Of the convulsive cough and asthma*[776] began the modern treatment of the latter condition. This work, like all but one of his writings, appears in translation in his *Practice of physick*[777], published in London in 1684 and providing one of the most fascinating insights into the rapid growth of seventeenth century descriptive medicine.

The strides made by English surgery are shown by the work of Richard Wiseman (1622–1676), the Royalist surgeon who ranks in surgery as does Sydenham in medicine. He gave the first description of tuberculosis of the joints ('tumor albus') and provided the first good account of 'the King's Evil' (scrofula or superficial tuberculosis, especially of the lymphatic glands). Wiseman also wrote one of the best accounts of the time of gunshot wounds and, in 1676, produced the important work called *Severall chirurgicall treatises*[778].

A major correction of an error which had stood since the days of Galen and which even Vesalius had continued to believe was achieved by the Cornishman, Richard Lower (1631–1691), who dispelled the ancient belief that the nasal secretions originated in the pituitary body and passed through the cribriform plate to cool the brain. Lower's teaching of 1670 on this subject ended the use of many medicines intended to purge the brain. The account was included in the *Tractatus de corde*[779] of 1669 in which Lower also demonstrated, for the first time, the special histological structure of the cardiac muscle. Lower's interest in the mechanisms of respiration led him to show that dark venous blood injected into insufflated lungs became bright red in colour, convincing him that the colour change was due to the blood absorbing air from the lungs. One of his studies which may have had a lasting effect upon surgery began with his report to the Royal Society of *The method observed in transfusing the blood out of one live animal into another* (1665–66)[780]. The first recorded[781] transfusion of blood into a human being was presented in Paris by Jean Baptiste Denis (*c.* 1625–1704) in 1667. Denis transfused the blood of a lamb into a young male subject, but his later transfusions failed. Within a few months, on 23rd November, 1667, the first blood transfusion of a human being in England was reported, again in the *Philosophical Transactions*, by Richard Lower and Sir Edmund King (1629–1707); this historic publication, of 1667, was called *An account of the experiment of transfusion , practised upon a man in London*[782].

Thomas Sydenham (1624–1689), 'The English Hippocrates', revolutionized clinical medicine by standing apart from Galenic dogma, speculative hypotheses of any sort, and even the scientific progress of his day, in order to concentrate on the careful, close observation of patients. He was born at Wynford Eagle in Dorset on September 10, 1624 and entered Magdalen Hall, Oxford in 1642; however, in support of the Parliamentary cause he soon left Oxford and did not obtain his medical degree until 1648.

This unacademic, practical background can be seen in his early writings on the treatment of fevers. These works arose from the detailed studies which Sydenham made of the epidemics he saw in London once he had set up practice in Westminster. The preliminary studies were so much admired by John Locke that he helped Sydenham expand the work into the *Observationes medicae circa morborum acutorum historiam et curationem*[783] – a book, now justifiably famous, which was published in London in 1676 and became a standard textbook of medicine until near the end of the nineteenth century.

Sydenham's favourite writers are said to have been Hippocrates, Cicero and Bacon; he seems to have held himself answerable for the care of his patients and his attitude illuminates, with a particular and clinical understanding, much of what he wrote. The '*Observationes medicae . . .*' of 1676 was really a third edition of his first work, the *Methodus curandi febres*[784] of 1666. In it he made important observations on dysentery, scarlet fever, measles and a number of febrile conditions. His description of scarlet fever is one of his finest and he produced the most careful and accurate account which had yet appeared of measles. His account differentiated these and related illnesses. In an almost Hippocratic manner he kept careful case records of individual cases and made his treatment straightforward and simple.

Today his name is perhaps most frequently remembered in relationship to gout and chorea. His masterpiece is usually considered to be the *Tractatus de podagra et hydrope* (1683)[785]. He suffered personally from gout and in this classic work differentiated this condition from rheumatism. Three years later he produced the *Schedula monitoria de novae febris ingressu*[786] of 1686. It is this work which contains the outstanding description of what we have come to call 'Sydenham's chorea'. His interest in epidemic illnesses continued and between the dates of these two books there appeared the 1685 edition[787] of his '*Observationes medicae . . .*' – this edition containing especially valuable accounts of the smallpox epidemics and malarial fevers common in London in the times of Sydenham.

There is an *Opera omnia*[788] of 1844 which restores to sight the now uncommon seventeenth century edition. Even more usefully there is a two volume *The works of Thomas Sydenham. Translated from the Latin . . . by R. G. Latham*[789] published by the Sydenham Society in 1848–50. This is reckoned the best translation and presentation of Sydenham and shows his fine disregard of theory and pragmatic, purely clinical approach to medicine. He discarded much of the filth and rubbish clogging the pharmacopoeias of the day and was a forceful advocate of fresh air in sickrooms and the use of a cooling, hygienic regime in the management of smallpox. He brought laudanum into practical English medical use, was one of the first to use iron in anaemia, and, even more importantly, he popularized the use of Peruvian bark, quinine, in the treatment of malaria. His version of the materia medica is, therefore, interesting and the listing of it given in the Latham translation is thoroughly worth consultation. From the same translation, the following is Sydenham's account[790] of measles in the year 1670:

1. The measles set in early as usual; i.e. at the beginning of January. They gained strength every day, until they reached their height, about the vernal equinox. After this they gradually decreased at the same rate; and by the month of July were wholly gone. As far as I have hitherto seen, I believe these measles to be the most perfect disease of their genus, for which reason I shall record their history with all the care and minuteness that the observations which I then made will warrant.

2. This disease begins and ends within the above-named period. It generally attacks infants, and, with them, runs through the whole family. It begins with shiverings and shakings, and with an inequality of heat and cold, which, during the first day, mutually succeed each other. By the second day, this has terminated in a genuine fever, accompanied with general disorder, thirst, want of appetite, white (but not dry) tongue, slight cough, heaviness of the head and eyes, and continued drowsiness. Generally there is a weeping from the eyes and nostrils; and this epiphora passes for one of the surest signs of the accession of the complaint. But to this may be added another sign equally sure; viz. the character of the eruption. Although measles usually shows itself by an exanthema upon the face, there appears upon the breast a second sort of breaking-out. This consists in broad red patches on a level with the skin, rather than true exanthemata. The patient sneezes as if from cold, his eyelids (a little before the eruption) become puffy; sometimes he vomits: oftener he has a looseness; the stools being greenish. This last symptom is commonest with infants teething, who also are more cross than usual. The symptoms increase till the fourth day. At that period (although sometimes a day later) little red spots, just like flea-bites, begin to come out on the forehead and the rest of the face. These increase both in size and number, group themselves in clusters, and mark the face with largish red spots of different figures. These red spots are formed by small red papulæ, thick set, and just raised above the level of the skin. The fact that they really protrude, can scarcely be determined by the eye. It can, however, be ascertained by feeling the surface with the fingers. From the face – where they first appear – these spots spread downwards to the breast and belly; afterwards to the thighs and legs. Upon all these parts, however, they appear as red marks only. There is no sensible protuberance by which they show themselves above the level of the skin.

3. In measles, the eruption has not the same effect in allaying the previous symptoms as it has in smallpox. The cough and fever still continue, so does the difficulty of breathing. The defluxion and the weakness still remain in the eyes. The continued drowsiness and want of appetite all keep on as before. The continuance, however, of the vomiting I have never yet observed. On the sixth day – there or thereabouts – the forehead and face grow rough, the cuticle being broken, and the pustules dying off. At the same time, the spots upon the rest of the body attain their greatest breadth and redness. By the eighth day the

spots have disappeared from the face, and show but faintly elsewhere. On the ninth day there are no spots anywhere. In place thereof, the face, trunk, and limbs are all covered with particles of loosened cuticle, so that they look as if they had been powdered over with flour, since the particles of broken cuticle are slightly raised, scarcely hold together, and, as the disease goes off, peel off in small particles, and fall from the whole of the body in the form of scales.

4. The measles most usually disappear about the eighth day, at which time, the vulgar (deceived by their reckoning in cases of smallpox) insist that they have *struck in*. In reality, however, they have finished their course. Thus it is believed that those symptoms which come on as the measles go off, are occasioned by their being struck in too soon; for it must be noted, that just at the time in question, the fever and the difficulty in breathing increase, and the cough becomes so harassing, that the patient can sleep neither night nor day. Infants, especially when they have been subjected to the hot regimen, and patients generally who have had recourse to hot remedies for the sake of promoting the eruption, are liable to these symptoms – symptoms which show themselves just as the measles give way. Hence, they may be thrown into a peripneumony, and this kills more patients than either the smallpox itself, or any symptom connected therewith. Yet, provided that the measles are properly treated, they are free from danger. A diarrhœa is a frequent symptom. This may succeed the disease, and run on for weeks, after every other symptom has departed; and it is of great danger to the patient, from the loss of spirits referable to the profuseness of the evacuation. Sometimes, too, after the more intense kinds of the hot regimen, the eruption grows first livid, and afterwards black. This happens to adults only; and when it *does* happen, all is over with the patient, unless, immediately upon the blackness, he be assisted by means of bloodletting and the cooling effects of a more temperate method.

5. The treatment of measles, like their nature, is nearly the treatment of smallpox. Hot medicines and the hot regimen are full of danger, however much they may be used by ignorant old women, with the intention of removing the disease as far as possible from the heart. This method, above others, has been most successful with me. The patient is kept to his bed for no more than two or three days after the measles have come out. In this way the blood may gently, and in its own way, breathe out, through the pores of the skin, those inflamed particles which are easily separable, but which offend it. He has, therefore, neither more blankets nor more fire than he would if well. All meats I forbid; but I allow oatmeal-gruel, and barley-broth, and the like; sometimes a roasted apple. His drink is either small beer, or milk boiled with three parts of water. I often ease the cough, which is constant in this disease, with a pectoral decoction, taken now and then, or with linctus, given with the same view. Above everything else, I take care to give diacodium every night throughout the disease.

> R︣ Pectoral decoction, lb.ss;
>   Syrup of violets,
>   Syrup of maidenhair, āā ℥iss.
> Mix, and make into an apozem. Take three or four ounces three
>   or four times a day.

> R︣ Oil of sweet almonds, ℥ij;
>   Syrup of violets,
>   Syrup of maidenhair, āā℥j;
>   White sugar-candy, q.s.
> Mix, and make into a linctus. To be taken frequently; especially
>   when the cough is distressing.

259

R⨯ Black-cherry-water, ℥iij;
      Syrup of white poppy, ℥j.
   Mix, and make into a draught; to be taken every night.

If the patient be an infant, the dose of the pectoral and anodyne must be lessened according to his age.

6. He that uses this remedy rarely dies; nor, with the exception of the necessary and inevitable symptoms of the disease, is he afflicted with any superadded disorders. It is the cough which is the most distressing. However, it is not dangerous, unless it continue after the disease is gone. And even then, if it last a week or a fortnight, by the use of fresh air, and the proper pectoral remedies, it is got rid of with no great difficulty. Nay, it may go off of its own accord.

7. But if, however, the patient, from the use of cordials, or from a hot regimen, be in a condition which is by no means unfrequent after the departure of the measles; i.e. if his life be endangered from the violence of a fever, from difficulty of breathing, or from any other symptom of a peripneumony, I take blood from the arm, and I do it with remarkable success. The bleeding is proportionate to the age; but it can be applied even to infants. At times I have even repeated it. Under Divine Providence, I have saved many infants in this way, and I know of no other. The symptoms themselves occur with infants at the recession of the eruption; and they are so fatal, that they do more to fill Charon's boat than the smallpox itself. Further – the diarrhœa, which has been stated to follow the measles, is equally cured by bloodletting. It arises (as in pleurisies, peripneumonies, and other inflammatory diseases) from the vapours of inflamed blood rushing upon the bowels, and so forcing them to the secretion. Nothing but venesection allays this. It makes a revulsion of the sharp humours, and reduces the blood to its proper temperature.

8. Let no one wonder that I recommend bleeding with tender infants. As far as I have observed, it is as safe with them as with adults. Indeed, so necessary is it in some cases, that, in respect to these particular symptoms, and in respect to some others as well, infants cannot be cured without it. For instance, how could we ease the convulsions of the teething-time of infants – which take place about the ninth or tenth month, and are accompanied with pain and swelling of the gums, compression and irritation of the nerves, and paroxysms that arise therefrom – without venesection? In such cases it is better by far than all the most vaunted specifics; be they what they may. Some of these, indeed, add to heat, and do mischief; and, however much they may have the credit of arresting the disorder by means of some occult property, frequently kill the little sufferer. At present, too, I say nothing about the immense relief afforded in the *pertussis* – or the hooping-cough – of infants by venesection. Here it leaves far behind it all pectoral remedies whatsoever.

9. What has been said concerning the cure of those symptoms which occur during the going-off of measles, occasionally applies to the treatment of them at their height. It does so when they are occasioned by the adscititious and artificial heat. In 1670, I was called in to see a maid servant of the Lady Anne Barrington's, suffering under this disease, together with a fever and difficulty of breathing, with purple spots discolouring the whole of her body, and with other symptoms of the most dangerous kind. I put down all this to the hot regimen, and the abundant hot medicines which she had used; and so I bled her at the arm, and ordered a cooling pectoral ptisan to be taken frequently. By the help of this, and by a more attempered regimen, the purple spots and the other bad symptoms gradually disappeared.

10. This disease, as stated above, began in the month of January, and increased every day until the vernal equinox. From that time forwards it decreased, and wholly disappeared in July. With the exception of a few places, where it showed itself in the following spring, it never returned during any of the years in which the present constitution prevailed. So much for the measles.

Sydenham (Figure 78) established no school of medicine during his lifetime and had few clinical pupils. The small number that he did teach included Thomas Dover (1660-1742), ultimately famous as a buccaneer and as the originator of 'Dover's Powder' (Ipecacuanha and Opium Powder, BPC[791], and Hans Sloane (1660-1753), founder of the British Museum.

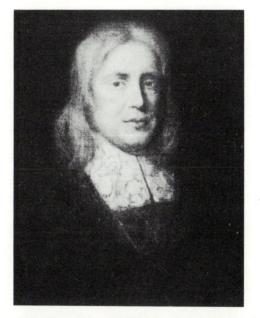

Figure 78   Thomas Sydenham (1624-1689). [*From: Joseph Frank Payne. Thomas Sydenham. London, Unwin, (1900).*]

There are a number of other seventeenth century names still used in the medical language of today. These include Pierre Gassendi (1592-1655) who demonstrated the vestigial foramen ovale of the adult heart, thereby putting to rest the vexed question of the perviousness of the septum of the heart, and Leonardo Botallo (born *c.* 1530) who in 1660 described the ductus arteriosus ('Botallo's duct') and the foramen ovale ('Botallo's foramen'). The names of those born after Sydenham include William Croone (1633-1684), whose widow endowed the Croonian Lectures of the Royal College of Physicians; Niels Stensen (1638-1686), who discovered the duct of the parotid gland ('Stensen's duct') and recognized the muscular nature of the heart; and the Dutchman, Regner de Graff (1641-1673), who was the first to study the pancreas and use fistulae in animals for this purpose and after whom the Graffian follicles are named in recognition of his work on the ovary.

Following these was Antonj Nuck (1650–1692), whose name is attached to the salivary glands and duct which he described; Johann Conrad Peyer (1653–1712), whose name is commemorated in the 'Peyer's patches', the lymphoid tissue of the small intestine which is so important in the pathogenesis of typhoid; Johann Brunner (1653–1727), who designated the duodenal glands that bear his name (they were discovered by Johann Wepfer, 1620–1695, who was his father-in-law) and Caspar Bartholin (1655–1738) of 'Bartholin's duct' and 'Bartholin's gland'.

Many of these names are now remembered because of the seventeenth century descriptions of anatomical structures. The continued interest of the greatest of painters, as well as medical people, in the features of anatomy is well illustrated by the famous painting of 'Doctor Nicolaas Tulp demonstrating the anatomy of the arm' (Figure 79). In this work Rembrandt (1606–1669) clearly shows the date of his painting, 1632, in the background. Human dissection remained, with the exception of Italy, a somewhat uncommon event and the Anatomy Book of the Amsterdam Guild of Surgeons records only one such dissection for the year 1632. The canvas, showing Dr Tulp, was the one with which Rembrandt van Rijn established his reputation. Now in the Hague, it hung until 1828 in the Theatrum Anatomicum of the Amsterdam Guild but, as only two foremen of that Guild are clearly shown as being present, it is possible that the work was a private commission.

It has some curious features and provides a series of puzzles which have recently been reviewed by William Schupbach[792]. Most dissections began with the abdomen, which decomposed first, and attended to the chest before the limbs; in the early dissections the corpse was decapitated to avoid the sacrilege of violating the brain case. In this painting Tulp is shown dissecting the arm first, the dissection having proceeded to the deep muscles with, it seems, Flexor digitorum profundus and Flexor pollicis longus being displayed. Tulp's left hand appears to be demonstrating the function of these muscles but Schupbach's analysis goes beyond this to suggest that Tulp is demonstrating the implications of anatomy in the form of a metaphysical paradox.

Nicolaas Tulp (1593–1674) is himself interesting. In his *Observationes medicae* (1652)[793] he gave such a fine account of the ileocaecal valve that this is often known as 'Tulp's valve'. More importantly, in the same book, he gave one of the earliest accounts ever written of beriberi – a condition the first scientific description of which had been provided 10 years before by Jacobus Bontius (1592–1631). Bontius had seen cases of the disease in the East Indies and gave a remarkable account of it in his *De medicina Indorum*[794] of 1642 (English translation, 1769).

There were other accounts of tropical diseases and their treatments and of deficiency diseases, stemming from the beginning of the century. George Wateson (b. 1544), in his *The cures of the diseased, in remote regions. Preventing mortalitie, incident in forraine attempts, of the English nation*[795], published in London in 1598, provided the earliest study of tropical medicine to appear in English. There is a facsimile edition of 1915. The first really important work on diseases of the tropics, giving good accounts of malaria, typhoid, and scurvy and early descriptions of yellow fever, amoebiasis, and a number of parasitic infesta-

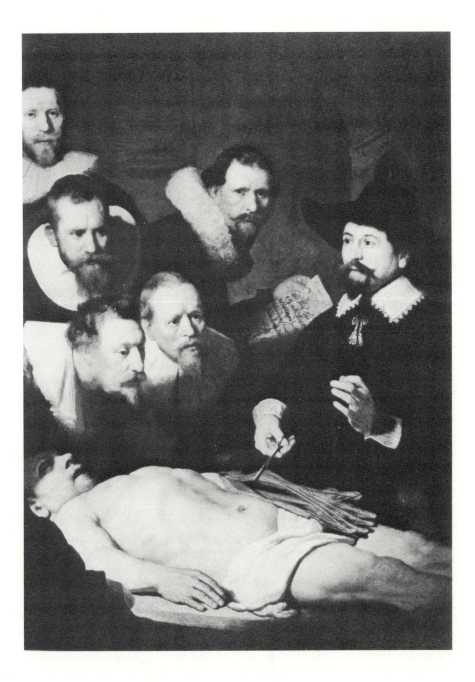

Figure 79   Rembrandt van Rijn. Nicolaas Tulp demonstrating the anatomy of the arm
(Detail).

263

tions, was the *Tratado de las siete enfermedades*... [796] produced by Alexo de Abreu (1568–1630) in 1623.

Of the deficiency diseases, scurvy attracted very early attention. Simple descriptions stretch back to the middle of the thirteenth century. Vasco da Gama noticed it at sea in his voyages of 1497–1502. The first medical account, recording how sailors cured themselves by eating citrus fruits as soon as they got back to the soil of Spain, was given by Balduinus Ronsseus (1525–1597) in his *De magnis Hippocratis lienibus, Pliniique stomacace, ac sceletyrbe, scu vulgo dicto scorbuto, libellus*[797], of 1564. This was followed by a significant early work of 1595[798] by Peter van Foreest (1522–1597) and by *The surgions mate* (1617)[799] of John Woodall (1556–1643), surgeon to St. Bartholomew's Hospital. Woodall, like writers on this subject before him, understood the usefulness of lemons and oranges in the treatment of scurvy and it is of some importance to realize that, even at this early date, the value of citrus fruits in this condition was understood. Abreu, in the *Tratado*... [796] of 1623, used fresh milk and rose syrup in the treatment of scurvy and Daniel Sennert (1572–1637), whose *Opera*[800] was first published in 1641 but which appeared in a better edition of 1676, added to the clinical knowledge of scurvy, alcoholism, and the diseases, such as dysentery, which were frequently seen under conditions of service.

Tulp, usually considered to have been the foremost anatomist of his day in Holland, was a direct academic descendant of Vesalius whose '*Fabrica*'[646] of 1543 carried the anatomical woodcut to what most would agree was its greatest degree of perfection. During the seventeenth century anatomy was displayed in brilliant copper-plates, some of which were not later excelled. The *Tabulae anatomicae lxxiix*[801] of Giulio Casserio (*c.* 1561–1616) provides fine examples and was published in 1627; Casserius was one of the teachers of Harvey at Padua. The splendid anatomies of later in the century included the *Anatomia humani corporis, centum et quinque tabulis per artificiosiss* (1685)[802] of Govert Bidloo (1649–1713), which has 105 magnificent copper-plates, and the 1691 *Anatomia*... [803] of Bernardino Genga (1655–1734) which is frequently chosen for study by artists due to the special quality of its engravings. These works found their fruition in the outstanding dissections and preparations of Frederik Ruysch (1638–1731), professor of anatomy at Leyden and Amsterdam, who perfected a method of injecting, and therefore visualizing, the blood vessels. The recipe for his injection has not been disclosed but the technique enabled him to provide the first description of the bronchial blood vessels and the finer ramifications of the vascular supply to the heart. He embodied many of his discoveries in his *Thesaurus anatomicus. i–x*[804] published in Amsterdam in 1701–16. The following century saw, well over 100 years after its author's death, the curiously delayed 1773 publication of the *Théorie de la figure humaine*[805] of the great artist and anatomist, Peter Paul Rubens (1577–1640); this study of the human figure is a work treasured for its copper-plates.

Late seventeenth century developments in other fields show their less advanced state of achievement: in physiology, Giovanni Borelli (1608–1679), in *De motu animalium* (1680–81)[806], began the neurogenic concept of the action of the heart and became the first to emphasize that the heart beat is due to simple muscular contraction. At much the same time, John Mayow (1643–1679), in a publication of 1674[807], became the first to place the location of animal heat in the

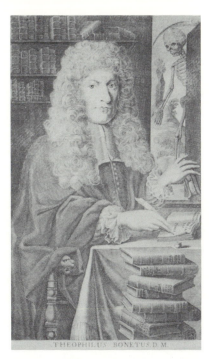

Figure 80 Théophile Bonet (1620-1689). [*From: Thomas Joseph Pettigrew (1838-1840).*]

muscles of the body; he was also the first to propose in a clear fashion that it is only a special fraction of the air which is used in the process of respiration. His *Tractatus quinque medico-physici* (1674)[807] forms one of the landmarks of English medical literature and was published in translation in Edinburgh in 1907. In the related field of medical biology Francesco Redi (1626-1697), in works dated 1684[808] and 1668[809] (and in an *Opere*[810] of 1762), delivered the first real blow to the theory of spontaneous generation; Redi also laid the groundwork of systematic parasitology by describing over 100 species of parasites. In the field of drug treatment itself, Sylvius (Franciscus de Le Boë; 1614-1672) advanced a number of new concepts in his *Praxeos medicae idea nova* (1671-74)[811]; Le Boë also established, at Leyden, the very first chemical laboratory in Europe. At much the same time Johann Major (1634-1693), professor of medicine at Kiel, became the first[812] to successfully inject drugs into the veins of man.

Events of even more far-reaching importance took place in the area in which organized pathology was to form a basis for much that is now everyday medicine. Le Boë (Sylvius) has an *Opera medica*[813] of 1679 which changed the understanding of tuberculosis by showing that the tuberculous lung contained tubercules which broke down to form cavities. Ten years later, in London, Richard Morton (1637-1698) produced his valuable *Phthisiologia, seu exercitationes de phthisi* (1689; English translation 1694)[814] in which he gave a fine description of tuberculosis and noted that tubercules are always present but that they can heal as well as soften and caseate.

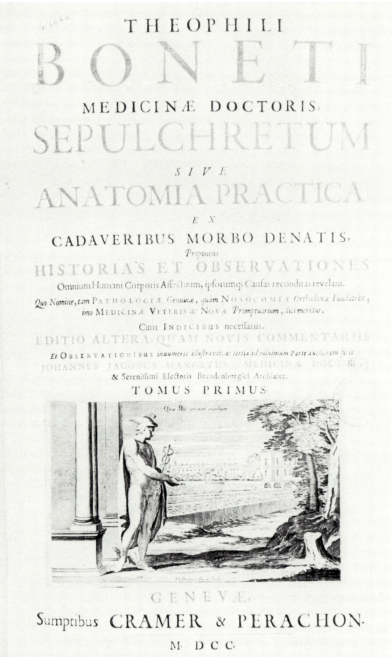

Figure 81   Théophile Bonet. Title page from: *Sepulchretum, sive anatomia practica ex cadaveribus morbo denatis*. Genevae, *L. Chouët* (1679). Edition of 1700. [*Royal Society of Medicine library, London.*]

266

These works had been preceded by the earliest works on general pathology. Amongst these must be numbered the *Observationum medicarum*...[815] of Johann Schenck (1530–1598), a book published in the year 1600 but giving access to important teachings on pathology by Vesalius and Sylvius, and the *De recondita abscessuum natura* (1632)[816] of Marco Aurelio Severino (1580–1656); the latter book is the first to provide illustrations of the conditions described in its text and gave the earliest organized classification of tumours of the breast.

Beyond these, the credit for having begun systematic morbid anatomy and much of scientific pathology must be given to Théophile Bonet (1620–1689). Bonet's *Sepulchretum, sive anatomia practica ex cadaveribus morbo denatis*[817] was published in Geneva in 1679. Taken from the edition of 1700, Figure 80 reproduces the portrait ('Theophilus Bonetus DM') and Figure 81 the title page. The work itself is a careful and detailed study providing clinical and pathological descriptions of almost 3000 autopsies gathered from the literature since the time of Hippocrates. Most of the material does, of course, come from the sixteenth and seventeenth centuries when thoughts on pathology were becoming more organized. The unique nature of this collection still provides access to some of the most ancient accounts of the physical nature of disease. The whole assembled the then known knowledge of its subject and provided an intellectual beginning to the study of the processes of human illness.

The Materia Medica

Sir Walter Raleigh (1554–1618), who was the first to settle colonists in Virginia and who became the brilliant favourite of Elizabeth, has his own special place in the history of seventeenth century therapeutics and the materia medica of today. Following the death of the Queen, and during the reign of the superstitious James I and VI, Raleigh – by then accused of treason by plotting in favour of Spain – was beheaded in 1618. His place in medicine is that in 1584 he brought back from Guiana, the territory which he had been the first to open to the enterprise of the British, the vitally important drug, curare.

This drug is the South American arrow poison (also primitively called 'wourara' or 'urari' amongst a number of names) which the natives of the Upper Amazonian and other regions had found could be extracted from the bark of a certain tree. It appeared as a gummy substance which would paralyse an animal if driven through its skin on the head of an arrow but which was harmless if taken by mouth. Thus, the meat of animals killed by its use was also harmless.

Modern accounts of the fascinating story of curare have been written by Archibald McIntyre (1947)[818], Kenneth Thomas (1964)[819] and J. Vellard (1965)[820]. The most fundamental piece of scientific work on the substance was the demonstration by Claude Bernard (1813–1878), in a publication of 1856[821], that curare acted by preventing transmission of the motor nerve impulses to the voluntary muscles. Curare itself appeared in the BPC 1934[822] and is the unstandardized extract obtained mainly from the bark of various species of *Strychnos* and *Chondodendron*; it varies a great deal in composition and appearance and is made by evaporation of a watery decoction or infusion of the woody vines forming its source. The great secret of its botanical origin was finally unravelled by B. A. Krukoff[823] of the New York Botanical Garden, who identified it as *Chondodendron tomentosum*. This is still the usual plant source of the alkaloid.

The native hunters stored it in a variety of pots and receptacles – hence the original names of 'calabash', 'pot', or 'tube' curare. The chemical composition of these different forms varied, and still does. The physiologically active substance, (+)-tubocurarine chloride has been isolated in crystalline form – the isolation of d-tubocurarine chloride from curare first being reported by Harold King (1887–1956) in 1935[824]. The introduction of curare into anaesthetic practice was described shortly afterwards in a notable paper (*The use of curare in general anaesthesia*)[825] by Harold Griffith and G. Enid Johnson (1942).

The contemporary use of the neuromuscular blocking agents, a vital part of today's anaesthesia, stems therefore from developments during and since World War II. Tubocurarine chloride is standardized chemically and, with its successors, is used in preference to curare. It is still sometimes called 'curare' in the literature of anaesthetics – and the use provides perhaps as dramatic an example as any of prehistoric drug lore reaching into the heart of twentieth century therapeutics.

One of the minor medicinal products of the seventeenth century was sodium sulphate (Glauber's salt) which, like copper sulphate and a number of other salts, was discovered by Johann Glauber (1604–1688). Glauber was probably the best chemical analyst of the century and was responsible for a number of processes, including the reaction of sulphuric acid with sea-salt to produce hydrochloric acid.

The two most important drugs introduced into England during the century were cinchona bark and ipecacuanha. Osler[826] gives an account of the discovery of the bark which, interesting in its own right, leads back to the earlier *A Memoir of the Lady Ana de Osorio Countess of Chinchon and Vice-Queen of Peru (AD 1629–39)*...[827] – a little work, now not particularly common, published by Clements R. Markham in 1874. Markham gives this record of events[828]:

> But the most notable historical event in this Viceroy's time was the cure of his Countess, in the year 1638, of a tertian fever, by the use of Peruvian bark. The news of her illness at Lima reached Don Francisco Lopez de Cañizares, who was then Corregidor of Loxa, and who had become acquainted with the febrifuge virtues of the bark. I have convinced myself that the remedy was unknown to the Indians in the time of the Yncas. It is mentioned neither by the Ynca Garcilasso nor by Acosta, in their lists of Indian medicines, nor is it to be found in the wallets of itinerant native doctors, whose *materia medica* has been handed down from father to son for centuries. It appears, however, to have been known to the Indians round Loxa, a town in the Andes, about 230 miles south of Quito. A Jesuit is said to have been cured of fever at Malacotas, near Loxa, by taking the bark given to him by the Indians, as long ago as 1600, and in about 1636 an Indian of Malacotas revealed the secret virtues of the *quinquina* bark to the Corregidor Cañizares. In 1638, therefore, he sent a parcel of it to the Vice-Queen, and the new remedy, administered by her physician, Dr Don Juan de Vega, effected a rapid and complete cure. It is known by tradition amongst the bark collectors, that the particular species from which the bark was taken which cured the Countess of Chinchon, was that known to them as *Cascarilla* (bark) *de Chahuarguera*.

A little later in his account Markham describes the carrying of the bark to Europe[829]:

> The Countess of Chinchon returned to Spain in the spring of 1640, with her husband, and bringing with her a supply of that precious *quina* bark which had worked so wonderful a cure upon herself, and the healing virtues of which she intended to distribute amongst the sick on her lord's estates, and to make known generally in Europe. The bark powder was most appropriately called Countess's powder (*Pulvis Comitissæ*), and by this name it was long known to druggists and in commerce. Dr Don Juan de Vega, the learned physician of the Countess of Chinchon, followed his patient to Spain, bringing with him a quantity of *quina* bark, which he sold at Seville at 100 reals the pound. The bark continued to have the same high value and the same reputation, until the trees became scarce, and the collectors began to adulterate it.
>
> After their return from Peru, the Count and Countess of Chinchon usually resided at the Castle of Chinchon, which was built by the Count's father in about 1590. The Countess administered Peruvian bark to the sufferers from tertian agues on her lord's estates, in the fertile but unhealthy *vegas* of the Tagus, the Jarama, and the Tajuña. She thus spread blessings around her, and her good deeds are even now remembered by the people of Chinchon and Colmenar, in local traditions.

The story of cinchona is of special interest for, unless one counts the use of mercury in syphilis, it provided – as the source of quinine with which to treat malaria – the first real specific treatment for disease to be discovered. This is Osler's summary of the naming of the bark after the Countess, and the later events which led to its also being called 'the Jesuits' bark'[826]:

> In 1638, the wife of the Viceroy of Peru, the Countess of Chinchon, lay sick of an intermittent fever in the Palace of Lima. A friend of her husband's, who had become acquainted with the virtues, in fever, of the bark of a certain tree, sent a parcel of it to the Viceroy, and the remedy administered by her physician, Don Juan del Vego, rapidly effected a cure. In 1640, the Countess returned to Spain, bringing with her a supply of quina bark, which thus became known in Europe as "the Countess's Powder" (*pulvis Comitissæ*). A little later, her doctor followed, bringing additional quantities. Later in the century, the Jesuit Fathers sent parcels of the bark to Rome, whence it was distributed to the priests of the community and used for the cure of ague; hence the name of "Jesuits' bark." Its value was early recognized by Sydenham and by Locke. At first there was a great deal of opposition, and the Protestants did not like it because of its introduction by the Jesuits. The famous quack, Robert Talbor, sold the secret of preparing quinquina to Louis XIV in 1679 for two thousand louis d'or, a pension and a title. That the profession was divided in opinion on the subject was probably due to sophistication, or to the importation of other and inert barks. It was well into the eighteenth century before its virtues were universally acknowledged.

In 1742 Linnaeus came to name the genus which provided the healing bark and, wishing to honour the Countess who had first made its virtues known to Europe, settled on the name *Chinchona*. Markham[827] devotes a large part of his book of 1874 to an explanation of the way in which Linnaeus, taking the name from a French variant spelling, frustrated his intention by writing the name of the genus as *Cinchona*. Thus, somewhat sadly, it has remained, although Markham has not been the only one who has tried to restore the lady's name to fame.

Although cinchona bark and quinine are effective used properly in malaria, the most devastating and widespread of the world's serious diseases, not all would agree with the traditional account of the drug's discovery. In an article *Fundamental errors in the early history of Cinchona* (1941)[830] A. W. Haggis held that the story was nothing but a fable. Holmstedt and Liljestrand (1963)[831] say that 'It is possible that it was the Count himself who carried the drug to Spain, but there is no proof of this. The Jesuits have also been mentioned in this connexion.'

The details of the curious beginnings of the drug are less important than its effects. It provided a powerful means of treating a very serious disease – and this was especially so once its confusion with other remedies (such as Peruvian balsam) ceased and once clinical malaria was differentiated from the fevers that were not responsive to quinine. The Italian pharmacologist, Francesco Torti (1658–1741)[832] did much to show the curative specificity of the cinchona bark in malaria and to distinguish the pernicious forms of the disease, which do not respond to it, from the varieties that do. Although Sydenham grasped only part of the truth, the advent of an effective drug to treat a major disease, and the consequent weakening of the long-held doctrine of the four humours was perhaps the most important single medical event of Sydenham's time. It is a happy accident that Sydenham, known for his fine descriptions of disease and for his having been a diligent student of Hippocrates, should have been of influence in bringing about the judicious use of the first practical remedy for such a grave condition.

The other notable drug of the seventeenth century was ipecacuanha. According to Garrison[833] this was first mentioned by a Portuguese friar in Purchas' *Pilgrimes* of 1625; the drug was taken to Paris in 1672. William Woodville[834] not only provides the illustration forming Figure 82 but also gives the following account of the plant and its history. He mentions the first recorded use (by Piso in 1649) and the events, once the drug reached Paris and was introduced into common practice by Helvetius, patronized by Louis XIV[834]:

> Piso divides this root into two sorts, the white and the brown, or according to Geoffroy, the Peruvian and Brazilian Ipecacuanha; but three sorts are evidently distinguishable in our shops, viz. ash-coloured or grey, brown, and white. The ash-coloured is brought from Peru, and "is a small wrinkled root, bent and contorted into a great variety of figures, brought over in short pieces full of wrinkles and deep circular fissures, down to a small white woody fibre that runs in the middle of each piece: the cortical part is compact, brittle, looks smooth and resinous upon breaking: it has very little smell; the taste is bitterish and subacrid, covering the tongue as it were with a kind of mucilage. The brown is small, somewhat more wrinkled that the foregoing; of a brown or blackish colour without, and white within; this is brought from Brazil (and corresponds with our specimen). The white sort is woody, has no wrinkles, and no perceptible bitterness in taste. The first, the ash-coloured or grey Ipecacuan, is that usually preferred for medicinal use. The brown has been sometimes observed, even in a small dose, to produce violent effects. The white, though taken in a large one, has scarce any effect at all." Dr. Irving has ascertained by experiments, that this root contains a gummy and resinous matter, and that the

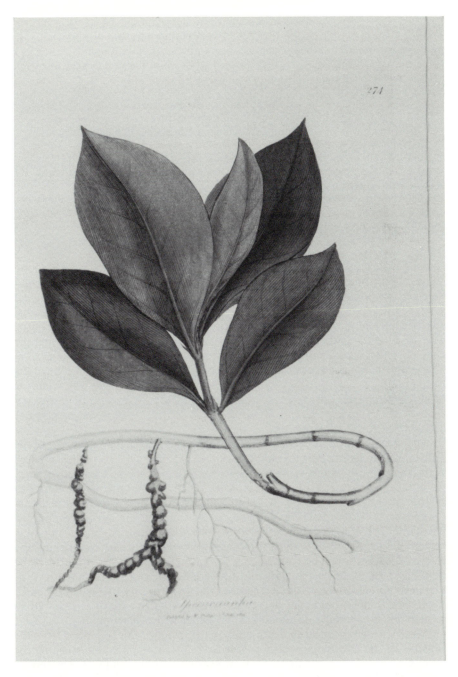

Figure 82 Cephaëlis ipecacuanha (= *Uragoga ipecacuanha*) or *C. acuminata.* Ipecacuanha. [*From: William Woodville. Medical botany... London, William Phillips, (1810). Vol. IV, Plate 274.*]

gum is in much greater proportion, and is more powerfully emetic than the resin: that the cortical part is more active than the ligneous, and that the whole root manifests an antiseptic and astringent power. He also found its emetic quality to be most effectively counteracted by means of the acetous acid, insomuch that thirty grains of the powder taken in two ounces of vinegar, produced only some loose stools.

The first account we have of Ipecacuan is that published by Piso, in 1649; but it did not come into general use till thirty years afterwards, when Helvetius, under the patronage of Louis XIV employed it at the Hotel de Dieu, and introduced this root into common practice; and experience has proved it to be the mildest and safest emetic with which we are acquainted, having this peculiar advantage, that if it does not operate by vomit, it readily passes off by the other emunctories.

It was first introduced to us with the character of an almost infallible remedy, in dysenteries and other inveterate fluxes, as diarrhœa, menorrhagia, and leucorrhœa, and also in disorders proceeding from obstructions of long standing: nor has it lost much of its reputation by time.

Woodville's specimen came to him from Sir Joseph Banks but he shows himself a little uncertain of its identification. The use he mentions – as an emetic – soon became popular, the drug being much safer than the toxic antimony emetics in vogue early in the seventeenth century. The Helvetius, whose name he records, was the Dutch physician Hadrianus Helvetius (1685–1755) to whom the use of the drug in dysentery of the amoebic type is largely attributed. Having cured the dauphin with ipecacuanha, Helvetius sold the secret of the remedy to Louis XIV, whereupon its use as a specific became general. The final disclosure of 'one of the best specifics in medicine' was contained in a work (*Recueil des methodes de Monsieur Helvetius, Medecin de S.A.R.M. le Duc d'Orleans, & Inspecteur General des Hôpitaux de Flandres. Pour la Guerison de diverses maladies*)[835] published at the Hague in 1710.

The specific within ipecacuanha was emetine, later to be isolated as part of the brilliant researches of Pelletier and Magendie (1817)[836]. The use of this alkaloid against amoebic dysentery is part of the story of nineteenth and twentieth century therapeutics. The emetic use of the extract of the plant substance continues today in the emergency treatment of poisoning: the new-style British National Formulary (1981)[837] describes the use, in appropriate circumstances, of the Paediatric Ipecacuanha Emetic Mixture and this must be about the only seventeenth century drug which the modern general practitioner might choose to carry for special use. The formula is a very simple one based on Ipecacuanha Liquid Extract[838]. Ipecacuanha Root is the dried root, or rhizome and roots, of *Cephaëlis ipecacuanha* of the Rubiaceae (Rio or Brazilian ipecacuanha) or *C. acuminata* (from Columbian and other sources); either way it is required to contain not less than 2% of total alkaloids, calculated as emetine[839].

Much of the rest of seventeenth century therapeutics can be judged from the contents of the *Pharmacopoeia Londinensis*[840] of 1618. This was issued by the College of Physicians, the first edition appearing on May 7th but containing so many typographical errors that a corrected version was published on December 7th, 1618. There is a readily available facsimile of both editions, with an introduction written by G. Urdang, which was produced in Madison in 1944.

The London Pharmacopoeia appeared 7 years after the Authorized Bible of 1611 and 2 years after the death of Shakespeare in 1616. The then known world was expanding when it was written: The East India Company's Charter of 1600 was 18 years old; the Settlement of Virginia (1607) was no longer new; the Pilgrim Fathers were to sail in the Mayflower in 2 years (1620). Ten years after this book with its strange contents appeared and was corrected, Harvey, in 1628, discovered the first copies of 'De Motu Cordis'[743] amongst his possessions. The Lumleian Lecture[741] of 1616, so important in relationship to the discovery of the circulation, was heard by Harvey's audience 2 years before the first edition of the Pharmacopoeia Londinensis became available.

When it did appear, it contained some 1960 remedies. Of these, 1028 were simples (medicines of one constituent, in contrast to the compound galenicals). The simples included 91 of animal and 271 from vegetable sources. The lungs of foxes were considered good for asthma and oil of ants, lozenges of dried vipers, and the bodies of earthworms, were all pharmacopoeial. Many of the 932 compound remedies still retained the names of their Greek or Arabian originators. They included Vigo's plaster, compounded from the flesh of vipers and the bodies of live frogs and earthworms. They also included mithridates and theriacs containing scores of ingredients.

The Codex medicamentarius seu pharmacopoeia Parisiensis. Lutetiae Parisiorum[841] was the first Paris pharmacopoeia and appeared in 1639. The Pharmacopoeia Londinensis, in its edition of 1650, contained what Garrison[842] listed as 'cochineal, antimonial wine, the red and white mercurial precipitates, moss from the skull of a victim of violent death, and Gascoyne's powder, compounded of bezoar, amber, pearls, crabs' eyes, coral, and black tops of crabs' claws.' Eight years later, in his De Indiae utriusque re naturali et medica libri quatuordecim[843] of 1658, Willem Piso (1611–1678) introduced ipecacuanha into Europe.

The London Pharmacopoeia of 1677 dropped many of the Greek and Arabic names and, amongst the substances we would still recognize as useful, introduced cinchona bark, digitalis and aqua vitae Hibernorum sive usquebaugh (Irish whisky). Providing one of his irresistable lists, Garrison[842] notes that 'contained in the three London Pharmacopoeias of the period were the blood, fat, bile, viscera, bones, bone-marrow, claws, teeth, hoofs, horns, sexual organs, eggs, and excreta of animals of all sorts; bee-glue, cock's-comb, cuttlefish, fur, feathers, hair, isinglass, human perspiration, saliva of a fasting man, human placenta, raw silk, spider-webs, sponge, sea-shell, cast-off snake's skin, scorpions, swallow's nests, wood-lice, and the triangular Wormian bone from the juncture of the sagittal and lambdoid sutures of the skull of an executed criminal (ossiculum antiepilepticum Paracelsi).'

The 1677 edition was a little later than the Anastasis corticis Peruviae, seu chinae defensio[844] in which, in 1663, Sebastiano Bado (fl. 1640–1676) produced a spirited defence of the virtues of the bark of the 'fever-tree' – the Peruvian bark. It is also a little later than the Pharmacopoeia Londinensis Collegarum[845] of 1668 from which the title page is reproduced as Figure 83 and pages 176 and 177, giving the formula for a mithridatium, are illustrated in Figures 84 and 85. The 1677 edition appeared just over 20 years before the publication of 1701, Censura medicamentorum officinalium[846], of Augustus Rivinus (1652–1723) which

PHARMACOPOEIA
LONDINENSIS
COLLEGARUM.

*Hodie viventium ſtudiis ac Sym-
belis ornatior.*

LONDINI,
Typis *W. Bentley,* impenſis
L. Sadler, & *R. Beaumont.*
An. 1668.

Figure 83 Title page of the *Pharmacopoeia Londinensis Collegarum...* London (1668). [*Royal Society of Medicine library, London.*]

marked the turn of the century and, perhaps significantly, listed not only officially recognized drugs but also, and in a European pharmacopoeia, incompatibilities between drugs and their unwanted and undesirable properties.

We have now reached almost 200 years since the time of the earliest medical work printed in English. It has been said[847] that this was a small quarto tract of 12 leaves with the title *A Passing Gode Lityll Boke Necessarye and Behovefull Agenst the Pestilence*; it was published without the printer's name or date but is attributed to the press of William de Machlinia, in London, and was printed about 1480. Perhaps, at the time of that first printed English medical work we would not have been too surprised at the contents of the London Pharmacopoeia. It is more amazing that the contents of the seventeenth century London apothecary's shop remained the wherewithal of primitive magic, relieved only by two or three specifics, when Harvey had written '*De Motu Cordis*'[743], Hooke had

274

176   *Electuaria.*

Boli Armenæ unciam unam femis.
Terræ figillatæ Lemniæ unciam dimi‹
diam.
Piperis longi,
Zingiberis ana drach. duas.
Mellis albi defpumati lib. duas femis.
Sacchari rofati lib. unam.
Vini Canarini Aromatici uncias de‹
cem.
Fiat Electuarium fecundùm Artem.

Mithridatium.

℞. Myrrhæ Arabicæ,
Croci,
Agarici,
Zingiberis,
Cinnamomi,
Spicæ Nardi,
Thuris,
Sem. Thlafpios ana drach. decem.
Sefeleos,
Opobalfami feu Olei Nucis Mofchatæ
per expreffionem.
Junci odorati,
Stœchados,
Cofti veri,
Galbani,
Terebinthinæ,
Piperis longi,
Caftorei,
Succi Hypociftidos,
Styracis Calamitæ,
Opopanacis,
Fol. Malabathri recentium, feu ejus de‹
fectu,

Figure 84   Formula for a mithridatium from the *Pharmacopoeia Londinensis Collegarum* (1668), p. 176.

described the cell, Boyle had discovered his law, Newton had published the 'Principia'[723], and Sydenham was practising medicine.

A figure of very different proportions was the curious and provocative early apothecary, Nicholas Culpeper (1615-1654); Culpeper served in the Parliamentary army, was wounded at Newbury, and aroused the wrath of the College of Physicians by translating the *Pharmacopoeia Londinensis* into the vernacular. He produced a substantial number of works, many with robust and quaint additions to the orthodox body of knowledge, but is of interest as providing readily available English translations of the seventeenth century pharmacopoeia. An example is the *Pharmacopoeia Londinensis: or the London Dispensatory. Further adorned by the studies and collections of the Fellows, now living, of the said Colledg...by Nicholas Culpeper* (1654)[848]. There is also a work, *Mr Culpeper's Ghost...*[849] one edition of which is dated 1656, in which after his

275

Electuaria. 177

fectu, Macis, ana unciam unam.
Casiæ ligneæ veræ,
Polii montani,
Piperis albi,
Scordii,
Sem. Dauci Cretici,
    Carpobalsami vel Cubebarum,
Trochisch. Cypheos,
Bdelli ana drach. septem.
Nardi Celticæ purgatæ,
Gummi Arabici,
Sem. Petroselini Macedonici,
Opii,
Cardamomi minoris,
Sem. Fœniculi,
Gentianæ,
Fol. Rosar. rubrarum.
Dictamni Cretensis ana drach. quinq;
Sem. Anisi,
Asari,
Acori, seu Calami Aromatici,
Ireos,
Phu majoris,
Saganeni ana drach. tres.
Mei Athamantici,
Acaciæ,
Ventrium Scincorum,
Summitatum Hyperici ana drach. duas
    semis.
Vini Malvatici quantum sufficit ad so-
    lutionem gummi, & succorum.
Mellis deinde despumati triplum ad
    omnia, præter vinum.
Fiat Electuarium secundum Artem.

Figure 85 Formula for a mithridatium (continued) from the *Pharmacopoeia Londinensis Collegarum* (1668), p. 177.

death his wife vindicates his reputation. From this divertissment the title page provides Figure 86 and the portrait of Culpeper Figure 87. Sibly[850] later (1813) published an expanded and illustrated Culpeper edition with a fine plate of the Jesuits' bark – and this is reproduced in Figure 88.

Plague, fever and smallpox

The decimating mediaeval plague epidemic of 1348–49 and the manner in which, from that time, plague became endemic in Europe, has already been discussed (p. 180). These epidemics continued and that of 1563, the first year for which there are authentic figures for the weekly plague deaths in London, soon became one of the most severe outbreaks that the city had known. It began in midsummer and,

MR CULPEPERS GHOST,

Giving Seasonable

ADVICE to the LOVERS

OF HIS

WRITINGS.

Before which is prefixed,

Mris. Culpepers EPISTLE
in Vindication *of her Husband's*
Reputation.

LONDON:
Printed for *Peter Cole*, and are to be sold at his Shop,
at the sign of the Printing-Press in Corn-hil,
neer the Royal Exchange.   1 6 5 6.

Figure 86   Mrs Culpeper. Title page from: *Mr Culpeper's ghost* ... London, P. Cole,
(1656).

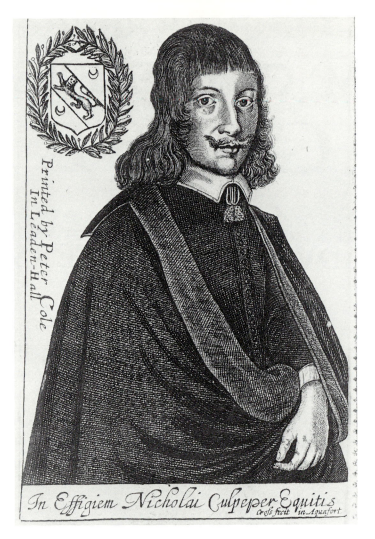

Figure 87 Nicholas Culpeper (1615–1654). *Cross portrait from: Mrs Culpeper (1656).*

at its peak, caused 1626 deaths in the one week of September 17; gradually, as the cold months of the winter came on, the severity of the epidemic declined.

Deriving much of his data from Graunt's *Natural and Political Observations mentioned in a following index, and made upon the Bills of Mortality*[728], of 1662, Charles Creighton (1891)[851] provides the details given in Table 2. This shows the deaths for the period 1629–1666; thus, it ends the year after the onslaught of the Black Death in 1665 and reaches to the year, 1666, of the Great Fire of London.

278

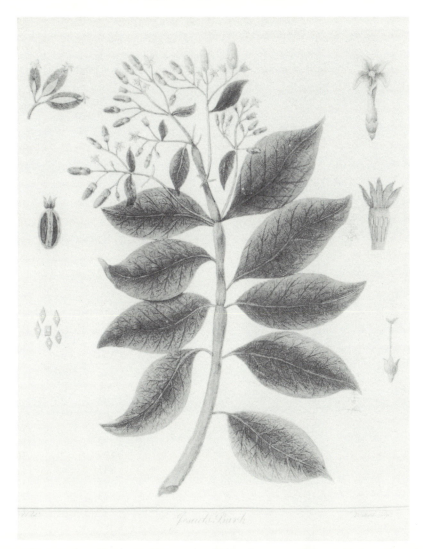

Figure 88   Cinchona calisaya. The Jesuit's Bark. [*From: Culpeper's English Physician and complete herbal . . . Sibly 15th edition. London, W. Lewis, (1813), Vol. I, Plate II.*]

The average annual figure for 'Total deaths' for the period 1630–1664, both years included, is 12 370. The missing figures in the Table for 'Fever' and 'Smallpox' are due to their having been found 'inconsistent with the capacity' of Graunt's sheet of paper. As all of the original documents prior to 1658 seem to have been lost in the Great Fire of 1666, Creighton adds the characteristic comment that: 'Graunt's omission cannot now be made good. One could wish that the worthy citizen had made no difficulty about the size of his paper. The

Table 2   London mortality, 1629–1666. From Charles Creighton (1891)

Year	Plague	Fever	Smallpox	Total deaths
1629	0	956	72	8771
1630	1317	1091	40	10554
31	274	1115	58	8562
32	8	1108	531	9535
33	0	953	72	8393
34	1	1279	1354	10400
35	0	1622	293	10651
36	10400	2360	127	23359
37	3082	—	—	11763
38	363	—	—	13624
39	314	—	—	9862
1640	1450	—	—	12771
41	1375	—	—	13142
42	1274	—	—	13273
43	996	—	—	13212
44	1492	—	—	10933
45	1871	—	—	11479
46	2365	—	—	12780
47	3597	1260	139	14059
48	611	884	401	9894
49	67	751	1190	10566
1650	15	970	184	8754
51	23	1038	525	10827
52	16	1212	1279	12569
53	6	282	139	10087
54	16	1371	832	13247
55	9	689	1294	11357
56	6	875	823	13921
57	4	999	835	12434
58	14	1800	409	14993
59	36	2303	1523	14756
1660	13	2148	354	12681
61	20	3490	1246	16665
62	12	2601	768	13664
63	9	2107	411	12741
64	5	2258	1233	15453
65	68596	5257	655	97306
1666	1998	741	38	12738

omitted years are not only those of great political revolution, which may have had an effect upon the public health, but they are of special interest for the beginning of that great period of fever and smallpox in London which continued all through the 18th century.'[852]

The average number of deaths of 12370 for the 35 years before the plague pandemic of 1665 has to be compared with the appalling total of 97306 in that year itself. Of this total, plague alone was held responsible for 68596 deaths in 1665. There were reasons for hiding plague as a cause of death, and that this may have not infrequently happened is suggested by the fact that deaths in the rather non-specific column headed 'Fever' were higher in 1665 than in any other year given in the Table. Creighton's figures also show the lesser plague epidemic of 1636 and the curious 12 year tail of the mortality due to the disease in the years immediately following 1636. Then there was a long span of 16 years with few plague deaths – before the outburst of the great plague year, the Black Death.

There is a steady mortality from 'Fever' (which we can no longer define in diagnostic terms) running throughout Table 2 – and there are 7 years in which smallpox caused over 1000 deaths. The latter finding is, perhaps, not unexpected. One would not guess though that there would have been just as many years, clustered before the outbreak of the Black Death, in which 'Fever' (whatever it was) would have carried off the same or more than twice that number.

Only in modern times has it been possible to inflict upon populations a holocaust like that which the plague brought upon the seventeenth century cities and nations of Europe. The pandemics of the century started in 1601–03 in Russia, where Moscow suffered over 125000 deaths from plague and famine. Pandemics started successively in England (1603), France, Holland, Italy, Denmark, Germany, Sweden, Switzerland, and led eventually to Spain (1677). The Black Death that caused the total already given of 68596 deaths in London in 1665, caused almost the same number of deaths in Vienna four years later and another 83000 deaths in Prague in 1681.

The effects of the London pandemic were witnessed by Samuel Pepys (1633–1703) who wrote his own well-known and first-hand account. They were also vividly described by Daniel Defoe (1660–1731); Defoe was a child of 4 or 5 when the plague raged in London and wrote his *A Journal of the Plague Year* (1722)[853] from his memories as the son of a butcher in St. Giles's, Cripplegate (one of the worst affected parishes) and from the records and memories of those who survived. He is likely also to have been helped by the accounts of the Marseilles plague of 1720 which reached its height while he was writing.

Using these sources and the original material, Defoe provides human and unforgettable descriptions of the sudden onset and symptomology of the disease in both its fulminant, pandemic and bubonic forms. He describes the ordinances of the Mayor and Aldermen intended to limit the spread of the infection – and gives one account of these precautions stumbling close to a means of controlling the vector of the disease[853]:

> (We) were ordered to kill all the Dogs and Cats: But because as they were domestick Animals, and are apt to run from House to House, and from Street to Street; so they are capable of carrying the Effluvia or Infectious Steams of Bodies infected, even in their Furrs and Hair; and therefore it was that in the

beginning of the Infection, an Order was published by the Lord Mayor, and by the Magistrates, according to the Advice of the Physicians; that all the Dogs and Cats should be immediately killed, and an Officer was appointed for the Execution.

It is incredible, if their Account is to be depended upon, what a prodigious Number of those Creatures were destroy'd: I think they talk'd of forty thousand Dogs, and five times as many Cats, few Houses being without a Cat, and some having several, and sometimes five or six in a House. All possible Endeavours were us'd also to destroy the Mice and Rats, especially the latter; by laying Rats-Bane, and other Poisons for them, and a prodigious multitude of them were also destroy'd.

Throughout the country local history collections provide less well-known but equally interesting descriptions – the following is of *The Great Plague in Chichester in 1665* and is originally from a record of J. Low Warren[854]:

The story is not a new one, yet in the present day few people know to what terrible suffering the good people of the City were put. How the plague ever reached it in the first instance is not known, but it was supposed that a traveller who came from London, introduced the malady. He came in the evening as well as man could be, but in the morning the inn keeper found him dead. The body bore every indication of the terribly agony the man had undergone; and when the surgeon had examined it, he said that the man had died of the plague. That same night he was buried by torchlight in the Churchyard of S. Pancras. Here the evil did not stop, for within a few hours it spread rapidly and well-known faces were soon missed from amongst the good folk of Chichester. Before long things became so serious that the Mayor called together a meeting of his *confreres*, and it was decided to rigidly enforce those regulations, which had been adopted in London. The inhabitants were warned of the infected streets, and when the examiners declared a death, the house in which it had occurred was shut up, a watchman placed at the door, to prevent ingress or egress, and the awful but familiar words, with the sign of the Cross, *Lord have mercy upon us*, were painted on the door. The Angel of Death was making wider and wider gaps in the ranks of the good citizens, and still there appeared no signs of abatement, and so the Mayor called another meeting to consider on this sad state of affairs. At this meeting it was decided to shut up the City; and so a cordon was drawn around the walls. As long as the provisions lasted this answered very well, but the plague continued longer than they had calculated upon, and soon famine began to stare them in the face. The Council then resolved to declare the pitiable state of affairs on the different gates of the City, in the hopes that someone would read the notices thereon affixed. A Bosham villager who had been tending his cattle in one of the meadows close to the walls, was attracted by those who were standing on the western tower, and impelled by curiosity he approached sufficiently near to learn the cause of the assemblage. A few words sufficed to make known to this man the sad state of affairs within the City walls, and he, after condoling with them, promised to return on the following morning with what food and assistance he could. Before sunrise the next day a cavalcade of carts laden with meat and grain, poultry and vegetables, was seen by the citizens to be approaching, and long before the procession of men and boys reached the gates, the western walls were crowded by an eagerly expectant throng. The cavalcade then made a halt in the road to the west of the gate, and signalled to the citizens that they had brought provisions. Then came the difficulty of dealing for the articles. The fisher-folk were afraid to come into close contact with the fever-stricken in-habitants of the City, and so the plan of laying the provisions on a flat stone and marking the price on them was adopted; the cautious people from Bosham retiring whilst those, who stood so sadly in need of the edibles, came and inspected. The provisions selected, the money was placed in a bucket of water; and so the chances of contagion were minimised, and later on as their fears abated, the Bosham folk helped the citizens to bury their dead; and in many other ways they proved good friends to the afflicted inhabitants.

The Londoner can, by contemporary documents point out the spots where the old plague pits existed, but unfortunately from lack of evidence, the exact site of the Chichester pits will never be known. It has been surmised – with what accuracy we know not – that some of the fields around the old S. James' Hospital, on the Arundel Road, were the most likely place, and in this there may be some reason.

But to return to our story. Day after day the men of Bosham brought provisions to the City so long as the plague lasted. As soon, however, as the sultry weather ceased, the awful disease, which had wrought such terrible havoc in the ranks of the citizens was carried away, as it were on the wings of the storm. The heavy rain which fell seemed to purge the air of its impurities, and the streets and houses of their filth and garbage. So soon as the storm died away, the sickness began to lessen, and soon, very soon, the plague ceased, and the citizens came out of their houses to remove the dread sign of the Cross, and the words of such awful import which covered their doors.

Services of thanksgiving were held in all the Churches and those who were left thanked their Maker that He had seen fit to spare them from the dread sickness and famine.

The medical records, as such, include the valuable study *London's dreadful visitation, or, a collection of all the Bills of Mortality for the present year: beginning the 27th of December 1664, and ending the 19th of December follow-ing . . . By the Company of Parish Clerks of London*[855]. This was published in London in 1665. There is also an important work, *Loimographia. An account of the great plague of London in the year 1665. By William Boghurst* (1631-1685). The work was written in 1666 by Boghurst, a London apothecary who dis-tinguished plague from typhus, and was published, entitled as above and with a useful introduction by J. F. Payne, in 1894[856]. But probably the best medical account of the Black Death of 1665 is the John Quincy, 1720 edition of the Λοιμολογία *sive pestis nuperae apud populum Londinensem grassantis narratio historica*[857] of Nathaniel Hodges; this work, published in 1672, was written by Hodges (1629-1688) who was not only physician to the City of London but who laboured throughout, and achieved a great reputation during, the great epidemic.

Collectively these different accounts show how the infection travelled from one part of London to another, from the western suburbs of the City to those in the east, so that it faded in its intensity in one of the parishes before flaring up in another. The final epidemic began with a single death in a house in or near Long Acre in December, 1664. This seemed not very different from previous epidemics and there was probably little that was unusual – apart from our having access to first-hand and well-written accounts – about the beginning of the 1665 outbreak. As it built to its total of deaths it became unique – devastating the parishes of

Cripplegate, Whitechapel, Stepney, St. Martin's in the Fields, St. Giles's, Southwark and Westminster. The epidemiologically important point is that the City itself escaped lightly compared with the parishes in the eastward path of the disease. Thus, the one thing that can be considered certain is that the old explanation of the schoolbooks – that the Great Fire of London burnt out and put an end to the disease – is not to be believed.

Northern and western Europe have been substantially free from plague – apart from the isolated and violent outbreak in Marseilles in 1720 – since 1665. It has not been so in the East where the last great wave, which started in 1894 (when there were 100 000 or more deaths in Canton) may not yet be exhausted. But in England, in the 200 years after the 1665 pandemic, there were only two deaths from plague, and these were in Cornwall. The signs are that the disease died back to sylvan proportions, emerging only in one curious, isolated outbreak in Suffolk between 1906 and 1918.

A great deal has been written in various attempts to explain why, in 1666, plague disappeared after being endemic in Britain for 300 years and frequently reaching epidemic proportions. It has often been asked if the disease could sweep back, as it once swept back after an absence of 800 years, to begin another such 300-year endemic period. All that is certain is that when plague disappeared nothing was known of the causative organism or the means of transmission – and the change, when it came, took place without any form of medical understanding or intervention. The lesson has to be in the power and rate of change of disease and the misleading variations of its natural history.

Smallpox, the other specific disease given in Creighton's table of the London mortality 1629–1666, behaved differently. It seems to have crept only gradually into prominence and not to have been one of the great causes of death until the reign of James I and VI. This was unlike either plague or the strange, influenzal-like 'sweating-sickness': both of these showed themselves fearsome from the beginning, retained their virulence over a long period of years, and ended in epidemics that were as severe in their effects as any that had occurred in their history. With plague, the final outbreak was, in fact, the most violent the country had recorded. Creighton says that 'in the Elizabethan period the Latin name *variolae* was rendered by measles, and ... smallpox, where distinguished from measles, was not reputed a very serious malady.'[858] If this was true in the sixteenth century, then it seems clear that things changed in the 100 years that followed.

The first smallpox epidemic in London for which weekly mortality figures of some reliability exist was 1628. In that year there were 79 deaths from smallpox in the last two weeks of May. Such a figure, in a population of about 300 000, and over such a short period, represents a major epidemic. We have already noted, from Table 2, that smallpox deaths exceeded 1000 in at least 7 of this span of years that covered the central parts of the seventeenth century. The Restoration in 1660 was followed by two deaths in the Royal Family, both from smallpox, within a few months. The late years of the century, after the Great Fire of London, experienced further major epidemics in 1681 and 1699. Between these two dates the London epidemic of 1694 was marked by the death of the Queen from the haemorrhagic form of the disease.

There was great controversy following the death, on December 28th, 1694, of the Queen – Mary II (1662–1694), joint ruler of Great Britain with William III –

and Walter Harris (1647–1732), physician to both William and Mary, was permitted to publish a descriptive account. This appears in the 1720 edition of his *De morbis acutis infantum*[859] – first published in 1689 and thereafter serving as a standard textbook on paediatrics for almost a century. Famous for having used calcium salts in the treatment of infantile convulsions in a way that anticipates the modern treatment of tetany, Harris's account of the death of the Queen, as rendered by Creighton, is this[860]:

> The symptoms of illness on the first day did not prevent the queen from going abroad; but, as she was still out of sorts at bedtime, she took a large dose of Venice treacle, a powerful diaphoretic which her former physician, the famous physiologist Dr Lower, had recommended her to take as often as she found herself inclined to a fever. Finding no sweat to appear as usual, she took next morning a double quantity of it, but again without inducing the usual effects of perspiration. Up to that time she had not asked advice of the physicians. To this severe dosing with one of the most powerful alexipharmac or heating medicines, the malignant type of the ensuing smallpox was mainly ascribed by Harris, who was a follower of Sydenham and a partizan of the cooling regimen. On the third day from the initial symptoms the eruption appeared, with a very troublesome cough; the eruption came out in such a manner that the physicians were very doubtful whether it would prove to be smallpox or measles. On the fourth day the smallpox showed itself in the face and the rest of the body "under its proper and distinct form." But on the sixth day, in the morning, the variolous pustules were changed all over her breast into the large red spots "of the measles"; and the erysipelas, or rose, swelled her whole face, the former pustules giving place to it. That evening many livid round petechiae appeared on the forehead above the eyebrows, and on the temples, which Harris says he had foretold in the morning. One physician said these were not petechiae, but sphacelated spots; but next morning a surgeon proved by his lancet that they contained blood. During the night following the sixth day, Dr Harris sat up with the patient, and observed that she had great difficulty of breathing, followed soon after by a copious spitting of blood. On the seventh day the spitting of blood was succeeded by blood in the urine. On the eighth day the pustules on the limbs, which had kept the normal variolous character longest, lost their fulness, and changed into round spots of deep red or scarlet colour, smooth and level with the skin, like the stigmata of the plague. Harris observed about the region of the heart one large pustule filled with matter, having a broad scarlet circle round it like a burning coal, under which a great deal of extravasated blood was found when the body was examined after death. Towards the end, the queen slumbered sometimes, but said she was not refreshed thereby. At last she lay silent for some hours; and some words that came from her shewed, says Burnet, that her thoughts had begun to break. She died on the 28th of December, at one in the morning, in the ninth day of her illness.

By the end of the sixteenth century leprosy had largely died out and syphilis, having ceased to assume an epidemic form, was treated by the barber-surgeons with mercury applied either by fumigation or inunction. If, as we have seen, smallpox changed and during the seventeenth century became much more severe, it still remained, especially in the latter parts of the century, a less common cause of death than 'Fever'. Most of this was probably typhus and some of it typhoid.

In central Europe, especially after the terrible events of the Thirty Years' War, dysentery, scurvy, famine, violence and lawlessness added to the causes of deaths.

It is possible that leprosy dwindled due to the draconic measures taken to prevent its spread in the community. It is clear that we do not really know why plague so suddenly and completely disappeared – but that this dramatic change for the better was not due to human intervention. Thus, the disease and its history remain one of the more awesome examples of the forces involved in the natural history of disease. Smallpox, which in the seventeenth century produced its quota of deaths amongst rich and poor alike, is quite the opposite – an example of a lethal disease the epidemiology of which was to be transformed by a specific act of medical intervention.

But if the seventeenth century was, as it has often been called, an 'Age of Enlightenment', then its light shone very largely in a number of brilliant, and frequently privileged, minds. It did not much illuminate the lives of the everyday people. The most common illnesses remained the infectious diseases, hygiene was everywhere primitive, and the great mass of the population lived under poor conditions indeed. Some idea of these conditions, and the almost complete absence of the effective prevention or treatment of disease, can be gained from the statistics on infant mortality: Garrison[861] provides the comment that 'In Restoration England, sometimes half the births were obliterated by disease and two-fifths of the total deaths were of infants under two years. In the hot summers of 1669–71, 2000 babies died of diarrhea in eight or ten weeks. The dense London population had swarmed to the waterside and the alleys of Wapping, Lambeth, Whitechapel, and Spitalfields, living in filthy, overcrowded tenements...'

The beginnings of medical care in a form in which it might reach the everyday people arose from a specialization in what was, essentially, a means of trade.

Oriental and other spices and herbs were used for both medicinal and culinary purposes and this continued, in the hands of the powerful Grocers' Company, long after the Act of 1518 by which the Physicians had been incorporated by Henry VIII as a College. While the Physicians continued to enjoy their learned status and the surgeons tried to free themselves from the barbers that encumbered them in the Barber-Surgeons Guild, the apothecaries – or those of them especially interested in the medicinal use of herbs and spices – strove to free themselves from the less medically-inclined Grocers. In 1607 they achieved a very limited measure of success and managed to incorporate themselves as a separate section within, but still very much part of, the huge Grocers' Company.

On December 6th, 1617 they were finally rewarded and, by Charter of James I and VI, were enabled to establish their own independent organization – the Worshipful Society of Apothecaries of London. The real champion of the piece, who had led the King to say: 'Grocers are but merchants, the business of an Apothecary is a Mistery...'[862], was Gideon de Laune (1565–1635), the son of a refugee French protestant clergyman who made a living by practising medicine in London. De Laune himself achieved such success at this art that he rose to become apothecary to Anne of Denmark (1574–1619), Queen of James I and VI. In this capacity he led the whole fraternity of expert apothecaries from the time of the partial separation of 1607 but, technically still a foreigner, he could not become Master of the newly-chartered Society until 1628.

At the beginning the young Society of Apothecaries had lamentably few friends. The Grocers, presumably fearing competition in a lucrative branch of the trade, tried hard to reabsorb them. They were prevented in doing this only by the intervention of the King. The Physicians, who were reluctant to give licences to any who did not have a university degree, and would certainly admit none but graduates to their Fellowship, steadily and with great ingenuity opposed the growth of the Apothecaries. The new Society flourished only because its members acted as the general medical practitioners of the time.

Within the ranks of the Apothecaries different activities arose. Some, as opportunity and interest came together, occupied themselves with the wholesale or retail distribution of drugs – so forming the beginnings of the group, keen on pharmacy, which 200 or so years later broke away from the Apothecaries to establish today's Pharmaceutical Society. Others were interested in the more botanical and scientific aspects of the materia medica, thereby providing for the ultimate growth of the science of pharmacology – and providing recruits for the ranks of the medical botanists. A third group of the early expert apothecaries, attending to patients, found themselves, by force of circumstances or design or both, giving advice to accompany the remedies they dispensed and sold. It was this third group which soon found itself in direct conflict with the College of Physicians who, perhaps rightly, feared for their monopoly of the practice of medicine.

Some of the early apothecaries are now very famous. They included the magnificent Royal Herbalists – amongst them John Parkinson (1567–1650), who was practising at the time of the granting of the Society's Charter in 1617 and whose works included the *Theatrum botanicum: The theater of plants. Or, an herball of a large extent*[637] of 1640, and Thomas Johnson (1604–1644), whose much improved and expanded version of Gerard's *The herball or generall historie of plantes*[635] appeared in 1633.

The Charter of the Apothecaries came the year before the College of Physicians published the first edition of the *Pharmacopoeia Londinensis*[840] in 1618; it divided the Apothecaries from the Grocers a year after Shakespeare's death in 1616. Thus, the Charter came at a period when, as in the lifetime of Shakespeare, there were no general practitioners of medicine and when ordinary people must have sought medical care wherever, in its impoverished state, they could find it. At this time the antagonism between the physicians – few and far between and demanding heavy fees, usually the gold coin then known as the Angel – and the apothecaries was very real. One of these early members of the Society was the colourful Nicholas· Culpeper (1615–1654) whom William Copeman credits with the statement that the 'physicians were like Balaam's ass – they would only speak when they saw an Angel.'[863] Copeman, one of the more recent historians of the Society and its Master 1958–59, provided the very readable *The Worshipful Society of Apothecaries of London, A History 1617–1967*[862] which appeared in the latter year, marking the period of 350 years which had passed since the granting of the King James Charter.

In 1632 the young Society had funds enough to allow it to move to the site of the Dominican monastery in Blackfriars Lane which it occupies now. The first Hall to be built was destroyed in the Great Fire of London in 1666 but was

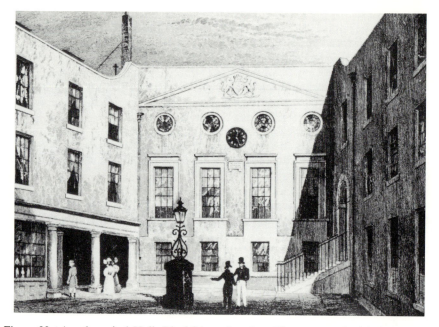

Figure 89 Apothecaries' Hall, Blackfriars, London. The courtyard with the Apothecaries' shop, about 1815. [*The Beadle: Worshipful Society of Apothecaries.*]

replaced by the present magnificent Hall which, despite damage all around it during the bombing of London in World War II, is almost unchanged. Figure 89 shows the paved courtyard outside the Great Hall with the well, still untouched, which was used by the thirteenth century Dominican monks.

From its earliest days the Society involved itself in the quality of medicines and, in 1623, established a laboratory for the production of galenical and vegetable substances, some of these being used in the training of apprentices. In 1671 a chemical laboratory was added to handle the simple chemical medicines that were, by then, being more and more used. This was one of the first chemical laboratories to be set up in Britain; it permitted a greater control of the purity of the drugs used by members of the Society, as well as reducing the cost of medicines which could be both produced and tested on a larger scale than before. At this stage the Society already had a monopoly for the supply of drugs to the Navy but its increased facilities allowed it to create similar monopolies for the supply of the Army, the Crown Colonies, and the East India Company. Ultimately, this experience led some of the Apothecaries to found pharmaceutical houses, such as Allen and Hanbury, and pharmaceutical chemists, such as John Bell and Croyden or Savory and Moore, which remain with us today.

As the seventeenth century became well advanced, the Apothecaries, in 1673, founded the Chelsea Physic Garden on the riverside site where it still stands between Royal Hospital Road and Swan Walk. Linnaeus visited the Garden in 1733 and it became a source of tuition not only to the contemporaries of

Linnaeus, but also to a number of generations as the profession of medicine organized itself in an orderly fashion in Britain.

For the Society of Apothecaries the century in which it achieved its Charter ended, and the new century opened, with the bitter dispute with the College of Physicians coming to a head. In 1701, William Rose, a Liveryman of the Society with his shop in St. Martin-in-the-Fields, was chosen by the College and sued by them for treating a butcher, named Seale, without using a physician as an intermediary. The action, in the Queen's Bench Division, was won by the College of Physicians. In 1703 the House of Lords, on appeal, reversed the decision, declaring it both contrary to established custom and the public interest that an apothecary should be prevented from accompanying his remedy with medical advice. The monopoly of the College was broken – but over 100 years were to pass before the apothecary was allowed to charge for his advice, as well as for the remedy. During the whole of that century the apothecary who did not sell a drug went without fee. The apothecary was everyman's doctor and, due to this seventeenth and eighteenth century accident of history, both doctor and patient alike came to expect that each consultation would end with the act of prescription.

At the time this was a matter of little, if any, consequence. What might matter most about the Age of Enlightenment, and about the span of the seventeenth century, was that some of the finest of its minds achieved great distinction, and that by the middle of the century, as Osler in his lectures delivered at Yale University on the Silliman Foundation wrote[864]: the profession was 'far on its way – certain objective features of disease were known, the art of careful observation had been cultivated, many empirical remedies had been discovered, the coarser structure of man's body had been well worked out, and a good beginning had been made in the knowledge of how the machinery worked – nothing more. What disease really was, where it was, how it was caused, had not even begun to be discussed intelligently.' Finally, that – largely to the credit of the Society of Apothecaries – trained practitioners of medicine, members of an organized body, were increasingly available to everyday people and reaching through their social surroundings toward them.

References

721. Locke, John. An essay concerning humane understanding. London, *by Eliz. Holt, for Thomas Basset*, 1690. Also An essay concerning human understanding, Ed. John W. Yolton, 2 vols., London, *Dent*, 1961
722. James I & VI. Demonology, 1597. *Vide* Willson, D.H., James VI and I, 1956
723. Newton, Sir Isaac. Philosophiae naturalis principia mathematica 1687. *Vide* The mathematical principles of natural philosophy, by Sir Isaac Newton, translated into English by Andrew Motte..., 3 vols., London, *Sherwood & others*, 1819. Also, Opticks or, a treatise of the reflections, refractions, inflections and colours of light. 2nd edn., London, *W. & J. Innys*, 1718
724. Santorio, Santorio (Sanctorius). Ars...de statica medicina. Venetiis, *apud N. Polum*, 1614. English translations 1676, 1712, 1842
725. Santorio, Santorio (Sanctorius). Commentaria in primam fen primi libri canonis Avicennae. Venetiis, *apud M.A. Brogiollum*, 1625

726. Floyer, Sir John. The physician's pulse-watch. 2 vols. London, *S. Smith & B. Walford*, 1707–10

727. Martine, George. Essays medical and philosophical. London, *A. Millar*, 1740

728. Graunt, John. Natural and political observations mentioned in a following index, and made upon the Bills of Mortality. London, *T. Roycroft for J. Martin, J. Allestry and T. Dicas*, 1662

729. Petty, Sir William. Several essays in political arithmetic. London, *Robert Clavel and Henry Mortlock*, 1699

730. Halley, Edmund. An estimate of the degrees of mortality of mankind, drawn from curious tables of the births and funerals at the city of Breslaw, with an attempt to ascertain the price of annuities upon lives. *Phil. Trans.*, 1693, **17**, 596–610

731. Boyle, Robert. A defence of the doctrine touching the spring and weight of the air. London, *J. G. for Thomas Robinson*, 1662

732. *Vide* J. F. Fulton, Selected readings in the history of physiology (2nd edn.), 1966, pp. 8–10

733. Boyle, Robert. New experiments physico-mechanicall touching the spring of the air. Oxford, *H. Hall for T. Robinson*, 1660

734. Boyle, Robert. Memoirs for the natural history of humane blood, especially the spirit of that liquor. London, *S. Smith*, 1683

735. Fabrizzi, Girolamo (Fabricius ab Aquapendente). De formato foetu. Venetiis, *per F. Bolzettam*, 1600. English trans. H. B. Adelmann, 1942

736. Fabrizzi, Girolamo (Fabricius ab Aquapendente). De formatione ovi et pulli. Patavii, *ex off. A Bencÿ*, 1621

737. Fabrizzi, Girolamo (Fabricius ab Aquapendente). De venarum ostiolis. Patavii, *ex typ. L. Pasquati*, 1603. English trans. ed. K. J. Franklin, 1933. Also Hieronymi Fabricii ab Aquapendente, Opera omnia anatomica & physiologica, Lipsiae, *J. F. Gleditschii*, 1688

738. Cesalpino, Andrea (Caesalpinus). As ref. 710

739. Cesalpino, Andrea (Caesalpinus). As ref. 711

740. Gilbert, William. De magnete, 1600. *Vide* William Gilbert of Colchester, physician of London. On the magnet, magnetick bodies also, and on the great magnet the earth; a new physiology, demonstrated by many arguments & experiments. London, *Chiswick Press*, 1900

741. Harvey, William. Praelectiones anatomiae universalis. London, *J. Churchill*, 1886. Edited and translated, G. Whitteridge, 1964

742. Osler, Sir William (1921). As ref. 19 but p. 166

743. Harvey, William. Exercitatio anatomica de motu cordis et sanguinis in animalibus. Francofurti, *sumpt. Guilielmi Fitzeri* 1628. English trans. G. Whitteridge, 1976

744. Harvey, William. The works of William Harvey. Translated from the Latin, with a life of the author, by Robert Willis. London, *Sydenham Society*, 1847

745. Harvey, William (1847 edn.). As ref. 744 but p. 22

746. Harvey, William (1847 edn.). As ref. 744 but pp. 45–46

747. Harvey, William (1847 edn.). As ref. 744 but p. 62

748. Harvey, William (1847 edn.). As ref. 744 but pp. 64–67

749. Harvey, William. Exercitationes de generatione animalium. Londini, *O. Pulleyn*, 1651

750. Stelluti, Francesco. Persio tradotto. Roma. *G. Mascardi*, 1630

751. Borel, Pierre (Borellus). Historiarum, et observationum medico-physicarum, centuria. Castris, *apud A. Colomerium*, 1653

752. Borel, Pierre (Borellus). De vero telescopii inventore. Hagae-Comitum, *A. Vlacq*, 1655

753. Kircher, Athanasius. Scrutinium physico-medicum contagiosae luis, quae pestis dicitur. Romae, *typ. Mascardi*, 1658

754. Needham, Marchmont. Medela medicinae. London, *R. Lownds*, 1665

755. Ford, Brian J. Revelation and the single lens. *Br. Med. J.*, 1982, **285**, 1822–1824

756. Leeuwenhoek, Antonj van. Ontledingen en ontdekkingen. 6 vols. Leiden, 1693–1718

757. Leeuwenhoek, Antonj van. Arcana naturae. (4 vols.), Delphis Batavorum, *H. a. Krooneveld*, 1695–1719

758. Leeuwenhoek, Antonj van. Microscopical observations concerning blood, milk, bones, the brain, spittle, and cuticula, etc. *Phil. Trans.*, 1674, **9**, 121–8

759. (Leeuwenhoek, Antonj van.) The select works of Antony van Leeuwenhoek, containing his microscopical discoveries in many of the works of nature. Translated from the Dutch

and Latin editions published by the author, by Samuel Hoole. 2 vols., London, *Henry Fry*, 1798-1807

760. (Leeuwenhoek, Antonj van.). As ref. 759 but Vol. I, pp. 92-93

761. Malpighi, Marcello. De pulmonibus observationes anatomicae. Bononiae, *B. Ferronius*, 1661

762. Malpighi, Marcello (1661). As ref. 761 but English trans. by J. Young, *Proc. R. Soc. Med., Sect. Hist. Med.*, 1929-30, **23**, 1-11

763. Malpighi, Marcello. De viscerum structura exercitatio anatomica. Bononiae, *ex typ. J. Montij*, 1666

764. Malpighi, Marcello. De ovo incubato observationes. Londini, *J. Martyn,* 1673

765. Malpighi, Marcello. Dissertatio epistolica de formatione pulli in ovo. Londini, *J. Martyn*, 1673

766. Malpighi, Marcello. Anatome plantarum. 2 pts. Londini, *J. Martyn*, 1675-79

767. Malpighi, Marcello. Opera omnia. 2 vols. Londini, *R. Scott*, 1686

768. Hooke, Robert. Micrographia, or some physiological descriptions of minute bodies made by magnifying glasses; with observations and inquiries thereupon. London, *J. Martyn & J. Allestry*, 1665

769. Hooke, Robert. An account of an experiment of preserving animals alive by blowing through their lungs with bellows. *Phil. Trans.*, 1667, **2**, 539-40

770. Helmont, Jean Baptiste van. Ortus medicinae. Amsterodami, *apud L. Elzevirium*, 1648

771. Glisson, Francis. De rachitide sive morbo puerili, qui vulgo The Rickets dicitur. Londini, *typ. G. Du-gardi*, 1650. English trans., 1651

772. Glisson, Francis. Anatomia hepatis. Londini, *typ. Du-Gardianis*, 1654

773. Glisson, Francis. Tractatus de ventriculo et intestinis. Londini, *H. Brome*, 1677

774. Willis, Thomas. Cerebri anatome: cui accessit nervorum descriptio et usus. Londini, *typ J. Flesher, imp. J. Martyn & J. Allestry*, 1664

775. Willis, Thomas. Opera omnia. 2 vols. Genevae, *apud Samuelem de Tournes*, 1676-80

776. Willis, Thomas. Of the convulsive cough and asthma. In his: *Practice of physick*, London, *T. Dring, etc.*, 1684, Treatise VIII, pp. 92-96

777. Willis, Thomas. Practice of Physick. London, *T. Dring, C. Harper and J. Leigh*, 1684

778. Wiseman, Richard. Severall chirurgicall treatises. London, *R. Royston*, 1676

779. Lower, Richard. Tractatus de corde. Londini, *J. Allestry*, 1669

780. Lower, Richard. The method observed in transfusing the blood out of one live animal into another. *Phil. Trans.*, 1665-66, **1**, 353-58

781. Denis, Jean Baptiste (Denys). Lettre . . . touchant deux expériences de la transfusion faites sur des hommes. Paris, *J. Cusson*, 1667

782. Lower, Richard and King, Sir Edmund. An account of the experiment of transfusion, practised upon a man in London. *Phil. Trans.*, 1667, **2**, 557-64

783. Sydenham, Thomas. Observationes medicae circa morborum acutorum historiam et curationem. Londini, *G. Kettilby*, 1676

784. Sydenham, Thomas (1676). Ref. 783 is the third edition of Sydenham's Methodus curandi febres of 1666

785. Sydenham, Thomas. Tractatus de podagra et hydrope. Londini, *G. Kettilby*, 1683

786. Sydenham, Thomas. Schedula monitoria de novae febris ingressu. Londini, *G. Kettilby*, 1686

787. Sydenham, Thomas. Observationes medicae circa morborum acutorum historiam et curationem. Ed. quarta. Londini, *G. Kettilby*, 1685

788. Sydenham, Thomas. Opera omnia. Ed. Gulielmus Alexander Greenhill. London, *Sydenham Society*, 1844

789. (Sydenham, Thomas) The works of Thomas Sydenham. Translated from the Latin edition of Dr Greenhill with a life of the author by R. G. Latham. 2 vols. London, *Sydenham Society*, 1848-50

790. Sydenham, Thomas (1848-50 edn.). As ref. 789 but Vol. I, pp. 182-186

791. BPC (1973). As ref. 78 but p. 777

792. Schupbach, William. The paradox of Rembrandt's 'Anatomy of Dr'Tulp'. *Med. Hist.*, Suppl. No. 2, 1982

793. Tulp, Nicolaas. Observationes medicae. Amstelredami, *apud. L. Elzevirium*, 1652

794. Bontius, Jacobus. De paralyseos quadam specie, quam indigenae beriberii vocant. In his:

De medicina Indorum. Lugduni Batavorum, 1642, pp. 115–120. English trans., 1769

795. Wateson, George. The cures of the diseased, in remote regions. Preventing mortalitie, incident in forraine attempts, of the English nation. London, *F. K(ingston) for H. L(ownes)*, 1598. Facsimile edition, 1915

796. Abreu, Alexo de. Tratado de las siete enfermedades, de la inflammacion universal del higado, zirbo, pyloron, y riñones, y de la obstrucion, de la satiriasi, de la terciana y febre maligna, y passion hipocondriaca. Lleva otros tres tratados, del mal de Loanda, del guzano, y de las fuentes y sedales. Lisboa, *P. Craesbeeck*, 1623

797. Ronsseus, Balduinus (Ronsse, (Boudewijn));. De magnis Hippocratis lienibus, Pliniique stomacace, ac sceletyrbe, seu vulgo dicto scorbuto, libellus. Antverpiae, *apud viduam Martini Nutii*, 1564

798. Foreest, Peter van (Forestus). Observationum et curationum medicinalium liber xix de hepatis malis ac affectibus; et xx de lienis morbis: ubi de scorbutto. Lunduni, Batavoram, *ex off. Plantiniana*, 1595

799. Woodall, John. The surgions mate. London, *E. Griffin*, 1617

800. Sennert, Daniel. Opera. 6 vols. Lugduni, *J. A. Huguetan*, 1676

801. Casserio, Giulio (Julius Casserius *Placentinus*). Tabulae anatomicae lxxiix. Venetiis, *apud E. Deuchinum*, 1627

802. Bidloo, Govert. Anatomia humani corporis, centum et quinque tabulis, per artificiosiss. G. de Lairesse ad vivum delineatis. Amstelodami, *vid. J. à Someren*, 1685. English trans. 1698

803. Genga, Bernardino. Anatomia per uso et intelligenza del disegno ricercata non solo su gl'ossi, e muscoli del corpo humano. Roma, *G. J. de Rossi*, 1691

804. Ruysch, Frederik. Thesaurus anatomicus. i–x. Amstelaedami, *J. Wolters*, 1701–16

805. Rubens, Pierre Paul. Théorie de la figure humaine. Paris, *C. A. Jombert*, 1773

806. Borelli, Giovanni Alfonso. De motu animalium. 2 pts. Romae, *ex typ. A. Bernabo*, 1680–81

807. Mayow, John. Tractatus quinque medico-physici. Oxonii, *e theatro Sheldoniano*, 1674. English trans. 1907

808. Redi, Francesco. Osservazioni . . . intorno agli animali viventi che si trovano negli animali viventi. Firenze, *per P. Matini*, 1684

809. Redi, Francesco. Esperienze intorno alla generazione degl'insetti. Firenze, *all'Insegna della Stella*, 1668

810. Redi, Francesco. Opere. 7 vols. Venezia, *Remondini*, 1762

811. Le Boë, Franciscus de [Sylvius]. Praxeos medicae idea nova. 4 vols. Lugduni Batavorum, *apud viduam J. Le Carpentier* (Hagae Comitum, *apud Henricum Scheuleer*), 1671–74

812. Major, Johann Daniel. Chirurgia infusoria. Kiloni, *J. Reumannus*, 1667

813. Le Boë, Franciscus de (Sylvius). Opera medica. Amstelodami, *apud D. Elsevirium et A. Wolfgang*, 1679

814. Morton, Richard. Phthisiologia, seu exercitationes de phthisi. Londini, *imp. S. Smith*, 1689

815. Schenck, Johann, von Grafenberg. Observationum medicarum, rararum, novarum, *etc.* 2 vols. Francofurti, *sumpt. J. Rhodii*, 1600

816. Severino, Marco Aurelio. De recondita abscessuum natura. Neapoli, 1632

817. Bonet, Théophile. Sepulchretum, sive anatomia practica ex cadaveribus morbo denatis. Genevae, *L. Chouët*, 1679. Also 2 vol. edn. (Vol. I = Tomus I; Vol. II = Tomus II & III), Genevae, *Cramer and Perachon*, 1700

818. McIntyre, Archibald Ross. Curare, its history, nature, and clinical use. Chicago, *University Press*, 1947

819. Thomas, Kenneth Bryn. Curare, its history and usage. London, *Pitman*, 1964

820. Vellard, J. Histoire du carare. Les poisons de chasse en Amérique du Sud. Paris, *Gallimard*, 1965

821. Bernard, Claude. Analyse physiologique des propriétés des systèmes musculaires et nerveux au moyen du curare. *C. R. Acad. Sci (Paris)*, 1856, **43**, 825–829

822. BPC (1934). As ref. 120 but pp. 378–379

823. Krukoff, B. A. Cited by Leake, Chauncey D. (1975). As ref. 1461 but p. 22

824. King, Harold. Curare. *Nature (Lond.)*, 1935, **135**, 469–70

825. Griffith, Harold Randall and Johnson, G. Enid. The use of curare in general anesthesia. *Anesthesiology*, 1942, **3**, 418–20
826. Osler, Sir William (1921). As ref. 19 but pp. 183–184
827. Markham, Clements R. A memoir of the Lady Ana de Osorio, Countess of Chinchon and Vice-Queen of Peru (AD 1629–39) with a plea for the correct spelling of the chinchona genus. London, *Trübner*, 1874
828. Markham, Clements R. (1874). As ref. 827 but pp. 40–41
829. Markham, Clements R. (1874). As ref. 827 but pp. 44–45
830. Haggis, Alec William James. Fundamental errors in the early history of cinchona. *Bull. Hist. Med.,* 1941, **10**, 417–59, 568–92
831. Holmstedt, B. and Liljestrand, G. (1963). As ref. 626 but p. 42
832. Torti, Francesco. Therapeutice specialis ad febres quasdam perniciosas, inopinato, ac repente lethales, una vera china china, peculiare methodo ministrata, sanabiles. Mutinae, *typ. B. Soliani*, 1712
833. Garrison, Fielding H. (1929). As ref. 179 but p. 290
834. Woodville, William (1810). As ref. 129 but Vol. IV, pp. 810–813
835. Helvetius, J. C. A. Recueil des methodes pour la guerison de diverses maladies. The Hague, *A. Moetjens*, 1710, pp. 280–282
836. Pelletier, Pierre Joseph and Magendie, François. Recherches chimiques et physiologiques sur l'ipécacuanha. *Ann. Chim. Phys.*, (Paris), 1817, **4**, pp. 172–185
837. British National Formulary 1981 Number 1. *British Medical Association and The Pharmaceutical Society of Great Britain.* 1981, p. 21
838. BNF 1981 No. 1. As ref. 837 but p. 338
839. Martindale, 27th edn. (1977). As ref. 1 but p. 601
840. Pharmacopoeia Londinensis (1618). As ref. 629
841. Codex medicamentarius seu pharmacopoeia Parisiensis. Lutetia Parisiorum, *sumpt. Olivarii de Varennes*, 1639
842. Garrison, Fielding H. (1929). As ref. 179 but p. 289
843. Piso, Willem (Le Pois, (Guillaume)). De Indiae utriusque re naturali et medica libri quatuordecim. Amstelaedami, *apud L. et D. Elzevirios*, 1658
844. Bado, Sebastiano (Baldi). Anastasis corticis Peruviae, seu chinae defensio. Genuae, *typ. P. I. Calenzani*, 1663
845. Pharmacopoeia Londinensis Collegarum, hodie viventium findiss ac symbolis ornatior. London, *L. Sadler & R. Beaumont*, 1668
846. Rivinus, Augustus Quirinus. Censura medicamentorum officinalium. Lipsiae, *J. Fritsch*, 1701
847. Payne, J. F. The earliest medical work printed in English. *Br. Med. J.*, 1889, **1**, 1085–1086
848. (Culpeper, Nicholas). Pharmacopoeia Londinensis: or the London Dispensatory, further adorned by the studies and collections of the Fellows, now living, of the said College . . . by Nich. Culpeper. London, *Peter Cole*, 1654
849. (Culpeper, Mrs). Mr Culpeper's ghost, giving seasonable advice to the lovers of his writings, before which is prefixed Mrs Culpeper's epistle in vindication of her husband's reputation. London, *Peter Cole*, 1656
850. Culpeper, Nicholas (Sibly's edn. of 1813). As ref. 99
851. Creighton, Charles (1891, but 1965 edn.). As ref. 586 but Vol. I, p. 533
852. Creighton, Charles (1891, but 1965 edn.). As ref. 586 but Vol. I, p. 532
853. Defoe, Daniel. A journal of the plague year: being observations or memorials, of the most remarkable occurrences, as well publick as private, which happened in London during the last great visitation in 1665. Written by a citizen who continued all the while in London. London, *E. Nutt, etc.*, 1722
854. Warren, J. Low. The great plague in Chichester in 1665. From J. Low Warren, Chichester: past and present, 1901. In Records of Chichester . . . compiled by Thomas Gordon Willis, Chichester, *T. G. Willis*, 1928, pp. 350–351
855. London's dreadful visitation, or, a collection of all the Bills of Mortality for the present year: beginning the 27th of December 1664, and ending the 19th December following . . . By the Company of Parish Clerks of London. London, *E. Cotes*, 1665
856. Boghurst, William. Loimographia. An account of the great plague of London in the year 1665. By William Boghurst. Now first printed from the British Museum Sloane Ms. 349,

for the Epidemiological Society of London. Edited by J. F. Payne, London, *Shaw & Sons*, 1894

857. Hodges, Nathaniel. Ασιμολογια sive pestis nuperae apud populum Londinensem grassantis

858. Creighton, Charles (1891, but 1965 edn.). As ref. 586 but Vol. II, p. 434

859. Harris, Walter. De morbis acutis infantum. Londini, *Samuel Smith*, 1689. English trans. 1693, 1742

860. Creighton, Charles (1891, but 1965 edn.). As ref. 586 but Vol. II, p. 459

861. Garrison, Fielding H. (1929). As ref. 179 but p. 307

862. Copeman, William Sydney. C. The Worshipful Society of Apothecaries of London, a history 1617-1967. London, *Pergamon*, 1967

863. Copeman, William S. C. (1967). As ref. 862 but p. 44

864. Osler, Sir William (1921). As ref. 19 but p. 184

5

The Eighteenth Century

The Age of Attainment
Linnaeus and the binomial classification

The eighteenth century began as part of the seventeenth century pastoral world, the population growing only slowly, and ended with the Industrial Revolution fully established and the population of Great Britain not much over ten million – it was 10 505 100 in the year 1801, the time of the First English Census.

If we look for a landmark standing for the turn of the century we might settle upon St. Paul's Cathedral – built between 1675 and 1710 by Sir Christopher Wren, and finished before the first full reign (1702–1714, that of Queen Anne) of the eighteenth century came to an end. Her death carried the Elector of Hanover, as George I (1660–1727), to the throne of Great Britain and Ireland – so beginning the Hanoverian dynasty with a king who could not speak English and who allowed his ministers power to a degree which began the cabinet system and the rise to strength of the great political parties.

The century was not much advanced when in 1733, in a world that knew few if any machines, John Kay (1704–*c.* 1764), the son of a Lancashire manufacturer of woollen goods, invented what the patent called a 'New Engine or Machine for Opening and Dressing Wool'. It included a newly invented shuttle and spurred the invention of spinning machines. The century had passed beyond mid-way when these improvements included the 1764 spinning jenny of James Hargreaves (1745–1778); it was not far from its close when Samuel Crompton (1753–1827) brought out, in 1779, the spinning mule. Together these inventions provided the means to clothe the massive nineteenth century expansion of the population.

We would recognize the face of medicine and the world around us far more at the end of the eighteenth century than at the close of the century before. As the Industrial Revolution began, power began to be harnessed allowing much that we would recognize: in 1763 the Scot, James Watt (1736–1819) conceived the idea of a separate condenser, leading to the development of the steam engine, which can be dated from 1769. New means of transport arose: James Brindley (1716–1772) being called, in 1759, by the Duke of Bridgwater to drive a canal from Worsley to Manchester. The success of this canal led to the construction of 360 miles of canal waterways, all designed and, with one exception, executed by Brindley.

These events were of the times of the loss of the American colonies (the War of Independence being 1775–83) and of the 1768–79 voyages of James Cook

295

(1728–1779), – voyages that Jenner (the discoverer of vaccination) was invited, as a London pupil of John Hunter's, to join. The tolerance of dissent and the rationalism won since the Renaissance thus allowed medicine to begin to change as the world changed round it.

No small part of the change was a response to the eighteenth century discoveries in physical science. Many of these discoveries had great impact on the growing knowledge of physiology – perhaps most remarkably the theory of animal electricity (galvanism) by Aloysio Luigi Galvani (1737–1798) whose *De viribus electricitatis in motu musculari commentarius*[865], of 1791, appeared from Bologna the year before Galvani was made lecturer in anatomy at that unversity. The electric battery, as the first source of continuous electrical current, was invented by Alessandro Volta (1745–1827), after whom the volt is named. Volta was appointed to the newly created chair of physics at Pavia in 1779 and showed that Galvani's 'animal electricity' was identical with the electricity generated from non-living materials.

The physical sciences were coming to resemble those of the early part of our own century: the late eighteenth century discoveries included hydrogen, isolated in 1766 by the English chemist Henry Cavendish (1731–1810). Cavendish also discovered the constituents of water and atmospheric air[866] and combined oxygen and hydrogen into water. The British chemist, Joseph Priestley (1733–1804) included oxygen, nitric oxide, hydrochloric acid and sulphur dioxide amongst his discoveries – but is most famous for his paper *Observations on different kinds of air*[867] of 1772 and for demonstrating that plants immersed in water give off oxygen which is essential for the support of animal life. In these experiments Priestley came close to understanding the essential physiological secret of respiration – for he certainly achieved the first isolation of oxygen – but it was left for Lavoisier to discover the real nature of gaseous interchange in the lungs. Antoine Laurent Lavoisier (1743–1794) published a *Mémoire sur la nature du principe qui se combine avec les métaux pendant leur calcination, et qui en augmente le poids*[868] in 1778. This work demonstrated his real understanding of the significance of oxygen and did away with the 'phlogiston' theories which had held sway for so many decades. Many others were involved in completing the modern understanding of the mechanisms of respiration – an understanding which represents the greatest achievement of eighteenth century physiology – but it is to Lavoisier that the ultimate credit for this advance must be given. It is a sad comment on history that he was guillotined during the worst excesses of the French Revolution. Much of this work had begun almost a quarter of a century before with the investigations on the function of the intercostal muscles in respiration published[869] by Albrecht von Haller (1708–1777) in 1746–47 – and the isolation[870] in 1754 of carbon dioxide by the brilliant Scot, Joseph Black (1728–1799). It had been paralleled by the discovery of nitrogen by Daniel Rutherford (1749–1819) whose *De aëre fixo dicto, aut mephitico*[871] appeared in Edinburgh in 1772. There is also the *Mémoire sur la chaleur*[872] of 1784 in which Lavoisier, with Pierre La Place (1749–1827), announced the invention of the ice calorimeter and measured the respiratory quotient of a pig; this work drew an analogy between the processes of respiration and those of combustion.

The advances continued with Armand Séguin (1768–1835) publishing, in 1793, the *Premier mémoire sur la respiration des animaux*[873]; this paper, in which

Lavoisier was co-author, reported metabolic measurements made on Séguin himself. By means of measurements thoroughly modern in style, it was shown that the degree of oxidation in the body of man is a function of food, the temperature of the environment and the amount of physical work imposed.

Close to the end of the century, the 1795 corrected edition of the *Experiments on the insensible perspiration of the human body*[874], first published in 1779 by William Cruikshank (1745–1800), demonstrated that carbon dioxide is given off by the skin. At much the same time the extraordinary Johann Christian Reil (1759–1813) founded the *Archiv für die Physiologie* – the world's first journal of physiology.

A further and far-reaching eighteenth-century achievement was the development of methods of classification which would allow new knowledge to be added to that already available without producing confusion. The pinnacle of this work was the binomial nomenclature of the great Swedish physician and biologist, Carl von Linné (Linnaeus; 1707–1778) whose life spanned much of the length of the century and forms the principal subject of the Linné museum at Uppsala.

Morton (1970)[875] says that the binomial nomenclature (genus and species) 'was probably devised in the first place by Joachim Jung, about 1640'. In the hands of Linnaeus, a man of vast industry, this sytem was used to organize natural science in a way that formed a basis for later, improved methods of classification. Linnaeus classified plants, mainly on the characteristics of their stamens and pistils, and provided the most logical and complete description then available.

His most famous work is the *Systema naturae*[876] first published in Leyden in 1735 and classifying plants, animals and minerals. The most prized version is the tenth edition published in 1758 in which Linnaeus first used the specific names for the zoological species which he described. He provided his botanical classification in the *Genera plantarum*[877] of 1737, dedicated to Hermann Boerhaave, which forms the real starting point of modern systematic botany. Of this work there is an important English translation of 1771.

Perhaps mistakenly (for without any real understanding of the nature and causes of infective and metabolic disease the attempt was premature) Linnaeus produced a classification of disease. This was the *Genera morborum in auditorum usum*[878] of 1763 but the system, based largely on the symptoms of disease, themselves varying from patient to patient and being almost always nonspecific, was not a success. Others made similar attempts and François Boissier de Sauvages de la Croix (1706–1767) produced a five volume *Nosologia methodica, sistens morborum classes, genera et species*[879], published in 1768, in which he recorded some 2400 different diseases.

The botanical classification based on the features of the sexual organs of plants was a different matter and relied on features that were constant, easily visible, and readily described. It dominated botany for over a century and established the use of a binomial classification for all time. The system of Linnaeus was extended and varied by others within the eighteenth century but it was left to Augustin Pyrame de Candolle (1778–1841), who studied at Geneva but settled in Paris in 1796, to lessen the emphasis on the sexual organs and flowers of plants and produce a morphological system based on the form and development of all the organs of plants. Later in life de Candolle returned to Geneva to occupy the chair of natural history in the University of his birthplace. His son, Alphonse (1806–1893) succeeded to his father's chair in 1842 and in collaboration with his own son Casimir (1836–1918) made a vital contribution to the development of the natural and more modern botanical classification.

Following the three generations of the family Pyrame de Candolle almost to the dawn of the twentieth century does perhaps emphasize the achievement of Linnaeus, upon whose work the whole enterprise was based and whose *Systema naturae*[876] formed one of the chief monuments of the eighteenth century.

Others who influenced biology included Lazaro Spallanzani (1729–1799), one of the first to dispute[880] the doctrine of spontaneous generation and the first (in 1768)[881] to advance the doctrine of the regeneration of the spinal cord; he also recorded important observations on the gastric juice[882]. From the ranks of the botanical chemists, Jan Ingen-Housz (1730–1799) showed that in photosynthesis the green parts of plants exposed to the light fix carbon dioxide extracted from the atmosphere – a power which they lose in the absence of light[883]. Ingen-Housz also demonstrated that animals ultimately depend upon plants for their food – so beginning the concept of the 'food-chain' so important in modern ecology. Erasmus Darwin (1731–1802), grandfather of Charles Darwin, produced *Zoonomia; or the laws of organic life* (1794–96)[884] – thereby demonstrating the interests in natural science that came to fruition in the work of his grandson; he also wrote a treatise on the nature of generation and an outline system of pathology. Born during the century but publishing after its close was Robert Brown (1773–1858), who made the vitally important discovery of the cell nucleus in 1831 and whose *Observations on the organs and mode of fecundation in Orchideae and Asclepiadeae*[885], including the great discovery, appeared in 1829–32. American science is represented amongst the biologists of this time by John Bartram (1699–1777), a botanist profoundly admired by Linnaeus, who produced his *Descriptions, virtues, and uses of sundry plants of these northern parts of America*[886] in 1751 and, at Kingsessing, founded the first botanical garden in America.

Boerhaave and physiological medicine

Although the eighteenth century was riddled with non-experimental theorizing and plagued by attempts to introduce philosophical systems of a general type into medicine, it also saw, principally in the person of Hermann Boerhaave (1668–1738) of Leyden, the establishment of bed-side clinical teaching in the modern manner.

The decade that began with the year 1660 and witnessed the birth of Boerhaave was rich in clinicians who were more and more aware of physiology and pathology as sciences fundamental to clinical medicine. The first to distinguish between smooth and striped muscle was Giorgio Baglivi (1668–1707), Professor of Anatomy in Rome but also a fine experimental physiologist, whose *Opera omnia medico-practica et anatomica*[887] appeared in 1704. Giovanni Lancisi (1654–1720), physician to Pope Clement XI and the ultimate publisher of the beautiful anatomical copper-plates originally made by Eustachius in 1552 was not only the first to describe cardiac syphilis[888] but was also a notable epidemiologist who understood the nature of contagion. Friedrich Hoffman (1660–1742) – whose works include the *Fundamenta physiologiae*[889] of 1718 and an *Opera omnia physico-medica . . .*[890] of 1740–53 – was probably the first to bring pathology and physiology fully together, seeing disease in an organ as being influenced by the function and nature of the organ. His theoretical ideas included the concept of a 'vital fluid' present in the nervous system and acting on muscles to preserve their tone and influence their contraction. Hoffmann was, in fact, a leader of the Iatromechanist school.

Others born in the fertile decade that began in 1660 were much more encumbered with theory. An example is Georg Ernst Stahl (1660–1734) whose *Theoria medica vera*[891] of 1708 and later works[892] assembled long after his death revived the concept of the 'sensitive soul' earlier put forward by van Helmont. Stahl developed this, as leader of the Animistic school, into a belief that the innervation of the body by the soul provides the essential nature of life itself, disease being a perturbation of the activities of the soul.

Boerhaave, probably the finest medical consultant of the day, was a skilled chemist as well as teacher of medicine. His greatest written work is probably his *Elementa chemiae*[893] published at Leyden in 1732. His medical works include the *Institutiones medicae in usus annuae exercitationis domesticos digestae* (1708)[894], which contains a substantial section on physiology emphasizing the digestive system; the *Aphorismi de cognoscendis et curandis morbis* (1709)[895] – the Aphorisms forming one of the best parts of Boerhaave's writings and available in an English translation of 1715 – and the *Opera omnia medica*[896] of 1742.

Boerhaave, appointed professor of botany and medicine at Leyden in 1709, was allocated only 12 beds in the hospital of the town. The more famous of his pupils include Albrecht von Haller, William Cullen, John Pringle, Gerhard van Swieten and Anton de Haen – all of whom played an important part in the developing science of therapeutics.

Leyden was already famous for the teaching of anatomy at the time of Boerhaave's appointment. Given the practicalities of his chemistry (and his book was by far the best of the eighteenth century and was used throughout Europe), his 12 beds, and the resources of his reading, Boerhaave soon built for Leyden an outstanding reputation in clinical teaching. He was helped by his mastery of languages – he had the main European tongues and both Hebrew and Chaldean available to him – and by his dual innovations of bed-side teaching and demonstrating the relationship between the symptoms and signs of disease as seen clinically and the causative lesions as exhibited in the postmortem room. This is the basic technique of clinical instruction today and, more than to any other person, must be attributed to Boerhaave of Leyden.

The limitations of Boerhaave's work, and he transmitted a number of traditional errors in some parts of physiology, arise from his not having been involved in the experimental aspects of all parts of the subject. What was missing in Boerhaave, as an experimentalist, was provided by his pupil Albrecht von Haller (1708–1777; Figure 90), frequently remembered as 'the Prince of Physiologists'.

After graduation at Leyden, von Haller, soon to become one of the greatest figures in the history of medicine and already established as both poet and botanist, migrated to the new University of Göttingen. There he laid the

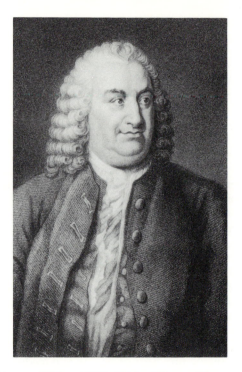

Figure 90 Albrecht von Haller (1708–1777). [*From: Thomas Joseph Pettigrew (1838–1840).*]

foundation of his reputation as the master physiologist of his time. In 1753 he returned to his birthplace, Bern, with his poem *Die Alpen* (1729) already recognized as one of the finest celebrations of the beauty and culture of his native Alpine Switzerland.

He wrote prodigiously and is credited with having produced over 1300 papers in science. His book, *Primae lineae physiologiae in usum praelectionum academicarum*[897], published in Göttingen in 1747 when he was still only 39 years old, embodies so much in physiology that many later ideas and so-called discoveries can be traced back to it. There is a good English edition of 1754 and the work contains Haller's well-known theory of sound resonance – anticipating that put forward by Helmholtz over a century later.

His greatest single contribution to physiology was probably his differentiation, said to have been based on over 500 experiments, of the nerve impulse and the contractility of muscle. In 1677 Glisson had brought in the concept of 'irritability' as a property of all tissues, but von Haller clearly distinguished between the sensibility of the nerve impulse and the 'irritability' of the contraction of muscle. These findings were contained in his *De partibus corporis humani sensibilibus et irritabilibus*[898] of 1753 – and this preceded the eight volume *Elementa physiologiae corporis humani*[899] (1757–66) in which von Haller assembled together the entire knowledge of physiology of the time.

The systematic nature of his reading is shown by his having become the founder of modern medical bibliography. He produced an outstanding anatomical bibliography but his *Bibliotheca botanica*[900] of 1771-72 is of such excellence that it is universally regarded as the best work of its kind of the eighteenth century. The range of his writings is shown by the anatomical descriptions included in the 1757-66 master summary[899] of physiology, already mentioned, and by the accurate and beautiful drawings which formed his *Icones anatomicae*[901] of 1743-56.

All of these accomplishments in science are additional to von Haller's place in German literature. Apart from this, the strength of his medical learning can be seen from the *Methodus studii medici* (1751)[902] – a work which earned Garrison's[903] accolade that he was the 'best historian of medicine after Guy de Chauliac' – a writer whose work had stood the test of time since the fourteenth century. It can be seen also from the *Bibliotheca anatomica* (1774-77, reprinted 1969)[904]; the *Bibliotheca chirurgica* (1774-75, reprinted 1971)[905], and the four volume *Bibliotheca medicinae practicae* (1776-88, re-presented 1805)[906], which concluded his four great bibliographies. Together, these volumes put forward von Haller's classified analysis of more than 52 000 publications from the world literature on medicine and the allied sciences. It must be remarked that there have indeed been few personal achievements of such proportions.

The developments stemming from Boerhaave in Leyden soon began to affect medical training in Britain. In 1700, John Munro, an army surgeon in Scotland but of good family, settled in Edinburgh where the 'College of Edinburgh' had been founded by Charter of James VI in 1582. The Charter made no mention of granting the full privileges usually associated with a university but in 1621 the Scots Parliament bestowed the rights already enjoyed by the older universities in Scotland – and this grant was ratified when the parliaments of England and Scotland were united. The Act of Union of England and Scotland was dated 1707, so forming one of the principal events of the beginning of the eighteenth century.

Edinburgh also had the benefit of the College of Physicians of Edinburgh, founded by Robert Sibbald – a student who had spent the years 1660-61 at Leyden. It was against this background, and wanting to further the interests of his son Alexander (1697-1767; Munro *primus*) that John Munro conceived the idea of establishing, on non-denominational and international lines like those of the University of Leyden, a medical school which could be associated with either the University of Edinburgh or the College of Physicians in the city.

For this purpose Munro *primus* was sent to Leyden to study under Boerhaave; to Paris, and to London where he worked under the enlightened guidance of William Cheselden (1688-1752) of St. Thomas's Hospital. Following this splendid training Munro *primus* returned to Edinburgh in 1719 and was examined and qualified by the Surgeon's Guild. In 1720, when he was still only 22 years of age, he was elected Professor of Anatomy in the newly-established University.

He taught the subject so well that the number of students in anatomy rose from just under 60 to something like treble that number by the middle of the century. At that point Munro *primus* was succeeded in the chair by his equally carefully trained son, also called Alexander (1737-1817; Munro *secundus*), who with the passage of time excelled his own father and produced the *Observations on the structure and functions of the nervous system* (published in Edinburgh in

1783)[907]. Munro *secundus* discovered the communication between the lateral ventricles and the third ventricle of the human brain – so identifying the 'foramen of Munro'. In turn, Munro *secundus* was succeeded in the same chair by his own son, also called Alexander (1773–1859; Munro *tertius*). This apostolic succession resulted in three generations of the Munro family holding the anatomy chair at Edinburgh for 126 consecutive years – 1720–1846 – during which time they played a major part in establishing Edinburgh as one of the greatest teaching centres in Britain.

In the time of Munro *primus*, in 1736, George II granted a Charter of Incorporation to the Edinburgh Royal Infirmary; the Charter linked the Infirmary with the University from its beginning. The primary intention was to provide a clinical teaching school and in this way the Infirmary differed from other eighteenth century foundations. The abundance of clinical cases, the highly qualified teaching provided by the professors of the university, the excellence of anatomical demonstration and the long association with the medical traditions of Leyden, combined to make Edinburgh unique: students flocked to its courses even though the qualifications of Scotland were not recognized as licences for the practice of medicine in England.

The tradition was spread to Glasgow largely by the kindly and erudite William Cullen (1710–1790), a physician who is remembered for the personal care which he devoted to his students and for his being the effective founder of the fine school

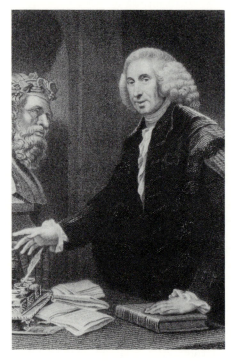

Figure 91 William Cullen (1710–1790). [*From: Thomas Joseph Pettigrew (1838–1840).*]

of medicine in Glasgow. Cullen (Figure 91), a pupil of Munro *primus*, held chairs of both chemistry and medicine at Edinburgh and Glasgow; he was amongst the very small original group who gave bed-side clinical instruction in Britain and has the distinction of having, in 1757, given the first lectures of this sort in the vernacular instead of in Latin.

The reputation of Cullen was first established with the *Synopsis nosologiae methodicae*[908] published in Edinburgh in 1769. There are a number of English translations of this work (in which Cullen divided the diseases into fevers, nervous illnesses, cachexias and local disorders) and these give the full flavour of mid-eighteenth century medicine at its most perceptive. Cullen believed that the vital force of the body rests in its nervous energy, that this is continuous between the muscle and nerve, and that aberrations of the conduct of this energy resulted in many forms of disease. He thus sought, in the functioning of the nervous system, an explanation for many of the phenomena of disease. Today, when we speak of an illness being 'nervous' or 'due to nerves' we revisit some of these concepts of Cullen.

He was keenly interested in therapeutics and gave a well-known series of lectures which were expanded into *A treatise of the materia medica* (1789)[909] – a work which remains informative. Probably his most widely read book today is *The Works of William Cullen, MD*[910] in the two volume edition edited by John Thomson and published in 1827. Years ahead of his time, Cullen, in these writings, provides a totally modern emphasis[911]:

> Medicine is the art of preventing and of curing diseases – The common language is that, 'Medicine is the art of preserving health and of curing diseases;' but I have said 'the art of preventing diseases;' for although I do not deny that the preserving of health is the object of a physician's care, yet I maintain that there is truly no other means of preserving health but what consists in preventing diseases...

By the mid-eighteenth century medicine was becoming much more practical and less like divinity or philosophy conducted in Latin. Real knowledge was being added to that already available and the great clinicians and teachers of the day included figures such as John Fothergill (1712–1780), a Quaker from Yorkshire and another pupil of Munro *primus*. Fothergill became a successful and respected London practitioner whose natural history collection passed eventually to William Hunter. He is now remembered for his writings *On a painful affection of the face* (1776)[912], the first description of facial neuralgia, and for the 1777–84 *Remarks on that complaint commonly known under the name of the sick headach*[913] which provided the first worthwhile description of migraine. His somewhat earlier *An account of the sore throat attended with ulcers*[914] (1748) gave the first good account of both diphtheria and scarlatinal angina (although Fothergill failed to differentiate the two conditions); his often quoted *Observations on the weather and diseases of London* (1783)[915] is a report, of 1751–54, which shared with Hippocrates an interest in the effects of climate on the pattern of disease. Fothergill's accounts of migraine, and especially that of facial neuralgia, form examples of the fine clinical descriptions which added to the knowledge of the time.

These descriptions included the classical account of sciatica by Domenico Cotugno (1736–1822) in 1764[916]; the recognition of the grave consequences of diseases of the spinal cord by Johann Frank (1745–1821) in 1792[917]; and the first account of facial nerve paralysis, by Nicolaus Friedreich (1761–1836), in 1797[918]. Edinburgh remained represented in these advances and Robert Whytt (1714–1766), a famous neurophysiologist in the city, produced his mid-century *An essay on the vital and other involuntary motions of animals* (1751)[919] in which he became the first to prove that the response to light of the pupils is a reflex action; this is known as 'Whytt's reflex', its author having given a good account of its afferent and efferent pathways.

The mixing of the old and the new can be shown in the life of the notable London physician, Richard Mead (1673–1754), whose *A short discourse concerning pestilential contagion, and the methods to be used to prevent it*[920], of 1720, contrasts with a work written *to* Mead – *An Epistle to Dr Richard Mead, concerning the epidemical diseases of Virginia, particularly, a pleurisy and peripneumony . . . by John Tennent* (1742)[921]. Mead's own discourse was written in response to a demand for his advice on the means of dealing with the plague – his treatise foreshadows, in its good sense, the establishment of the modern public health system. Tennent's epistle to Mead includes a 'cut of that most valuable plant' (Figure 92), which he calls the 'Seneca Rattle-snake Root', and of which he says[922]:

> . . . the *Indians*, and others, when hunting in the Woods, carried this Root powdered in their Shot-Bags, to be ready to take in the most expeditious Manner, in case they should have the Misfortune to be bit by that terrible Creature; That he himself had been bit by that Snake, when the Poison was at its greatest Height, and was recovered by taking the *Seneca Rattle-snake Root*; and that these *Indians* deduced the Efficacy of the Plant from the Resemblance which the Flowers and Root have to the Rattles of the Snake.

There are few better examples of the Paracelsian 'Doctrine of Signatures' in English. That such a vivid example of believing that a drug carries a sign showing its properties, and that such a belief could be of the mid-eighteenth century, seems quite remarkable – even more so that it could be addressed to one of London's most eminent physicians who himself wrote so rationally on plague.

The humanity that had shown in Cullen showed also in John Pringle (1707–1782), a pupil of Boerhaave, who became Physician-General to the British Army from 1744 to 1752 and to whom must be given the credit for having become the founder of modern military medicine. Pringle's *Observations on the diseases of the army* (1752)[923] is justifiably famous and pioneered sensible ventilation and effective methods of hygiene amongst large concentrations of people. It was due to Pringle that foot-soldiers were given blankets when on active service and it is largely as a result of his writings that sensible measures of sanitation became part of military organization. He gave a well-known description of typhus and showed this and jail fever and hospital fever to be the same. In *A discourse upon some late improvements of the means for preserving the health of mariners* (1776)[924] he extended the humane effect of his teachings and began the improvement in conditions at sea, and in hospital ships, that marked the work of James Lind.

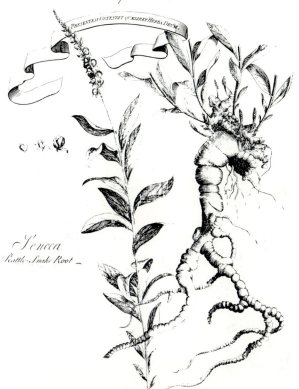

Figure 92 The 'Seneca Rattle-snake Root'. From: *An epistle to Dr. Richard Mead, concerning the epidemical diseases of Virginia, particularly, a pleurisy and peripneumony . . .* by John Tennent. Edinburgh, (1742).

Lind (1716–1794), author of the famous *A treatise of the scurvy* (1753) [925], brought together the cause, circumstances, and cure of a disease in a way seldom equalled before. Lind's book, reprinted in 1953, is a classic account of scurvy and records his numerous experiments on the disease. He became the founder of effective naval hygiene in British ships and it was due to Lind, and his urging of the issue of lemon juice and the use of citrus fruits, that scurvy was eventually eradicated from the fleets.

Lind was physician to the Royal Naval Hospital at Haslar from 1758 to 1783 and saw no less than 350 cases of scurvy in a voyage of only 10 weeks' duration. Remembered for his work on this disease, he also wrote one of the more important early books on tropical diseases: in *An essay on diseases incidental in Europeans in hot climates* (1768) [926] he came close to understanding the place of the mosquito in malaria. He entered deeply into the concepts of preventive medicine in what is, from some points of view, his most important work – *An essay on the most effectual means, of preserving the health of seamen, in the*

305

Royal Navy (1757)[927]. The reading of this book shows Lind's concern with the unbelievable conditions under which the crews of naval vessels lived and worked; it puts forward also his advocacy of improved ventilation, hygiene, and the means of preventing the transmission of disease afloat.

The message spread, Richard Brocklesby (1722–1797) producing, in 1764, one of the best books[928] of the century on military sanitation, and Captain James Cook (1728–1779) showing, in the historic *The method taken for preserving the health of the crew of H.M.S. the Resolution during her late voyage round the world* (1776)[929] that in voyages lasting several years scurvy could be prevented by the modifications to the diet suggested by Lind. It was carried to America by Benjamin Rush (1745–1813) – one of the earlier of the great physicians of North America – who wrote *Directions for preserving the health of soldiers:*

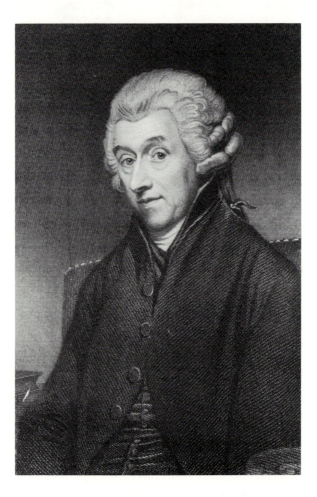

Figure 93 William Heberden (1710–1801). [*From: Thomas Joseph Pettigrew (1838–1840).*]

306

recommended to the consideration of the officers of the Army of the United States ... (1778)[930].

The Admiralty order on the use of lemon juice was not issued until 1795 but even at the time of Lind's early writings on scurvy the idea was not new. His own works show that orange and lemon juice had been used by the Dutch in 1564 but Lind's application of this information and his study of it by well-designed experiments were in keeping with the best of the eighteenth century practical tradition.

Another of Boerhaave's pupils, John Huxham (1692–1768), in *De morbo colico Damnoniensi* (1739)[931] wrote a fine account of 'Devonshire colic' (which he thought to be due to tartar involved in the making of cider, rather than to lead poisoning). His most important work is on fevers and suggests (*An essay on fevers*, 1750)[932] that he appreciated the difference between typhoid and typhus. He wrote importantly on diphtheria and was the first English physician to use the word 'influenza'. In a work of 1757[933] he also became the first to record, in diphtheria, the sign of paralysis of the soft palate. He has an *Opera physico-medica* (1764)[934] recording many of these valuable observations.

The best of eighteenth century clinical realism is provided by the writings of William Heberden (1710–1801) whose life spanned most of the length of the century and turned, by one year, into the decade that followed. His portrait forms Figure 93. Heberden was an outstanding Cambridge classicist whose first, brilliant, published medical writing Αντιθηριακά; *An essay on mithridatium and theriaca* (1745)[935] did the subject of therapeutics a vast service by ridding it of some of its superstition and a little of its dependence on the gross polypharmacy typified by theriac.

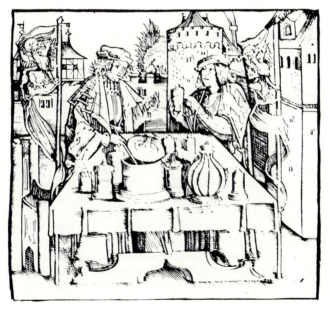

Figure 94 The preparation of theriac in Strasbourg at the beginning of the sixteenth century. From: Hieronymus Brunschwig, *Liber de arte distillandi* (1512). [*Royal Society of Medicine library, London.*]

There is a modern study of these ancient medicines, their history, and their vast number of ingredients (*Theriac and mithridatium, a study in therapeutics*)[936] by Gilbert Watson (1966). This reproduces the charming woodcut (Figure 94), showing the preparation of a theriac in Strasbourg at the beginning of the sixteenth century, and taken from the *Liber de arte distillandi* (1512)[937] of Hieronymus Brunschwig. The somewhat restricted list of contents from a fairly late mithridatium in the *Pharmacopoeia Londinensis Collegarum* of 1668 has already been given in Figures 84 and 85. The reasons for the civic ceremonies in mediaeval times included the cost of some of the precious ingredients and the great importance ascribed to the finished product by the community.

Heberden presents a pungent and lucid argument against the efficacy of these mixtures and adds[938]:

> If our objections stopped here, and these grand antidotes were only good for nothing; it would hardly be worth while to censure or take any notice of them: but we may justly fear that their use is attended with a good deal of danger. As many people busy themselves with the practice of Physic . . . it may be advisable . . . to discountenance a medicine, which, upon the tradition of it's sovereign virtues, or as a sudorific, is often applied at random, and, by means of the Opium, does much mischief.

He goes on with the statement that 'Opium or any powerful drug, mixed up into an electuary with so many other things, is against all rules of pharmacy . . . '[939]; he ends his attack on 'this medley of discordant Simples' by saying that it has[940]:

> no better title to the name of *Mithridates*, than as it so well resembles the numerous, undisciplined forces of a barbarous King, made up of a dissonant crowd collected from different countries, mighty in appearance, but in reality, an ineffective multitude, that only hinder one another.

It was an attack that, in the grand style, succeeded – and Heberden drove the formulae for theriac and mithridatium from the pharmacopoeia. In doing so, he advanced sound principles regarding the need for both safety and efficacy in drugs, the folly of including potent remedies in mixtures or overlooking the likelihood of incompatibilities, and the equal folly of failing to challenge superstition or disbelieve that which is authenticated only by authority or tradition.

Fairly shortly he read three papers before the College of Physicians. One was a classical description, a report of one case only, of nyctalopia (*Of the nightblindness or nyctalopia*, 1768)[941]; the second was of the same year (*On the chickenpox*)[942], a classic paper which presents the first clear differentiation of chickenpox from smallpox; the third, now that the pattern of disease has changed, seems even more important. It was *Some account of a disorder of the breast*[943], a paper of 1772, which like the other two, appeared in the *Medical Transactions of the College of Physicians of London*, but which gave the classical description of angina pectoris. This paper did not just mention the shortness of breath recorded by other and earlier writers giving accounts of what might have been this condition but it used the term 'angina pectoris' and spoke of the paroxymal retrosternal oppression which is so characteristic a feature of the disease.

The account is totally modern in its definition of one of the most important of the diagnoses of medicine.

Any one of these three papers would have made Heberden's name memorable – but it is usually associated with the rheumatic lesion, Heberden's nodes, of the interphalangeal joints described in *De nodis digitorum*[944] which forms part of the most notable of all his written works, the *Commentarii de morborum historia et curatione*[945] published for him by his son and printed in London in 1802. It included all the papers which had given Heberden his great reputation as one of the most singular figures of British clinical medicine and it at once acquired a European reputation. It was the last really important treatise on medicine written in Latin and a translation in English appeared in the same year as the original. This is the *Commentaries on the history and cure of diseases by William Heberden, MD*, of which the third edition appeared in 1806[946]. This edition contains an appendix, seeking to foster the publications of others, which is missing from the 1962 facsimile[947] of the first edition.

Not having become too solemn he starts his preface with the passage[948]:

> Plutarch says, that the life of a vestal virgin was divided into three portions; in the first of which she learned the duties of her profession, in the second she practised them, and in the third she taught them to others. This is no bad model for the life of a physician...

In the appendix just mentioned he adds characteristically[949]:

> Fact, and repeated experiments, have alone informed us that jalap will purge, and ipecacuanha vomit, that the poppy occasions sleep, that the bark will cure an ague, and that quicksilver will salivate. If we examine the whole materia medica, and the whole practice of physic, we shall not find one efficacious simple, nor one established method of cure, which were discovered, or ascertained, by any other means.

Morgagni and pathology

The cardiovascular physician of today has one of his ancestors in the eighteenth century physiologist, Stephen Hales (1677–1761). A practical application of Hales's physiology and humane interests was given in his *A description of ventilators*[950] – a book published in London in 1743 and giving an account of the ventilator Hales had invented and by means of which fresh air could be directed into the holds of ships, hospital buildings, gaols, mines and other crowded areas where it could improve the health of the employed. With this work Hales became the inventor of artificial ventilation and his devices were soon widely used. He became the forerunner of today's cardiologist, routinely involved with quantitative measurements of haemodynamic function, with the publication of his *Statical essays, containing haemastaticks* (Volume 2)[951] in 1733. This work is the first great landmark in cardiovascular science after Harvey's discovery of the circulation of the blood and ranks second only to von Haller's *Elementa physiologiae corporis humani*[899] of 1757–66 as a contribution to eighteenth century physiology. Hales provides a fascinating description of his invention of the manometer and of his making the first measurements of the blood pressure. The technique used was to insert a tall glass tube in an artery of a horse and, by these means, determine not only the blood pressure but also the capacity of the heart. Hales, in a manner perhaps a little unexpected in an English clergyman, also estimated the velocity of the arterial blood flow and, as a result of these studies, began the development of the blood pressure measuring instruments now in world-wide use.

The modern haematologist has a parallel eighteenth century predecessor in the person of William Hewson (1739–1774) who showed that fibrinogen is the natural substrate of blood coagulation and was the first to describe the lymphocyte. Hewson, born in Northumberland, is remembered as the colleague John Hunter left in charge of his dissecting room when, to recover from his anatomical exertions, Hunter left London to spend a period with the army. Earlier in the century the discovery of iron in the blood had been made by Vincenzo Menghini (*De ferrearum particularum sede in sanguine*, 1746)[952] but Hewson's own work on blood clotting is contained in his important *An experimental inquiry into the properties of blood*[953] of 1771. He gave the first complete account of the anatomical features of the lymphatics and described the leukocytes as being derived from the lymphatic glands and thymus (*Experimental inquiries: Part the second. Containing a description of the lymphatic system in the human subject and in other animals. Together with observations on the lymph, and the changes which it undergoes in some diseases*, 1774)[954]. There is also, of this brilliant writer, *The works Edited with an introduction and notes by G. Gulliver*[955] – a volume published by the Sydenham Society in 1846 and showing the remarkable degree to which Hewson, student and companion to both of the Hunters, produced studies which form the beginnings of much of present-day haematology.

Before this work blood had been thought to clot by some process, akin to setting, which occurred as it cooled and became immotile. Others thought that it solidified as the red cells set into rouleaux. Hewson, quite brilliantly, demonstrated that if the clotting of the blood is delayed, either by its being cooled or by the use of neutral salts, then a plasma could be skimmed off – and this plasma was not only clottable but, prior to being coagulated, contained a substance which could be precipitated or removed by gentle heating. Hewson thought, therefore, that blood clotting was due to the natural condensation of an insoluble form of this factor, which he called the 'coagulable lymph' of the plasma. Much later work, showing that in blood coagulation the soluble fibrinogen of plasma is precipitated as an insoluble mesh-work of fibrin, has added a great deal of interest to the logical set of studies undertaken by Hewson.

Hales, Hewson, and a number of other eighteenth century pioneers can be thought of as having begun present-day specialities but the beginnings of organized pathology are perhaps even more fundamental. Just before the century started Théophile Bonet (1620–1689) published, in his *Sepulchretum, sive anatomia practica ex cadaveribus morbo denatis*[817] of 1679, a record of the 3000 or so autopsies which had been described by physicians since the earliest times. To these records he added his own observations – thereby leaving behind him the most useful reference we have of the early descriptions of pathology dating back to the days of Hippocrates. Even though the work is richest in the descriptions of the sixteenth and seventeenth centuries, it ensured that the eighteenth century began with all of the worthwhile knowledge of pathological anatomy carefully systematized. The work had been preceded by the 1584–97 studies of Schenck[815] and the 1632 publication on surgical pathology of Severino[816] which have been previously mentioned.

It was followed by a book[956], published in 1731 by Friedrich Hoffmann (1660–1742) which provided the first insight into functional pathology, and then by one of the most important of all books in the history of medicine. This was the *De sedibus, et causis morborum per anatomen indagatis libri quinque*, 1761[957], of Giovanni Battista Morgagni (1682–1771). It was this work which brought pathology to the degree of advancement at which it could form the basis of virtually the whole of modern medical science.

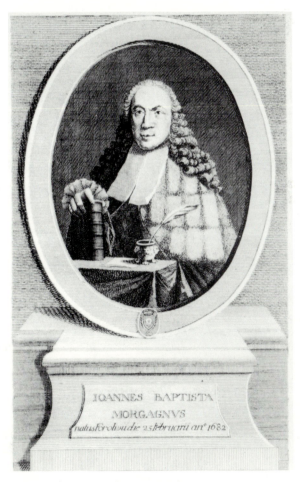

Figure 95 Giovanni Battista Morgagni (1682–1771). [*From: Thomas Joseph Pettigrew (1838–1840).*]

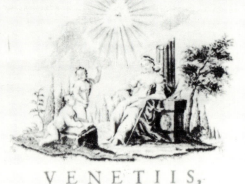

JO. BAPTISTÆ
MORGAGNI
P. P. P. P.

DE SEDIBUS, ET CAUSIS
MORBORUM
PER ANATOMEN INDAGATIS
LIBRI QUINQUE.
DISSECTIONES, ET ANIMADVERSIONES, NUNC PRIMUM EDITAS
COMPLECTUNTUR PROPEMODUM INNUMERAS, MEDICIS,
CHIRURGIS, ANATOMICIS PROFUTURAS.

Multiplex præfixus eſt Index rerum, & nominum
accuratiſſimus.

TOMUS PRIMUS
DUOS PRIORES CONTINENS LIBROS.

VENETIIS,
MDCCLXI.
EX TYPOGRAPHIA REMONDINIANA.
SUPERIORUM PERMISSU, AC PRIVILEGIO.

Figure 96   Giovanni Morgagni. Title page from: *De sedibus, et causis morborum per anatomen indagatis*... Venetiis (1761). [*Royal Society of Medicine library, London.*]

312

Morgagni (Figure 95 is the portrait from the 1779 edition) was appointed Professor of Anatomy at Padua in 1715 and occupied that chair for 56 years; he published '*De sedibus*' in his 79th year. The work consists of 70 letters reporting about 700 necropsies and correlating the clinical record with the postmortem findings. It is this correlation which is the whole point of the work and the reason for its importance – but Morgagni also made very extensive additions to morbid anatomical knowledge. He demonstrated that, in stroke, the cerebral lesion is on the opposite side of the body to the resulting paresis. He related the clinical features of pneumonia to the stages of hepatization of the lungs, described many of the visceral lesions of syphilis, gave the first description of cerebral gummata and provided an early account of syphilitic aneurysm. These and many other observations were important but, standing out as one of the greatest medical contributions of the century, was the idea which compared the clinical appearances during life with the findings in the organs after death.

The title page of the first edition forms Figure 96. There is a fine three volume translation by B. Alexander published in London in 1769 (*The seats and causes of diseases investigated by anatomy, in five books, containing a great variety of dissections, with remarks...*); there are also modern translated selections and a facsimile of the Alexander translation dated 1960 – a further facsimile appeared in 1980.

The following, from the translation by Alexander, is Morgagni's account of the death and dissection of a young tailor[958]. The clinical features (not very complex in this instance) are described in a way that considers the circumstances of the wounding and the death from internal haemorrhage. The state of the blood in the body cavities is described as 'so fluid that very few coagula could be observed therein...' – providing one of the first accounts of the fluid state of the blood in some cases of sudden death. The excellence of the anatomy is shown by the description of the track of the wound and the emphasis on the arched nature of the diaphragm:

> A taylor, of twenty years of age, was wounded by a foreigner, for a reafon of very little confequence, by a double-edg'd and pretty broad knife, in the lower part of his right fide. This happen'd on the 24th of March, in the year 1742; that is, on the very day when the refurrection of our Saviour was celebrated; a circumftance that made the fact more heinous.
>
> He did not fall down after receiving the wound. But being immediately brought into the hofpital, which was at fome diftance from thence, he vomited in the way, and difcharg'd the excrements both of the intestines and bladder. When he came thither, he was cold all over his body; he had no ftrength, and no pulfe; or, at leaft, his pulfe was very obfcure; and he fcarcely could mutter over a few pious words. As the blood was difcharg'd in very fmall quantity, the wound was for that reafon dilated; but he fhow'd not the leaft fign of feeling. Therefore, after an hour, or a little more, from the infliction of the wound, he died without any difficulty of breathing, or any difcharge of blood from the mouth.
>
> Two days after the death of this patient, we began to diffect the body, accurately, in the fame place, and continu'd the diffection the fix following days; as it was very proper for our purpofe by reafon of the fize and habit, which you could neither call fat nor lean. I fhall take notice here only of what relates to the wound, and any thing elfe which occurr'd unexpectedly.

313

The abdomen, which was neither tumid nor tenfe, and contain'd, neverthe-lefs, fuch a quantity of blood as I fhall mention, being cut into, and laid open, the furface of all the vifcera appear'd to be flightly bloody. In obferving the fituation of thefe vifcera, and among the others of the omentum, we found that, as it defcended from the right fide obliquely to the middle of the belly, it was drawn up on the left fide, and roll'd together, fo as to cover the ftomach; and then we immediately went on to the examination of the wound.

The knife had enter'd the lower fide of the right cavity of the thorax, betwixt the ninth and tenth rib; and after having pierc'd through the flefhy part of the diaphragm, near to thofe ribs, and pafs'd through the neareft fide of the liver, having enter'd it on the convex furface, at fome diftance from the lower edge, by a fiffure about two inches in length; but having come out on the con-cave furface at a fiffure fomewhat lefs: fo that the whole paffage of the knife through the liver was not longer, in general, than two inches.

After it had come out from the liver, it was forc'd through the right kidney, at fome diftance from the upper part, paffing obliquely, in like manner, from the anterior to the pofterior furface, as in the liver; by a fiffure which was almost one-half lefs in length than that in the liver. Finally, it had again per-vaded the diaphragm, and had gone quite to the lower part of the cavity of the thorax, through the flefhy part of this mufcle that lies behind the kidney: and, after having injur'd the trunk of the intercoftal nerve, at the fide of the twelfth vertebra dorfi, and a certain branch of the vena fine pari; and after having gone through fuch a number of other parts; it laft of all wounded the neighbouring mufcles which pafs by the fide of the fpine: and thefe to the depth of an inch, or rather more, notwithftanding fo many parts had been already pierc'd through at one ftroke. Therefore, altho' neither in the intercoftal mufcles, nor in the diaphragm, nor in the liver, nor the kidney, nor in the fide of the fpine, nor in thofe mufcles which I laft of all mention'd, it had wounded any veffel of a confiderable fize; yet it had cut into fo many fmaller veffels, that within the fhort time for which life continu'd, no lefs a quantity of blood feem'd to have been effus'd, than if the emulgent veffels, or the vena portarum, or rather the trunk of the vena cava itfelf, all of which we found to be unhurt, had been wounded.

For, upon lifting up the inteftines with the hands, a quantity of black blood was feen under them, and ftill more in the cavity of the pelvis; fo that moft of the perfons who were prefent at the diffection, feem'd to think that there were twenty pounds at leaft: although, as it was fo fluid that very few coagula could be obferv'd therein, and as nothing of a polypous appearance was feen in the diffection of the whole body, either in the veffels, or in the heart itfelf, it is probable that it had alfo continu'd to flow from the incis'd veffels after death, and that it had increas'd the quantity of that which had been extravafated before death. This, at leaft, is certain, that, at the end of the fourth day after the death of the man, we faw, even then, blood difcharg'd from the very extremity of the wound which we have defcrib'd, at the fide of the fpine.

But whether part of the blood defcended from thence, through the tranffix'd diaphragm, into the belly; or whether, on the other hand, it afcended into the thorax of the fupine carcafe from the belly; it is not eafy to determine. This, however, is certain, that before the thorax was open'd; when, after removing the vifcera of the belly, and exhaufting the blood, we examin'd the diaphragm; blood iffu'd forth from the laft wound of this part; and, by preffing the hand upon that part of the diaphragm, fomething was perceiv'd to fluctuate above this place: and a kind of croaking and found was heard, fimilar to that which arifes from flatus included in the inteftines. And, finally, when the thorax was open'd, fome quantity of blood was found in the cavity on that fide; and the lobe of the lungs therein was drawn upwards to a confiderable degree.

For this lobe was every-where unconnected to the pleura; whereas the left lobe was connected thereto anteriorly, and at the fide, but particularly on the back-part. Befides thefe things, there was nothing either in the thorax, or in the belly, that deferves to be taken notice of here. For it was to no purpofe that we look'd whether there was any thing bloody contain'd in the bladder, by reafon of the wounded kidney; as the fmall quantity of urine that was contain'd therein, was without any mixture of blood. But as to what we obferv'd in the tunica albuginea of one of the teftes, this has been already faid on a former occafion.

Of the appearances, however, that I faw in the diffection of the head, thefe things ought not to be pafs'd over; I mean, that the right vertebral artery, at leaft within the cranium, was four times as wide as the left: and that within the dura mater, not only externally, but where it invefts the lateral ventricles of the brain alfo, the veffels were not diftended with a fmaller quantity of blood, than if the man had died of a phrenzy. So, also, in thofe ventricles, each of which contain'd about a fpoonful of clear water, the plexus choroides were of a blackifh colour inclining to red.

So in whatever part the medullary fubftance was cut into, fmall bloody drops diftill'd here and there; and if you wip'd thefe away, and comprefs'd the cerebrum, other larger drops immediately burft forth: and we thought it altogether furprifing, what fhould prevent the return of the blood from the cranium, unlefs we fuppos'd fome convulfive contractions to have been excited; in confequence of the injury done to the trunk of the intercoftal nerve; which retain'd the blood there, in fpite of the great extravafation thereof into the belly. And to thefe contractions you may alfo attribute the vomiting; although you, perhaps, have fufficient caufes in the wounds of the kidney and diaphragm, from whence to account for the exiftence of this fymptom.

But however thefe things might be; this you will, in particular, gather from the obfervation in queftion, (and from others fimilar thereto) that if any furgeons happen to be not very well fkill'd in anatomy, they may fall into very grievous miftakes, by fuppofing that wounds which enter betwixt the ribs, belong only to the thorax. That is to fay, they are led afide by not being well acquainted with the arch'd fituation of the diaphragm; and never obferving that the upper part of the belly is, therefore, contain'd betwixt the ribs, they do not, in the leaft, fufpect, that the vifcera of this cavity may, at the fame time, be injur'd by thofe wounds.

This danger is so much the more increas'd, if there be any caufe in the belly, which drives the diaphragm up higher than ufual: whether this be, as I have taken notice of in a fat woman, a quantity of pinguedinous matter, or of flatus, or of water, or even the bulk of the diftended uterus, or of any other vifcus; as, for inftance, of the liver; whereby, even in a natural ftate, as I have already admonifh'd, the right fide of the diaphragm is frequently rais'd up. And the danger is ftill greater, if the wound is inflicted upon a perfon when in a recumbent pofture, inftead of ftanding upright.

Nor do wounds of this kind occur fo rarely, but I can remember four inftances at leaft; which you may add to the Sepulchretum; befides one of Gliffon's, that certainly fhould have been inferted there, by thofe who compil'd and made additions to the Sepulchretum. The firft is that of Mauchart, which is fimilar to the one produc'd above, from Valfalva, in

315

THE

MORBID ANATOMY

OF

SOME OF THE MOST IMPORTANT

PARTS

OF THE

HUMAN BODY

BY

MATTHEW BAILLIE, M.D. F.R.S.

FELLOW OF THE ROYAL COLLEGE OF PHYSICIANS, AND
PHYSICIAN OF ST. GEORGE'S HOSPITAL.

LONDON:

PRINTED FOR J. JOHNSON, ST. PAUL'S
CHURCH-YARD; AND G. NICOL,
PALL-MALL.

1793.

Figure 97 Matthew Baillie. Title page from: *The morbid anatomy of some of the most important parts of the human body*. London, (1793).

this circumftance, that as much blood as was exhaufted from the thorax, fo much immediately flow'd in thither, by the wound of the diaphragm, from the belly.

The fecond is that of Goetzius. The third, of the celebrated Heifter. And the fourth is that of Cramerus. And in all thefe cafes, in fact, the wound defcended from the thorax, which it had firft enter'd, through the diaphragm into the belly, and had perforated the liver. Moreover, on account of the fame confirmation, and pofition, of the diaphragm, which I have mention'd, and its declivity towards the pofterior parts; it alfo happens, that if the wounds, inflicted upon the upper part of the abdomen, are continued to any confiderable extent, not only the vifcera of the belly, but thofe of the thorax alfo, will be wounded together with the diaphragm.

However, you fee that wounds of this kind muft be referr'd by us to the next letter; as we here attend to the part from whence they begin. You may therefore expect this letter fhortly; and, in the mean while, farewel.

The significance of the finding that, in such circumstances, the blood should appear fluid and virtually free from coagula was soon to arouse the interest of John Hunter and has been discussed elsewhere[959].

The type of work undertaken by Morgagni was continued by Matthew Baillie (1761-1823), the nephew of William Hunter. Just before Baillie's principal works were published Eduard Sandifort (1742-1814) produced his finely illustrated *Observationes anatomicae-pathologicae* (1777-81)[960] which not only showed how far the art of pathological illustration had advanced but also provided good accounts of aortic endocarditis, kidney stones, ankylosis of bone and a number of congenital malformations. Within a few years Baillie wrote his *An account of a remarkable transposition of the viscera* (1788)[961]. This was followed by *The morbid anatomy of some of the most important parts of the human body*[962] – first published in 1793 – which was illustrated by the magnificent copper-plates of William Clift, John Hunter's factotum and friend. The title page of this very significant work provides Figure 97.

The book was the first systematic textbook of morbid anatomy to concentrate on the viscera and brain and describe the pathological appearances, organ by organ, in the manner of a modern study; throughout it Baillie correlated the post-mortem appearances with the details of the clinical history during life – in the manner of Morgagni. Baillie gave the first accurate definitions of the types of hepatic cirrhosis and carefully described the stages of pneumonic hepatization of the lung. He differentiated the focal and infiltrating types of tuberculous lesions and gave an account of the pulmonary pathology of this disease which makes sensible reading today. He provided the first clear correlation of the symptoms and morbid anatomy of gastric ulcer and wrote descriptions of pulmonary conditions which compare in quality with the classical accounts of mitral stenosis, heart block and angina pectoris which Morgagni had included in '*De sedibus*'.

Baillie's '*Morbid anatomy*' appeared in a second edition[963] in 1797 and this contained (derived, by repute, from Baillie's autopsy of Samuel Johnson) the first clinical description of chronic pulmonary emphysema. The work was completed by the publication, in 1799-1802, of an atlas[964] of morbid anatomy – the title page of this remarkable volume forming Figure 98. Perhaps due to his time as physician to George III, perhaps due to the fact that he was the last and most

SERIES OF ENGRAVINGS,

ACCOMPANIED WITH

EXPLANATIONS,

WHICH ARE INTENDED TO ILLUSTRATE

THE MORBID ANATOMY

OF SOME OF THE MOST IMPORTANT PARTS OF THE

HUMAN BODY.

FASCICULUS I.

COMPREHENDING

THE CHIEF MORBID APPEARANCES OF THE HEART, AND OF THE AORTA NEAR ITS ORIGIN.

By MATTHEW BAILLIE, M.D. F.R.S.

FELLOW OF THE ROYAL COLLEGE OF PHYSICIANS, AND PHYSICIAN TO ST. GEORGE'S HOSPITAL.

LONDON:

PRINTED BY W. BULMER AND CO.

AND SOLD BY J. JOHNSON, ST. PAUL'S CHURCH-YARD;
AND G. NICOL, PALL-MALL.

1799.

Figure 98 Matthew Baillie. Title page from: *A series of engravings, accompanied with explanations, which are intended to illustrate the morbid anatomy of some of the most important parts of the human body.* London, (1799–1803).

eminent owner of the gold-headed cane of the Physicians, Baillie was honoured with a memorial in Westminster Abbey. Knowledge of pulmonary diseases advanced along with Baillie's own studies – an example being the first description of bronchitis by Charles Badham (1780–1845), whose *Observations on the inflammatory affections of the mucous membrane of the bronchiae*[965], published in 1808, followed soon after the close of the century.

The two Hunters

Paris, at the beginning of the eighteenth century, was the only place where surgery could be properly studied. It was here that surgical skill had advanced to a degree that gave supremacy to the school of France; but in both obstetrics and operative surgery the lives of William and John Hunter and some of their contemporaries were soon to change this profoundly.

William Hunter (1718–1783) became the most sought-after and successful accoucheur of his day. His own contributions were immense, but the eighteenth century also saw a great improvement in the sciences supporting obstetrics. In embryology, even though as late as 1762[966] Charles Bonnet (1720–1793) was recording his belief in the preformation of the embryo, the century saw the firm foundation laid for the modern view of the growth of the conceptus. This view has its foundation in the work of Caspar Friedrich Wolff (1733–1794) who observed in fine detail the early processes of embryonic differentiation and published his observations in his *Theoria generationis*[967] of 1759. With this work Wolff effectively ended the preformation theory and, by showing that the parts of the body are evolved from embryonic leaf-like layers, he produced the basis of the germ-layer theory which was shortly to achieve for Carl Ernst von Baer (1792–1876) recognition 'as the father of modern embryology'. Wolff's second major work, *De formatione intestinorum praecipue*[968], appeared in three contributions of 1768–69 and described the formation of the intestinal tract of the chick by the development of a leaf-like layer of the embryonic blastoderm. These observations went a long way towards proving the theory of epigenesis and formed the ultimate groundwork for Carl von Baer's *Ueber Entwicklungsgeschichte der Thiere*[969] – the three volumes of which, published between 1828 and 1888, not only finally established the modern understanding of embryonic development but also showed Baer's discoveries of the notochord and the human ovum. The latter momentous discovery was first announced in Baer's *De ovi mammalium et hominis genesi*[970] of 1827 but – even if the germ-layer concept ceased to be merely a theory and became acknowledged as fact during the nineteenth century – its foundations lay in the classical contributions to embryology made by Caspar Wolff soon after the middle of the century before.

In the clinical world progress in the care of women in labour had been made by the beginning of the eighteenth century. The milestones which had been passed included the 1549 publication[684] by which Ambroise Paré revived podalic version and made the procedure practicable. Abnormal labour remained a hazardous event, often mismanaged, and the *Heel-konstige aanmerkkingen betreffende de gebreeken der vrouwen*[971], a work published in Amsterdam in 1663 by Hendrik van Roonhuyze (1622–1672), is commonly accounted the first textbook of operative obstetrics and gynaecology in any modern sense. There is an English edition of this book dated 1676 and it shows that Roonhuyze used retractors in operations like the repair of a vesico-vaginal fistula and that he recorded several successful caesarean sections.

The book which is credited with having established obstetrics as a science is the *Des maladies des femmes grosses et accouchées*[972]. Published in Paris in 1668 by François Mauriceau (1637–1709), the greatest obstetrician of his day, it was translated into English by Hugh Chamberlen in 1673. This notable treatise gives an account of the conduct of normal labour, the use of version, and the management of placenta praevia. Mauriceau was the French obstetrician who began the practice of sending women to bed to be delivered, instead of using the obstetric chair, and it was to him that Chamberlen tried to sell the long-kept secret of the obstetric forceps.

The turn of the century was marked by the publication in 1701, of the *Operationes chirurgicae novum lumen exhibentes obstetricantibus*[973] of Hendrik van Deventer (1651–1724) – the great Dutch obstetrician of the Hague who became known as the 'father of modern midwifery'. Deventer provided the first accurate descriptions of the female pelvis and gave the first practical accounts of the effects of its deformities on the progress of labour.

Compared with these rational and scientific items of progress, the story of the discovery of the obstetric forceps is curious in the extreme. It involves the descendants of the Huguenot refugee, William Chamberlen, who reached England in 1569. His son, Peter Chamberlen the elder (d. *c.* 1631), became a member of the Barber-Surgeons' Company and attended the Queens of both James I and VI and Charles I. He became the most famous of the accoucheurs of his time – probably because of his invention and secretive use of the obstetric forceps. This invention remains impressive: ultimately it resolved the shape of the fetal head and its need for protection with the diameters of the maternal pelvis, leaving the operator to guide the protected head through the birth canal. At the beginning it must be presumed to have been a much more simple instrument. Peter the elder had a brother (Peter Chamberlen the younger; 1572–1626) who was also a famous man-midwife and who probably shared the secret. The son of Peter the younger, also called Peter (1601–1683) was one of the physicians to Charles II.

Hugh Chamberlen the elder (b. *c.* 1630), son of the third Peter Chamberlen, also an accoucheur at court, is the member of the family who is thought to have sold the secret of the forceps. Some accounts say that it was sold, about 1693, to Rogier, the son of Hendrik van Roonhuyze, whose book has already been mentioned; others say that it was sold to Mauriceau. The son of Hugh the elder, also called Hugh Chamberlen (1664–1728), has a bust in Westminster Abbey. The brother of Hugh the elder, Paul Chamberlen (1635–1717) was also a renowned London accoucheur but was the last of importance in this remarkable family.

The Chamberlens seem to have kept their secret for over a century. After the death of Hugh the younger and Paul Chamberlen the forceps were lost sight of for almost another century. Then, in 1813, at Woodham Mortimer Hall, near Maldon, Essex, four sets of the forceps were found in a box hidden under the floorboards of the house which, in the days of Charles II, Peter Chamberlen had occupied.

The dominating figure among eighteenth century obstetricians was William Smellie (1697–1763), born in Lanarkshire soon after the Chamberlen secret had been sold. Smellie was of the same county as his eventual student, William Hunter, but studied midwifery in Paris before settling in London in 1739. He taught students within his own house, using a pliable manikin and an actual pelvis in a thoroughly modern manner. In his important *Treatise on the theory and practice of midwifery*[974] of 1752 he described the mechanisms of labour far more accurately than any previous writer. He provided the first safe rules for the use of the obstetric forceps, taught the differential diagnosis of the normal, contracted, and deformed pelvis by actual measurement, and himself introduced the steel-lock, the curved, and double curved forceps. His book, reprinted by the New Sydenham Society in 1876–78, contains the first illustration of a rachitic pelvis and was followed by two volumes (1754 and 1764) of informative case reports. It is to Smellie that the credit must be given for the great advance of introducing the double-curved forceps offering both cephalic and pelvic conformity. The natural successor to Smellie was John Harvie who taught the expression of the placenta by gentle external compression (so anticipating Credé by nearly a century) and who embodied his experience in the *Practical directions, shewing a method of preserving the perinaeum in birth, and delivering the placenta without violence*[975] published in 1767.

William Hunter (1718–1783), perhaps the most distinguished of Glasgow's medical graduates, became pre-eminent as both anatomist and obstetrician. William and John Hunter, his younger brother by 10 years, were born in Long Calderwood, East Kilbride, Lanarkshire. They were, respectively, the seventh and tenth children of a large family of Ayrshire descent. William, in almost all ways the more cultured – his portrait forms Figure 99 – matriculated in 1731 at

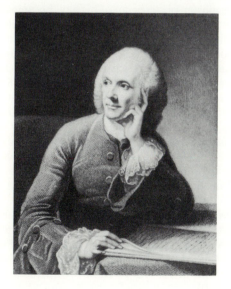

Figure 99   William Hunter (1718–1783). Frontispiece from: *Anatomia uteri humani gravidi tabulis illustrata . . . Birmingham* (1774).

Glasgow and, for his medical studies, resided with William Cullen at Hamilton. He attended the course at Edinburgh, reading medicine in 1739 and the following year, and then went to London to reside with William Smellie and then James Douglas. The rest of his early career involved equally famous names: in 1741 he was a surgical pupil at St. George's Hospital under James Wilkie; he became the tutor of his illustrious brother, John, and the associate of the pathologist, Matthew Baillie.

The development of William's career was such that he began to teach only a year or so after William Cheselden had, in 1745, secured the separation of the surgeons from the barbers from whose fraternity they had grown; William was also a master of the school which produced men of the calibre of Charles Bell (1774–1842; after whom is named Bell's palsy and who occupied the Edinburgh chair of surgery) and Peter Mark Roget (1779–1869, writer of the *Thesaurus*).

The school of the Hunters was at 16 Great Windmill Street, London and taught not only practical anatomy but also chemistry, medicine and the practice of surgery. William's lectures on anatomy were polished and erudite and by these means, and by providing for the painstaking dissection of the cadaver, he revived the teaching of anatomy in London. He amassed also a magnificent museum of anatomical and pathological specimens and these, on his death, formed the nucleus of the fine Hunterian Museum and Library of the University at Glasgow.

Increasingly he concentrated his practice on obstetrics and from about 1756 devoted his clinical work almost completely to this favourite subject. He was consulted by Queen Charlotte during her first pregnancy in 1762 and seems to have become an exponent of non-invasive, physiological methods of childbirth. Many accounts are given of his showing his midwifery forceps with rust upon them to indicate how little use he had for such instruments. There is no doubt that William Hunter, the master-obstetrician of his day, became the mentor of British obstetrics, raising the subject from the prerogative of unskilled midwives to make it the branch of medicine and sophisticated midwifery which it has become today.

Over a period of years he published a number of papers on a variety of anatomical, pathological, and obstetric subjects. Of these, the account *On retroversion of the uterus* (1772)[976] is typical and the paper of 1784 *On the uncertainty of the signs of murder, in the case of bastard children*[977] is interesting as providing an early and important British contribution to the science of forensic medicine. But these works are less than William Hunter's *Anatomia uteri humani gravidi tabulis illustrata. The anatomy of the human gravid uterus exhibited in figures*[978]. This, one of the finest anatomical atlases ever to be produced, was published in 1774 and (apart from a little book by J. Dalby of 1762) is the only medical work to come from the famous Baskerville Press. Following the death of Jane Douglas in 1744, Hunter seems to have become restrained, frugal, and preoccupied with anatomy and obstetrics. Perhaps something of this remoteness shows in the text, which is in both Latin and English, of the work. But to the excellence of its 34 copper-plates and its presentation Hunter devoted much of the effort of 30 years and great expense. The title page of its original edition (the Sydenham Society published a good reprint in 1851) is given in Figure 100 and one of its plates is represented in Figure 101.

One of William Hunter's visitors in London in 1778, when the great atlas was available, was Samuel Soemmerring (1755–1830). Hunter's illustrations dealt

A N A T O M I A
UTERI HUMANI GRAVIDI.
T A B U L I S   I L L U S T R A T A.

AUCTORE

GULIELMO HUNTER,

SERENISSIMÆ REGINAE CHARLOTTAE MEDICO EXTRAORDINARIO,

IN ACADEMIA REGALI ANATOMIAE PROFESSORE,

ET SOCIETATUM, REGIAE ET ANTIQUARIAE, SOCIO.

BIRMINGHAMIAE excudebat JOANNES BASKERVILLE, MDCCLXXIV.

LONDINI prostant apud S. BAKER, T. CADELL, D. WILSON, G. NICOL, et J. MURRAY.

THE ANATOMY
OF THE
HUMAN GRAVID UTERUS
EXHIBITED IN FIGURES,

BY

WILLIAM HUNTER,

PHYSICIAN EXTRAORDINARY TO THE QUEEN, PROFESSOR OF

ANATOMY IN THE ROYAL ACADEMY, AND FELLOW OF THE

ROYAL AND ANTIQUARIAN SOCIETIES.

PRINTED AT BIRMINGHAM BY JOHN BASKERVILLE, 1774.

SOLD IN LONDON BY S. BAKER AND G. LEIGH, IN York-Street; T. CADELL IN THE Strand; D. WILSON AND G. NICOL,
OPPOSITE York-Buildings; AND J. MURRAY, IN Fleet-Street.

Figure 100   William Hunter. Title page from: *Anatomia uteri humani gravidi tabulis illustrata*... Birmingham (1774).

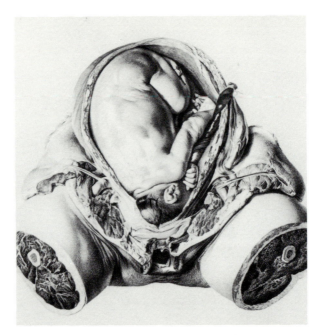

Figure 101   William Hunter. Plate VI from: *Anatomia uteri humani gravidi tabulis illustrata* . . . Birmingham (1774).

with the appearances of the last part of pregnancy. Soemmerring, resolved to produce a companion volume depicting the first half of pregnancy, achieved his aim with the *Icones embryonum humanorum*[979] published in 1799. Both atlases remain of permanent value due to their fine engravings and anatomical accuracy.

The eighteenth century saw not only these splendid works representing the functional anatomy of obstetrics – it saw also the appearance, in 1742, of *A treatise in midwifry*[980] by Sir Fielding Ould (1710–1789). This was the first text-book of any real importance on its subject in English. Earlier than this there is almost nothing of note to reflect, in English, the medical care of the pregnant woman of the time. It provides, therefore, a base-line from which to estimate progress and the changing practices in obstetric care.

Apart from Fielding Ould there were others whose attitudes would, in time, begin to affect both maternal and infant mortality rates. These included John Burton (1697–1771), whose publication[981] of 1751 was the first to propose that puerperal fever is contagious, and John Leake (1729–1792) whose *Practical observations on the child-bed fever* (1772)[982] was emphatic about the contagious-ness of the fever that had such a mortality in the postpartum period. The physician who carried these ideas into practice was Charles White (1728–1813) who published *A treatise on the management of pregnant and lying-in women* (1773)[983] – a tract of the utmost importance advocating cleanliness in obstetrics and beginning many of the later developments in aseptic midwifery.

Few families in the history of medicine have produced brothers as notable,

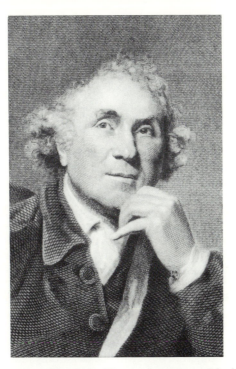

Figure 102   John Hunter (1728–1793). [*From: A treatise on the blood, inflammation, and gun-shot wounds . . . by . . . Everard Home. London, (1794).*]

and yet different from one another, as the Hunters. By contrast with his elder brother, William, the education of John Hunter (1728–1793; Figure 102) was undistinguished. He never completed a full course of studies in any university and, in 1748, seems to have come down to London only to assist William in the anatomy teaching which had been begun 2 years before. Once in London his curious and unusual ability at the art of dissection became obvious and William was eventually able to prevail on Cheselden to teach him surgery at Chelsea. There were probably also later periods of surgical training at St. Bartholomew's in 1751 and at St. George's in the years around 1754. John seems to have become House Surgeon at St. George's in 1756 and to have been made a member of the Corporation of Surgeons in 1768. He taught anatomy not only in the school at Windmill Street but also as Master of Anatomy at Surgeon's Hall and when on the staff of St. George's. His ability to teach this subject became renowned and his students included many of the most famous men of medicine of the next generation: Edward Jenner, who established preventive vaccination against smallpox; John Abernethy (1764–1831), the first surgeon to ligate the external iliac artery for aneurysm; and Astley Cooper (1768–1841), the surgeon whose habit of dissecting nearly every day led to a surgical brilliance which has presented Guy's with a treasured tradition, were all students of John Hunter; others were of importance in the early progress of surgery in North America; these included John Morgan (1735–1789) of Philadelphia, a pupil of both of the Hunters, two of the Munros, and of Cullen, who became Director General of Military Hospitals and Physician in Chief of the American Army; and William Shippen (1736–1808), who became successor to Morgan as Surgeon General in 1777 and who is remembered as having been the first great teacher of obstetrics in the rapidly growing American states.

Like his brother, John became an avid collector – but one with a vast and surprising range of interests: the whole of biology seemed to fascinate him and he is said to have dissected over 500 animal species. It is typical of him that when Jenner asked his advice on overcoming a personal problem which Jenner suffered on returning to his native Gloucestershire, Hunter imposed upon him the responsibility of studying the hibernation physiology of the hedgehog. His own early work was detailed and exacting and included *The natural history of the human teeth*[984] of 1771 and *A practical treatise on the diseases of the teeth, intended as a supplement to the natural history of those parts*[985] – the latter published in London in 1778. These are classical works and virtually began the organized study of dental surgery. Hunter devised the classification of the teeth into incisors, cuspids, bicuspids, molars and so on. He gave instructions regarding the transplantation of teeth and can be remembered as having begun the orderly study of an important and neglected subject.

He made an original observation in his paper giving an *Account of a woman who had the smallpox during pregnancy, and who seemed to have communicated the same disease to the foetus* (1780)[986] but tragically confounded two diseases in his work of 1786, *A treatise on the venereal disease*[987]. Working at a time when venereal disease was thought to be due to one cause only, and wanting to test this belief, Hunter inoculated himself with pus from a patient who had gonorrhoea and unsuspected syphilis. The resulting syphilis seemed to confirm Hunter's opinion. The hard (Hunterian) chancre eponymized Hunter's name – but this experiment held back understanding of the venereal diseases for many years and, even though Hunter, in this same work, provided the first suggestion that lymphogranuloma venereum is a separate disease, it was left to Benjamin Bell (1749–1806) to differentiate gonorrhoea from syphilis for the first time. Bell recorded this important differentiation in his *A treatise on gonorrhoea virulenta, and lues venerea* (1793)[988] – a work which appeared almost two decades before René Bertin (1757–1828) produced, in 1810, the first systematic study[989] of congenital syphilis.

In the same year that Hunter published his work on venereal diseases he produced a collection of papers, gathered into a book, entitled *Observations on certain parts of the animal oeconomy* (1786)[990]. This work contains a number of original observations including a description of the olfactory nerves and gives an account of the secondary sexual characteristics in birds, the descent of the testis, and the structure of the placenta.

Running throughout all of these works is a great sense of curiosity – a sense which showed in the early essay *On the digestion of the stomach after death*[991] of 1772 and lasted throughout the writings just mentioned. Nowhere is it more evident than in the important posthumous *A treatise on the blood, inflammation, and gun-shot wounds*[992] published in London in 1794, the year after Hunter had died. Hunter collected the material for this unique and original study while serving with the army at Belle Isle during the Seven Years' War. His accounts of the process of inflammation are among the first and best of their kind and are fundamental to the science of modern pathology. The 1794 edition is prefixed by a short account of Hunter's life written by his brother-in-law, Everard Home, and this provides one of the most readable insights into the medical life of London and the growth of anatomy and surgery of the time. The same work provides the fine portrait of Hunter which forms Figure 102. But it is the body of the work which shows the precision of Hunter's observations. In a manner which suggests that he knew of the earlier accounts by Morgagni of the events which sometimes follow sudden or traumatic death, John Hunter wrote[993]:

> As the coagulation of the blood is a natural process, and as all natural processes have their time of action, unless influenced by some exciting causes, and since cold is not a cause of the blood's coagulation, even when removed out of the circulation, the blood may be frozen much more quickly than it can coagulate, by which change its coagulating power is suspended. To prove this by experiment, I took a thin leaden vessel, with a flat bottom, of some width, and put it into a cold mixture below o, and allowed as much blood to run from a vein into it, as covered its bottom. The blood froze immediately, and when thawed, became fluid, and coagulated, I believe, as soon as it would have done had it not been frozen.
>
> As the coagulation of the blood appears to be that process which may be compared with the action of life in the solids, we shall examine this property a little further, and see if this power of coagulation can be destroyed; if it can, we shall next inquire, if by the same means life is destroyed in the solids; and if the phænomena are nearly the same in both. The prevention of coagulation may be affected by electricity, and often is by lightning: it takes place in some deaths, and is produced in some of the natural operations of the body; all of which I shall now consider.
>
> Animals killed by lightning, and also by electricity, have not their muscles contracted: this arises from death being instantaneously produced in the muscles, which therefore cannot be affected by any stimulus, nor consequently by the stimulus of death. In such cases the blood does not coagulate. Animals who are run very hard, and killed in such a state, or what produces still a greater effect, are run to death, have neither their muscles contracted, nor their blood coagulated; and in both respects the effect is in proportion to the cause.
>
> I had two deer run, till they dropped down and died; in neither did I find the muscles contracted, nor the blood coagulated.
>
> In many kinds of death, we find that the muscles neither contract, nor the blood coagulate. In some cases the muscles will contract while the blood continues fluid, in some the contrary happens; and in others the blood will only coagulate to the consistence of cream.
>
> Blows on the stomach kill immediately, and the muscles do not contract, nor does the blood coagulate. Such deaths as prevent the contraction of the muscles, or the coagulation of the blood, are, I believe, always sudden. Death from sudden gusts of passion, is of this kind; and in all these cases the body soon putrifies after death. In many diseases, if accurately attended to, we find this correspondence between muscles and blood; for where there is strong action going on, the muscles contract strongly after death, and the blood coagulates strongly.
>
> It is unnecessary, I imagine, to relate particular instances of the effects of each of those causes: I need only mention that I have seen them all. In a natural evacuation of blood, viz. menstruation, it is neither similar to blood taken

from a vein of the same person, nor to that which is extravasated by an accident in any other part of the body; but is a species of blood, changed, separated, or thrown off from the common mass, by an action of the vessels of the uterus, similar to that of secretion; by which action the blood loses the principle of coagulation, and I suppose life.

In this account Hunter's observation that the blood can be frozen quicker than it can coagulate shows his practical, experimental approach. Equally remarkable is his record that in animals run to death the blood is not coagulated. We might now explain this as being due to the outpouring of plasminogen activator from the venous wall and the consequent vast increase in blood fibrinolytic activity which accompanies intense exercise – this activity ensuring that any fibrin formed is rapidly lysed, leaving the blood incapable of further coagulation. But Hunter's observations anticipate modern knowledge in the same way that his comments on menstrual blood provide such an anticipation: he says that menstrual blood is a species which has lost the 'principle of coagulation' due to an 'action of the vessels of the uterus': the principle is the fibrinogen and fibrin, the vessels providing the plasminogen activator – this beginning the process which lyses the blood clot so that it is then incoagulable. These perceptive observations of John Hunter provide some of the earliest and clearest clues to our current understanding of the mechanisms of fibrinolysis.

There is also *The works of John Hunter, with notes*[994] – a four volume study accompanied by an atlas edited by J. F. Palmer and published in London betweeen 1835 and 1837. The scope of this work shows Hunter as the architect of the science of comparative anatomy; it shows also the impetus that he gave to the study of morbid anatomy and experimental pathology. Not only did Hunter become one of the greatest surgeons of all time but he amassed a collection of well over 10 000 anatomical, pathological and biological specimens. This collection was purchased by the government in 1799 and when, in 1800, the Corporation of Surgeons became The Royal College of Surgeons, the Hunterian Museum formed one of its greatest attributes. Sadly, much of the collection was destroyed during an air raid on London in May, 1941.

An example of Hunter's contributions to surgery, apart from his descriptions of surgical shock, phlebitis, intussusception, inflammation, gun-shot wounds, and a number of other conditions, is his development of the important surgical principle that aneurysms (which were common in his day as a manifestation of vascular syphilis) should be ligated high up, in the healthy tissues, by a single ligature. Such a ligature had been used before but Hunter's innovation was the deliberate adoption of a procedure intended to develop the collateral circulation. In doing this he established an important principle of physiology – learnt, it is said, from his observations on the changes in the capillary circulation in the antlers of the King's deer in Richmond Royal Park.

The two brothers grew apart as their lives progressed. John was survived by two of his four children, but both of these died without issue. Long after his death, in 1859, the remains of John Hunter were removed from St. Martin-in the-Fields and re-interred in Westminster Abbey, where they remain on the north side of the nave. Everard Home, in the 1794 edition of the great '*Treatise. . .*', says that: 'The symptoms of Mr Hunter's complaint, for the last 20 years of his life, may be considered as those of the angina pectoris; and form one of the most complete histories of that disease upon record.'[995] He gives this account of Hunter's death on October 16th, 1793, and of the morbid appearances underlying the condition[996]:

In the autumn of 1790, and in the spring and autumn 1791, he had more severe attacks than during the other periods of the year, but of not more than a few hours duration: in the beginning of October 1792, one, at which I was present, was so violent that I thought he would have died. On October the 16th, 1793, when in his usual state of health, he went to St. George's Hospital, and meeting with some things which irritated his mind, and not being perfectly master of the circumstances, he withheld his sentiments, in which state of restraint he went into the next room, and turning round to Dr. Robertson, one of the physicians of the hospital, he gave a deep groan, and dropt down dead.

It is a curious circumstance that, the first attack of these complaints was produced by an affection of the mind, and every future return of any consequence arose from the same cause; and although bodily exercise, or distention of the stomach, brought on slighter affections, it still required the mind to be affected to render them severe; and as his mind was irritated by trifles, these produced the most violent effects on the disease. His coachman being beyond his time, or a servant not attending to his directions, brought on the spasms, while a real misfortune produced no effect.

At the time of his death he was in the 65th year of his age, the same age at which his brother, the late Dr. Hunter, died.

Upon inspecting the body after death, the following were the appearances: the skin in several places was mottled, particularly on the sides and neck, which arose from the blood not having been completely coagulated, but remaining nearly fluid.

The contents of the abdomen were in a natural state, but the coats of the stomach and intestines were unusually loaded with blood, giving them a fleshy appearance, and a dark reddish colour; those parts which had a depending situation, as in the bottom of the pelvis, and upon the loins, had this in a greater degree than the others; this evidently arose from the fluid state of the blood. The stomach was rather relaxed, but the internal surface was entirely free from any appearance of disease; the orifice at the pylorus was uncommonly open. The gall-bladder contained five or six small stones of a light yellow colour. The liver and the other viscera exhibited nothing unusual in their appearance.

The cartilages of the ribs had in many places become bone, requiring a saw to divide them. There was no water in the cavity of the chest, and the lungs of the right side were uncommonly healthy; but those of the left had very strong adhesions to the pleura, extending over a considerable surface, more especially towards the sternum.

The pericardium was very unusually thickened, which did not allow it to collapse upon being opened; the quantity of water contained in it was scarcely more than is frequently met with, although it might probably exceed that which occurs in the most healthy state of these parts.

The heart itself was very small, appearing too little for the cavity in which it lay, and did not give the idea of its being the effect of an unusual degree of contraction, but more of its having shrunk in its size. Upon the under surface of the left auricle and ventricle, there were two spaces nearly an inch and half square, which were of a white colour, with an opaque appearance, and entirely distinct from the general surface of the heart: these two spaces were covered by an exudation of coagulating lymph, which at some former period had been the result of inflammation there. The muscular structure of the heart was paler and looser in its texture than the other muscles in the body. There were no coagula in any of its cavities. The coronary arteries had their branches which ramify through the substance of the heart in the state of bony tubes, which were with difficulty divided by the knife, and their transverse sections did not collapse, but remained open. The valvulæ mitrales, where they come off from the lower edge of the auricle, were in many places ossified, forming an imperfectly bony margin of different thicknesses, and in one spot so thick as to form a knob; but these ossifications were not continued down upon the valve towards the chordæ tendineæ.

The semilunar valves of the aorta had lost their natural pliancy, the previous stage to becoming bone, and in several spots there were evident ossifications.

The aorta immediately beyond the semilunar valves had its cavity larger than usual, putting on the appearance of an incipient aneurism; this unusual dilatation extended for some way along the ascending aorta, but did not reach so far as the common trunk of the axillary and carotid artery. The increase of capacity of the artery might be about one-third of its natural area; and the internal membrane of this part had lost entirely the natural polish, and was studded over with opaque white spots, raised higher than the general surface.

On inspecting the head, the cranium and dura mater were found in a natural state. The pia mater had the vessels upon the surface of the two hemispheres of the brain turgid with blood, which is commonly found to be the case after sudden death.

The internal structure of the brain was very carefully examined, and the different parts both of the cerebrum and cerebellum were found in the most natural and healthy state; but the internal carotid arteries as they pass by the sides of the cella tursica were ossified, and several of the ramifications which go off from them had become opaque and unhealthy in their appearance. The vertebral arteries lying upon the medulla oblongata had also become bony, and the basillary artery, which is formed by them, had opaque white spots very generally along its coats.

From this account of the appearances observed after death, it is reasonable to attribute the principal symptoms of the disease to an organic affection of the heart. That organ was rendered unable to carry on its functions, whenever the actions were disturbed, either in consequence of bodily exertion, or affections of the mind.

The stoppage of the pulse arose from a spasm upon the heart, and in this state the nerves were probably pressed against the ossified arteries, which may account for the excruciating pain he felt at those times.

John Hunter was preceded by only two British surgeons of great stature: these were William Cheselden (1688–1752) and Percivall Pott (1714–1788). William Cheselden (Figure 103), surgeon to St. Thomas's from 1718, was probably the greatest of the lithotomists but he also wrote two important books on anatomy. His *The anatomy of the humane body*[997], of 1713, went through 13 editions and was one of the great textbooks of the British schools of medicine. But he produced, in addition, the lovely *Osteographia, or the anatomy of the bones*[998], of 1733, probably the best production of the anatomists of the eighteenth century. The title page of this volume forms Figure 104; the front and rear views (both slightly oblique) of the human skeleton form Figures 105 and 106; the memorable view of the skeleton in the position of supplication forms Figure 107.

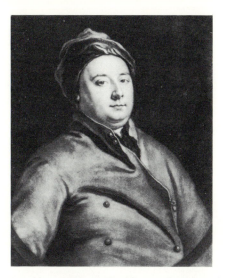

Figure 103   William Cheselden (1688–1752). [*From: Osteographia, or the anatomy of the bones. London, (1733)*.]

Cheselden was the first illustrator known to have used the camera obscura to achieve precision in his anatomical drawings. These were executed by Van der Gucht whose work, in the opinion of many, has not been bettered. The whole work, dating from one-third of the way through the eighteenth century, serves as a reminder of the excellence of the anatomy of the period.

The other great surgeon in England who preceded John Hunter was Percival Pott, surgeon to St. Bartholomew's from 1744 to 1787. He wrote his classical book on hernia – *A treatise on ruptures* (1756)[999] – while confined to bed suffering from the effects of a fall. In this book he did away with many of the old theories on the cause and treatment of ruptures, introduced a good deal of surgical sense into their management, and gave the first description of congenital hernia. His 1765 *Some few general remarks on fractures and dislocations*[1000] is one of the classical works of medicine: in this Pott gave an account of fractures and dislocations which led to the universal adoption of some of his methods; he emphasized the need for the muscles to be relaxed if proper reduction of a fracture was to be achieved and, in this book, described the fracture-dislocation of the ankle which is called 'Pott's fracture'. He gave the first account of what became known as 'Percivall Pott's puffy tumour' in the *Observations on the nature and consequences of wounds and contusions of the head, fractures of the skull, concussions of the brain*...[1001] – a work published in London in 1760 and displaying not only Pott's knowledge of the literature of surgery but also the range of head injuries even then being encountered. This notable book was followed by the classical description of hydrocele (*Practical remarks on the hydrocele or watry rupture*, (1762)[1002] and by Pott's *Chirurgical observations relative to the cataract, the polypus of the nose, the cancer of the scrotum*... (1775)[1003]. The latter is his great contribution to oncology, for Pott's report of scrotal cancer in chimney-sweeps was not only the first description of

OSTEOGRAPHIA,

OR THE

ANATOMY

OF THE

BONES.

BY WILLIAM CHESELDEN

SURGEON TO HER MAJESTY;

F. R. S.

SURGEON TO S^T THOMAS'S HOSPITAL,

AND MEMBER OF THE ROYAL ACADEMY OF SURGERY AT PARIS.

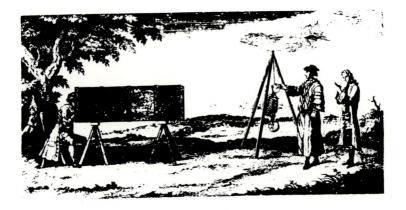

LONDON MDCCXXXIII.

Figure 104 William Cheselden. Title page from: *Osteographia, or the anatomy of the bones.* London, (1733).

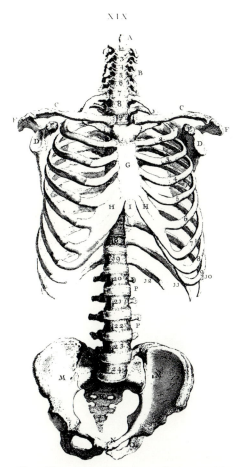

Figure 105   William Cheselden. Plate XIX from *Osteographia, or the anatomy of the bones.* London, (1733).

occupational cancer but was also the first demonstration of a cancer due to clearly identifiable external causes. It thus began the still incomplete process of ridding cancer of a little of its superstition. Pott did not recognize the tuberculous nature of the disease of the spine which he described in his *Remarks on that kind of palsy of the lower limbs, which is frequently found to accompany a curvature of the spine* (1779)[1004] but he did give the great classic account of the spinal curvature (due to tuberculous caries) which can result in paralysis of the lower limbs and has since been known as 'Pott's spine'. This account, like that of Pott's fracture, was reprinted in *Medical Classics* in 1936.

Hunter left surgery in the hands of men of the calibre of William Hewson, John Abernethy (1764–1831) and William Cruikshank (1745–1800). Cruikshank became the successor to Hewson as William Hunter's assistant and was the colleague who, with Matthew Baillie, eventually took over the Great Windmill Street anatomical and surgical school.

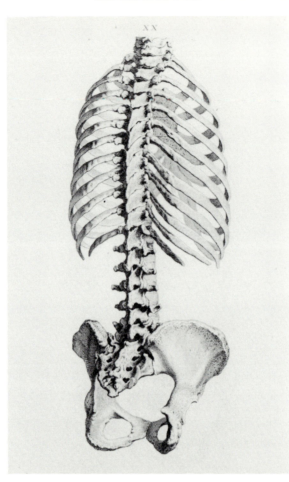

Figure 106   William Cheselden. Plate XX from *Osteographia, or the anatomy of the bones*. London, (1733).

Anatomy in the eighteenth century reached the accuracy and excellence of illustration achieved by Bernhard Albinus (1697–1770), one of the greatest of anatomists whose *Tabulae sceleti et musculorum corporis humani*[1005] of 1747 (English translation 1777) set a fine standard in the art of anatomical representation. The century ended with the *Anatomie générale, appliquée à la physiologie et à la médecine* (1801)[1006] in which Marie François Bichat (1771–1802) transformed descriptive anatomy by showing that separate tissues within anatomical organs, as well as the organs themselves, could become the seat of disease.

The successors of John Hunter were anatomists, comparative anatomists, physiologists and morbid pathologists – as well as surgeons. This broad and ample level of science carried into the practice of clinical surgery was, to no small extent, the result of the tuition of Hunter. Before Hunter's imprint had been set

334

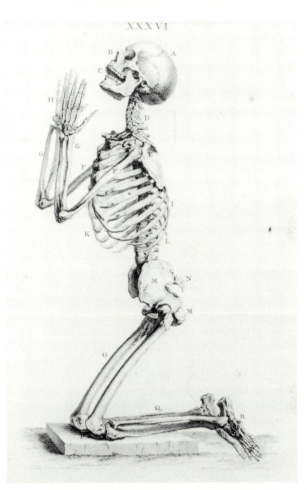

Figure 107   William Cheselden. Plate XXXVI from *Osteographia, or the anatomy of the bones.* London, (1733).

on the subject, advances in surgery were limited to the design of more rapid operative techniques, better methods of excision, and more reliable and safe methods of amputation – most of these advances coming from the French surgical school. Hunter was responsible for much of the intellect of British surgery. As Garrison puts it: 'It is no exaggeration to repeat that Hunter found surgery a mechanical art and left it an experimental science'[1007] – and such, at its best, it remained.

Edward Jenner

The eighteenth century had been spanned by the 1735 publication of the *Systema naturae*[876] of Linnaeus, the 1761 *De sedibus, et causis morborum* . . . [957] of Morgagni, the engraving of the *Anatomia uteri humani gravidi* . . . [978]in 1774 –

the great work of William Hunter – and the posthumous 1794 publication of the *Treatise on the blood, inflammation, and gun-shot wounds*[992] by John Hunter. The century also witnessed the life of William Heberden and closed with his epitome of medicine, the *Commentarii . . .* [945] of 1802.

Eighteenth century anatomy reached a memorable level of accomplishment. This included the masterly steel-plate illustrations in the 1733 *Osteographia . . .* [998] of Cheselden; the accurate depiction of the viscera and blood vessels in the *Icones anatomicae* (1743–56)[901] of the great physiologist, Albrecht von Haller; the beautiful atlases of the bones, muscles, visceral blood vessels, skeleton, skeletal muscles, and the gravid uterus, produced by Bernhard Albinus whose *Tabulae sceleti et musculorum corporis humani*[1005] of 1747 was especially notable; and finally, the splendid *Tabulae neurologicae, . . .* (1794)[1008] of Antonio Scarpa (?1747–1832). This splendid work provided the first accurate delineation of the nerves of the heart. It represented the acme of Scarpa's anatomical achievement.

Scarpa had been the first to consider arteriosclerosis as a lesion primarily of the inner layers of the arterial wall. But he is remembered as an anatomist – and his name is used (Scarpa's triangle) to describe the anatomy of the thigh.

In 1803 Scarpa gave the first accurate description[1009] of the pathological anatomy of congenital club-foot. This was followed by the *Sull'ernie. Memorie anatomico-chirurgiche*[1010] of 1809. These works were contemporaneous with *The anatomy and surgical treatment of abdominal hernia* (1804–07)[1011] – the study by Sir Astley Paston Cooper (1768–1841) which was the finest contribution to its subject of the nineteenth century: it not only described 'Cooper's ligament' and 'Cooper's hernia' but demonstrated the groundwork laid in the preceding century in the now mature science of anatomy.

Eighteenth century progress in Heberden's world and in internal medicine was perhaps more limited. Some of the more significant advances can be represented by the *De morbis artificum diatriba* (1700)[1012] of Bernardino Ramazzini (1633–1714) whose book, published in Modena, was the first satisfactory account of a range of occupational diseases. It was the first major work since the days of Paracelsus to raise the subject of industrial illnesses and describe pneumonoconiosis in a number of different forms. The work dealt with the subjects of lead poisoning in potters, occupational toxicities among metal workers and silicosis in stonemasons. It has long been recognized that this study was fundamental to a subject which became of increasing importance and there were translations into English in 1705 and 1940.

Real thought began to be given to other aspects of the general health of the community. Following in the earlier tradition of John Graunt, a German army chaplain, Johann Peter Süssmilch (1707–1767) produced a work[1013], published in Berlin in 1742, which made an important contribution to vital statistics. This book was marked by a humane interpretation of the data and Süssmilch demonstrated the need for a fit and industrious population if a nation was to expand and thrive.

The end of the eighteenth century and the beginning of the following century saw the work of Johann Peter Frank (1745–1821), one of the founders of modern public health hygiene. In these writings the medical mind can be seen to extend from the care of a small class in the community to the needs and opportunities of the body politic. Frank's first substantial publications, of 1792[1014] and 1794[1015], were concerned with such purely medical subjects as the great seriousness of diseases of the spinal cord and the first definition of diabetes insipidus. Between 1779 and 1827 Frank produced the nine volume *System einer vollständigen medicinischen Polizey*[1016], the first systematic treatise on public health and hygiene. There is a part-translation in English dated 1976 and this shows the range of Frank's political and medical thinking: he imposed virtually paternal responsibilities upon rulers and governments, expecting these to provide both laws for the care of the public health and the physical means of caring for the people. These concepts were further expanded in his *De curandis hominum morbis epitome*[1017] published between 1792 and 1825.

Similar concerns led to the report on *The state of the prisons in England and Wales*[1018] published by John Howard (1726–1790) in 1777. This now famous report disclosed the abuses and appalling conditions then prevalent in the prisons. Its appearance formed part of Howard's lifetime effort to reform conditions, secure appropriate legislation, and obtain a reasonable diet and level of prison cleanliness. This work has a modern reprint (1973).

Equally appalling conditions existed in the hospitals and, in France, these were disclosed by the *Mémoires sur les hôpitaux de Paris*[1019], written by Jacques René Tenon (1724–1816) and published in 1788. Tenon founded a unique hospital for children but his record of the dreadful conditions then existing in hospitals can be read only as an indictment of the authorities of the time. As the years went by Howard journeyed widely in Britain and continental Europe and wrote his travels and findings in the 1789 *An account of the principle lazarettos in Europe*[1020], published, like his first book, in England. This important work (again, reprinted in New York in 1973) did much to diminish, by improving conditions, the incidence of hospital-transmitted infection, just as Howard's other reforms had lessened the incidence of typhus fever in prisons.

Within the narrower confines of internal medicine, the work of Robert Whytt (1714–1766), another pupil of Boerhaave and Munro *primus*, shows the growth of the rational aspects of the subject. Whytt was a famous Edinburgh neuro-physiologist and was the first to show convincingly that the response of the pupils to light is a reflex action – a mechanism still known as 'Whytt's reflex'. He published *An essay on the vital and other involuntary motions of animals*[1021] in 1751 and followed this with the *Observations on the nature, causes, and cure of those disorders which have been commonly called nervous hypochondriac, or hysteric, to which are prefixed some remarks on the sympathy of the nerves* (1765)[1022]. Following comments made by Fielding Garrison[1023], this has come to be regarded as the first really important book on neurology to have appeared after Willis. The other notable writing of Robert Whytt is the *Observations on the dropsy in the brain*[1024]; this work, of 1768 (2 years after Whytt's death) was, like his other books mentioned, published in Edinburgh – it gives the classical first account of the clinical manifestations of tuberculous meningitis in children and shows that Whytt fully recognized that the course of the illness, invariably fatal, was due to the serous exudate covering and affecting the brain.

One of the most important developments in medicine in the late eighteenth century went almost unnoticed. It came to publication in the year (1761) that Frank Nicholls (1699–1778), physician to George II from 1753 to 1760, communicated to the Royal Society his paper entitled *Observations concerning the body of his late Majesty, October 26, 1760* [1025]. By means of this paper Nicholls became the first to describe the dissecting aneurysm of the aorta, the patient concerned having been the King. This historic and interesting observation was dwarfed in importance by the barely noticed *Inventum novum ex percussione thoracis humani ut signo abstrusos interni pectoris morbos detegendi* (1761) [1026] of the Austrian physician, Leopold Auenbrugger (1722–1809).

Auenbrugger, born at Graz, was the son of an innkeeper and it seems that he learnt in boyhood how, by percussing or tapping a barrel, the fluid level of its contents could be determined. He graduated in medicine at Vienna and probably first applied his boyhood knowledge to medicine when he was physician at the Spanish Military Hospital. He rapidly found that he could not only determine the fluid level in the chest but that he could percuss the outline of the heart. By deliberate experiments, often involving the injection of free fluid into the thorax of a cadaver, he built up enough knowledge to enable him to develop his system of thoracentesis and, of course, produce the now famous *Inventum novum . . .* of 1761.

Although this was the first monograph on the clinical use of percussion anywhere in the world it had little effect. A French translation by Rozière de la Chassagne in 1770 passed virtually unnoticed. Auenbrugger lived until, in 1808, 47 years after his book first appeared and nearly 40 years after the forgotten translation, Jean Nicolas Corvisart (1755–1821), the favourite physician of Napoleon, prepared a now-classical translation into French. It was this translation and Corvisart's generous recognition of the value of the technique which led to percussion becoming a universally adopted procedure. There is an English translation of 1824 reproduced in 1936 and 1941 – but there is no physician throughout the world who does not use Auenbrugger's informative eighteenth century technique.

Corvisart was one of the French masters of medicine. His greatest individual contribution was made at the beginning of the nineteenth century when he published his *Essai sur les maladies et les lésions organiques du coeur et des gros vaisseaux* [1027] in Paris in 1806. This work made clear the differentiation of cardiac and pulmonary conditions and formed the basis for many recent developments in both of these fields. There is an English translation of 1812 which shows Corvisart's recognition of cardiac failure as a mechanical event; the work gives this author's description of effort dyspnoea and provides one of the corner-stones of contemporary medicine.

Auenbrugger discovered percussion by applying an everyday observation to science. A somewhat similar application of a commonplace observation led Edward Jenner (1749–1823) to the discovery of vaccination – thereby making a huge contribution to the worldwide eradication of smallpox.

The sudden disappearance of bubonic plague left smallpox, already well established in the community, to become the most dreaded of diseases. Bubonic plague disappeared two-thirds of the way through the seventeenth century – smallpox then became more and more notable, its incidence presumably fostered by the close personal contacts of the expanding population. Virulent smallpox seems to have been noticed in Europe during the sixteenth century, perhaps imported along the expanding trade routes to the East. In its virulent form,

Variola major, it became fairly common in England by the time of James I and VI and then existed, frequently as a disease of adolescents and young adults, alongside the childhood disease, *Variola minor* or alastrim. We have already noted the increase in the incidence of smallpox and the severe epidemics of the late seventeenth century – the epidemic of smallpox in London in 1694 (page 284) being made memorable by the death of the Queen from the haemorrhagic form of the disease.

At the beginning of the eighteenth century the age incidence of smallpox seems to have changed. Coincident with London reaching what may well have been its peak of overcrowding, smallpox became the most common lethal disease of young children. There were severe epidemics in London in 1710 (3138 deaths), 1714 (2810 deaths), and 1719 (3229 deaths) – the comparable number of deaths from all causes in London being 25 to 28 000 in each of those years.

Little was done, or could be done, to relieve the overcrowding and the overall mortality remained so high that the population of the city was kept up only by recruitment from rural areas. The same situation existed in many of the cities of Britain. This increased incidence of the disease threatened the rich and poor together – the most privileged often being exposed to the infections of their servants. This led, in 1746, to the establishment of the first smallpox hospital – a centre in which those who carried 'subscribers' letters' could be treated (and in a way that reduced the risk to the subscribers). It seems likely that, at this stage, alastrim had almost died out, to be replaced by epidemics, of greater or lesser severity, of *Variola major*.

The idea that exposure to mild forms of a disease might protect against a lethal or near-lethal episode of the same illness was by no means new. From ancient times, in China and elsewhere, it formed the basis for deliberate inoculation to protect against virulent smallpox. The first report of this practice that came to notice in England was *An account, or history, of the procuring of the smallpox by incision or inoculation, as it has for some time been practised at Constantinople*[1028]. This was a letter, addressed by Emmanuel Timoni (d. 1718) to John Woodward and printed, under this title, in the *Philosophical Transactions* of 1714–16. The letter had been addressed to Woodward, Gresham Professor of Physic, by Timoni, who is known to have been in England in 1703 and who had been incorporated at Oxford in his doctorate degree on the basis of his Paduan qualification.

The communication in the *Philosophical Transactions* aroused the interest of Sir Hans Sloane (1660–1753) who obtained further information from another Greek physician, Giacomo Pylarini (1659–1718). In 1701 this physician had inoculated three children at Constantinople with smallpox virus, reporting his findings, again in the *Philosophical Transactions*, in a paper (*Nova et tuta variolas excitandi per transplantationem methodus; nuper inventa et in usum tracta*[1029]) of 1715. It is this work which establishes Pylarini's claim to his having been the first professional immunologist and which is the source of the first record, of a technical type, of variolation.

The non-technical records are lost in antiquity: it is said that the Chinese prevented smallpox by sniffing small desquamated crusts from mild cases of the disease.

Apart from the formal communications, an alternative means of news of the inoculation procedure reaching London was provided by Lady Mary Montagu (1689–1762), wife of the British Ambassador in Constantinople. Lady Montagu had her 3-year-old son inoculated in 1718 in Turkey and, on returning to England, had her 5-year-old daughter inoculated in 1721 in London in the presence of several physicians.

Whether the interest of Dr Woodward and Sir Hans Sloane, or the communications of Timoni and Pilarini in the *Philosophical Transactions*, or the social efforts of Lady Montagu were of greatest effect in spreading the popularity of inoculation has been much debated. Lady Montagu's intimates included the Princess of Wales who, for the sake of her own children, prevailed on George I to remit the capital sentences on six felons in Newgate Prison. These six were inoculated with smallpox matter in August, 1721, insertions of the material being made into both arms and the right leg of each. All six survived and showed only minimal eruptions. The same happened with a seventh convict, a young woman under sentence of death, in whom a pledget of cotton containing smallpox pus was inserted in the nose in imitation of the technique reputed to be used by the Chinese.

The practice of variolation – inoculation with matter from a very mild case of smallpox – became uncommon in Europe after 1728 but Garrison[1030] reports that in the Boston epidemic of 1752 some 2109 people were inoculated; nearly 20 000 received similar treatment in England in 1764–65 after the mid-century revival of the procedure. Inoculation was common during the American Revolution and, as a preventive measure, became so common in Britain that it was undertaken by 'inoculators', many of whom were not medically qualified. These inoculators used pustule material from the mildest cases available and re-used it from the mildest lesions produced; this technique, of 'removes', and the use of a very slight superficial scratch as an inoculation site, aimed at limiting the severity of the resulting infection.

Despite these precautions it was gradually recognized that inoculation produced a small incidence of severe, even lethal, smallpox – and these cases sometimes transmitted the virulent form of the disease. The difficulties could not be prevented by isolation or providing facilities where the poor could be inoculated. Such facilities included the London Smallpox and Inoculation Hospital (1746) and, when the limitations of establishments of this kind were realized, the whole method – widely prevalent in the second half of the eighteenth century – was gradually discontinued.

There is no known measure of its usefulness. That it failed to give certain and complete protection and that doubts about its safety persisted is clear. Even so, Cartwright[1031] quotes the poor-house account books of a Somerset village as showing payments to inoculators in 1798 – thus, at least in country areas, the method was still thought worthy of the restricted funds available in these institutions at that time. One estimate of its effect has been given by Peter E. Razzell in *Population in Industrialization*[1032], who suggests that the practice of variolation in the second half of the eighteenth century, when it was much used, diminished the mortality from smallpox to a degree which made it a significant factor in the massive rise of the population. The fact remains that the method could transmit full-blown smallpox and its decline – it was made illegal in 1840 – may have been largely for this reason. The greater factor is likely to have been the

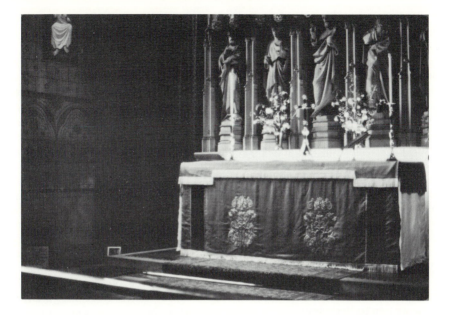

Figure 108   The chancel, containing the Jenner tomb, Berkeley Church, Gloucestershire.

growth in popularity of the far safer and surer technique of smallpox vaccination
developed by Jenner.

Edward Jenner (1749–1823) was the son of a family Dorothy Fisk has
described as comprising 'country gentlemen, parsons, farmers, doctors – well-
connected, well-respected and well-loved even before one of their number made
their name world-renowned' [1033]. His father was the Rev Stephen Jenner, rector of
Rockhampton and vicar of Berkeley in Gloucestershire. The parish church, with
its beautiful chancel and nave, has behind it a history of a Berkeley abbot and
abbey going back to the mid-eighth century. The church (the chancel, containing
the Jenner tomb, forms Figure 108) stands alongside the castle of Berkeley in
which, in 1327, Edward II was murdered at the instigation of his wife; the body
was later buried in Gloucester Cathedral.

Jenner's father died when he was 5; he was then cared for by an elder brother,
Stephen, and an aunt and sent to school locally before, at the age of 14, being
apprenticed to Daniel Ludlow, a surgeon in the small town of Sodbury, near
Bristol, at the head of the vale of Berkeley. It seems that while he was Ludlow's
apprentice Jenner was told by a young countrywoman that her rash could not be
smallpox because she had already had cowpox.

It is clear that there was some sort of West Country tradition that contact with
cows, or previous cowpox, protected against smallpox; part of this tradition was
that milkmaids formed one of the small group of young women then not
blemished by the healed pocks of the disease. Why some variant of this piece of
folklore should have stayed in Jenner's mind is not explained – but, on the farms
around him, if it was more than a myth, Jenner could have noticed its observable

consequence. At all events, Jenner, having learnt what he could with Ludlow, showed sufficient promise to become a student at St. George's Hospital and, in 1770, a house-pupil of the renowned John Hunter.

Jenner was at this time 21. Hunter was 42 and the owner of a menagerie at Brompton. This facility provided part of the means for Hunter's comparative anatomy; it was also an interest which Jenner, already an experienced field naturalist, readily shared. In 1771, while Jenner was still with Hunter, Captain Cook returned from the successful southern voyage during which he had surveyed the length of the east coast of Australia. Joseph Banks (1743–1820), afterwards President of the Royal Society, had furnished Cook's expedition – he now returned with a mass of natural history and botanical material, much of it collected at what was later named Botany Bay, 13 miles south of Sydney. Jenner's reputation was already such that he was asked to prepare Banks' specimens and he did this with such skill that he was offered a place as naturalist on Cook's next expedition. This was due to sail in 1772 but Jenner declined not only this offer but also a proposed partnership with Hunter. The reasons for this, perhaps striking, pair of decisions, and for Jenner's wish to return to Berkeley, have been discussed by Drewitt in his *The Life of Jenner* (1931)[1034].

Jenner and Hunter remained lifelong friends and wrote regularly to each other until Hunter's sudden death in 1793. Jenner's letters to Hunter are lost; those written to Berkeley form an important part of the priceless collection of the Royal College of Surgeons.

It is a mistake to think of Jenner as a country practitioner who made, largely by luck, one important discovery: he was, in fact, a well-trained and experienced practitioner, with a background of substance, who had mixed with and worked with several of the leading medical and scientific figures of the day. His clinical acumen was such that he gave one of the earliest papers on rheumatic illnesses as a cause of cardiac disease. David Pitcairn is usually credited with having first suggested this causal relationship in a lecture given in 1788 but Jenner read a paper on it the following year. The first published clinical report was that of Charles William Wells (1757–1817) – a communication *On rheumatism of the heart*[1035] printed in 1812.

Jenner's discovery of vaccination reflected his experience and experimental approach to natural history. He is remembered for his closely observed description of the special anatomical adaptation of the recently-hatched cuckoo which enables it to eject the eggs or young of its foster-parents from the nest. These observations, part of the long correspondence with Hunter, were included in a paper in the *Philosophical Transactions* (1788) for which Jenner was elected to the Fellowship in 1789. His remarkable observations on this subject were later confirmed by means of photography.

Thus, it was a person of some distinction who set out to investigate the story that cowpox, or some such factor, might protect against smallpox.

On May 14th, 1796 Jenner deliberately vaccinated a boy, James Phipps, with matter from a typical cowpox lesion on the hand of a dairymaid, Sarah Nelmes. There was a transient local lesion, like that following inoculation (variolation) but this rapidly healed. On 1st July, some 6 weeks later, Jenner inoculated the boy with matter from a suitable smallpox lesion. The ethics of this might now cause comment – if it is not realized that such variolation was then an everyday event. In

James Phipps the result was quite unusual: there was no local lesion and the 'vaccination' with vaccinia (cowpox) lymph seemed to have protected against the subsequent inoculation (variolation) with smallpox material.

The piece of folklore concerned had probably been explored before. Creighton[1036], whose later attack on Jenner and vaccination now seems to have blighted an assiduous career, in *A history of epidemics in Britain* of 1891, gives an account of a 'farmer at Yetminster, Dorset, named Benjamin Jesty,' who 'had used matter from that source for the inoculation of his wife and two young children in 1774, with the result that the arm of the former was much inflamed and had to be treated by a surgeon.' Creighton's 'that source' is what he describes as 'a pox bearing the name of a brute animal, which was, however, a true affection of brutes – the cowpox or pap-pox'. Creighton had a nineteenth century anthropomorphic view of giving man cowpox.

At a time when, in London, very few wanted to be vaccinated by means of the cowpox material, Jenner left some of the dried lymph with the surgeon Henry Cline. This material was used by Cline to vaccinate a boy who, in St. Thomas's Hospital, was suffering from hip disease: it was thought that vaccination, performed over the hip, might help by providing effective counter-irritation. When it was found that the boy showed subsequent resistance to smallpox inoculation, Cline and his associates became protagonists of Jenner's procedure.

Jenner, promised £10 000 a year to take a house in Grosvenor Square, delayed – hoping to find time to care for his sick wife, then in Cheltenham. He was troubled also by the fleeting and infrequent nature of cowpox and the resulting shortage of lymph. Confusion also arose because William Woodville (1752–1805) of the London Smallpox and Inoculation Hospital, and George Pearson (1751–1828) of St. George's, became enthusiasts – but their energies led to a second strain of the vaccine, originating with Woodville and the Smallpox Hospital, becoming widely distributed. It may be this strain which became most widely used during the greater part of the nineteenth century. The strain was supposed to have come from a dairy herd at Gray's Inn Lane in 1799 – Woodville having found two infected animals amongst this herd – but he vaccinated subjects at the Smallpox Hospital and then, as Cartwright relates[1037], 'inoculated all seven with matter from a smallpox pustule, three of them after an interval of only five days'. Woodville treated large numbers of patients, possibly giving most of them the smallpox inoculation strain, and certainly getting some severe reactions and adverse results. More importantly, in a way, he possibly contaminated the so-called cowpox vaccination lymph with attenuated or scarcely modified smallpox.

Jenner's *An inquiry into the causes and effects of the variolae vaccinae* ... (1798)[1038] had been far more straightforward: it described 23 successful vaccinations – thereby announcing a technique which was rapidly to become far more popular than the old method of variolation. Woodville had muddled the situation and, as the practical benefits of vaccination became clear in one location after another – a single, simple example is provided by Sir William Osler's chart of the effects of vaccination on smallpox mortality in the German Empire (1816–1910), Figure 109 – much official action and standardization of the vaccine and vaccination procedure was required.

In 1781, in Philadelphia, Benjamin Rush had written *The new method in inoculating for the small pox*[1039] – but he was unaware of Jenner's 'Inquiry' which

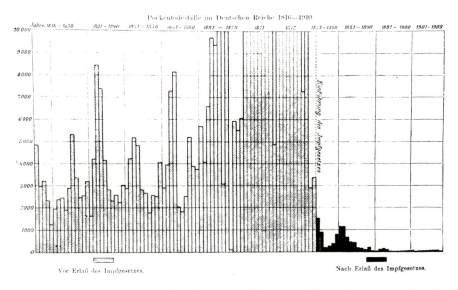

Figure 109 The effect of vaccination on smallpox mortality in the German Empire, 1816–1910. [*From: William Osler. The evolution of modern medicine... New Haven, Yale Univ. Press (1921).*]

was to come in 1798. Jenner's book incidentally gave what is probably the first account of anaphylaxis; it has been reissued, in facsimile, in 1923, 1949, 1966 and 1978. It announced a practice which was introduced into America by Benjamin Waterhouse (1754–1846) – the author of *A prospect of exterminating the smallpox* (1800–02)[1040].

In Britain, Jenner helped to establish a National Vaccine Establishment. Glycerinated calf lymph was eventually introduced to prolong the life of the vaccine and lessen the risks of transmitting syphilis or other extraneous infection. Despite opposition and convinced philosophical objections, the epidemic of 1837–40 (with 16000 smallpox deaths in 1838) awoke the public conscience, leading to the 1840 banning of variolation and the 1853 Act making the vaccination of infants compulsory. The massive epidemic of 1870, with 44079 deaths in England gave teeth to the earlier legislation. This experience was contemporaneous with the Franco-Prussian War and this showed that the French, amongst whom vaccination was not compulsory, fared far worse than the Germans, who had vaccination by edict. Gradually, the weight of experience showed that local outbreaks of smallpox could be contained by vaccination of the susceptible – and slowly, throughout the world, smallpox became a rare, exotic cause of death in highly-vaccinated communities. In 1980, the World Health Organization was able to announce, 184 years after Jenner's original experiments, that 'smallpox is dead'.

From Edward Jenner's studies the science of immunology has since emerged – but it is doubtful if the work of any one man has provided a greater benefaction. Its relic in Berkeley is the small building (Figure 110) in which, in Chantry Garden, Jenner used to vaccinate the poor of the community.

344

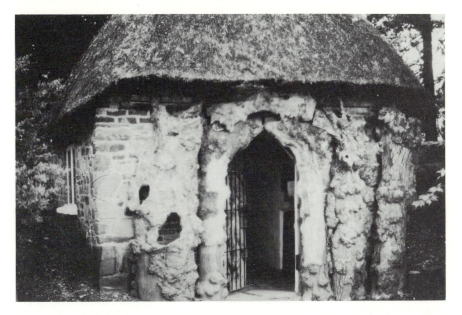

Figure 110   The building in Chantry Garden, Berkeley, used by Jenner for smallpox vaccination.

Despite the level of achievement, the nature of the vaccine itself remains unclear. The early workers had to consider only smallpox and the animal poxes they knew: these were cowpox and horsepox, which Jenner called 'grease'. Modern studies show that different strains of vaccine differ in virological detail fron one another and from both cowpox and smallpox. Horsepox is now extinct and smallpox is confined to a very few highly selected laboratories. The nature of vaccinia virus – the virus of the lymph used for clinical vaccination – and the enigma of the origin of this material has been reviewed by a number of workers, perhaps most interestingly by Derrick Baxby in his paper *Edward Jenner, William Woodville, and the origins of vaccinia virus* (1979)[1041] and his later *Jenner's smallpox vaccine – the riddle of vaccinia virus and its origin* (1981)[1042]. The subject is complex but the possibilities include cowpox, cowpox modified by passage, attenuated smallpox, a hybrid, a derivative of grease affecting cows, or even that vaccinia – the virus of the conventional clinical vaccine – was present from the beginning. It is an unsatisfying fact that we cannot be sure of the nature of the vaccine used to deal with this dreadful disease – and that, for this reason, we cannot be sure of the theoretical reason for the benign effect.

In America, John Redman Coxe became the first to practise the new technique in Philadelphia; he was also instrumental in eliminating some of the prejudice against vaccination. In this cause his *Practical observations on vaccination: or inoculation for the cow pock* (1802)[1043] was of marked effect.

Jenner's experiments were highly rational and the story of the early spread of vaccination and his efforts to secure a constant technique has been frequently recounted. The ultimate significance of his studies and findings, although confounded by our lack of knowledge of the changing natural history of smallpox, is that Garrison[1044] wrote of 'one of the greatest triumphs in the history of medicine'. That Jenner's work led to the first global effort to eradicate a lethal human disease, and that this effort united peoples and caused them to accept appropriate legislation, is itself a milestone.

Jenner must be credited with having explored a piece of folklore which had an observational basis; he showed that vaccination could be transmitted from person to person and that there was a practicable means of doing so. That his method could contain outbreaks of smallpox is open to no reasonable dispute. Even allowing for the possibilities that smallpox was entering on a benign phase of its natural history, or that its progress had been affected by variolation, or that social conditions and the general well-being of the community were much improved – or for all of these things affecting the outcome in more privileged countries – few would dispute that, on a global scale, the general effectiveness of vaccination has been amply proved. It is perhaps a cause for some satisfaction that, unlike plague, the vanquishing of smallpox can be credited to human intervention.

William Withering

Much of the eighteenth century increase in knowledge of the pharmacology of plant substances was provided by the old Vienna school of medicine which arose under Gerhard van Swieten (1700–1772) of Leyden. In medical terms this great school reflected the ascendancy of the Austrian Empire of Maria Theresa (1717–1780) and her eldest son, Joseph II (1741–1790) – the Holy Roman Emperor whose life, like that of many of his subjects, showed the effects of the ravages of smallpox: the Emperor's notably happy union with the Bourbon Princess Isabella of Parma was ended by Isabella's death from smallpox in 1763; his less happy second marriage to Maria Josepha of Bavaria ended when she too died of the disease in 1767.

Gerhard van Swieten had been a pupil of Boerhaave and he carried the latter's clinical methods of teaching to Vienna where they became the foundation of the Vienna school of medicine. He spent a great section of his life in preparing the fine *Commentaria in Hermanni Boerhaave aphorismos, de cognoscendis et curandis morbis*[1045], the six volume work of 1742–76 which forms his memorial; there is an excellent 18 volume translation into English of 1771–76. The volume of the *Commentaria . . .* for 1764 contains an essay on *Podagra*[1046] which is one of the early major contributions to the literature on this condition and did much to increase interest in it. The dissertation[1047] on the gout and related diseases, written by William Cadogan (1711–1797) in England, followed in 1771 and caused additional interest; this, in turn, was followed by the first usefully accurate description of rheumatoid arthritis – a description provided in a work[1048] published in Paris in 1800 by Augustin Jacob Landré-Beauvais (1772–1840).

The Vienna school included Anton de Haen (1704–1776) of The Hague who wrote the *Ratio medendi*[1049] of 1759; de Haen was a believer in witchcraft whose mid-eighteenth century study of hospital therapeutics in 15 volumes is well remembered, as is his record (*De cranii ustione*, in his book of 1759) of amenorrhoea occurring in connection with a pituitary tumour. This was one of the earlier specific observations of endocrinology and dates from a generation before the work of Anton Stoerck (1731–1803) of Swabia. Stoerck, one of the great figures of the Vienna school, undertook careful pharmacological and toxicological studies on plant substances, including hemlock (1760–1); stramonium, hyoscyamus, and aconite (1762); colchicum (1763) and pulsatilla (1777). These studies allowed far more rational recommendations than had been previously available for the use of the plant drugs; they also antedate the isolation of the active plant principles and alkaloids a century or so later.

Most notable of all of those who dealt with the medicinal plants was William Withering (1741–1799) – a man whose reputation has been vastly enhanced by modern advances in clinical pharmacology: Withering can now be seen not just as the discoverer of the safe and effective means of using digitalis, still one of the most essential of medicines, but also as a pioneer in demanding drug standardization as a basis for effective control of dosage; dose-titration when the therapeutic ratio of a drug is narrow, and the study of dose–response relationships. In each of these respects, and in the effort to use the minimum effective dose individualized in order to secure the best benefit-to-risk ratio for the particular patient, Withering's increasing understanding of the drug he had discovered serves as a model for today's therapeutics. Thus, those who wrote 50 years ago, before the present range of potent but often toxic drugs were discovered, and before modern principles of pharmacology were extensively applied to medicine, saw Withering as one of the finest of medical botanists and as the source of the clinical use of digitalis. Today we might see him as something more – as one who established principles extending far beyond the one important drug he discovered.

Withering was born in 1741 at Wellington, Shropshire, about 70 miles from Berkeley where Jenner was born 8 years later. His father, Edmund Withering, was an apothecary in Wellington and his mother's brother was a physician at nearby Lichfield. He was educated at home but in 1762 entered the University of Edinburgh; he received his MD in 1766. His friends at Edinburgh included Fowler, who later played a main part in the introduction of arsenic into British therapeutics. His teachers at Edinburgh included Whytt in medicine; Munro *secundus* in anatomy (he was at Edinburgh when his tutor discovered the foramen of Munro in 1764), and Cullen who went to Edinburgh as Professor of Chemistry in 1755 and who lectured on the materia medica in 1760–61. Cullen's teaching and example were of profound and useful influence on Withering.

His graduation thesis was on *De angina gangrenosa* and its acceptance was followed by visits to London and Oxford and a tour of France and Paris. He returned to England at the end of 1766 and began to practise in the small town of Stafford the following year. Here, with only a small practice, he began to study botany, his interest arising from opportunities to provide specimens for the water-colour drawings of a patient, Helena Cook, who later became his wife.

In matters of science he seems to have been more than ordinarily perceptive from the beginning. Holmstedt and Liljestrand[1050] quote his paper of 1779 (*An account of the scarlet fever and sore throat, or scarlatina anginosa; particularly as it appeared at Birmingham in the year 1778*)[1051] as containing what they rightly call 'this remarkable statement':

But whether the disease is caused by animalcula capable of generating their kind, or by certain miasmata which have their own nature, by some mode of fermentation hitherto but little understood, there can be no doubt but it is contagious, and perhaps so in a degree nearly equal to the small-pox and measles.

Withering, after his marriage, moved (in 1775) to Birmingham. There he was able to find a larger practice and associate with Dr John Ash of the General Hospital. Soon after his move he published his first book: *A botanical arrangement of all the vegetables naturally growing in Great Britain with descriptions of the genera and species according to Linnaeus*[1052]; this work, of 1776, established his reputation as a botanist and it is worth remembering that Withering was one of the finest specialists, in this subject, of his century. He was also knowledgeable regarding minerals and there are two eponyms: *Witherite* is natural barium carbonate, a mineral discovered by Withering and named in his honour by the German geologist, Werner, in 1790; and the *Witheringia*, a genus of plants, the name having been given, again in honour of Withering, by the French botanist, L'Heritier de Brutelle. Withering's botany extended far beyond the materia medica and the medical aspects of the subject. This can be seen from Figure 111 – the plate from the section on the *Introduction to the study of botany* in the fourth (four volume) edition of Withering's book, this edition having been corrected and enlarged by William Withering, his son, and published in 1801. The plate illustrates part of the botanical classification of the time and, incidentally, the systematic approach which he brought to descriptive botany.

Withering's home became a meeting-place for scientists and colleagues and in the year of his textbook he joined the Lunar Society of Birmingham. Amongst its members this Society included James Watt, Josiah Wedgewood, Erasmus Darwin and Joseph Priestley. At the age of 42, in 1783, he had to abandon his practice due to the onset of pulmonary tuberculosis (a condition that, far in advance of the views of the day, he considered infectious). He spent much of his time writing and within 2 years had recovered. By 1785, the year of the publication of the book which was to make his name famous, he was travelling widely – over 6000 miles a year by horseback and carriage – in support of a consultant practice that spread across large areas of central and western England and the adjacent parts of Wales. His home at this date was Edgbaston Hall; he was elected to the Fellowship of the Royal Society and honoured with the diploma of the Medical Society of London before, in 1790, being elected a Fellow of the Linnaean Society.

His health again deteriorated so that he spent the winter of 1792 in Portugal attempting to recover from a serious episode of pleurisy sustained the previous year. In 1796, aged 55, he retired from practice and on October 6th, 1799, died of pulmonary tuberculosis; he is buried at Edgbaston Church where there is a monument inscribed with his name and encircled with the Witheringia, which he had described, and with a carving of the purple foxglove on which he had written.

Withering's remarkable book, one of the classics of pharmacology, is *An account of the foxglove, and some of its medical uses: with practical remarks on dropsy, and other diseases*[1053]; it was published in Birmingham in 1785, almost exactly 200 years ago. A version (not totally accurate) appeared in *Medical Classics*[1054] in December, 1937 and there is a facsimile reprint of 1949.

It is clear that there was some sort of West Country tradition regarding the use

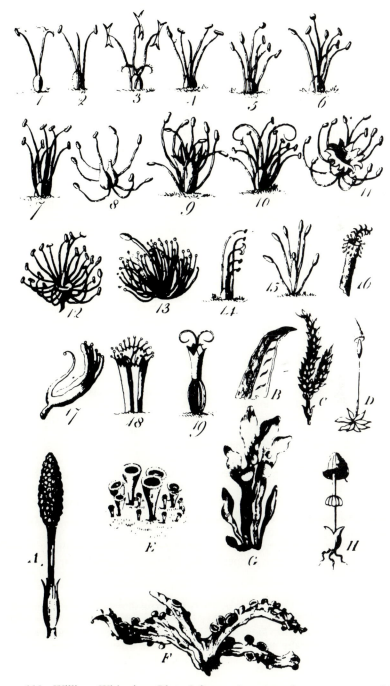

Figure 111 William Withering. Plate I from: *A systematic arrangement of British plants . . . by William Withering* (1801).

of herbs, particularly foxglove, in the treatment of dropsy. The plant had been mentioned as a possible remedy for a number of conditions in earlier writings. Most plants have been written of in this way by scores of authors and given an impressive list of curative properties. The foxglove was no exception, but it would seem that what may have attracted Withering to this piece of folklore was its observational basis, and perhaps a specific episode. The situation is remarkably similar to the experience of Jenner, who was also able to pick out from the mass of 'old wives' tales' a piece of tradition worth investigating. Withering made his discovery during his early years in practice at Stafford and, talking of the means of investigating animal and vegetable substances, gave this account of the beginnings of his study [1055]:

> we have hitherto made only a very small progress in the chemistry of animal and vegetable substances. Their virtues must therefore be learnt, either from observing their effects upon insects and quadrupeds; from analogy, deduced from the already known powers of some of their congenera, or from the empirical usages and experience of the populace.
>
> The first method has not yet been much attended to; and the second can only be perfected in proportion as we approach towards the discovery of a truly natural system; but the last, as far as it extends, lies within the reach of every one who is open to information, regardless of the source from whence it springs.
>
> It was a circumstance of this kind which first fixed my attention on the Foxglove.
>
> In the year 1775, my opinion was asked concerning a family receipt for the cure of the dropsy. I was told that it had long been kept a secret by an old woman in Shropshire, who had sometimes made cures after the more regular practitioners had failed. I was informed also, that the effects produced were violent vomiting and purging; for the diuretic effects seemed to have been over-looked. This medicine was composed of twenty or more different herbs; but it was not very difficult for one conversant in these subjects, to perceive, that the active herb could be no other than the Foxglove.

The methods Withering describes for the detection of new active pharmacological substances are interesting: the choices, as he sees them, are pharmacological tests in insects and quadrupeds, comparison with the known activities of congenera (for which, he recognizes, knowledge is inadequate), or from such sources as the wisdom of folklore.

His early experience demonstrated that the drug had a previously unrecognized and important diuretic property but, falsely reasoning from the squill, he got the dose wrong [1056]:

> I soon found the Foxglove to be a very powerful diuretic; but then, and for a considerable time afterwards, I gave it in doses very much too large, and urged its continuance too long; for misled by reasoning from the effects of the squill, which generally acts best upon the kidneys when it excites nausea, I wished to produce the same effect by the Foxglove.

The attempt to standardize the condition of the plant to produce a measured dose from an adequately reliable formulation is described in the following passage[1057] (the spelling modernized, as in these other quotations of the original text):

> (I . . .) was too well aware of the uncertainty which must attend on the exhibition of the *root* of a biennial plant, and therefore continued to use the *leaves*. These I had found to vary much as to dose, at different seasons of the year; but I expected, if gathered always in one condition of the plant, viz. when it was in its flowering state, and carefully dried, that the dose might be ascertained as exactly as that of any other medicine; nor have I been dis-appointed in this expectation. The more I saw of the great powers of this plant, the more it seemed necessary to bring the doses of it to the greatest possible accuracy. I suspected that this degree of accuracy was not reconcileable with the use of a *decoction*, as it depended not only upon the care of those who had the preparation of it, but it was easy to conceive from the analogy of another plant of the same natural order, the tobacco, that its active properties might be impaired by long boiling. The decoction was therefore discarded, and the *infusion* substituted in its place. After this I began to use the leaves in *powder*, but I still very often prescribe the infusion.

Withering had, at this stage, learnt that 'the diuretic effects of this medicine do not at all depend upon its exciting a nausea or vomiting . . .'[1058] These effects (previously thought to be the main properties of the remedy) were now seen to be adverse effects which are 'far from being friendly or necessary . . .'[1059].

In February, 1779 a colleague communicated to the Medical Society at Edinburgh the results of Withering's studies of the foxglove. Not only in Edinburgh but also elsewhere the drug began to be used – not always carefully, and sometimes with the kind of results which would bring it into disrepute; efforts intended to avoid this misfortune occupied Withering and provided the main reason for the 1785 publication of his book. The foxglove was included in the 1783 edition of the Edinburgh Pharmacopoeia, this appearance preceding Withering's publication by some 2 years. The drug was then taken up by many doctors and became widely used – such use being guided by the notably objective case reports forming the bulk of Withering's book (and reporting successes and failures equally).

Withering's Case IV, of which he gives the following account[1060], provides both a record of his early use of digitalis and an interesting illustration of medicine, at what is likely to have been its best, late in the eighteenth century:

> *July* 25th. Mrs. H—, of A—, near N—, between forty and fifty years of age, a few weeks ago, after some previous indisposition, was attacked by a severe cold shivering fit, succeeded by fever; great pain in her left side, short-ness of breath, perpetual cough, and, after some days, copious expectoration. On the 4th of *June*, Dr. Darwin, was called to her. I have not heard what was then done for her, but between the 15th of *June*, and 25th of *July*, the Doctor, at his different visits, gave her various medicines of the deobstruent, tonic, anti-spasmodic, diuretic, and evacuant kinds.
>
> On the 25th of *July* I was desired to meet Dr. Darwin at the lady's house. I found her nearly in a state of suffocation; her pulse extremely weak and irregular, her breath very short and laborious, her countenance sunk, her arms of a leaden colour, clammy and cold. She could not lye down in bed, and had

neither strength nor appetite, but was extremely thirsty. Her stomach, legs, and thighs were greatly swollen; her urine very small in quantity, not more than a spoonful at a time, and that very seldom. It had been proposed to scarify her legs, but the proposition was not acceded to.

She had experienced no relief from any means that had been used, except from ipecacoanha vomits; the dose of which had been gradually increased from 15 to 40 grains, but such was the insensible state of her stomach for the last few days, that even those very large doses failed to make her sick, and consequently purged her. In this situation of things I knew of nothing likely to avail us, except the Digitalis: but this I hesitated to propose, from an apprehension that little could be expected from anything; that an unfavourable termination would tend to discredit a medicine which promised to be of great benefit to mankind, and I might be censured for a prescription which could not be countenanced by the experience of any other regular practitioner. But these considerations soon gave way to the desire of preserving the life of this valuable woman, and accordingly I proposed the Digitalis to be tried; adding, that I sometimes had found it to succeed when other, even the most judicious methods, had failed. Dr. Darwin very politely, acceded immediately to my proposition and, as he had never seen it given, left the preparation and the dose to my direction. We therefore prescribed as follows:

> R. Fol. Digital. purp. recent. oz. iv. coque ex
>   Aq. fontan. purae lb iss ad lb i. et cola.
> R. Decoct. Digital. oz. iss.
>   Aq. Nuc. Moschat. dr. ii. M. fiat, haust. 2dis horis sumend.

The patient took five of these draughts, which made her very sick, and acted very powerfully upon the kidneys, for within the first twenty-four hours she made upwards of eight quarts of water. The sense of fulness and oppression across her stomach was greatly diminished, her breath was eased, her pulse became more full and more regular, and the swellings of her legs subsided.

26th. Our patient being thus snatched from impending destruction, Dr. Darwin proposed to give her a decoction of pareira brava and guiacum shavings, with pills of myrrh and white vitriol; and, if costive, a pill with calomel and aloes. To these propositions I gave a ready assent.

30th. This day Dr. Darwin saw her, and directed a continuation of the medicines last prescribed.

August 1st. I found the patient perfectly free from every appearance of dropsy, her breath quite easy, her appetite much improved, but still very weak. Having some suspicion of a diseased liver, I directed pills of soap, rhubarb, tartar of vitriol, and calomel to be taken twice a day, with a neutral saline draught.

9th. We visited our patient together, and repeated the draughts directed on the 26th of *June*, with the addition of tincture of bark, and also ordering pills of aloes, guiacum, and sal martis to be taken if costive.

September 10th. From this time the management of the case fell entirely under my direction, and perceiving symptoms of effusion going forwards, I desired that a solution of merc. subl. corr. might be given twice a day.

19th. The increase of the dropsical symptoms now made it necessary to repeat the Digitalis. The dried leaves were used in infusion, and the water was presently evacuated, as before.

It is now almost nine years since the Digitalis was first prescribed for this lady, and notwithstanding I have tried every preventive method I could devise, the dropsy still continues to recur at times; but is never allowed to increase so as to cause much distress, for she occasionally takes the infusion and relieves herself whenever she chooses. Since the first exhibition of that medicine, very small doses have been always found sufficient to promote the flow of urine.

I have been more particular in the narrative of this case, partly because Dr. Darwin has related it rather imperfectly in the notes to his son's posthumous publication, trusting, I imagine, to memory, and partly because it was a case which gave rise to a very general use of the medicine in that part of Shropshire.

Acknowledging that the activity of the different parts of the plant varied and that, within one part, there were seasonal and other variations, Withering gathered the foxglove at one time, the time of its flowering. He made these notes on the drying of the leaves and the doses that he came to regard as typical[1061]:

> If well dried, they readily rub down to a beautiful green powder, which weighs something less than one-fifth of the original weight of the leaves. Care must be taken that the leaves be not scorched in drying, and they should not be dried more than what is requisite to allow of their being readily reduced to powder.
>
> I give to adults, from one to three grains of this powder twice a day. In the reduced state in which physicians generally find dropsical patients, four grains a day are sufficient. I sometimes give the powder alone; sometimes unite it with aromatics, and sometimes form it into pills with a sufficient quantity of soap or gum ammoniac.
>
> If a liquid medicine be preferred, I order a dram of these dried leaves to be infused for four hours in half a pint of boiling water, adding to the strained liquor an ounce of any spirituous water. One ounce of this infusion given twice a day, is a medium dose for an adult patient. If the patient be stronger than usual, or the symptoms very urgent, this dose may be given once in eight hours; and on the contrary in many instances half an ounce at a time will be quite sufficient. About thirty grains of the powder or eight ounces of the infusion, may generally be taken before the nausea commences.

Withering lived before the differentiation of cardiac from renal dropsy but he recognized that the foxglove was ineffective in some forms of oedema. He gives an account of the kinds of patients who seemed to respond and, at the end of his book, in separate paragraphs which are among the most aphoristic of any work on medicine, he lists the side-effects and signs of overdose, the method of securing the optimal dose by dose-titration against the onset of the first adverse effect in the individual patient and, finally, the inferences from his experience:

On overdose[1062]:

> The Foxglove when given in very large and quickly-repeated doses, occasions sickness, vomiting, purging, giddiness, confused vision, objects appearing green or yellow; increased secretion of urine, with frequent motions to part with it, and sometimes inability to retain it; slow pulse, even as slow as 35 in a minute, cold sweats, convulsions, syncope, death.

On dose-titration[1063]:

> (The directions require)... attention to the state of the pulse, and it was moreover of consequence not to repeat the doses too quickly, but to allow sufficient time for the effects of each to take place, as it was found very possible

to pour in an injurious quantity of the medicine, before any of the signals for forbearance appeared.

Let the medicine therefore be given in the doses, and at the intervals mentioned above:—let it be continued until it either acts on the kidneys, the stomach, the pulse, or the bowels; let it be stopped upon the first appearance of any one of these effects, and I will maintain that the patient will not suffer from its exhibition, nor the practitioner be disappointed in any reasonable expectation.

The inferences[1064]:

I. That the Digitalis will not universally act as a diuretic.

II. That it does do so more generally than any other medicine.

III. That it will often produce this effect after every other probable method has been fruitlessly tried.

IV. That if this fails, there is but little chance of any other medicine succeeding.

V. That in proper doses, and under the management now pointed out, it is mild in its operation, and gives less disturbance to the system, than squill, or almost any other active medicine.

VI. That when dropsy is attended by palsy, unsound viscera, great debility, or other complication of disease, neither the Digitalis, nor any other diuretic can do more than obtain a truce to the urgency of the symptoms; unless by gaining time, it may afford opportunity for other medicines to combat and subdue the original disease.

VII. That the Digitalis may be used with advantage in every species of dropsy, except the encysted.

VIII. That it may be made subservient to the cure of diseases, unconnected with dropsy.

IX. That it has a power over the motion of the heart, to a degree yet unobserved in any other medicine, and that this power may be converted to salutary ends.

Several of Withering's digitalis-treated patients may have suffered from auricular fibrillation (Case IV, with an 'irregular' pulse is one of them) but his 'Inference' IX seems to anticipate later knowledge with his comment that the drug 'has a power over the motion of the heart'; his singular use of the word 'converted' (? restored to normal rhythm) is just as striking.

The life of Withering, one of the greatest embellishments of English medicine, has attracted the interest of generations of physicians. Among those who felt special interest was Sir William Osler who, commenting on the paper *William Withering, MD, FRS*[1065] delivered in London in March, 1915, by A. R. Cushney, observed that 'Withering . . . discovered the secret of the use of digitalis; and the indications which he relied upon for its employment did not differ much from those enumerated in the present day.'[1066] Certainly, Withering's remarkable piece of work stood the test of time to Osler's day, and beyond.

Osler's bequest to the Royal Society of Medicine was a volume catalogued as 7637 in his *Bibliotheca Osleriana*[1067]. This collection of Withering's letters, papers and a diploma granted to Withering by the Society of Students of Medicine of Edinburgh, March 31st, 1764, forms the subject of the paper *The Withering*

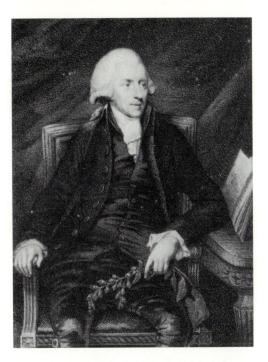

Figure 112 William Withering (1741–1799).

letters in the possession of the Royal Society of Medicine[1068] by Sir William Hale-White and included in the *Proceedings* of the Society for 1928–29. There is also an unpublished *Catalogue of the Withering letters drawn up by W. Hale White in 1928*[1069] and kept with the collection of the 134 letters from and to Withering. The copy of the Withering portrait engraved by W. Bond from the painting by C. F. Breda and included at the front of the collection of letters is reproduced in Figure 112.

The letters of the Osler bequest include one dated August 11th, 1785 and written from London by the scientist Jean Hyacinthe de Magellan (1723–1790) and expressing his profuse thanks to Withering for a copy of his book on the fox-glove. The collection then includes a letter of March 14th, 1786 from B. P. van Lilyveld who writes from The Hague to Magellan giving a long and interesting account of his asthma and asking if Magellan will find out whether Dr Withering thinks the foxglove would be beneficial. This act was performed by Magellan, so bringing about the handwritten essay on 'The spasmodic asthma' by Withering (Figures 113–115) and van Lilyveld's reply, from The Hague, of June 8, 1786 (Figures 116–118). Both of these interesting and previously unpublished letters are reproduced by the generous permission of the Librarian of the Royal Society of Medicine, London.

Withering's advice, in the letter [1069] ascribed by Hale-White to his hand, repays careful study. His suggestion that asthma can be cured by a long sea voyage, a prolonged change of scene, or constant exercise strikes a familiar modern note, as

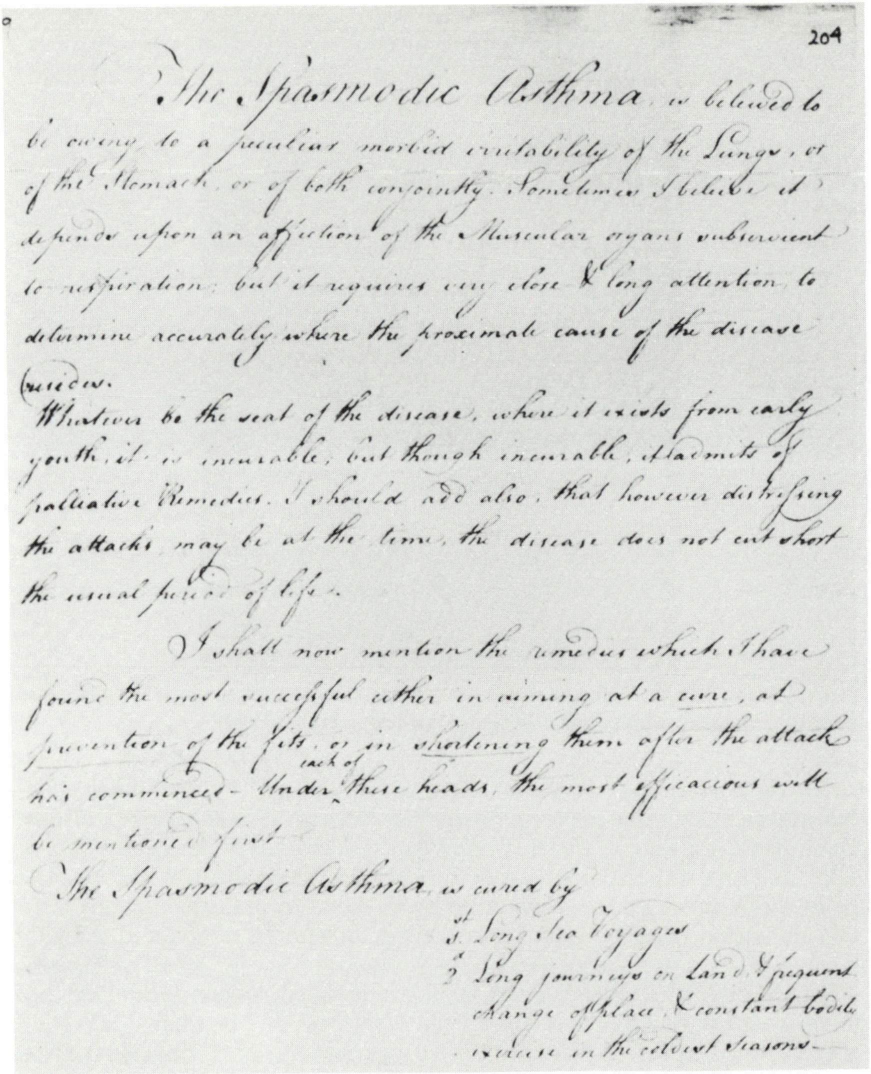

Figure 113 William Withering. 'The spasmodic asthma...' Previously unpublished holograph forming part of the Osler bequest. [*By permission, Librarian, Royal Society of Medicine, London.*]

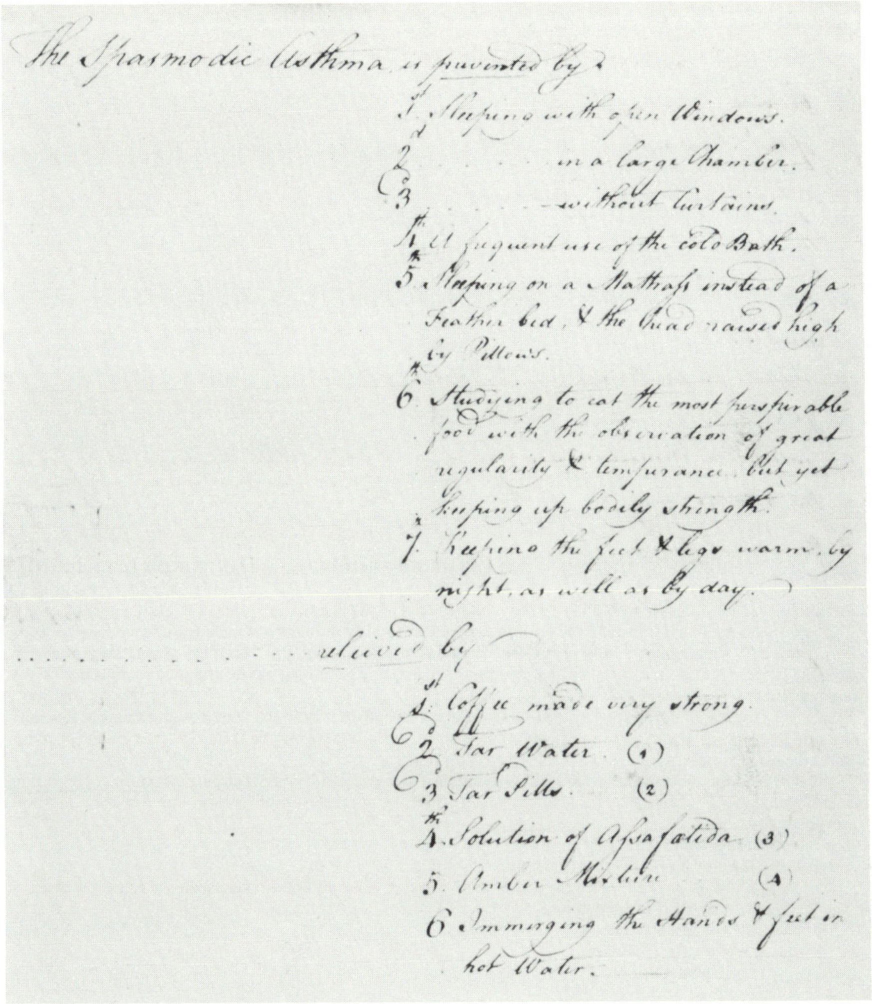

Figure 114   William Withering. 'The spasmodic asthma...' Holograph (continued).

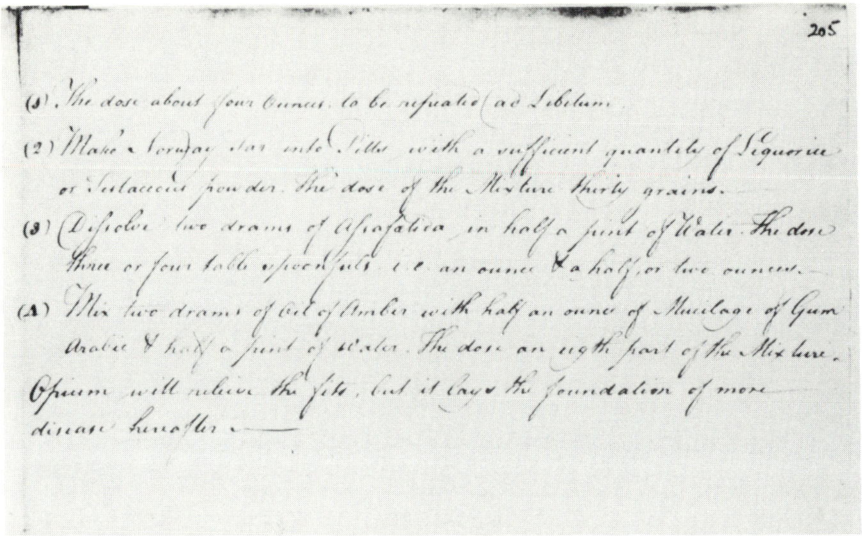
205

(1). The dose about four Ounces to be repeated ad Libitum.

(2) Make a Norway Tar into Pills with a sufficient quantity of Liquorice or Testaceous powder. The dose of the Mixture thirty grains.

(3) Dissolve two drams of Assafoetida in half a pint of Water. The dose three or four table spoonfuls i.e. an ounce & a half, or two ounces.

(4) Mix two drams of Oil of Amber with half an ounce of Mucilage of Gum Arabic & half a pint of Water. The dose an eigth part of the Mixture.

Opium will relieve the fits, but it lays the foundation of more disease hereafter.

Figure 115 William Withering. 'The spasmodic asthma . . .' Holograph (concluded).

Transcript:

The Spasmodic Asthma is believed to be owing to a peculiar morbid irritability of the Lungs, or of the Stomach, or of both conjointly. Sometimes I believe it depends upon an affection of the Muscular organs subservient to respiration; but it requires very close & long attention to determine accurately where the proximate cause of the disease resides.

Whatever be the seat of the disease, where it exists from early youth, it is incurable; but though incurable, it admits of palliative Remedies. I should add also, that however distressing the attacks may be at the time, the disease does not cut short the usual period of life.

I shall now mention the remedies which I have found the most successful either in aiming at a cure, at prevention of the fits, or in shortening them after the attack has commenced – Under each of these heads, the most efficacious will be mentioned first.

The Spasmodic Asthma is cured by

1st. Long Sea Voyages

2d. Long journeys on land, & frequent change of place, & constant bodily exercise in the coldest seasons.

The Spasmodic Asthma is prevented by

1st. Sleeping with open Windows.

2d. .... in a large Chamber.

3d. .... without Curtains.

4th. A frequent use of the cold Bath.

5th. Sleeping on a Mattrass instead of a Feather bed, & the head raised high by Pillows.

6th. Studying to eat the most perspirable food with the observation of great regularity & temperance, but yet keeping up bodily strength.

7th. Keeping the feet & legs warm by night, as well as by day.

....relieved by

1st. Coffee made very strong.

2d. Tar Water. (1)

3d. Tar Pills (2)

4th. Solution of Assafoetida (3)

5. Amber Mixture (4)

6. Immerging the Hands & feet in hot Water.

(1) The dose about four Ounces; to be repeated ad Libitum.

(2) Make a Norway Tar into Pills with a sufficient quantity of Liquorice or Testaceous powder. The dose of the Mixture thirty grains.

(3) Dissolve two drams of Assafoetida in half a pint of Water. The dose three or four table spoonfuls. i.e. an ounce & a half, or two ounces.

(4) Mix two drams of Oil of Amber with half an ounce of Mucilage of Gum Arabic & half a pint of Water. The dose an eigth part of the Mixture.

Opium will relieve the fits, but it lays the foundation of more disease hereafter.

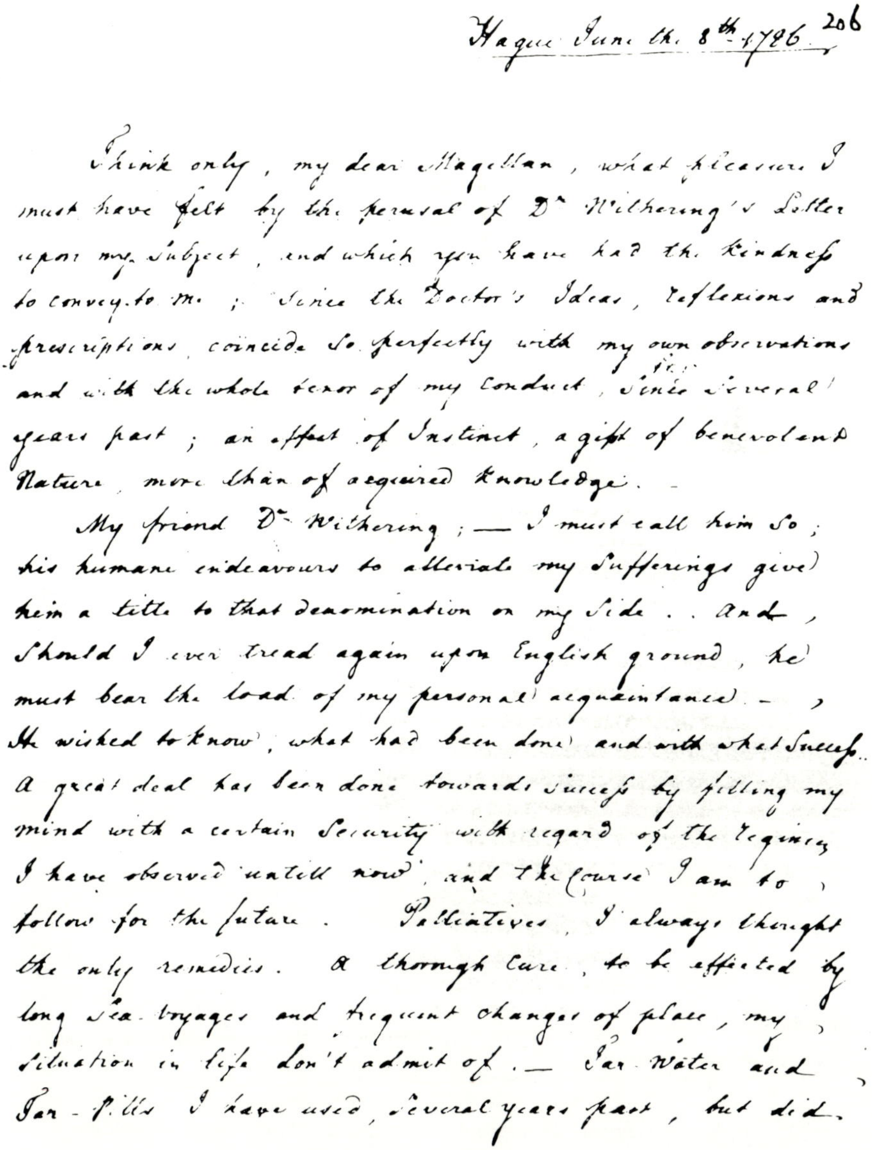

Hague June th. 8th 1786 206

Think only, my dear Magellan, what pleasure I must have felt by the perusal of Dr Withering's Letter upon my Subject, and which you have had th. kindness to convey to me; Since the Doctor's Ideas, reflexions and prescriptions, coincide so perfectly with my own observations and with the whole tenor of my Conduct, Since several years past; an effect of Instinct, a gift of benevolent Nature more than of acquired knowledge.

My friend Dr Withering; — I must call him So; his humane endeavours to alleviate my Sufferings give him a title to that denomination on my Side.. And, should I ever tread again upon English ground, he must bear the load of my personal acquaintance. —, He wished to know, what had been done and with what Success. A great deal has been done towards Success by filling my mind with a certain Security with regard of the regimen I have observed untill now, and the Course I am to follow for the future. Palliatives, I always thought the only remedies. A thorough Cure, to be effected by long Sea voyages and frequent changes of place, my Situation in life don't admit of. — Tar Water and Tar-Pills I have used, several years past, but did.

Figure 116   B. P. van Lilyveld. Holograph letter to Jean Hyacinthe de Magellan, dated June 8th, 1786. [*By permission, Librarian, Royal Society of Medicine, London.*]

not agree with me .. The Coffee still maintains his ground, tho' its virtue is lessening, by having been put to the tryal too often. In vindication however of its qualities, and out of gratitude, I will add, that I am confident, the frequent recurrency of my disorder since a twelvemonth is owing a good deal to the disorder of my nerves, which at present are irritable to a degree—. As soon as the Weather will allow it, I shall take the cold Baths again — they have allways proved friendly to my constitution, but when under the actual influence of the Asthma — I used to take them in the open air, getting out of bed, even in the Severest Colds, and felt the greatest — benefit by them. — Amongst the Doctor's Prescriptions, I don't meet with Chearfulness; Indeed He knew very well, no such thing was Sold in the Apothecary's Shops, and that it is easier to Say, Be wise and merry, than to make any body be So. — I have allways thought myself better, after I had been chearfull, which is not often the Case. — I have often been told by way of Consolation, asthmatic people live long .. Aye, very well ; My great maxim is, Satis diu qui Satis bene . — I could never bring myself to think Seriously of the end of

Figure 117 B. P. van Lilyveld. Holograph letter to Jean Hyacinthe de Magellan, dated June 8th, 1786, (continued).

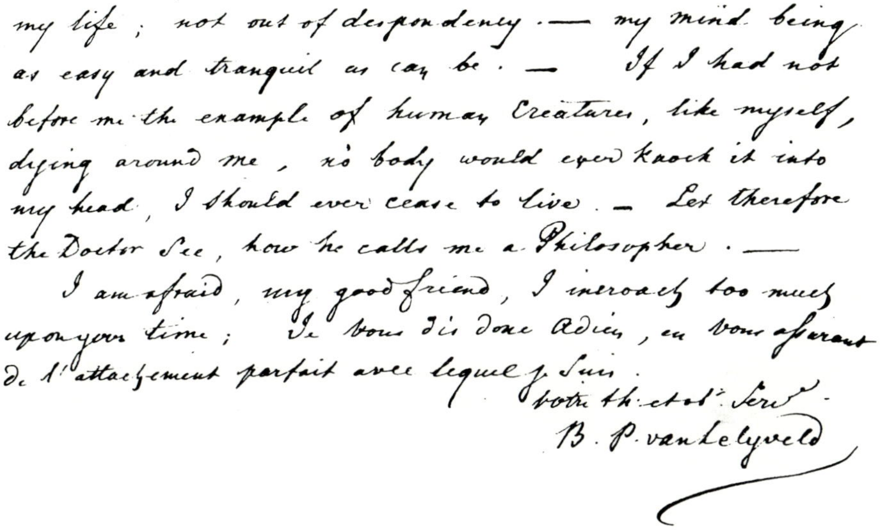

my life; not out of despondency.— my mind being as easy and tranquil as can be.— If I had not before me the example of human Creatures, like myself, dying around me, no body would ever knock it into my head, I should ever cease to live.— Let therefore the Doctor See, how he calls me a Philosopher.—

I am afraid, my good friend, I incroach too much upon your time; Je vous dis donc Adieu, en vous assurant de l'attachement parfait avec lequel j. Suis.

votre th: et obt. Serv.

B. P. van Lelyveld

Figure 118 B. P. Van Lilyveld. Holograph letter to Jean Hyacinthe de Magellan, dated June 8th, 1786, (concluded).

does his advice that episodes of the disease can be prevented by fresh air, open uncluttered windows, avoiding the feather bed, and paying sensible attention to the general bodily well-being. Of his drugs – tar, assafoetida, and amber mixture, the modern pharmacopoeias and sources know next to nothing. It is remarkable that Withering's regime for the management of asthma is so prudent – for it has the merit of being free of the bleedings, purges, vomits, blisterings, cuppings and toxic substances beloved by previous generations of physicians and many of Withering's contemporaries.

Such good sense as Withering had written did not everywhere prevail – and may, in fact, have relatively seldom done so. George Washington (1732-1799) died the same year as Withering. The hero of the American Revolution, chosen in 1788 as first President of the United States of America, is recorded as having awoken one night with fever, laboured breathing and obvious signs of a major respiratory tract infection. He was bled, at his own instigation, during the night and then, in the care of his physicians, blistered upon the throat, given repeated bleedings, given an enema, three doses of calomel (the last of ten grains), administered antimony (as tartar emetic) and subjected to such frantic medical efforts that, despite his being already seriously ill and 67 years of age, he was deprived of a significant part of his circulating blood volume.

The authoritative source-book of the history of medicine in the United States is the two volume work [1070] by Francis Packard (1931). There is also *Amerika und die Medizin* (1933) by Henry Sigerist, the great medical historian who became resident in North America and whose book was published in an English translation (*American Medicine*) [1071] in New York in 1934. Neither Packard nor Sigerist has a great deal to say on the medical treatment given to Washington in his short, terminal illness but his own physicians published a letter (reproduced by Wyndham Blanton in *Medicine in Virginia in the eighteenth century*, 1931) [1072] which gives the following account of these events:

"Messrs. J. and D. Westcott,

"Presuming that some account of the late illness and death of General Washington will be generally interesting, and particularly so to the professors and practitioners of medicine throughout America, we request you to publish the following statement.

James Craik,   Elisha C. Dick."

The statement was as follows:

"Some time in the night of Friday, the 13th inst., having been exposed to rain on the preceding day, General Washington was attacked with an inflammatory affection of the upper part of the windpipe, called in technical language, cynanche trachealis. The disease commenced with a violent ague, accompanied with some pain in the upper and fore part of the throat, a sense of stricture in the same part, a cough, and a difficult rather than painful deglutition, which were soon succeeded by fever and a quick and laborious respiration. The necessity of blood-letting suggesting itself to the General, he procured a bleeder in the neighborhood, who took from the arm in the night, twelve or fourteen ounces of blood; he would not by any means be prevailed upon by the family to send for the attending physician till the following morning, who arrived at Mount Vernon at eleven o'clock on Saturday morning. Discovering the case to be highly alarming, and foreseeing the fatal tendency of the disease, two consulting physicians were immediately sent for, who arrived, one at half past three and the other at four in the afternoon. In the interim were employed two copious bleedings; a blister was applied to the part affected, two moderate doses of calomel were given, an injection was administered which operated on the lower intestines, but all without any perceptible advantage, the respiration becoming still more difficult and distressing. Upon the arrival of the first of the consulting physicians, it was agreed, as there were yet no signs of accumulation in the bronchial vessels of the lungs, to try the result of another bleeding, when about thirty-two ounces were drawn, without the smallest apparent alleviation of the disease. Vapours of vinegar and water were frequently inhaled, ten grains of calomel were given, succeeded by repeated doses of emetic tartar, amounting in all to five or six grains, with no other effect than a copious discharge from the bowels. The powers of life seemed now manifestly yielding to the force of the disorder. Blisters were applied to the extremities, together with a cataplasm of bran and vinegar to the throat. Speaking, which was painful from the beginning, now became almost impracticable, respiration grew more and more contracted and imperfect, till half after eleven o'clock on Saturday night, when, retaining the full possession of his intellect, he expired without a struggle.

"He was fully impressed at the beginning of his complaint as well as through every succeeding stage of it, that its conclusion would be fatal, submitting to the several exertions made for his recovery, rather as a duty than from any expectation of their efficacy. He considered the operation of death upon his system as coeval with the disease; and several hours before his decease, after repeated efforts to be understood, succeeded in expressing a desire that he be permitted to die without interruption.

"During the short period of his illness he economized his time in the arrangement of such few concerns as required his attention, with the utmost serenity, and anticipated his approaching dissolution with every demonstration of that equanimity for which his whole life had been so uniformly and singularly conspicuous."

The statement was signed by "James Craik, Attending Physician," and "Elisha C. Dick, Consulting Physician."

There seem to have been differences between those attending Washington on the wisdom or otherwise of the final substantial venesection – but the hawks carried the day. That, in the few weeks that followed, they may have had second thoughts has frequently been suggested. Blanton P. Seward, for example, in an attractive article on *Pioneer Medicine in Virginia* (1938)[1073] has a paragraph in which he says[1074]:

A notable example is found in George Washington's last illness, when Elisha Cullen Dick, one of the consultants, urged his confreres not to bleed the General again, but they did not heed his advice. Gustavus R. Brown, the other consultant, acknowledged in a letter dated January 2, 1800, to James Craik, the personal physician and intimate friend of Washington, that they were wrong in bleeding him so much.

Today we would have no doubt that Washington's treatment was injurious. It suggests that little real progress had been made in therapeutics, though there are not all that many well-observed and closely documented earlier cases with which comparison can be made. One such case, although it takes us back nearly 200 years before the death of Washington, is the death, probably from typhoid, of Henry Frederick, Prince of Wales (famed as 'The Darling of England'), eldest son of King James and Queen Anne. An excellent account of this particular illness and its treatment is given by Thomas Gibson in a paper *Doctor Theodore Turquet de Mayerne's account of the illness, death and post-mortem examination of the body of His Royal Highness, Prince Henry of Wales*[1075]. The substance of Gibson's paper was his translation from the French version in Browne's '*Opera medica*'; the paper was published in 1938. De Mayerne, who died in 1655, enjoyed an extensive practice at the court of Henry IV in Paris before becoming chief physician at the court of James I and VI in London. Thus, he became the principal medical attendant to the young Prince of Wales who fell ill at Richmond on October 10th, 1612 and who, to use De Mayerne's phrase, 'departed this life at St. James, London, on November, 6th, 1612'. Part of the record for November 5th includes the following[1076]:

> *Nov. 5th*: During the whole of the eleventh day things went from bad to worse, and the majority of his attendants decided to await the crisis, far off as that appeared to be. During the night cupping glasses were applied, with scarifications, over his shoulders, and some split pigeons were laid upon his shaven head.
>
> The next day a cock, split down the back, was applied, and the cordials were given in double doses and twice as often, all without any advantage.
>
> By this time it was plain that the issue so long dreaded, must now be regarded as inevitable. To obviate this, so far as medical art might do so, and in such a way as the state of the illness seemed to indicate, the Doctors de Mayerne, Hammon, Atkins and Butler decided to have recourse once more to bleeding. It seemed that the blood was being determined upwards with great force upon the brain and surcharging it. This state of things placed His Highness in imminent danger more than the drowsiness, which was due to the hot and bilious blood disordering the ventricles and membranes of the brain. Hence there was no other possible resource than to open a vein. The patient's condition did not seem to contraindicate this, for the pulse was strong enough and His Highness was still able to rise and go to the commode, and sit there some time without faintness, just as he had done throughout the illness.

On the same day the assembled physicians decided, the outlook appearing hopeless, that the diascordium was to be administered, 'tempered by cordials less warm in nature'. Gibson provides as full and satisfactory a record of the diascordium as appears in any readily available source[1077]:

> The diascordium prescribed for the Prince, after serious consultation, was introduced by Hieronymus Fracastorius, and called after him "Confectio Fracastorii." On page 92 of the pharmacopœia section of Doctor Browne's "Opera Medica" there are descriptions of several diascordia. The first has the formula of Fracastorius' Confection. The second is a variant by Riverius, Mayerne's master at Montpellier, and colleague on the staff of the King's physicians at Paris. The third he calls by the name of Guenault, but in a side note he says that he himself gave it to the Paris pharmacopœia on June 28, 1627. The "Diascordium Magistrale" is the last example, containing no fewer

than twenty-nine drugs mixed in honey and malmsey wine. They all contained opium in some form; the last contained "my own Laudanum."

The Confection of Fracastorius contained: cinnamon, cassia ligna, of each half an ounce; scordium (water germander) an ounce; dittany of Crete, tormentilla, bistort, galbanum, gum arabic, of each half an ounce; Armenian bole an ounce and a half; Lemnian earth, half an ounce; long pepper, ginger, of each two drachms; clarified honey, two pounds and a half; sugar of roses, one pound; canary wine, eight ounces. In Dr. Hooper's "Lexicon medicum" it is described as "cordial and astringent, and was formerly much used in dysentery." In the Prince's case it appears to have acted as a slight sedative, perhaps owing to the opium it contained.

Armenian bole was clayey earth of a red color due to its iron content. Lemnian earth was a similar substance. These clays were often made into cakes and stamped with certain impressions, which gave rise to the term "terrae sigillatae" or sealed earths.

The Dittany (Figure 38), which formed one ingredient of the Confection of Fracastorius, is an item of which Mrs Grieve (*A modern herbal*, 1931) wrote that: 'The leaves of a plant growing in Crete and Candy were used by the Ancients for wounds, and it is still known as Dictamnus or Dittany of Crete, being *Origanum Dictamnus* of the Labiatae family.' [1078] In his *Medical botany . . .* of 1810 William Woodville noted that 'Both the Greek and Roman writers have fabled this plant into a great celebrity.' [1079] He says, 'The leaves of this plant are apparently very warm and aromatic; of an agreeable smell, and hot biting taste.' [1080] As a drug, Dittany had largely fallen from use by Woodville's day – but it remains well known and is still favoured as a herbal tea and sold dried to be used for that purpose in Crete.

The cock 'split down the back' [1076] and applied to the Prince in his grave illness on November 5th, 1612 is an example of the Court's belief in the most primitive magic only 300 years before the beginning of the modern age of chemotherapy. Things were hardly more rational when Washington died, aided by his physicians, close on 200 years later. Woodville's account of the Dittany of Crete provides an example of the, perhaps surprising, longevity of items of folklore and legend. Out of this folklore Withering had drawn digitalis. The rest of the late eighteenth century pharmacopoeia can be examined in Cullen's splendid *A treatise of the materia medica* [909] of 1789.

Amongst his remedies and means of preventing and treating disease, Cullen included a great range of fruits, dried fruits, roots, vegetables, cereals, nuts, mushrooms, wines, milks, meats, birds, plants and mineral substances. The list was free of obviously noxious and foul materials and contained many usefully active botanical drugs. Amongst its more toxic and, as we might now see them, less desirable remedies it included butter of antimony, quicksilver, and arsenic. Amongst its drugs that, in difficult circumstances, we might still choose to use, it included opium, Peruvian bark and the foxglove.

The *Materia medica Americana, potissimum regni vegetabilis* [1081] published in 1787 by Johann Schoepff (1752–1800) is the nearest equivalent to Cullen's work in the materia medica of eighteenth century America. Schoepff went to that country as an army surgeon accompanying the British Forces in 1777. He later returned to Germany and in the years that followed wrote his account of the

American pharmacopoeia. Cullen's own work, excellent as it is, shows the influence of the time – perhaps most visibly in his essay on mercury. Of this, then widely used, toxic material he says: 'I shall treat of this medicine as fully as I can, as it is one of the most useful and universal medicines known . . . '[1082] He adds that, 'Universally mercury in its active state seems to be a stimulus to every sensible and moving fibre of the body to which it is immediately applied; and in consequence, it is particularly a stimulus to every excretory of the system to which it is externally or internally applied.'[1083] To a profession versed since time immemorial in coaxing or forcing the noxious elements of disease from the body a 'stimulus to every excretory of the system' was of such virtue that Cullen ended his pages on the subject with this paragraph[1084]:

> To conclude the fubject of the medicinal powers of mercury, it will readily appear, that whoever confiders the general deobftruent powers mentioned above, and at the fame time the various effects of it when employed as a purgative, will fully apprehend its very extenfive ufe in the practice of phyfic.

Discussion

The eighteenth century was a time of affluence amongst its most celebrated physicians; it was also a period of fashionable quacks many of whom became as well known as the doctors. Physicians and quacks alike ministered to the gullible and credulous rich, largely ignoring the rest of the population which must be assumed to have contained an increasing proportion of the poor – this proportion reflecting the results of the Industrial Revolution and urbanization.

The difficulties which had to be tackled with the limited knowledge of the time, the level of public awareness which existed, and the materia medica which we have briefly reviewed, were not just due to a bigger population and urbanization. In the country districts poor housing, miserable sanitation and hygiene, low wages, indifferent nutrition and a host of problems added their quota. The effects are best measured in the appalling infant mortality rate and the data showing the short mean expectation of life.

In the large cities the Industrial Revolution generated not only problems but, at times, the impetus that provided the means of improvements in hygiene. Westminster obtained an Improvement Act in 1762, Birmingham in 1765, the City of London in 1766 and Manchester in 1776. Many of the towns in the provinces gradually followed. As a result of these and related Acts, drains were covered in the cities, streets were lighted and paved, and many of the towns, by the late eighteenth century, came to look much as they look now.

Beneath the superficial elegance all was less well. In most towns continuous water supply was unknown. Most of London's water supply, for instance, came from surface wells and rivers exposed to pollution. Cesspits remained in widespread use and it is hard to remember that even as late as the early part of the nineteenth century typical London houses had only intermittent water supplies and no adequate means of sewage disposal: even in the better class houses water-closets were not general until about 1830–1840. Thus, we reach almost to the discovery of inhalational anaesthesia before we reach anything like a uniformly accessible provision of the means of hygiene.

During the period when the facilities fundamental to the public health were slowly being provided, an increasing number of new hospitals were built. These aimed to relieve the problems of the towns but, at their best, were hardly a match for the problems around them. The first voluntary hospital was the Westminster, founded in 1719. The other London hospitals included Guy's (1725), St. George's (1733), the London (1740), the Middlesex (1745), the London Smallpox and Inoculation Hospital (1746), and the rebuilding of St. Bartholomew's (1730–53). The picture of urban illness was to some extent relieved by the building of provincial hospitals – those at York (1710), Salisbury (1716), and Cambridge (1719) being among the earlier ones in England; Edinburgh and its Royal Infirmary (1729, 1736) became the forerunner of such developments in Scotland and Cork (1720) provided one of the first of such new hospitals in Ireland. Attention began to be given to doing something about the obvious ravages of tuberculosis, the Royal Sea-Bathing Infirmary for Scrofula being founded in Margate in 1791.

Tragically, conditions in some of the great hospitals sank to the level at which they provoked the vivid *Mémoires sur les hôpitaux de Paris* (1788)[1019] of Jacques Tenon. This account was contemporaneous with the equally disturbing report on *The state of the prisons in England and Wales* (1777)[1018] and *An account of the principle lazarettos in Europe* (1789)[1020] by the reformer, John Howard. Contemporary with these calls for reform was the founding of the Quaker retreat, at York, in 1794 – the attempt of William Tuke to provide for the humane treatment of the insane.

Few things are more striking than the rate of change in many of the departments of medicine since the middle and late eighteenth century. In England, about 1740, the infant mortality rate was such that roughly 75% of children born alive died before they were 5 years of age. In the institutions caring for the unwanted and for orphans the losses were higher: Garrison[1085] quotes a figure showing that at the Dublin Foundling Asylum, during 1775–96, only 45 out of 10 272 children survived – a 99.66% mortality. By the end of the century attempts to improve child care had resulted in the invention of artificial feeding, the virtual abolition of dry feeding of very small children, and the displacement of the wet-nurse with the use of boiled cow's milk diluted with barley-water. The cow's horn, previously recommended, was replaced by the glass feeding bottle and, by 1800, the infant mortality rate had improved so that only 41% of children born alive died before they were 5.

Apart from the infectious fevers and tuberculosis in its different forms, the most characteristic disease of town children in the earlier parts of the eighteenth century seems to have been rickets. It is suggested that this disease diminished as the winter feeding of cattle became widespread with the resulting year-round improvement in human nutrition. Over much of Europe malaria, dysentery, influenza and scarlet fever remained common, sometimes reaching pandemic proportions, and smallpox, diphtheria and pertussis caused well-recorded epidemics. Outbreaks of typhus fever were associated with the wars of the century and this illness ('jail fever') at the Black Assize of the Old Bailey in 1750 resulted in the deaths of the Lord Mayor, three judges, eight jurymen, and many others.

It remains hard to imagine the ravages of uncontrolled disease under the conditions which then existed. One example of the scale of the calamities that marked the earlier centuries is the Irish disaster in which, in 1740, typhus combined with the failure of the potato harvest to cost the lives of 80 000 people.

Despite these rates of disease the whole of the eighteenth century was spanned by the implementation of a piece of legislation which saw few equals until the Finance Act of 1972 imposed a tax on the repair or maintenance (but not the alteration or demolition) of houses and suchlike. The 1696 window-tax, firmly enforced in the eighteenth century, produced what Garrison[1086] called 'a tyrannous tax on light and air' and 'an activator of infection, in dark houses throughout the entire 18th century'. It was not until 1803 that houses and their windows were, as before, rated as a whole. It was not until 1851 that the window-tax, in all its forms, was finally abolished.

Other legislation had a more benign effect. William Cheselden, in June, 1745, secured the separation of the surgeons from the barbers, establishing the 'Masters, Governors, and Commonalty of the Art and the Science of Surgeons of London'. In 1800, the Corporation of Surgeons became, by Charter of George III, the Royal College of Surgeons of London; in 1843 this body became the Royal College of Surgeons of England.

These careful steps forward were accompanied by improved facilities for clinical teaching in Britain and, one by one, hospital medical schools were established. Notable institutions included schools at Guy's (1723), the Edinburgh Hospital (1736), and the Meath Hospital, Dublin (1756). Private instruction continued, sometimes providing the best tuition available – as with the anatomy teaching of the two Hunters, Cullen's instruction in internal medicine, Smellie's coaching in obstetrics, and the chemistry classes of Joseph Black.

The eighteenth century exhibit of the Apothecaries is the Chelsea Physic Garden, the site of which has been previously mentioned (p. 288). The centre of the garden (Figure 119) has a statue of Hans Sloane who, having bought the Manor of Chelsea from Charles Cheyne in 1712, owned the freehold of the Garden. He had studied at this site in the early part of his medical training and, once master of the property, leased it to the Society of Apothecaries for the sum of 5 pounds a year in perpetuity, so long as it was kept as a 'physic garden'. The other great benefit conferred on the Society by Sloane was the instigation of the appointment of Philip Miller (1691–1771), who became Gardener in 1722. Under Miller's care the botanical garden at Chelsea became the finest in eighteenth century Europe. Miller also produced the famous *The Gardener's Dictionary* (1731) which was praised by Linnaeus and, in its eighth edition, adopted the binomial nomenclature which had been introduced by Linnaeus almost 20 years before. It is this edition which remains of practical use now that the Garden has passed from the care of the Apothecaries to be maintained, since 1899, by Trustees who have preserved it as a centre of botanical research and study.

Other, perhaps less helpful, changes affected the Apothecaries. In 1748 Parliament refused to confirm their original monopoly of compounding prescriptions and selling drugs. As a result, retail trade in medicines slipped from the hands of the apothecary to those of the unqualified chemist and druggist. Those who resented the prices charged by the earlier apothecaries may have been unworried by the change – but it left the purveying of drugs in trade hands controlled by neither the College of Physicians nor the Society of Apothecaries. The

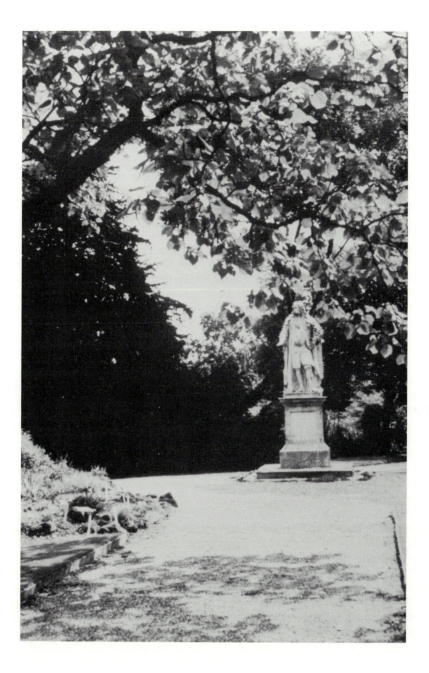

Figure 119   The Chelsea Physic Garden and the statue of Sir Hans Sloane, London.

harm done to the pharmaceutical apothecary was such that only the apothecary practising medicine could readily survive and, in 1774, the Society restricted its livery to those of its members who were practitioners of medicine. In 1841 the pharmaceutical apothecaries, after a difficult period, joined forces with the better unqualified chemists and druggists – so establishing the Pharmaceutical Society of Great Britain and leaving the Society of Apothecaries as a purely medical body.

As the hospitals and organs of professional life of the eighteenth century were assembled, the gap remained between knowledge at its best and the level of care which could be applied to the lives of the great mass of people. Eighteenth century anatomy was far advanced. The best of the physiology of the century can be represented by the versatile and important writings of Friedrich Hoffman (1660–1742) whose successive contributions to the early part of the century included the *Fundamenta physiologiae* of 1718[1087], the *De metastasi sive sede morbo mutata* of 1731[956], the *De genuina chlorosis indole, origine et curatione*, also of 1731[1088], and a series of observations leading to the *Opera omnia physico-medica* of 1740–53[1089]. The first of these works was an outstanding treatise on the whole of physiology; the second shows Hoffmann's approach to pathology seen from its functional, physiological aspect. The third work provides Hoffmann's classical description of chlorosis – a condition first described by Johann Lange (1485–1565) in 1554[1090] and called 'De morbo virgineo' before being given its English account (*Hints respecting the chlorosis of boarding schools*)[1091] in 1795 by John Lettsom (1744–1815). The later achievements in physiology of the eighteenth century include the brilliant writings[868] of 1778 in which Antoine Lavoisier demonstrated his understanding of the respiratory significance of oxygen.

There are many highlights in eighteenth-century medicine. A favourite is *A new theory of consumptions: more especially of a phthisis, or consumption of the lungs*[1092], this was published in 1720 by Benjamin Marten (1704–1782) and suggests that a micro-organism, a parasite, might be the cause of tuberculosis. In this writing Marten anticipated the discovery of the tubercule bacillus by over 160 years. The century also saw the first full clinical and pathological account of emphysema, this being given by Sir William Watson (1715–1787) in *An account of what appeared on opening the body of an asthmatic person* (1746)[1093]. Francis Home (1719–1813) in 1765 published in Edinburgh one of the best early descriptions[1094] of the clinical manifestations of diphtheria; this was followed by *An enquiry into the nature, cause and cure, of the angina suffocativa, or, sore throat distemper, as it is commonly called by the inhabitants of this city and colony*[1095] – an American classic, published in New York in 1771, in which Samuel Bard (1742–1821) gave his own account of this terrible infection. Knowledge of deficiency diseases advanced, pellagra first being given its present-day name by the Italian, Francesco Frapolli (?died 1773) who published his *Animadversiones in morbum, vulgo pellagram* in 1977[1096]. The first major work on the subject of skin diseases to provide an acceptable nomenclature and to be illustrated by coloured plates was *On cutaneous diseases* (1796–1808)[1097], by Robert Willan (1757–1812). Willan, whose book was published in London, died when Volume One only had appeared but the contribution was such that modern dermatology can be said to have begun with his name.

The sciences close to medicine also made worthwhile advances. As might be expected they come late in the century; examples, are the first major attempt at a systematic classification of bacteria by Otto Müller (1730–1784)[1098] in 1786, the first modern proposal of the nature of fermentation by Giovanni Fabbroni (1752–1822)[1099] in 1787, and what was almost certainly the first attempt to stain bacteria (with carmine and indigo) -- the 1778 contribution to bacteriology of Wilhelm von Gleichen (1717–1783)[1100]. In biochemistry the century saw the discovery of urea by Hilaire Rouelle (1718–1779), whose *Observations sur l'urine humaine*[1101] appeared in 1773, and the discovery of uric acid by Carl Scheele (1742–1786), whose findings were announced in 1776[1102].

Thus, it is clear that more than the mere outlines of some of these subjects was available to the best eighteenth century minds. Special departments of medicine had begun to organize themselves and their practitioners started to systematize the available body of knowledge. One such department was in the hands of Daniel Le Clerc (1652–1728) whose *Histoire de la médecine*[1103] first appeared in 1696 (English translation 1699); the later editions of this, the first major history of medicine, include the 1729 version which is still consulted today. The best English work of the period was designed in the Tower of London. This notable two volume study, *The history of physick; from the time of Galen to the beginning of the sixteenth century*[1104], was published by John Friend (1675–1728) in 1725–26 when Friend had been released from his charge of high treason following the intervention of his associate Richard Mead who had been called to relieve Robert Walpole, Prime Minister of the time, of his urinary problems from stone.

The great and the lowly of the eighteenth century could receive little from the physicians of the day apart from the materia medica. This, for the later part of the century, can be taken from the absorbing *A new translation of the pharmacopoeia of the Royal College of Physicians of London, of the year 1787 . . . by an Apothecary*[1105] – a work published in London in 1789. It was dedicated to 'His Most Sacred Majesty George the Third, King of Great Britain, France, and Ireland, Defender of the Faith, Duke of Brunswic and Lunenburgh, Arch-Treasurer and Elector of the Holy Roman Empire, &c'. The Preface acknowledges that 'medicine has not perhaps kept pace in its progress with other useful arts, yet it has received assistances and improvements from various sources, which are neither few, nor of little value or estimation; and more particularly from chemistry, which being lately studied with greater zeal and accuracy, and deeper judgment and attention, is well known to be much more, and better understood.'[1106] Throughout the book, although something of the modern approach to therapeutics has crept in and the work is far less credulous than earlier pharmacopoeias, there is evident the fact that knowledge had advanced only slowly in the forming of remedies – and that chemical substances had become important amongst them. There had been conscious rationalization[1107]:

> Particular care has been taken that there fhall not remain any veftiges of medicines whofe virtues are grounded on no better foundation than old womens tales. If, however, there may be found here and there remedies or prefcriptions which may appear fuperflous, or of no ufe, it is to be afcribed to our rather wifhing to leave them to be corrected, or totally thrown out by our fucceffors, than to obftinately fet our faces againft opinions, which, although

not true, are neverthelefs harmlefs. We have been particularly attentive to fimplicity in prefcription, and careful that medicines fhould not be mixed together, which would not readily coalefce, and which did not co-operate to the fame purpofe. Hence thofe pompous antidotes, compofed of an enormous quantity of fimples, huddled together without judgment, and for no reafon, as being formed of fubftances collected together from all parts and all fources, of virtues totally repugnant, heaped together in an incongruous mafs, are at length totally rejected. Even by this it appears, that we are no longer governed by a blind attachment to authority derived from inveterate habit, nor unbounded reverence for the antients.

In reading the pharmacopoeias of the seventeenth and eighteenth centuries it is necessary to bear in mind the systems of weights and measures used in the handling of medicines. The 1789 translation of the Pharmacopoeia of the Royal College of Physicians [1105] gives the following details; to these, the so-called 'medicinal characters' most commonly used are added:

WEIGHTS AND MEASURES.

Two kinds of weights are ufed in this kingdom, one for gold and filver, the other for other merchandifes; the firft we call Troy weight, the other Avoirdupois weight. The pounds are differently divided. The pound troy into twelve ounces, avoirdupois into fixteen. Thefe weights differ both in their pounds and ounces; the avoirdupois pound is greater, the ounce lefs than the troy*. We ufe the troy pound, but we divide it differently from goldfmiths, to wit:

A pound			twelve ounces
An ounce			eight drachms.
A drachm	contains		three fcruples.
A fcruple			twenty grains

The meafures are alfo of two kinds in this kingdom, ale meafure and wine meafure. We ufe wine meafure, of which

| A pint | | | fixteen ounces, |
| An ounce | contains | | eight drachms, |

according to our divifion; and a gallon contains eight pints.

To avoid ambiguity, wherever we ufe the words ounces or drachms, we put W and M to diftinguish weight and meafure, in as much as an ounce and a drachm meafure bear no general proportion to an ounce and a drachm weight.

Twenty *Grains*			a *Scruple*.	Э
Three *Scruples*			a *Drachm*.	Ʒ
Eight *Drachms*	make		an *Ounce*.	Ʒ
Twelve *Ounces*			a *Pound*.	℔

The items provided in the materia medica of the 1789 pharmacopoeia are given in the Appendix (p. 717).

To the present-day doctor the most dramatic inclusion in the 1789 translation of the College Pharmacopoeia is probably *Cissampelos pareira*. This is translated

*The troy ounce contains 480 grains, the avoirdupois 437½ grains.

as *Pareira brava* and the use of the root is specified. The drug disappeared from use and is not mentioned in the mid-nineteenth century *The elements of materia medica*[1108] – the fine, two volume study by Jonathan Pereira (1804–1853) which was the first great English work on the subject. Pereira was Professor of Materia Medica in the School of Pharmacy established by the Pharmaceutical Society of Great Britain and his book remains, for the English reader, the most informative of its period. *Cissampelos pareira* remained absent from the BPC (1934) prepared one-third of the way through the twentieth century.

At about the time that the BPC omitted reference to the drug, Mrs M. Grieve (*A modern herbal*)[1109] not only showed *Cissampelos Pareira* and *Pereira Brava* as synonyms for *Chondrondendron tomentosum* of the Menispermaceae but she provided the following brilliant description of the plant for which she gave the habitat as 'West Indies, Spanish Main Brazil, Peru.'[1109]

> A woody vine, climbing a considerable height over trees; very large leaves, often 1 foot long with a silky pubescence, on the inner side grey colour; flowers diœcious in racemes; in the female plant the racemes are longer than the leaves, bearing the flowers in spike fascicles; the berries, first scarlet, then black, are oval, size of large grapes in commerce. The root is cylindrical in varying lengths from ½ inch to 5 inches in diameter and from 2 or 3 inches to several feet long; externally blackish brown, longitudinally furrowed, transversed knotty ridges; it is hard, heavy, tough, and when freshly cut has a waxy lustre; interior woody, reddy yellow; transversed section shows several successive eccentric and distinctly radiate concentric zones of projecting secondary bundles fibrovascular. Stem deeply furrowed; colour grey and covered with patches of lichen; odour, slight, aromatic, sweetish flavour, succeeded by an intense nauseating bitterness, yielding its bitterness and active properties to water or alcohol.

It is perhaps not surprising that the travellers who sent back exotic plants that featured in the seventeenth and eighteenth century pharmacopoeias should select so notable a vine. That interest in it waned does not alter the fact that those familiar with the materia medica of 1789 handled, without knowing its modern pharmacology, the vine of which the BPC (1959) says[1110]:

> Tubocurarine Chloride is the chloride of an alkaloid, (+)-tubocurarine, obtained from extracts of the stems of *Chondodendron tomentosum* Ruiz et Pav. (Fam. Menispermaceæ) and possessing the specific biological activity of curare on neuromuscular transmission.

Tubocurarine chloride remains in the BP (1980)[1111] and serves as an exemplar of the modern use of the neuromuscular blocking agents, of especial value in anaesthesia, which developed from the South American arrow poison.

There are many toxic substances in the 1789 translation. Hemlock, *Conium maculatum* (Figure 120), of which the translator specified the use of the whole herb as well as the flower and seed, is well known for its toxic properties. The features of this poison are shown in this account of the sacrifice of Socrates[1112]:

> ... Then Crito made a sign to his slave who was standing by; and the slave went out, and after some delay returned with the man who was to give the

poison, carrying it prepared in a cup. When Socrates saw him, he asked, You understand these things, my good sir; what have I to do?

You have only to drink this, he replied, and to walk about until your legs feel heavy, and then lie down. and it will act of itself. With that he handed the cup to Socrates, who took it quite cheerfully, Echecrates, without trembling, and without any change of colour or of feature, and looked up at the man with that fixed glance of his, and asked, What say you to making a libation from this draught? May I, or not? We only prepare so much as we think sufficient, Socrates, he answered. I understand, said Socrates. But I suppose that I may, and must, pray to the gods that my journey hence may be prosperous: that is my prayer; be it so. With these words he put the cup to his lips and drank the poison quite calmly and cheerfully. Till then most of us had been able to control our grief fairly well; but when we saw him drinking, and then the poison finished, we could do so no longer: my tears came fast in spite of myself: it was not for him, but at my own misfortune in losing such a friend. Even before that Crito had been unable to restrain his tears, and had gone away; and Apollodorus, who had never once ceased weeping the whole time, burst into a loud cry, and made us one and all break down by his sobbing and grief, except only Socrates himself. What are you doing, my friends? he exclaimed. I sent away the women chiefly in order that they might not offend in this way; for I have heard that a man should die in silence. So calm yourselves and bear up. When we heard that we were ashamed, and we ceased from weeping. But he walked about, until he said that his legs were getting heavy, and then he lay down on his back, as he was told. And the man who gave the poison began to examine his feet and legs, from time to time: then he pressed his foot hard, and asked if there was any feeling in it; and Socrates said, No: and then his legs, and so higher and higher, and showed us that he was cold and stiff. And Socrates felt himself, and said that when it came to his heart, he should be gone. He was already growing cold about the groin, when he uncovered his face, which had been covered, and spoke for the last time. Crito, he said, I owe a cock to Asclepius; do not forget to pay it. It shall be done, replied Crito. Is there anything else that you wish? He made no answer to this question; but after a short interval there was a movement, and the man uncovered him, and his eyes were fixed. Then Crito closed his mouth and his eyes.

Such was the end, Echecrates, of our friend, a man, I think, who was the wisest and justest, and the best man that I have ever known.

The description given[1112] is an accurate account of the effects of the alkaloid, coniine, the active principle of hemlock. There is paralysis of both the motor and sensory peripheral nerve endings then the central nervous system is affected producing death when the medullary respiratory centre is reached.

Another two interesting drugs were the Lousewort and the Coughwort – both of which appeared in the 1789 listing and in the BPC (1934). The Lousewort, *Delphinium Staphisagria*, provided the 1934[1113] pharmacopoeial item Staphisagriae Semina, or Stavesacre Seeds. *Delphinium Staphisagria*, of the family Ranunculaceae, provided the seeds, which in their pharmacopoeial form contained about 1% alkaloids, of which the most important was delphinine. Staphisagria, a highly toxic material, was used in an ointment to destroy pediculi – the BPC 1934 thereby recognizing the traditional use indicated by the rural name of the Lousewort.

The Coughwort, *Tussilago Farfara* or Coltsfoot, appeared in the 1934 BPC[1114] as Tussilaginis Flos, the Coltsfoot flower, and as Tussilaginis Folium, the

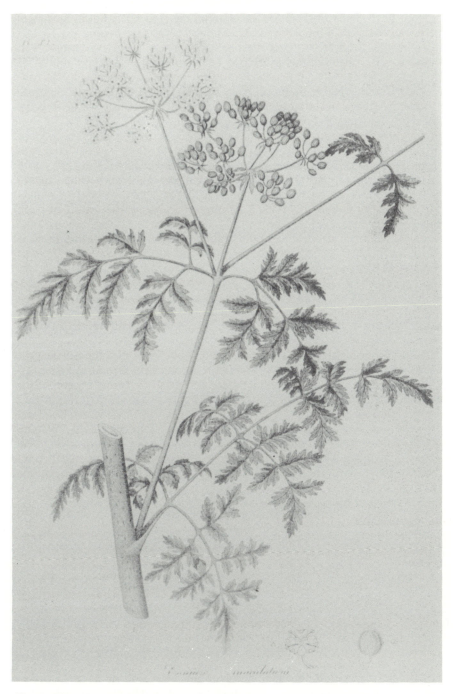

Figure 120 Conium maculatum (The Hemlock). [*From: Jacob Bigelow. American medical botany. Boston (1817–20). Vol. I, Plate XI.*]

Coltsfoot Leaf. The Coltsfoot, of the Compositae, was said to yield mucilage, tannin and traces of a bitter glycoside. The yield was put to good use for the *Codex*[1114] said 'Coltsfoot leaf is used as a demulcent to relieve chronic and irritable cough. A decoction (1 in 20) may be taken in doses of 2 fluid ounces, or more, several times daily.' It is another example of the use indicated by the centuries-old Country Name finding a place in the modern semi-official pharmacopoeias. Another plant, traditionally of useful activity and listed in 1789, is the Dandelion, *Leontodon Taraxacum* or *Taraxacum officinale*, of which the root and the whole herb was used. Because this tradition has been explored by modern pharmacognosy and experimental pharmacology, this drug is considered subsequently – as is the Elecampane, *Enula* or *Inula Helenium*, the Scabwort, which relates to a period soon after Koch's discovery of the tubercule bacillus, against which the drug was studied and then, seemingly, forgotten.

The 1789 translation contained a number of fruits and foodstuffs of great utility, such as oats, barley, wheat and sugar. It contained also, amongst the previously described drugs that would still be recognized as of utility (even if obsolete) a number of substances including *Colchicum autumnale, Digitalis purpurea, Dryopteris felix-mas, Psychotria ipecacuanha, Papaver somniferum, Cinchona officinalis, Artemisia cina, Scilla maritima* and *Cassia acutifolia* – sources of colchicine, digitalis, Male Fern extract, ipecac, opium, quinine, santonin, squill, and senna with which to do something about gout, cardiac failure, worm infestation, amoebic dysentery, and some forms of malaria.

The 1789 version of the Pharmacopoeia almost bisects the time between the First London Pharmacopoeia of 1618 and the current British Pharmacopoeia of 1980. It is considerably less Mesopotamian than the 1618 second version of the first edition, the animal parts of which included horn of a unicorn or rhinoceros, the bone from the heart of a stag, elephant tusk, bezoar stone, vipers' flesh, nest of swallows and oil of foxes. Of the 1618 College Pharmacopoeia, William Brockbank has a splendid modern study entitled *Sovereign Remedies, a critical depreciation of the 17th-century London pharmacopoeia*[1115]; this paper, published in 1964, gives the following analysis of the 1190 ingredients of the pharmacopoeia:

CONTENTS OF THE FIRST EDITION

Roots	138	Juices	29
Barks	34	Plant excrements	7
Woods	16	Animals	31
Leaves	292	Animal parts or excrements	162
Flowers	85	Things from the sea	25
Fruits & Buds	93	Salts	11
Seeds or Grains	144	Metals	73
Tears, fluid extracts, gums, resins	50		
Total	1190		

From Brockbank, W. (1964)

This list shows that the ingredients of the 1618 College Pharmacopoeia comprised 888 botanical items, 218 of animal origin, and 84 chemical substances – a total of 1190.

The list of the materia medica given in the Appendix and derived from the 1787 College Pharmacopoeia amounts to 188 botanical species, 17 items of animal origin, and 36 chemicals – a total of 241.

The change over the 169 years between the First London Pharmacopoeia and the 1787 edition at the end of the eighteenth century had been considerable; it had eliminated many noxious, foul and ineffective substances – unpleasant even if most of them were earlier used only in poultices and topical applications.

But the useful means of therapy, even at the end of the eighteenth century, were limited. Faced with the huge gap between the privileged and the poor, the presence of a great deal of absolute poverty and the prevalence of infectious disease, there was little that the doctor could usefully use beyond mercury, iron, the natural salicylates, opium, quinine, a range of anthelmintics and purgatives – and those magnificent additions to the eighteenth century pharmacopoeia, digitalis and smallpox vaccine. With this rather limited range of drugs the doctors and apothecaries of the day had to face the appalling infant mortality rate, the poor conditions in hospitals, prisons and ships, the deficient standard of hygiene and the short expectation of life characteristic of the social circumstances of their community.

The only specific amongst these drugs was mercury, apart from quinine in some forms of malaria. It is important to remember the toxicity of many of these remedies as well as their limited efficacy. Mercury is the classic example – used, because there was so little else that was effective, but toxic to a degree which has left a number of vivid accounts. Its use as calomel, mercurous chloride, the subchloride of mercury, soon became popular as this was one of the forms in which toleration seemed best. The toxicity, especially in small doses and for limited periods, remained unnoticed; in higher doses, for syphilis in particular, it was tolerated for lack of other drugs that were considered effective.

However, even from the early days, there were some who were perceptive and recognized that calomel could produce very serious intoxication, sometimes causing gastrointestinal disturbance, emaciation, dental loss and decay, intense salivation, debility, mental changes, and death. James Hamilton (1749–?1833), of Edinburgh, wrote his *Observations on the use and abuse of mercurial medicines in various diseases* (1819)[1116] and in this, probably the first serious study in medical science of the side-effects of drugs, he opposed the use of calomel for trivial conditions suggesting that, especially in children, the drug was a cause of debilitating chronic intoxication.

Despite this the abuse continued and the BPC 1934 entry describing the indications for calomel now makes curious reading and shows how long its employment in trivial conditions persisted[1117]:

Action and Uses. – Mercurous chloride is practically non-corrosive to the alimentary canal. It is excreted partly unchanged and partly as sulphide in the fæces. In small, repeated doses, it is useful for disinfecting the bowel in the treatment of common bilious attack, especially as its mildly irritant properties produce a slight purgative effect. As a purgative in large doses, when constipation is due to obstruction, mercurous chloride should be used with care, since, if its elimination is delayed, absorption may take place causing toxic symptoms. When given as a purgative, it is advisable to administer mercurous chloride at night, and to give a saline purgative before breakfast the following morning to minimise the possibility of the absorption of the mercurial. Repeated doses of 0·01 gramme ($\frac{1}{6}$ grain) of mercurous chloride are useful in follicular tonsillitis. It has also been used in acute dysentery, often with ipecacuanha, and in cholera and enteric fever. It exerts a marked diuretic action in some cases of cardiac dropsy. As a purgative, mercurous chloride is often combined with colocynth, as in Pilulæ Hydrargyri Subchloridi, Colocynthidis et Hyoscyami and Pilulæ Hydrargyri Subchloridi et Colocynthidis. In the form of ointment, it is used as an anti-pruritic in the treatment of eczema, psoriasis and pruritus ani.

Like all mercurials, mercurous chloride has an antisyphilitic action. Ointments containing 30 to 50 per cent. of mercurous chloride are used as prophylactics against syphilis, and are said to be effective when applied within four hours of contact. In the form of Injectio Hydrargyri Subchloridi it is used intramuscularly for syphilis; it is very slowly absorbed, and may give rise to pain. Preparations for **injection** should be made by suspending the mercurous chloride in an oily medium which has been heated at 150° for one hour, and the final containers should be sterilised by tyndallisation.

The later parts of the eighteenth century saw the growth to adult stature of Wordsworth, Beethoven, Constable, Turner and their contemporaries. Those

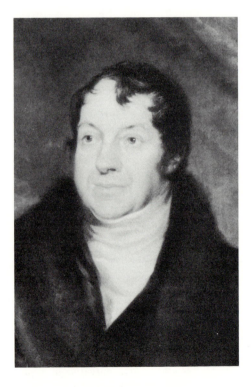

Figure 121   Edward Jenner (1749–1823). *William Hobday portrait, copy in possession of the Royal Society of Medicine, London.*

378

who attended them had no anaesthetics, no blood transfusion, no surgery of the cavities of the body, and only a range of drugs based upon the materia medica which the 1789 translation of the College Pharmacopoeia has listed. It can probably be regarded as one of the lesser accomplishments of the century.

Perhaps, in medicine, and with gathering momentum, the ten great accomplishments of the century were the 1735 *Systema naturae* of Linnaeus, the 1745 ... *Essay on mithridatium and theriaca* of Heberden, the 1757–66 *Elementa physiologiae*... of von Haller, the 1761 *De sedibus*... of the aged Morgagni, the 1761 *Inventum novum*... of the Austrian innkeeper's son Auenbrugger, the splendid *Anatomia uteri humani gravidi*... published in 1774 by William Hunter and the vastly important 1785 *An account of the foxglove*... by William Withering; these were followed, at the very close of the century, by John Hunter's posthumous *A treatise on the blood, inflammation, and gun-shot wounds* (1794), the epoch-making *An inquiry into the causes and effects of the variolae vaccinae*... (1798) of Edward Jenner (Figure 121) and, to begin the next century with an epitome of medicine, the *Commentaries on the history and cure of diseases* by William Heberden, whose mid-century 'Essay' had helped to clean up the pharmacopoeia and whose posthumous 'Commentaries', published in Latin then in English, appeared in 1802.

References

865. Galvani, Aloysio Lugi. De viribus electricitatis in motu musculari commentarius. *Bonon. Sci. Art. Inst. Acad. Comment.*, Bologna, 1791, **7**, 363–418. Trans. R.M. Green, 1953

866. Cavendish, Henry. Experiments on air. *Phil. Trans.*, 1784, **74**, 119–53

867. Priestley, Joseph. Observations on different kinds of air. *Phil Trans.*, 1772, **62**, 147–264

868. Lavoisier, Antoine Laurent. Mémoire sur la nature du principe qui se combine avec les métaux pendant leur calcination, et qui en augmente le poids. *Hist. Acad. R. Sci.*, (1775), 1778, 520–26

869. Haller, Albrecht von. De respiratione experimenta anatomica, quibus aëris inter pulmonem et pleuram absentia demonstratur et musculorum intercostalium internorum officium adseritur. 2 pts. Gottingae, *A. Vandenhoeck*, 1746–1747

870. Black, Joseph. Dissertatio medica inauguralis de humore acido a cibis orto, et magnesia alba. Edinburgi, *G. Hamilton & J. Balfour*, 1754

871. Rutherford, Daniel. De aëre fixo dicto, aut mephitico. Edinburgi, *Balfour & Smellie*, 1772

872. Lavoisier, Antoine Laurent and La Place, Pierre Simon de. Mémoire sur la chaleur. *Hist. Acad. R. Sci. (Paris)*, (1780), 1784, 355–408

873. Séguin, Armand and Lavoisier, Antoine Laurent. Premier mémoire sur la respiration des animaux. *Hist. Acad. Sci. (Paris)*, (1789), 1793, 566–84

874. Cruikshank, William Cumberland. Experiments on the insensible perspiration of the human body. London, *G. Nicol*, 1795. 1st. edn. 1779

875. Morton, Leslie T. (1970). As ref. 610 but p. 28

876. Linné, Carl von (Linnaeus). Systema naturae. Lugduni Batavorum, *apud Theodorum Haak*, 1735

877. Linné, Carl von (Linnaeus). Genera plantarum. Lugduni Batavorum, *apud Conradum Wishoff*, 1737. English trans. 1771

878. Linné, Carl von (Linnaeus). Genera morborum in auditorum usum. Upsaliae, *C. E. Steinert*, 1763

879. Sauvages de la Croix, François Boissier de. Nosologia methodica, sistens morborum classes, genera et species. 5 vols. Amstelodami, *frat. de Tournes*, 1763

880. Spallanzani, Lazzaro. Saggio di osservazioni microscopiche relative al sistema della generazione. Modena, 1767

881. Spallanzani, Lazaro. Prodromi sulla riproduzione animali. Riproduzione della coda del girino. Modena, 1768.
882. Spallanzani, Lazaro. Opusculi di fisica animale e vegetabile. 2 vols. Modena, *Soc. tipografica*, 1776
883. Ingen-Housz, Jan. Experiments on vegetables, discovering their great power of purifying the common air in the sun-shine, and of injuring it in the shade at night. To which is joined, a new method of examining the accurate degree of salubrity of the atmosphere. London, *P. Elmsley and H. Payne*, 1779
884. Darwin, Erasmus. Zoonomia; or the laws of organic life. 2 vols. London, *J. Johnson*, 1794–96
885. Brown, Robert. Observations on the organs and mode of fecundation in Orchideae and Asclepiadeae. *Trans. Linn. Soc.*, 1829–32, **16**, 685–746
886. Bartram, John. Descriptions, virtues, and uses of sundry plants of these northern parts of America. (Philadelphia), 1751
887. Baglivi, Giorgio. Opera omnia medico-practica et anatomica. Lugduni, *Anisson & J. Posuel*, 1704
888. Lancisi, Giovanni Maria. Opera quae hactenus prodierunt omnia. 2 vols. Genevae, *J. A. Cramer et fil.*, 1718
889. Hoffmann, Friedrich. Fundamenta physiologiae. Halle, 1718
890. Hoffmann, Friedrich. Opera omnia physico-medica (Supplementum, *etc.*) 9 vols. Genevae, *fratres de Tournes*, 1740–53
891. Stahl, Georg Ernst. Theoria medica vera. Halae, *lit. Orphanotrophiei*, 1708 (1707)
892. Stahl, Georg Ernst. Œuvres médico-philosophiques et pratiques. 6 vols. Paris, *J. B. Baillière*, 1849–64
893. Stahl, Georg Ernst. Elementia chemiae (2 vols.). Leiden, 1732
894. Boerhaave, Herman. Institutiones medicae in usus annuae exercitationis domesticos digestae. Lugduni Batavorum. *J. van der Linden*, 1708
895. Boerhaave, Herman. Aphorismi de cognoscendis et curandis morbis. Lugduni Batavorum, *J. vander Linden*, 1709. English trans. 1715
896. Boerhaave, Herman. Opera omnia medica. Venetiis, *apud L. Basilium*, 1742
897. Haller, Albrecht von. Primae lineae physiologiae in usum praelectionum academicarum. Gottingae, *A. Vandenhoeck*, 1747. English trans. 1754
898. Haller, Albrecht von. De partibus corporis humani sensibilibus et irritabilibus. *Comment. Soc. Reg. Sci. Getting.* (1752), 1753, 2, 114–58. English trans. *Bull. Hist. Med.* 1936, **4**, 651–699
899. Haller, Albrecht von. Elementa physiologiae corporis humani. 8 vols. Lausanne, Berne, 1757–66
900. Haller, Albrecht von. Bibliotheca botanica. 2 vols. Tiguri, *apud Orell, Gessner, Fuessli, et socc.*, 1771–72
901. Haller, Albrecht von. Icones anatomicae. 8 pts. Gottingae, *A. Vandenhoeck*, 1743–56
902. Haller, Albrecht von. Methodus studii medicin. Amsterdam, 1751
903. Garrison, Fielding H. (1929). As ref. 179 but p. 318
904. Haller, Albrecht von. Bibliotheca anatomica. 2 vols. Tiguri, *apud Orell, Gessner*, etc., 1774–77
905. Haller, Albrecht von. Bibliotheca chirurgica. 2 vols. Bernae & Basileae, *Haller & Schweighauser*, 1774–75
906. Haller, Albrecht von. Bibliotheca medicinae practicae. 4 vols. Basle, *J. Schweighauser*; Berne, *E. Haller*, 1776–88
907. Monro, Alexander, *Secundus*. Observations on the structure and functions of the nervous system. Edinburgh, *W. Creech*, 1783
908. Cullen, William. Synopsis nosologiae methodicae. Edinburgi, 1769
909. Cullen, William. A treatise of the materia medica. 2 vols. Edinburgh, *C. Elliot*, 1789
910. Cullen, William. The works. 2 vols. Edinburgh, *W. Blackwood*, 1827
911. Cullen, William (1827). As ref. 910 but p. 3
912. Fothergill, John. On a painful affection of the face. *Med. Obs. Inqu.*, 1776, **5**, 129–42
913. Fothergill, John. Remarks on that complaint commonly known under the name of the sick head-ach. *Med. Obs. & Inqu.*, London, 1777–84, **6**, 103–37
914. Fothergill, John. An account of the sore throat attended with ulcers. London, *C. Davis*, 1748

915. Fothergill, John. Observations on the weather and diseases of London. In his *Works*. London, 1783, **1**, 145–240
916. Cotugno, Domenico. De ischiade nervosa commentarius. Neapoli, *apud frat. Simonios*, 1764. English version, 1775
917. Frank, Johann Peter. De vertebralis columnae in morbis dignitate. In his *Delectus opusculorum medicorum*, Ticini, 1792, **11**, 1–50
918. Friedreich, Nicolaus Anton. De paralysi musculorum faciei rheumatici. Wirceburgi, 1797
919. Whytt, Robert. An essay on the vital and other involuntary motions of animals. Edinburgh, *Hamilton, Balfour & Neill*, 1751
920. Mead, Richard. A short discourse concerning pestilential contagion, and the methods to be used to prevent it. London, *S. Buckley*, 1720
921. Tennent, John. An epistle to Dr Richard Mead, concerning the epidemical diseases of Virginia, particularly, a pleurisy and peripneumony: wherin is shewn the surprising efficacy of the Seneca Rattle-Snake Root, in diseases owing to a viscidity and coagulation of the blood; such as pleurisies and peripneumonies these being epidemick, and very mortal in Virginia, and other colonies on the continent of America, and also the Lee-Ward Islands . . . by John Tennent. Edinburgh, P. Matthie, 1742
922. Tennent, John (1742). As ref. 921 but p. 5
923. Pringle, Sir John. Observations on the diseases of the army. London, *A. Millar & D. Wilson*, 1752
924. Pringle, Sir John. A discourse upon some late improvements of the means for preserving the health of mariners. London, *Royal Society*, 1776
925. Lind, James. A treatise of the scurvy. Edinburgh, *Sands, Murray & Cochran*, 1753. Reprinted Edinburgh, 1953
926. Lind, James. An essay on diseases incidental in Europeans in hot climates. London, *T. Becket & P. A. De Hondt*, 1768
927. Lind, James. An essay on the most effectual means, of preserving the health of seamen, in the Royal Navy. London, *A. Millar*, 1757
928. Brocklesby, Richard. Oeconomical and medical observations . . . tending to the improvement of military hospitals, and to the cure of camp diseases, incident to soldiers. London, *T. Becket & P. A. De Hondt*, 1764
929. Cook, James. The method taken for preserving the health of the crew of H.M.S. the Resolution during her late voyage round the world. *Phil. Trans.*, 1776, **66**, 402–06
930. Rush, Benjamin. Directions for preserving the health of soldiers: recommended to the consideration of the officers of the Army of the United States. Published by order of the Board of War. Lancaster, *John Dunlap*, 1778
931. Huxham, John. De morbo colico Damnoniensi. Londini, *S. Austen*, 1739
932. Huxham, John. An essay on fevers. London, *S. Austen*, 1750
933. Huxham, John. A dissertation on the malignant, ulcerous sore-throat. London, *J. Hinton*, 1757
934. Huxham, John. Opera physico-medica. Lipsiae, *J. P. Kraus*, 1764
935. Heberden, William, Snr. Αντιθηριακα; an essay on mithridatium and theriaka. (London), 1745
936. Watson, Gilbert. Theriac and mithridatium, a study in therapeutics. London, *Wellcome Historical Medical Library*, 1966
937. Brunschwig, Hieronymus. Liber de arte distillandi, 1512
938. Heberden, William (1745). As ref. 935 but p. 14
939. Heberden, William (1745). As ref. 935 but pp. 14–15
940. Heberden, William (1745). As ref. 935 but p. 19
941. Heberden, William, Snr. Of the night-blindness or nyctalopia. *Med. Trans. Coll. Phys. Lond.*, 1768, **1**, 60–63
942. Heberden, William, Snr. On the chickenpox. *Med. Trans. Coll. Phys. London.*, 1768, **1**, 427–36
943. Heberden, William, Snr. Some account of a disorder of the breast. *Med. Trans. Coll. Phys. Lond.*, 1772, **2**, 59–67
944. Heberden, William, Snr. De nodis digitorum. In his *Commentarii de morborum historia*. Londini, *T. Payne*, 1802, p. 130
945. Heberden, William, Snr. Commentarii de morborum historia et curatione. Londini, *T. Payne*, 1802

946. Heberden, William, Snr. Commentaries on the history and cure of diseases. 3rd edn., London, *T. Payne*, 1806

947. (Heberden, William, Snr.) Commentaries on the history and cure of diseases by William Heberden, MD with an introduction by Paul Klemperer. New York, *Hafner*, 1962

948. Heberden, William (1806). As ref. 946 but p. vii

949. Heberden, William (1806). As ref. 946 but p. 488

950. Hales, Stephen. A description of ventilators. London, *W. Innys*, 1743

951. Hales, Stephen. Statical essays, containing haemastaticks. Vol. 2. London, *W. Innys & R. Manby*, 1733

952. Menghini, Vincenzo. De ferrearum particularum sede in sanguine. *Bonon. Sci. Art. Inst. Acad. Comment.*, 1746, **2**, pt. 2, 244–66

953. Hewson, William. An experimental inquiry into the properties of the blood. Part III. A description of the red particles of the blood. London, *T. Cadell*, 1771

954. Hewson, William. Experimental inquiries: Part the second. Containing a description of the lymphatic system in the human subject and in other animals. Together with observations on the lymph, and the changes which it undergoes in some diseases. London, *J. Johnson*, 1774

955. Hewson, William. The works. Edited with an introduction and notes by G. Gulliver. London, *Sydenham Society*, 1846

956. Hoffmann, Friedrich. De metastasi sive sede morbo mutata. Halae, 1731

957. Morgagni, Giovanni Battista. De sedibus, et causis morborum per anatomen indagatis libri quinque. 2 vols. Venetiis, *typog. Remondiniana*, 1761. English trans. B. Alexander, 3 vols., London, 1769

958. Morgagni, Giovanni Battista (1761, but trans. of 1769). As ref. 957 but Vol 3, Book IV, pp. 196–199

959. Mann, Ronald David. Inhibitory aspects of the fibrinolytic system of human plasma. Thesis, MD, London, 1969, p. 60

960. Sandifort, Eduard. Observationes anatomicae-pathologicae. 4 vols. Lugduni Batavorum, *P. v. d. Eyk & D. Vygh*, 1777–81

961. Baillie, Matthew. An account of a remarkable transposition of the viscera. *Phil. Trans.*, 1788, **78**, 350–63

962. Baillie, Matthew. The morbid anatomy of some of the most important parts of the human body. London, *J. Johnson & G. Nicol*, 1793

963. Baillie, Matthew. The morbid anatomy of some of the most important parts of the human body. 2nd edn. London, *J. Johnson & G. Nicol*, 1797, vol. 2, p. 72

964. Baillie, Matthew. A series of engravings, accompanied with explanations, which are intended to illustrate the morbid anatomy of some of the most important parts of the human body. London, *W. Bulmer & Co.*, 1799–1803

965. Badham, Charles. Observations on the inflammatory affections of the mucous membrane of the bronchiae. London, *J. Callow*, 1808

966. Bonnet, Charles. Considérations sur les corps organisés. 2 vols. Amsterdam, *M. M. Rey*, 1762

967. Wolff, Caspar Friedrich. Theoria generationis. Halae ad Salam, *lit. Hendelianis*, 1759

968. Wolff, Caspar Friedrich. De formatione intestinorum praecipue. *Novi Comment. Acad. Sci. Petropol.*, 1768, **12**, 43–7, 403–507; 1769, **13**, 478–530

969. Baer, Carl Ernst von. Uber Entwicklungsgeschichte der Thiere. 3 vols. Königsberg, *Bornträger*, 1828–88

970. Baer, Carl Ernst von. De ovi mammalium et hominis genesi. Lipsiae, *L. Vossius*, 1827. English trans. *Isis*, 1956, *47*, 117–153

971. Roonhuyze, Hendrik van. Heel-konstige aanmerkkingen betreffende de gebreeken der vrouwen. Amsterdam, *weduwe van T. Jacobsz*, 1663. English edn. 1676

972. Mauriceau, François. Des maladies des femmes grosses et accouchées. Paris, *chez l'Auteur*, 1668. English trans. 1673

973. Deventer, Hendrik van. Operationes chirurgicae novum lumen exhibentes obstetricantibus. Lugduni Batavorum, *A. Dyckhuisen*, 1701

974. Smellie, William. A treatise on the theory and practice of midwifery. London, *D. Wilson*, 1752

975. Harvie, John. Practical directions, shewing a method of preserving the perinaeum in birth, and delivering the placenta without violence. London, *D. Wilson & G. Nicol*, 1767

976. Hunter, William. On retroversion of the uterus. *Med. Obs. Inqu.*, 1772, **4**, 400–09; 1776, **5**, 388–93

977. Hunter, William. On the uncertainty of the signs of murder, in the case of bastard children. *Med. Obs. & Inqu.*, London, 1784, **6**, 266–90

978. Hunter, William. Anatomia uteri humani gravidi tabulis illustrata. The anatomy of the human gravid uterus exhibited in figures. Birmingham, *John Baskerville*, 1774

979. Soemmerring, Samuel Thomas. Icones embryonum humanorum. Francofurti ad Moenum, *Varrentrapp u. Wenner*, 1799

980. Ould, Sir Fielding. A treatise of midwifry. Dublin, *O. Nelson & C. Connor*, 1742

981. Burton, John. An essay towards a complete new system of midwifery, theoretical and practical. London, *J. Hodges*, 1751

982. Leake, John. Practical observations on the child-bed fever. London, *J. Walter*, 1772

983. White, Charles. A treatise on the management of pregnant and lying-in-women. London, *E. & C. Dilly*, 1773

984. Hunter, John. The natural history of the human teeth. London, *J. Johnson*, 1771

985. Hunter, John. A practical treatise on the diseases of the teeth, intended as a supplement to the natural history of those parts. London, *J. Johnson*, 1778

986. Hunter, John. Account of a woman who had the smallpox during pregnancy, and who seemed to have communicated the same disease to the foetus. *Phil. Trans.*, 1780, **70**, 128–42

987. Hunter, John. A treatise on the venereal disease. London, 1786

988. Bell, Benjamin. A treatise on gonorrhoea virulenta, and lues venerea. 2 vols. Edinburgh. *J. Watson & G. Mudie*, 1793

989. Bertin, René Joseph Hyacinthe. Traité de la maladie vénérienne chez les enfans nouveau-nés, les femmes enceintes et les nourrices. Paris, *Chez Gabon*, 1810

990. Hunter, John. Observations on certain parts of the animal oeconomy. London, 1786

991. Hunter, John. On the digestion of the stomach after death. *Phil. Trans.*, 1772, **62**, 447–54

992. Hunter, John. A treatise on the blood, inflammation, and gun-shot wounds, by the late John Hunter. To which is prefixed, a short account of the author's life, by his brother-in-law, Everard Home. London, *G. Nicol*, 1794

993. Hunter, John (1794). As ref. 992 but pp. 87–88

994. Hunter, John. The works of John Hunter. With notes. Edited by J. F. Palmer. 4 vols. and atlas. London. *Longman*, (1835)–37

995. Hunter, John (1794). As ref. 992 but p. xlv

996. Hunter, John (1794). As ref. 992 but pp. lxi–lxiv

997. Cheselden, William. The anatomy of the humane body. London, *N. Cliff & D. Jackson*, 1713

998. Cheselden, William. Osteographia, or the anatomy of the bones. London, 1733

999. Pott, Percivall. A treatise on ruptures. London, *C. Hitch & L. Hawes*, 1756

1000. Pott, Percivall. Some few general remarks on fractures and dislocations. London. *L. Hawes, W. Clarke, R. Collins*, 1765

1001. Pott, Percivall. Observations on the nature and consequences of wounds and contusions of the head, fractures of the skull, concussions of the brain, etc. London, *C. Hitch & L. Hawes*, 1760

1002. Pott, Percivall. Practical remarks on the hydrocele or watry rupture. London, *C. Hitch & L. Hawes*, 1762

1003. Pott, Percivall. Chirurgical observations relative to the cataract, the polypus of the nose, the cancer of the scrotum, *etc.* London, *Hawes, Clarke & Collins*, 1775

1004. Pott, Percivall. Remarks on that kind of palsy of the lower limbs, which is frequently found to accompany a curvature of the spine. London, *J. Johnson*, 1779

1005. Albinus, Bernhard Siegfried. Tabulae sceleti et musculorum corporis humani. Lugduni Batavorum, *J. & H. Verbeek*, 1747

1006. Bichat, Marie François Xavier. Anatomie générale, appliquée à la physiologie et à la médecine. 4 vols. [in 2]. Paris, *Brosson, Gabon & Cie.*, an X [1802]. English trans. Boston, 1822

1007. Garrison, Fielding H. (1929). As ref. 179 but p. 347

1008. Scarpa, Antonio. Tabulae nevrologicae, ad illustrandum historiam anatomicam cardiacorum nervorum, noni nervorum cerebri, glossopharyngaei et pharyngaei ex octavo cerebri. Ticini, *apud B. Comini*, 1794

1009. Scarpa, Antonio. Memoria chirurgica sui piedi torti congenita dei fanciulli, Pavia, *G. Comini*, 1803. English trans. Edinburgh, 1818

1010. Scarpa, Antonio. Sull' ernie. Memorie anatomico-chirurgiche. Milano, *d. reale Stamperia*, 1809

1011. Cooper, Sir Astley Paston, Bart. The anatomy and surgical treatment of abdominal hernia. 2 pts. London, *Longman & Co.*, 1804–07

1012. Ramazzini, Bernardino. De morbis artificum diatriba. Mutinae, *A. Capponi*, 1700. English trans. 1705

1013. Süssmilch, Johann Peter. Die göttliche Ordnung in denen Veränderungen des menschlichen Geschlechts. Berlin, *D. A. Gohl*, 1742

1014. Frank, Johann Peter (1792). As ref. 918

1015. Frank, Johann Peter. De curandis hominum morbis epitome. Liber V. Mannheim, *C. F. Schwann & C. G. Goetz*, 1794

1016. Frank, Johann Peter. System einer vollständigen medicinischen Polizey. 9 vols. Mannheim, Tübingen, Wien, 1779–1827. Part English trans. 1976

1017. Frank, Johann Peter. De curandis hominum morbis epitome. 7 vols. (in 10). Mannhemii, Tubingae, Viennae, Taurini, 1792–1825

1018. Howard, John. The state of the prisons in England and Wales. Warrington, *W. Eyres*, 1777

1019. Tenon, Jacques René. Mémoires sur les hôpitaux de Paris. Paris, *P. D. Pierres*, 1788

1020. Howard, John. An account of the principle lazarettos in Europe. Warrington, *T. Cadell*, 1789

1021. Whytt, Robert (1751). As ref. 919

1022. Whytt, Robert. Observations on the nature, causes, and cure of those disorders which have been commonly called nervous hypochondriac, or hysteric, to which are prefixed some remarks on the sympathy of the nerves. Edinburgh, printed for *T. Becket and P. Du Hondt, London*, and *J. Balfour, Edinburgh*, 1765

1023. Garrison, Fielding H. (1929). As ref. 179 but p. 326

1024. Whytt, Robert. Observations on the dropsy in the brain. Edinburgh, *J. Balfour*, 1768

1025. Nicholls, Frank. Observations concerning the body of his late Majesty, October 26, 1760. *Phil. Trans.* (1761), 1762, **52**, 265–75

1026. Auenbrugger, Leopold, Edler von Auenbrugg. Inventum novum ex percussione thoracis humani ut signo abstrusos interni pectoris morbos detegendi. Vindobonae, *J. T. Trattner*, 1761. English trans. 1824

1027. Corvisart Des Marest, Jean Nicolas, Baron. Essai sur les maladies et les lésions organiques du coeur et des gros vaisseaux. Paris, *Métquignon-Marvis*, 1806. English trans. 1812

1028. Timoni, Emanuel. An account, or history, of the procuring of the smallpox by incision or inoculation, as it has for some time been practised at Constantinople. *Phil. Trans.*, 1714–16, **29**, 72–82

1029. Pylarini, Giacomo. Nova & tuta variolas excitandi per transplantationem methodus, nuper inventa & in usum tracta. *Phil. Trans.*, 1714–16, **29**, 393–99

1030. Garrison, Fielding H. (1929). As ref. 179 but p. 373

1031. Cartwright, Frederick F. (1977). As ref. 178 but p. 83

1032. Razzell, P. E. Population change in 18th. century England. In Drahe, M. (Ed.), Population in industrialization. London, *Methuen*, 1969, pp. 128–156

1033. Fisk, Dorothy. Dr. Jenner of Berkeley. London, *Heinemann*, 1959, p. 1

1034. Drewitt, F. Dawtrey. The life of Edward Jenner M.D., F.R.S., naturalist, and discoverer of vaccination. London, *Longmans*, 1931

1035. Wells, William Charles. On rheumatism of the heart. *Trans. Soc. Improve. Med. Chir. Knowl.*, 1812, **3**, 373–424

1036. Creighton, Charles. (1891–94, but 1965 reprint). As ref. 586 but Vol. II, p. 558

1037. Cartwright, Frederick F. (1977). As ref. 178 but p. 88

1038. Jenner, Edward. An inquiry into the causes and effects of the variolae vaccinae. London, *S. Low*, 1798

1039. Rush, Benjamin. The new method in inoculating for the small pox. Philadelphia, *C. Cist*, 1781

1040. Waterhouse, Benjamin. A prospect of exterminating the small-pox. 2 pts. Boston, *W. Hilliard*, (Cambridge, Mass., Univ. Press), 1800–02

1041. Baxby, Derrick. Edward Jenner, William Woodville, and the origins of vaccinia virus. *J. Hist. Med. Allied Sci.* 1979, **34** (2), pp. 134–162

1042. Baxby, Derrick. Jenner's smallpox vaccine, the riddle of vaccinia virus and its origin. London, *Heinemann*, 1981

1043. Coxe, John Redman. Practical observations on vaccination: or inoculation for the cow pock. Philadelphia, *J. Humphreys*, 1802

1044. Garrison, Fielding H. (1929). As ref. 179 but p. 372

1045. Swieten, Gerard L. B. van. Commentaria in Hermanni Boerhaave aphorismos, de cognoscendis et curandis morbis. 6 vols. Lugduni Batavorum, *J. & H. Verbeek*, 1742–76

1046. Swieten, Gerard L.B. van. Podagra. In his Commentaria in Hermanni Boerhaave aphorismos de cognoscendis et curandis morbis. Lugduni Batavorum, *J. & H. Verbeek*, 1764, **4**, 287–393. English trans. 18 vols., 1771–76

1047. Cadogan, William. A dissertation on the gout, and all chronic diseases, jointly considered, as proceeding from the same causes; what those causes are; and a rational and natural method of cure proposed. London, *J. Dodsley*, 1771. A reprint of the 10th edition of this essay appears in *Ann. Med. Hist.*, 1925, **7**, 67–90

1048. Landré-Beauvais, Augustin Jacob. Doit-on admettre une nouvelle espèce de goutte sous la dénomination de goutte asthénique primitive? Paris, *J. Brosson*, an VIII, (1800)

1049. Haen, Anton de. De cranii ustione. In Ratio medendi, Viennae Austriae, 1759, **6**, 264–72

1050. Holmstedt, Bo, and Liljestrand, Goran (1963). As ref. 626 but p. 55

1051. Withering, William. An account of the scarlet fever and sore throat, or scarlatina anginosa; particularly as it appeared at Birmingham in the year 1778. London, *T. Cadell*, 1779

1052. Withering, William. A botanical arrangement of all the vegetables naturally growing in Great Britain with descriptions of the genera and species according to Linnaeus. 2 vols. 1776. Botanical arrangement of British plants. 2nd edn., 3 vols., Birmingham, *Robinson*, 1787–1792. (Same) 3rd edn., 4 vols., Birmingham, The author, 1796. (Same) 4th edn., 4 vols., London, *Cadell & Davies*, 1801. (Same) 6th edn., corrected and considerably enlarged by William Withering, Jnr, London, *Cadell & Davies*, 1818

1053. Withering, William. An account of the foxglove, and some of its medical uses: with practical remarks on dropsy, and other diseases. Birmingham, *Robinson*, 1785. Facsimile, London, 1949. In German, 1786 and 1929

1054. Withering, William (1785). As ref. 1053 but reprint in Medical Classics, Vol. II, No. 4, 1937, Baltimore, *Williams & Wilkins*, 1937–38, pp. 294–439

1055. Withering, William (1785). As ref. 1053 but pp. 1–2

1056. Withering, William (1785). As ref. 1053 but pp. 2–3

1057. Withering, William (1785). As ref. 1053 but pp. 3–4

1058. Withering, William (1785). As ref. 1053 but p. 4

1059. Withering, William (1785). As ref. 1053 but p. 4

1060. Withering, William (1785). As ref. 1053 but pp. 12–16

1061. Withering, William (1785). As ref. 1053 but pp. 181–182

1062. Withering, William (1785). As ref. 1053 but p. 184

1063. Withering, William (1785). As ref. 1053 but p. 186

1064. Withering, William (1785). As ref. 1053 but pp. 191–192

1065. Cushny, A.R. William Withering, MD, FRS *Proc. R. Soc. Med.; Sect. Hist. Med.*, 1914–15, **8**, 85–94

1066. Cushny, A.R. (1914–15). As ref. 1065 but p. 94

1067. Osler, Sir William, Bart. Bibliotheca Osleriana. A catalogue of books illustrating the history of medicine and science, collected, arranged, and annotated by Sir William Osler, Bt. and bequeathed to McGill University. Oxford, *Clarendon Press*, 1929

1068. Hale-White, Sir William. The Withering letters in the possession of the Royal Society of Medicine. *Proc. R. Soc. Med.; Sect. Hist. Med.*, 1928–29, **22**, 1087–1091

1069. Hale-White, Sir William. Catalogue of the Withering letters drawn up by W. Hale-White in 1928. (Unpublished; a document in the possession of the Librarian, Royal Society of Medicine, London)

1070. Packard, Francis Randolph. History of medicine in the United States. 2nd edn. 2 vols. New York. *P. B. Hoeber*, 1931

1071. Sigerist, Henry Ernest. Amerika und die Medizin. Leipzig, *G. Thieme*, 1933. English trans. 1934

1072. Blanton, Wyndham Bolling. Medicine in Virginia in the seventeenth (eighteenth, nineteenth) century. 3 vols. Richmond, *W. Byrd Press; Garrett & Massie*, 1930–33

1073. Seward, Blanton P. Pioneer medicine in Virginia. *Ann. Med. Hist.* (New Series), 1938, X, 61–70; 169–188

1074. Seward, Blanton P. (1938). As ref. 1073 but p. 173

1075. Gibson, Thomas. Doctor Theodore Turquet de Mayerne's account of the illness, death and postmortem examination of the body of His Royal Highness, Prince Henry of Wales; translated from the French version in Browne's 'Opera Medica'. *Ann. Med. Hist.* (New Series), 1938, X, pp. 550–560

1076. Gibson, Thomas (1938). As ref. 1075 but p. 555

1077. Gibson, Thomas (1938). As ref. 1075 but p. 559

1078. Grieve, Mrs M. (1931). As ref. 124 but p. 147

1079. Woodville, William (1810). As ref. 129 but p. 357

1080. Woodville, William (1810). As ref. 129 but p. 357

1081. Schoepff, Johann David. Materia medica Americana, potissimum regni vegetabilis. Erlangae, *J. J. Palmii*, 1787

1082. Cullen, William (1789). As ref. 909 but Vol. II, p. 442

1083. Cullen, William (1789). As ref. 909 but Vol. II, p. 443

1084. Cullen, William (1789). As ref. 909 but Vol. II, p. 454

1085. Garrison, Fielding H. (1929). As ref. 179 but p. 402

1086. Garrison, Fielding H. (1929). As ref. 179 but p. 403

1087. Hoffmann, Friedrich (1718). As ref. 889

1088. Hoffmann, Friedrich. De genuina chlorosis indole, origine et curatione. Halis, 1731

1089. Hoffmann, Friedrich (1740–53). As ref. 890

1090. Lange, Johann. Medicinalium epistolarum miscellanea. Basileae, *J. Oporinus*, 1554

1091. Lettsom, John Coakley. Hints respecting the chlorosis of boarding schools. London, *C. Dilly*, 1795

1092. Marten, Benjamin. A new theory of consumptions: more especially of a phthisis, or consumption of the lungs. London, *R. Knaplock*, 1720

1093. Watson, Sir William. An account of what appeared on opening the body of an asthmatic person. *Phil. Trans.*, 1746, **54**, 239–45

1094. Home, Francis. An enquiry into the nature, cause, and cure of the croup. Edinburgh, *Kincaid & Bell*, 1765

1095. Bard, Samuel. An enquiry into the nature, cause and cure, of the angina suffocativa, or, sore throat distemper, as it is commonly called by the inhabitants of this city and colony. New York, *S. Inslee, & A. Car*, 1771

1096. Frapolli, Francesco. Animadversiones in morbum, vulgo pellagram. (Mediolani, *apud. J. Galcatium*), 1771

1097. Willan, Robert. On cutaneous diseases. Vol. 1. London, *J. Johnson*, (1796)–1808

1098. Müller, Otto Friedrich. Animalcula infusoria fluviatilia et marina, quae detexit, systematice descripsit et ad vivum delineari. Hauniae, *N. Mölleri*, 1786

1099. Fabbroni, Giovanni Valentino Mattia. Dell' arte de fare il vino. Firenze, 1787

1100. Gleichen, Willhelm Friedrich von (Russworm). Abhandlung über die Saamen- und Infusionsthierchen, und über die Erzeugung: nebst mikroskopischen Beobachtungen des Saamens der Thiere, und verschiedener Infusionen. Nürnberg, *A. W. Winterschmidt*, 1778

1011. Rouelle, Hilaire Marie. Observations sur l'urine humaine. *J. Méd. Chir. Pharm.*, 1773, **40**, 451–68

1102. Scheele, Carl Wilhelm. Undersökning om blåsestenen. *Kongl. Vetenskaps-Acad. Handl.*, 1776, **37**, 327–32. English trans. 1786

1103. Le Clerc, Daniel. Histoire de la médecine. A La Haye, *I. van der Kloot*, 1729. English trans. (of 1696 end.) 1699

1104. Friend, John. The history of physick: from the time of Galen to the beginning of the sixteenth century. 2 vols. London, *J. Walther*, 1725–26

1105. Anonymous. A new translation of the pharmacopoeia of the Royal College of Physicians of London, of the year 1787; with notes, critical and explanatory . . . together with Latin and English indexes. By an Apothecary. London, 1789

1106. (Pharmacopoeia of 1789). As ref. 1105 but p. vii
1107. (Pharmacopoeia of 1789). As ref. 1105 but p. ix
1108. Pereira, Jonathan, The elements of materia medica. 2 vols. London, *Longman*, 1839–40
1109. Grieve, Mrs M. (1931). As ref. 124 but p. 609
1110. BPC (1959). As ref. 499 but p. 804
1111. BP (1980). As ref. 79 but Vol. I, p. 469
1112. Plato. Phaedo. In Church, E. J. The trial and death of Socrates, London, *Macmillan*, 1896, pp. 211–213
1113. BPC (1934). As ref. 120 but p. 1007
1114. BPC (1934). As ref. 120 but p. 1083–1084
1115. Brockbank, William. Sovereign remedies, a critical depreciation of the 17th-century London Pharmacopoeia. *Med. Hist.*, 1964, **8,** 1–14
1116. Hamilton, James. Observations on the use and abuse of mercurial medicines in various diseases. Edinburgh, *Constable*, 1819
1117. BPC (1934). As ref. 120 but pp. 523–525

6

The Nineteenth Century

The understanding of disease and René Laennec

The nineteenth century saw a rapid expansion in most departments of knowledge; it was also characterized by a massive expansion in the size of the population. The century witnessed the final establishment of modern pharmacology; its medicine and surgery were transformed by the discoveries of inhalational anaesthesia and antisepsis. The nineteenth century understanding of the nature and cause of many diseases was revolutionized by the development of the cellular and germ theories and the discovery of the causative organisms of illnesses such as tuberculosis.

The Domesday Book estimate of the population of England was of about 1 500 000. The growth, although it increased steadily from the time of the Wars of the Roses, was so gradual that the population of Great Britain stood at only 10 505 100 at the time of the First English Census in 1801. Thus, it had taken some seven full centuries for the population to expand from about 1.5 to 10.5 million.

By 1821 the First UK Census showed an official population figure of 15 472 000. The Census of 1871 gave a figure close on 27.5 million. At the end of the century the population stood at 38 237 000 when it was counted in 1901. Thus, in the 80 years from 1821 to 1901 the population of Great Britain more than doubled and passed from 15.5 to over 38 million. The same rate of change continued into the present century but was of a totally different order than the slow, protracted growth which had typified the previous centuries.

Most of this growth took place during the life of Queen Victoria (1819–1901), Queen of the United Kingdom of Great Britain and Ireland from 1837 until her death and Empress of India from 1876. The Reform Bill of 1832 and the Abolition of slave owning in 1833 preceded the reign; the Industrial Revolution was virtually complete by the time in 1840 when the Penny Post was introduced, and the mid-part of the reign saw the passing of the Education Act of 1870.

The nineteenth century enclosed both the births and deaths of Charles Dickens (1812–1870), Charles Darwin (1809–1882) and Karl Marx (1818–1883). The inventions and developments of the century produced much of the environment familiar today; they included the miners' safety lamp (Davy) in 1815, McAdam's appointment as Inspector General of 1827 and the proliferation of macadamized roads, the growth of railways with Stephenson's Rocket in 1829, the development of the dynamo by Faraday in 1831, Brunel's transatlantic steamship in 1838, the iron, screw-driven steamship (also of Brunel) in 1844, Simpson's pioneering of the use of chloroform in 1847, Bessemer's steel making process of 1856, Bell's telephone of 1876, Parsons' steam turbine of 1884 and the Lanchester car and Marconi's wireless – both of 1895. If one imagines each of these discoveries and their later developments removed from the environment of today then, in the imagination, one has returned to a world something like that of the beginning of the nineteenth century – to the days of Trafalgar (1805), Waterloo (1815), and the mid-points of the lives of Turner, Constable, Wordsworth and Beethoven with the Industrial Revolution a little less than half-way complete.

In Britain the Industrial Revolution brought about changes typified by the steam engine, the railway train and the factory system. The process carried an agrarian society into the towns and cities and transformed its mobile segments into the modern industrial society. It occurred first in England, the crucial early stage coinciding with the French Revolution. The textile industry was the first to be industrialized, this industry usually being involved early as the process affected other countries. Thus, in the United States, Eli Whitney produced the cotton gin (1793) which more than trebled the amount of cotton a person could pick free from seeds in a day – the result was a vast increase in the cotton crop, from 1 500 000 lb in 1790 to 85 000 000 lb in 1810, as the beginnings of industrialization were adapted to the American situation.

The factory system, although there had been previous examples on a limited scale, grew out of and typified the growth of the textile industry. The changes, progressively affecting the lives of everyday people, required the development not only of industrial power but also of the means of transporting both raw materials and finished goods. From such needs arose the Stockton and Darlington railway (1825) in the North of England, designed to carry coal from the mines to the waterways, but which proved so immediately successful that within a few years England was covered by a network of railways. Steam was also applied to the transport of goods upon water and in 1807 Robert Fulton's steamboat was successfully used on the Hudson River. Despite this success it was many years before the steamship fully replaced the sailing vessel.

With these and a few additional exceptions the Industrial Revolution was confined to Britain during the period 1760–1830. In Germany, although there were vast reserves of iron and coal, industrial expansion did not really begin until the achievement of national unity in 1870. It then became linked with technological and scientific advances which enabled Germany to build a great chemical industry based on the discoveries taking place in the laboratories of the universities and organized industries.

Thus, the timing and character of the process of industrialization varied from country to country – but the ultimate effect has been to transform the lives of most populations in the Western World. Even though the pioneers of the change may have hoped that economic freedom would be achieved by both individuals and communities, this seldom took place. The average worker was employed for very long hours under miserable conditions which allowed only a few to escape from poverty. The town and city populations that endured these conditions were nourished by a rural work-force whose own habits and way of life had been almost equally changed. Considerable new problems of moral, physical and communal hygiene arose – and these provided many of the problems which nineteenth century medicine and science began to address.

Much of this early growth in medicine began in France, the century seeing not only the establishment of modern pharmacology by Magendi and Claude Bernard, but also the beginnings – largely in the hands of Corvisart, Bichat and René Laennec – of modern clinical medicine.

These men built upon an eighteenth century intellect typified at its best by Heberden and Withering. Although they have been previously mentioned, specific points made by these two pioneers in the attitudes of modern clinical pharmacology are worth revisiting – both men having written classical contributions which proved fundamental to nineteenth and twentieth century science.

Heberden's beautiful, slim treatise, *An essay on mithridatium and theriaca*, of 1745[935], includes the following passage containing a mid-eighteenth century teaching opposing the mixing of potent remedies with far less active substances[1118]:

> If our objections ftopped here, and thefe grand antidotes were only good for nothing; it would hardly be worth while to cenfure or take any notice of them: but we may juftly fear that their ufe is attended with a good deal of danger. As many people bufy themfelves with the practice of Phyfic, who are unqualified to know what they are doing; it may be advifable, for the fake of fuch as fall into their hands, to difcountenance a medicine, which, upon the tradition of it's fovereign virtues, or as a fudorific, is often applied at random, and, by means of the Opium, does much mifchief. But it's ufe may be of ill confequence not only in the hands of the vulgar, but even of a fkillful Phyfician; for Opium or any powerful drug, mixed up into an electuary with fo many other things, is againft all rules of pharmacy; the prefcriber lies too much at the mercy of the perfon who mixes the ingredients, whether what he gives for an ordinary dofe fhall not contain a dangerous or fatal quantity of opium: and indeed it is hardly to be expected, in fuch a multiplicity of ingredients, that the ufual dofe will contain a juft proportion of all of them, and of courfe the Phyfician will be greatly in the dark, whenever he prefcribes it.

Heberden's view, that such a practice is 'against all rules of pharmacy' is certainly true, but it is striking to see the danger of such poor science spelled out at this early date. The intellect that recognized this problem saw also the dangers of inadequately preserved, unstable formulations and wrote that[1119]:

> Laftly, this *farrago* is very apt to ferment; which fermentation, while it lafts, is faid to exalt the power of the Opium to a degree of ftrength three or four times as great as it had before; and a common dofe may by thefe means be fo much ftronger than was intended; which is a danger not commonly thought of nor eafily avoided, and cannot be balanced by any real virtues belonging to thefe medicines.

Heberden also strikes for the simple prescription, avoiding all unnecessary polypharmacy[1120]:

> Why then fhould we retain them any longer in our fhops? Can we not do every thing, that they can reafonably pretend to, in a much artfuller, fafer and

more fimple manner? I think that they are now chiefly given as Opiates and *Aromatics*; which intentions would furely be much better anfwered by mixing two or three of our many fpices, in which we fo far excell the Antients, with as much Opium added to every dofe as was thought proper; without loading a fick man's ftomach with fo many other ufelefs things, that muft accompany them, when given in the *Mithridatium* or *Theriaca*.

Withering's *An account of the foxglove, and some of its medical uses . . .* of 1785 describes the culmination of his experience with digitalis in the following paragraph[1121]:

> Let the medicine therefore be given in the dofes, and at the intervals mentioned above: – let it be continued until it either acts on the kidneys, the ftomach, the pulfe, or the bowels; let it be ftopped upon the firft appearance of any one of thefe effects, and I will maintain that the patient will not fuffer from its exhibition, nor the practitioner be difappointed in any reafonable expectation.

This paragraph follows that in which Withering has advised that the doses must be given paying considerable attention to the state of the pulse; it is of 'consequence not to repeat the doses too quickly, but to allow sufficient time for the effects of each to take place'[1122]. Thus, the intervals between doses are to be determined by the biological effect in the individual patient, the pulse being used as the sensitive and relevant indicator. In the paragraph quoted above what is probably the first account of dose-titration by biological effect appears – dosing being continued until either diuresis, nausea or vomiting, slowing of the pulse, or effects upon the bowel appear. Full digitilization having then been achieved, dosing is then to be reduced to maintenance levels. This account of the use of an essential but toxic drug with a narrow therapeutic ratio which varies from patient to patient is one of the great early landmarks of modern pharmacology.

The impetus then passed to France, and Garrison[1123] says that 'Up to the year 1850 and well beyond it, most of the advancements in medicine were made by the French. After the publication of Virchow's "Cellular Pathology" (1858), German medicine began to gain its ascendancy. The descriptions of new forms of disease, and the discoveries of anesthesia (1847) and antiseptic surgery (1867), were the special achievements of the Anglo-Saxon race.'

The arbitrary doctrines prevalent in continental medicine and the sanguinary and extreme methods of therapeutics in vogue at the beginning of the nineteenth century were typified by the views and practice of François Joseph Victor Broussais (1772–1838). Broussais graduated in medicine in 1803 and obtained his early surgical experience in the armies of Napoleon.

The reaction against these practices and the theorizing on which they were based came principally from Pierre Charles Alexandre Louis (1787–1872), who was the founder of medical statistics (as distinct from vital statistics), and René Théophile Hyacinthe Laennec (1781–1826, the most distinguished specialist in internal medicine of the early French school and one of the most important physicians in the history of medicine.

Pierre Louis based his practice upon incessant dissection, a factual and numerical expression of his observations, and a refusal to entertain speculative theory. Of his three important publications, the *Recherches anatomico-pathologiques sur la phthisie* (1825)[1124] was based on 358 dissections and 1960 clinical cases; there is an English translation by the Sydenham Society (1844) and this book not only described 'the angle of Louis' (the angle formed by the manubrium and the body of the sternum) but also showed the frequency of tuberculosis in the apex of the lung. His second work, *Recherches anatomiques, pathologiques et thérapeutiques sur la maladie connue sous les noms de gastroentérite; fièvre putride, adynamique, ataxique, typhoïde, etc.*[1125], was published in 1829 (English translation, 1836) and gave the first description of the rose-red spots characteristic of typhoid; the same studies provided the first satisfactory account of the pathological manifestations of this disease and gave it the modern name (fièvre typhoïde). The third work demolished the teachings of Broussais with a statistical demonstration that venesection is of little or no value in pneumonia; it is this study, the *Recherches sur les effets de la saignée dans quelques maladies inflammatoires, et sur l'action de l'émetique et des vésicatoires dans la pneumonie* (1835)[1126], which introduced statistical methods into medicine; this work, of which there is an English translation dated 1836, is therefore one of the fundamental texts of medical science.

The reason for the rise to such strength of the early French school is perhaps not too obscure. The idea that the anatomical alterations of organs or body structures in disease can be correlated with the clinical symptoms and signs during life had culminated in the splendid 1761 *De sedibus . . .*[957] of Morgagni. This concept established a new understanding of the nature of disease; in the minds of Bichat, Corvisart, and their colleagues pathology was brought to life. Baron Jean Nicolas Corvisart des Marest (1755–1821), whose translation of Auenbrugger's book on percussion resulted in the universal adoption of the technique, produced a work of 1806[1027] which provided the first full insight into cardiac symptomatology. Corvisart, who was the favourite physician to Napoleon, was the first to explain failure of the heart in mechanical terms and to describe dyspnoea of effort. Corvisart, half a century after Morgagni, perhaps looked for a student who could make an anatomical and pathological diagnosis in the living by understanding the physical signs arising from the internal organs still hidden from inspection.

Laennec enrolled in Corvisart's course at the Charité Hospital where these ideas were voiced. At the École Pratique he attended the lectures of Bichat (1771–1802; Figure 122) who seems to have been able to see beyond organs and their anatomy and pathology to understand the structure of the body in terms of the tissues which could be the seat of disease. He became the founder of tissue classification and pathology and of modern histology with the *Traité des membranes en général et diverses membranes en particulier* (1800)[1127]; of this work there is an English translation dated 1813. The functional approach to the problem was shown in the *Recherches physiologiques sur la vie et la mort*[1128], also of 1800 (English translation 1809). Bichat then produced the vitally important *Anatomie générale, appliquée à la physiologie et à la médecine* (of 1801)[1006] in which he showed how individual tissues, within organs, could be the site of disease (English version 1822). His five volume last work, unfinished at his death, was the *Traité d'anatomie descriptive* (1801–03)[1129] which began modern

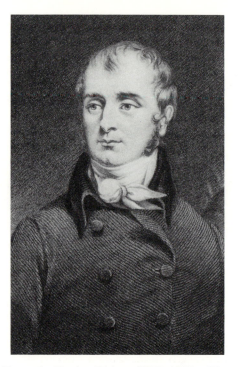

Figure 122 Marie François Xavier Bichat (1771–1802). [*From: Thomas Joseph Pettigrew (1838–40)*]

descriptive anatomy and which, in the volume of 1802, contains *Nerfs de la vie organique* introducing the concepts of the animal and vegetative systems. Bichat, as the originator of our understanding of the significance of the tissues as a site of the pathology of disease, made a contribution of the first order of importance.

The new attitude was fundamental to the thinking of René Laennec who attended Bichat's lectures and gained a lasting admiration for the intellect of their author. The translator of Laennec's own masterwork noted how far in advance of the facilities for the study of pathology in England, the schools of Paris had become in Laennec's formative years. Laennec's own achievement (a lesser one was the invention of the stethoscope in 1816) was to fuse the pathology of disease, in terms of both organs and tissues, with its physical manifestations – making diagnosis, unlike the generalizations of earlier generations, a display in which the hidden structure of the physical nature of the illness was revealed.

Laennec's *De l'auscultation médiate, ou traité du diagnostic des maladies des poumons et du coeur*[1130], published in Paris in 1819, was epoch-making. Auscultation, by instrumental means, began in the hands of Laennec as a stiff roll of paper applied to the chest to conduct sounds. It developed into the wooden stethoscope shown in Figures 1–6 of Plate 1 of the first 1819 edition of *De l'auscultation médiate . . .* ; of this historic edition Figure 123 shows the title page and Figure 124 illustrates Plate 1, giving the diagrams of the early stethoscope and a section of a cavitated tuberculous lung.

DE

L'AUSCULTATION

MÉDIATE

OU

TRAITÉ DU DIAGNOSTIC DES MALADIES

DES POUMONS ET DU COEUR,

FONDÉ PRINCIPALEMENT SUR CE NOUVEAU
MOYEN D'EXPLORATION.

PAR R. T. H. LAENNEC,

D. M. P., Médecin de l'Hôpital Necker, Médecin honoraire
des Dispensaires, Membre de la Société de la Faculté de
Médecine de Paris et de plusieurs autres sociétés nationales
et étrangères.

Μέγα δὲ μέρος ἡγεῦμαι τῆς τέχνης εἶναι
τὸ δύνασθαι σκοπεῖν.

Pouvoir explorer est, à mon avis, une
grande partie de l'art. HIPP., *Épid. III.*

TOME PREMIER.

A PARIS,

CHEZ J.-A. BROSSON et J.-S. CHAUDÉ, Libraires
rue Pierre-Sarrazin, n° 9.

1819.

Figure 123 René Théophile Laennec. Title page from: *De l'auscultation médiate...*
(1819).

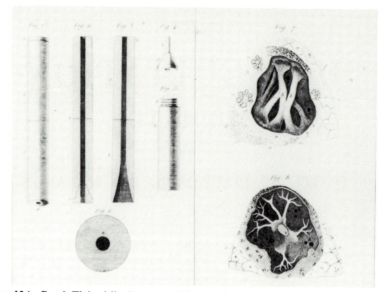

Figure 124 René Théophile Laennec. Plate I from: *De l'auscultation médiate...*
(1819).

Fig. 1.   This represents a section of the superior lobe of the lung, containing tubercles in different stages, and a vast tuberculous excavation. There are also, here and there, some pulmonary spots, more numerous between the excavation and top of the lung.

a.   Very large anfractuous excavation, produced by the softening of the tuberculous matter, which still lines it partially.

bb. Columnar bands crossing from one side of the excavation to the other, composed of the pulmonary tissue condensed, and covered with a thin layer of tuberculous matter.

cc.   Masses formed by the reunion of several immature tubercles, exhibiting, in the section of their substance, an indented appearance. The shaded parts represent the grey and semitransparent matter of the incipient tubercle, and the inner white portions point out the same where it has become yellow and opaque.

d.   The miliary granulations of M. Bayle.

ee.   Bronchial tubes opening into the excavation.

f.   Part of the exterior surface of the lungs.

Fig. 2.   A section of the upper lobe of the left lung, exhibiting a vast and very antient pulmonary fistula, traversed by obliterated blood vessels, and lined by a thin semi-cartilaginous membrane. Between this cavity and the top of the lung are seen spots of black pulmonary matter, tinging the substance of the lung quite black.

a.   Bottom of the fistula lined by the semi-cartilaginous membrane.

bbb.   Bronchial tubes opening into it.

ccc.   Obliterated blood vessels, crossing the cavity and then ramifying on its walls.

d.   Small excavations, or ulcerations, occupying only a portion of the thickness of the semi-cartilaginous membrane.

ee.   External surface of the lung.

396

T R A I T É

DE

L'AUSCULTATION

MÉDIATE

ET DES MALADIES

DES POUMONS ET DU COEUR,

Par R.-T.-H. LAENNEC,

Médecin de S. A. R. Madame duchesse de Berry , Lecteur et Professeur royal en Médecine au Collége de France , Professeur de Clinique à la Faculté de Médecine de Paris , Membre de l'Académie royale de Médecine, des Sociétés de Médecine de Stockholm , Bonn , Liége , et de plusieurs autres Sociétés savantes nationales et étrangères, Chevalier de l'ordre royal de la Légion-d'Honneur , etc.

Μίγα δὶ μίρος ἡγεῦμαι τῆς τίχνης εἶναι τὸ δύνασθαι σκοπεῖν.

Pouvoir explorer est, à mon avis, une grande partie de l'art. Hipp., Epid III.

SECONDE ÉDITION ENTIÈREMENT REFONDUE.

TOME PREMIER.

𝕻𝖆𝖗𝖎𝖘,

J.-S. CHAUDÉ, LIBRAIRE-ÉDITEUR,

RUE DE LA HARPE , N° 56.

1826.

Figure 125   René Théophile Laennec. Title page from: *De l'auscultation médiate...* (1826 edition).

The 1819 edition of this book transformed the study of diseases of the chest, but the second edition, of 1826[1131] (the title page forms Figure 125), was even more important. This edition described not only the various physical signs elicited in the chest but it added the diagnostic features, treatment, and underlying pathology of each of the diseases described. There is an English translation of the 1819 edition by John Forbes (1821)[1132] and this was reprinted (with an introduction by Paul Klemperer) in 1962. Laennec's account 'Of the essential, or anatomical, character of Tubercles of the Lungs' will serve to demonstrate the excellence of his knowledge of the morbid anatomy of the condition[1133]:

> The existence, in the lungs, of those peculiar productions to which the name of *Tubercles* has been restricted by modern anatomists, is the cause, and constitutes the true anatomical character, of Consumption.
>
> These bodies, when first observable in the substance of the lungs, have the appearance of small semi-transparent grains, greyish or colourless, and varying from the size of a millet seed to that of a hemp seed: in this, their first state, they may be called *Miliary Tubercles*. These gradually increase in size, and become yellowish and opaque, at first in the centre and successively throughout their whole substance. In their progressive and mutual increase, several unite together so as to form larger masses of the same kind, which, like the individual ones, are of a pale yellow, opaque, and of the consistence of very firm cheese: in this stage they may be named *crude* or *immature Tubercles*.
>
> It is in this stage of their progress that the substance of the lungs, which had been hitherto healthy, begins to grow hard, greyish, and semi-transparent around the tubercles, by means of a fresh production and seeming infiltration of tuberculous matter, in its first or transparent stage, into the pulmonary tissue. It also sometimes happens that considerable portions of the pulmonary tissue put on this character without any previous development of individual tubercles. Parts so affected are dense, humid, quite impermeable to air, and exhibit, when cut into, a smooth and polished surface. Gradually there are developed in these comparatively solid and pellucid masses, an infinity of very minute yellow opaque points, which, increasing in size and number, at length convert the whole diseased space into a tuberculous mass of the kind named *crude* or *immature*.
>
> In whatever mode the tubercles have first shown themselves, they at length, after a very uncertain period, become, first, softened, and finally liquefied. This change of consistence commences in the centre, and progressively approaches the circumference.
>
> In this stage the tuberculous matter is of two different kinds in appearance: – the one resembling thick pus, but without smell, and yellower than the immature tubercle; the other, a mixed fluid, one portion of it being very liquid, more or less transparent and colourless (unless tinged with blood), and the other portion opaque, of a caseous consistence, soft and friable. In this last condition, which is chiefly observable in strumous subjects, the fluid perfectly resembles whey having small portions of curd floating in it.
>
> When the softening of the tuberculous mass is completed, this finds its way into some of the neighbouring bronchial tubes; and as the opening is smaller than the diseased cavity, both it and the latter remain of necessity, fistulous, even after the complete evacuation of the tuberculous matter. It is extremely rare to find only one such excavation in a tuberculous lung. Most commonly the cavity is surrounded by tubercles in different stages of their progress,

which, as they successively soften, discharge their contents into it, and thus gradually form those irregular and continuous excavations so frequently observable, and which sometimes extend from one extremity of the lungs to the other.

Bands, composed of the natural tissue of the organ, condensed, as it were, and charged with the tuberculous degeneration, frequently cross these cavities, in a manner something resembling the *columnæ carneæ* of the ventricles: these are of less dimensions in their middle than at their extremities. These cross bands have often been mistaken for vessels; and M. Bayle himself seems to have fallen occasionally into this error, since, he says, that vessels *frequently* traverse such cavities; whereas this is, in my opinion, a very rare circumstance. Nay more, I have never even found a vessel of any consequence included within the substance of these bands. Neither is there any example of this in M. Bayle's work; and I only remember to have heard him mention one case where this took place, viz. in a fatal Hæmoptysis, where the ruptured vessel was found crossing a very large cavity. In the few cases where I have found blood vessels in such bands, they constituted only a small portion of their mass, and were, for the most part, obliterated. Generally, indeed, they can only be traced for a small space into these columns, being soon undistinguishable from the pulmonary tissue injected with the tuberculous substance. It would appear that the tubercles, during their increase, press on one side and separate the blood vessels, as we find these sometimes of considerable size, lining the internal surface of the cavities, and forming a part of them. These vessels are generally flattened, but rarely obliterated: their smaller ramifications, however, which stretch towards the tuberculous excavations, or towards unevacuated tubercles, are evidently so, as is proved by our abortive attempts to inject them. Baillie and Starck had already made the same observation. The ramifications of the bronchia, on the contrary, seem rather enveloped than pressed aside by the tuberculous matter; and it would appear that the pressure soon obliterates their canal, as they are hardly ever to be detected in the morbid substance. That they must, nevertheless, have originally traversed the spaces now occupied by the tubercles, seems proved by the fact, that in every excavation, even the smallest, we find one or more bronchial tubes opening into it. These tubes scarcely ever open sideways, but are cut directly across, on a line with the internal surface of the excavation; and their direction is such as shows them to have originally crossed this space.

In proportion as an excavation discharges its contents, its walls become covered with a species of morbid or false membrane, thin, smooth, white, nearly quite opaque, of a very soft consistence, and almost friable, so that it can readily be scraped off by the scalpel. This membrane is generally quite perfect, covering the whole internal surface of the cavity. Sometimes, in place of that just described, we find a membranaceous exudation, thinner, more transparent, less friable, more intimately connected with the walls of the cavity, and, for the most part, lining these only in part. When completely investing the cavity, it presents, in different parts of its surface, points here and there of greater prominence, as if the exudation had begun in these different spots at the same time. Frequently we find this second membrane beneath the first, which last is then quite loose and lacerated in several places. Occasionally, also, both these membranes are entirely wanting, and the walls of the cavity are directly formed by the natural tissue of the lungs, which, in this case, is commonly condensed, red, and charged with tuberculous degeneration in different stages of its development.

399

From these facts it appears to me that the second species of false membrane just mentioned is only the first stage of the first species; and that when this is fully formed it is apt to be detached and discharged in a greater or less degree, – forming one portion of the sputa expectorated by the consumptive.

Bayle thinks that this false membrane secretes the pus expectorated in this disease; – an opinion which is founded on the analogy existing between it and that which forms on the surface of blisters and ulcers. It seems certain, however, to me at least, that the greater part of the matter expectorated is the product of the bronchial secretion, augmented as this is by the irritated condition of the lungs. I do not assert that pus is not formed in these tuberculous excavations at all, but I certainly have observed that when these are lined by the soft membrane described above, they are often entirely empty, and that, when they do contain any puriform matter, this bears by no means so great a resemblance to the sputa, as that does which is contained in the bronchia.

If the disease remains long stationary, there are at length developed, in different points under this false membrane, patches of a greyish white colour, semi-transparent, of a texture like that of cartilage, but somewhat softer, and adhering closely to the pulmonary tissue. These patches coalesce as they grow in size, so as eventually to form a complete lining to the ulcerous excavation, and this lining seems to form one continuous surface with the internal coat of the bronchial tubes which open into it.

When this cartilaginous membrane is completely formed, it is commonly white or of a pearl-grey; or it has a slight reddish or violet tint, which latter colour is derived from the colour of the subjacent tissue being seen through it. Sometimes, however, even when the membrane is of considerable thickness, its internal surface is of a rose or red colour, which does not yield to washing, and which is therefore probably occasioned by the vascularity of the part, although, in such cases, we are unable to detect any distinct vessel.

In some very rare instances we find tubercles entirely, or almost entirely, softened, in a portion of lung in other respects quite healthy and crepitous; and, in such cases, (two or three of which only I have met with in eighteen years,) the walls of the cavity are smooth, and seem to be formed merely by the pulmonary tissue somewhat condensed, there being no accidental membranous production whatever.

Sometimes, but very rarely, the semi-cartilaginous membrane is perceptible before the softening of the tubercles, and, indeed, seems to be of the same date as themselves. This is the *encysted tubercle* of Bayle. The texture of these cysts is entirely cartilaginous, only a little less solid than cartilage, and they belong, therefore, to the class of *imperfect cartilages*, of which I have given an account in another place.* They adhere firmly, by their exterior surface, to the parts which surround them, so as only to be separable by the knife, or by forcible detraction. The tuberculous matter contained in these adheres strongly to their sides, which, when it is removed, are seen to be smooth and polished, though more or less uneven or rugged. These encysted tubercles are more frequent in the bronchial glands than in the substance of the lungs.

The above is the ordinary manner in which tubercles are developed; but there are two other modes which, although probably mere varieties of the former, are yet deserving notice. The one is where, in a lung containing tubercles in different stages, we find small portions of the pulmonary tissue seemingly infiltrated by a gelatinous-looking matter of a consistence inter-

* Dict. des Scienc. Med.

mediate between liquid and solid, transparent, and of a light greyish or sanguineous hue. In these diseased portions the cellular structure of the lung is quite destroyed; but we can perceive in them a multitude of very small points of a yellowish white colour and opaque, and which are evidently portions of the tuberculous matter which has reached the second stage of its progress, without there being any surrounding portion of the greyish substance which denotes the first stage.

The second mode of anomalous development of tubercles appears likewise to take place without any previous formation of grey matter: at least, if there be such, the transition from it to the second stage is so rapid that I have never been able to detect its presence. In this variety we find here and there in the lung tuberculous masses of a yellowish white colour, much paler, less clear, and differing less from the substance of the lung than the ordinary *immature* tubercle. These masses are irregular, angular, and have scarcely ever the rounded form of ordinary tubercles. They seem, like the variety described in the preceding paragraph, and like the diffused grey matter noticed before to be an infiltration of tuberculous matter into the pulmonary tissue, while the proper, or rounded, tubercles are foreign bodies which separate or press it aside, rather than penetrate it. These masses may, therefore, properly enough be named *tubercular infiltration of the lungs*. They occupy sometimes a considerable portion of one lobe. When they reach the surface they occasion no prominence on the part, nor in any degree alter its form. As they increase they assume the yellow colour of other tubercles, and terminate by softening in the same manner.

These three varieties of tuberculous degeneration are often found in the same lung. Sometimes I have found the last variety alone, in lungs affected with peripneumony, and this even in the *hepatised* portions. In these cases, the small number and extent of the diseased masses, and their deep pale colour, showed their formation to be recent. We must not, however, conclude that the tuberculous degenerations were here the effect of the inflammation, since – setting aside their infrequency compared with the frequency of this disease of the lungs – I have often had occasion to observe this variety of tubercle, and to the same extent, in subjects whose lungs were, in every respect, quite sound. Besides, M. Bayle has completely proved that tubercles cannot be regarded either as a termination, or consequence, of inflammation.

It cannot, indeed, be denied that peripneumony, both acute and chronic, sometimes co-exists with tubercles; it is even probable that this disease may, at one time, be the cause of their development in subjects predisposed to them, and at another, may itself be excited by the irritation produced by a numerous crop of these. Any person at all accustomed to the examination of bodies after death must admit these positions; yet it is, nevertheless, satisfactorily proved by a multitude of facts, that the growth of tubercles in the lungs most commonly takes place without any previous inflammation, and that, when inflammation is found contemporaneous with these, it is generally posterior in its origin.

To convince us of the truth of this observation, we have only to attend to the progress of tubercles in scrophulous glands, which we frequently find to remain swollen for a very long time, without the least redness, not only of the surrounding skin, but even of the gland itself. It is often not till after several years that inflammation comes on, which then seems to accelerate the softening of the tuberculous matter. Sometimes, however, this takes place, and the matter is even evacuated, without the supervention of what can properly be called inflammation. When this does occur it has evidently its seat in the tissues surrounding the scrophulous gland, and not in the gland itself.

Another proof, equally strong, of what has just been advanced, is afforded by, the simultaneous existence of tubercles in different organs of the same subject. In consumptive patients it is very uncommon to find the tubercles confined to the lungs: almost always they occupy the intestinal coats, at the same time, and are the cause of the ulceration and consequent diarrhœa so general in this disease. There is perhaps no organ free from the attack of tubercles, and wherein we do not, occasionally, discover them in our examination of phthisical subjects. The following are the parts in which I have met with these degenerations, and I enumerate them in the order of their frequency: the bronchial, the mediastinal, the cervical, and the mesenteric glands; the other glands throughout the body; the liver – in which they attain a large size, but come rarely to maturation; the prostate – in which they are often found completely softened, and leave, after their evacuation by the urethra, cavities of different sizes; the surface of the peritonæum and pleura, in which situations they are found small and very numerous, usually in their first stage, and occasion death by dropsy before they can reach the period of maturation; the epididymis, the vasa deferentia, the testicle, spleen, heart, uterus, the brain and cerebellum, the bodies of the cranial bones, the substance of the vertebræ or the point of union between these and the ligaments, the ribs, and, lastly, tumours of the kind usually denominated *schirrus* or *cancer*, in which the tuberculous matter is either intimately combined with, or separated in distinct patches from, the other kinds of morbid degeneration existing in these.

Tubercles are found more rarely in the muscles of voluntary motion than in any other part. The most remarkable case of this sort I have met with, was that of a consumptive patient who had. tubercles in almost every situation mentioned above, and who had, besides, the ureters so much dilated as to receive the thumb, and their internal coat converted into an adhesive layer of tuberculous matter. In this person the lower extremity of one of the sterno-mastoid muscles was converted into tuberculous matter, firm and consistent. In this case the muscular structure was still preserved in the parts most altered. In the parts least altered, and which passed by insensible gradation into the sound portion, the tuberculous matter was in its early stage, grey and semi-transparent. I had particularly attended to this man's case; he never complained of pain in the neck, but merely some difficulty in moving it. At the same time the cervical lymphatic glands were full of tubercles and much enlarged.

Almost all the cases given in M. Bayle's treatise, afford examples of the simultaneous development of tubercles in different parts of the body, without there being discoverable in the affected parts either pain or any symptom of inflammation. The same is true of the tubercles of the lungs, which scarcely ever occasion any disorder until they have become numerous and large.

From all this it follows, that we must either admit that tubercles are *not* a termination or a product of inflammation, or agree to receive this word in a sense as general and vague as that of *irritation*, or even to consider it as synonymous with *cause*: – a mode of proceeding which seems to possess no advantage whatever. There is sufficient obscurity already in the etiology of disease without augmenting this by forced relations. The above remarks respecting inflammation are equally applicable, as has been well shown by M. Bayle, to several other diseases, both general and local, which have been assigned as causes of consumption; – such, for instance, as Syphilis, Hooping Cough, Eruptions,

Hæmoptoe and Catarrh. These affections may accelerate the development of tubercles already existing; they may even sometimes be the occasion of their development, but this can only be in subjects primarily predisposed to them. The real cause, like that of all other diseases, is probably beyond our reach.

M. Bayle does not seem to have been well acquainted with the different modes of development of tubercles, as above described. This appears to be owing to his not having paid sufficient attention to the grey semi-transparent character of them in their early stage, and the true relation between these and the yellow opaque tubercles.

On the other hand, he has been, perhaps, too much struck with one variety of these tubercles, those, namely, which he has described under the name of *miliary granulations*. These are, no doubt, very remarkable by their want of colour, transparency, distinct round or oval shape, smooth and shining surface, great hardness, uniformity of size, and infinite number spread through the whole lungs, (healthy in other respects,) or a great part of them, without their being ever found united or grouped together. They look as if they had all been produced on the very same day, not one of them being more advanced than another.

M. Bayle has however evidently been deceived in considering these granulations as different from tubercles; still more so in classing them with morbid cartilaginous bodies (cart. accidentels). If this opinion were correct, we should see them occasionally converted into bone, which is never the case. But, indeed, an attentive examination shows them to be tubercles. In the centre of those least transparent we can discover a yellow opaque point, which is obviously the commencement of the passage to the second or mature stage. M. Bayle himself cites a strong example of this (case 4).

Besides, in some cases, we find the lungs completely filled with very small, equal-sized tubercles, but opaque, yellow, and occasionally in a well-marked state of maturation. M. Bayle gives also an example of this kind, (case 16), although he pretends to distinguish this variety from that of his *miliary granulations*. The only difference, in my opinion, between them, is the difference that exists between the green and ripe fruit. Besides, these miliary granulations are never found but in lungs which contain other and larger tubercles, whose advanced stage incontestibly proves their character.

The progress of tubercles in different organs affords a sufficient number of facts, to prove, that in their first and earliest stage, these foreign bodies are always diaphanous or semi-transparent, colourless, or at most slightly greyish. This is often the case with the tubercles observed on the surface of the pleura and peritonæum. On the contrary, these have sometimes an opaque yellow spot in the centre, and, on other occasions, they are converted into tuberculous matter more or less soft. All these varieties are observed on the same membrane. The same varieties of miliary tubercles are found in the bottom of the intestinal ulcers of consumptive patients. Lymphatic glands containing tubercles have often a slight degree of semi-transparency and pearl colour in the tissue surrounding these, a proof and sign of the ulterior degeneration of the whole gland. Bayle has found the spleen filled with small greyish bodies, which he himself considers as tubercles.

Besides the effect of the various degrees of development, other accidental causes may affect the colour of tubercles. Icterus renders them yellow, especially at the surface, and this is chiefly in the liver. Gangrene in their vicinity, and also the black pulmonary matter, blackens them in a greater or less degree. More especially those found in the bronchial glands are often tinged with a deep black, which is seen gradually fading into the natural colour of the tubercle. Most miliary tubercles, whether semi-transparent, or yellow and opaque, have a small dark spot in their centre, which disappears as they enlarge. This condition must not be confounded with *melanosis*, as will be shown more particularly hereafter.

When there exists a great number of tubercles, even very small ones, in the lungs, death will sometimes take place before any of them have arrived at the stage of maturation, and consequently before these can have formed any ulcerous excavation.

When, on the contrary, there is only a small number of tubercles, we sometimes find them all evacuated and hollow on examination after death. In the majority of cases, however, the development of tubercles is evidently successive, so that, on examination, we generally find these bodies in the different stages we have described, viz: 1. granular, grey or colourless, and semi-transparent; 2. grey, but larger, and yellow and opaque in the centre; 3. yellow and opaque throughout, but still hard; 4. soft, especially towards the centre; and, lastly, cavities more or less completely empty.

The whole of Laennec's book is marked by the factual, observational spirit of this quotation – given at some length because this is one of the prime texts of the beginning phase of modern medicine. In the same work Laennec gives this account of the historic discovery of the stethoscope[1134]:

In 1816, I was consulted by a young woman labouring under general symptoms of diseased heart, and in whose case percussion and the application of the hand were of little avail on account of the great degree of fatness. The other method just mentioned being rendered inadmissible by the age and sex of the patient, I happened to recollect a simple and well-known fact in acoustics, and fancied, at the same time, that it might be turned to some use on the present occasion. The fact I allude to is the augmented impression of sound when conveyed through certain solid bodies, – as when we hear the scratch of a pin at one end of a piece of wood, on applying our ear to the other. Immediately, on this suggestion, I rolled a quire of paper into a sort of cylinder and applied one end of it to the region of the heart and the other to my ear, and was not a little surprised and pleased, to find that I could thereby perceive the action of the heart in a manner much more clear and distinct than I had ever been able to do by the immediate application of the ear. From this moment I imagined that the circumstance might furnish means for enabling us to ascertain the character, not only of the action of the heart, but of every species of sound produced by the motion of all the thoracic viscera. With this conviction, I forthwith commenced at the Hospital Necker a series of observations, which has been continued to the present time. The result has been, that I have been able to discover a set of new signs of diseases of the chest, for the most part certain, simple, and prominent, and calculated, perhaps, to render the diagnosis of the diseases of the lungs, heart and pleura, as decided and circumstantial, as the indications furnished to the surgeon by the introduction of the finger or sound, in the complaints wherein these are used.

Laennec showed that all phthisis was due to tuberculosis and he became recognized as the greatest teacher and authority of the day on this subject. He clearly differentiated the clinical pictures of pneumonia, bronchitis in its various forms, and pleurisy; he also described pneummothorax and gave the classical account of chronic interstitial hepatitis ('Laennec's cirrhosis'). He suffered from the disease that he studied, dying from tuberculosis in 1826 but leaving behind him a body of work upon which the modern knowledge of diseases of the chest largely rests.

In the Place Saint-Corentin at Quimper there is a statue erected to the memory of Laennec in 1868 but his real memorials are the everyday terms of medicine which he invented ('pectoriloquy', sonorous and sibilant 'rales' and the like) and the splendid second (1826) edition of his book about which Garrison[1135] says 'the method is synthetic, each disease being described in detail in respect of diagnosis, pathology, and (most intelligent) treatment, so that this edition is, in effect, the most important treatise on diseases of the thoracic organs ever written.'

Unlike Auenbrugger's book, that of Laennec was rapidly taken up and widely translated. In Great Britain it was of great effect in the Irish school, several of whose physicians provided clinical accounts by which their names are still remembered. John Cheyne (1777–1836), one of the founders of the Dublin school of medicine, gave the first description of acute hydrocephalus (1808)[1136], wrote importantly on croup (1809)[1137], and in 1818 published *A case of apoplexy in which the fleshy part of the heart was converted into fat*[1138] – a work which gave the first accurate description of what is now known as 'Cheyne–Stokes respiration'.

Robert Adams (1791–1875), another of the founders of the Dublin school, gave a classical account of heart block with syncopal attacks (1827)[1139]. Thomas Spens (1764–1842) had reported what was almost certainly heart block in 1792[1140] but the credit for first satisfactorily describing this condition is usually given to Adams who also wrote of the palpable thrill from mitreal regurgitation and provided a reasonable record of tricuspid incompetence. In his *A treatise on rheumatic gout, or chronic rheumatic arthritis, of all the joints* (1857)[1141], Adams provided one of the most important accounts of these types of polyarthropathy.

Robert James Graves (1796–1853), another founder figure of the Irish schools of medicine, in 1835[1142] published so fine a description of exophthalmic goitre that the condition ('Graves' disease') has since been known by his name. He published *A system of clinical medicine*[1143] in Dublin in 1843 and this book, especially in its second edition of 1848, was widely admired and remains vivid and interesting.

Even before he had completed his medical qualification (at Edinburgh), William Stokes (1804–1878) demonstrated his understanding of the work of Laennec by publishing *An introduction to the use of the stethoscope* (1825)[1144]. He established a position of stature in the Irish schools of medicine with his *A treatise on the diagnosis and treatment of diseases of the chest*[1145], published in Dublin in 1837. After his notable paper (*Observations on some cases of permanently slow pulse*)[1146] of 1846 on heart block with syncopal attacks, this condition became universally known as the Stokes–Adams syndrome – a lasting tribute to the association of Stokes, who was a colleague of Graves at the Meath Hospital, and Adams, his companion at Dublin. The name of Stokes is also in current use, in the term 'Cheyne–Stokes respiration' which recalls the excellent account of periodic breathing given by Stokes in his *The diseases of the heart and aorta*[1147] of 1854.

The last of this extraordinary group who formed the early nineteenth century Irish school of medicine was Sir Dominic John Corrigan (1802–1880), author of the 1832 paper *On permanent patency of the mouth of the aorta, or inadequacy of the aortic valves*[1148]; this gives so lucid and clear an account of aortic insufficiency and the 'water-hammer pulse' that the sign has since become known as 'Corrigan's pulse'. Corrigan also recognized that the massive heart of aortic regurgitation represented a compensatory hypertrophy – thereby establishing a physiological principle of importance.

Bright, Addison and Hodgkin

The English clinicians of the early nineteenth century rapidly absorbed the ideas of Bichat and Laennec and began to look upon clinical medicine from the point of view of the pathology of disease in the living, correlating their findings during life with the morbid anatomy of the autopsy room.

Guy's Hospital enjoyed particular distinction in this process which represents the real establishment of modern medicine and the final release of the subject from the priestly tradition. The approach led to the clinical definition of many important conditions – Bright (Figure 126), Addison, and Hodgkin giving their

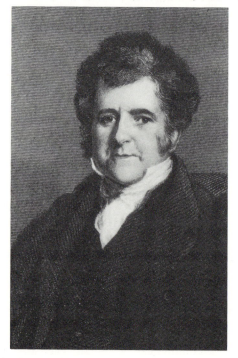

Figure 126   Richard Bright (1789–1858). [*From: Thomas Joseph Pettigrew (1838–40).*]

names to such important descriptions that they have provided some of the more permanent of medical eponyms.

Richard Bright (1789–1858), originally of Bristol, studied under Astley Cooper and James Currie and was physician to Guy's from 1820 to 1843. Just prior to this period William Charles Wells (1757–1817) became the first to observe the presence of blood and albumin in dropsical urine (*On the presence of the red matter and serum of blood in the urine of dropsy, which has not originated from scarlet fever*, 1812)[1149] and John Blackall (1771–1860) correlated albuminuria with dropsy, recording his findings in a work (*Observations on the nature and cure of dropsies*)[1150] of 1813 which also includes clinical accounts of cases of angina pectoris. Both of these works advanced the knowledge of dropsy beyond that available to William Withering but the epoch-making distinction between cardiac and renal dropsy, and the original description of essential nephritis was provided by Bright in his finely-illustrated *Reports of medical cases selected with a view of illustrating the symptoms and cure of diseases by a reference to morbid anatomy*[1151], published in two volumes in London in 1827–31. In this work Bright clearly associated dropsy, coagulable urine, and renal disease – showing that the latter was the cause of dropsy in some cases, whilst others were of cardiac origin. Bright described 24 'Cases illustrative of some of the Appearances observable on the Examination of Diseases terminating in Dropsical Effusion... and first of the Kidney', 11 cases in which the '... Dropsical Effusion has been connected with Disease of the Liver', and a further four cases '... where Disease connected with the Viscera of the Thorax has been followed by Dropsical Effusion.' The description of these 39 famous cases represents one of the greatest embellishments of English medicine and includes the classical account of chronic non-suppurative nephritis, or 'Bright's disease'. The following is part of Bright's original account of the three main types of morbid anatomical appearance seen in cases with albuminous or coagulable urine[1152]:

From the observations which I have made, I have been led to believe that there may be several forms of disease to which the kidney becomes liable in the progress of dropsical affection: I have even thought that the organic derangements which have already presented themselves to my notice, will authorise the establishment of three varieties, if not of three completely separate forms, of diseased structure, generally attended by a decidedly albuminous character of the urine. – In the *first*, a state of degeneracy seems to exist, which from its appearance might be regarded as marking little more than simple debility of the organ. In this case the kidney loses its usual firmness, becomes of a yellow mottled appearance externally; and when a section is made, nearly the same yellow colour slightly tinged with gray is seen to pervade the whole of the cortical part, and the tubular portions are of a lighter colour than natural. The size of the kidney is not materially altered, nor is there any obvious morbid deposit to be discovered. This state of the organ is sometimes connected with a cachectic condition of body, attended with chronic disease, where no dropsical effusion has taken place either into the cellular membrane or into the cavities of the body; I have found it in a case of diarrhœa and phthisis, and in a case of ovarian tumour. In the former it was connected with slight and almost doubtful coagulation of the urine by heat; in the latter I had omitted to examine the state of the urine. I also met with nearly the same condition of the kidney, with some opake yellow deposits interspersed through the structure, in the case of a man who died exhausted with diarrhœa brought on by hardships and intemperance, and in whose case the secretion of urine was very deficient, but whether coagulable or not I had no opportunity of ascertaining. When this disease has gone to its utmost, it has appeared to terminate by producing a more decided alteration in the structure; some portions becoming con-solidated, so as to admit of very partial circulation; in which state the surface has assumed a somewhat tuberculated appearance, the gentle projections of which were paler than the rest, and scarcely received any of the injection which was thrown in by the arteries. In this more advanced stage, if it be the same disease, dropsy has existed, and the urine has been coagulable (Sallaway).

The *second* form of diseased kidney is one in which the whole cortical part is converted into a granulated texture, and where there appears to be a copious morbid interstitial deposit of an opake white substance. This in its earliest stage produces externally, when the tunic is taken off, only an increase of the natural fine mottled appearance given by the healthy structure of the kidney; or under particular circumstances, gives the appearance of fine grains of sand sprinkled more abundantly on some parts than others. On making a longitudinal section, a slight appearance of the same kind is discovered internally, and the kidney is generally rather deficient in its natural firmness. After the disease has con-tinued for some time, the deposited matter becomes more abundant, and is seen in innumerable specks of no definite form thickly strewed on the surface; and on cutting into the kidney these specks are found distributed in a more or less regular manner throughout the whole cortical substance, no longer presenting a doubtful appearance, but most manifest to the eye without any preparation; and other cases less advanced, requiring maceration in simple spring water for a few days to render them more obvious. When this disease has gone on for a very considerable time, the granulated texture begins to show itself externally, in frequent slight uneven projections on the surface of the kidney; so that the morbid state is readily perceived even before the tunic is removed. The kidney is generally rather larger than natural; sometimes it is increased very much, but at other times it is little above the natural dimensions. Occasionally I have seen (Hobson) the kidney assume a good deal of the tuberous appearance observed in the advanced stage of the first disease, as shown in the representation of Sallaway's kidney: but then it has been manifest even by simple inspection, but much more so after maceration, that the whole is made up of small opake deposits. It is evident from the case of Hobson, that this state of kidney attended also with highly coagulable urine may exist without any marked appearance of anasarca.

The *third* form of disease is where the kidney is quite rough and scabrous to the touch externally, and is seen to rise in numerous projections not much exceeding a large pin's head, yellow, red, and purplish. The form of the kidney is often inclined to be lobulated, the feel is hard, and on making an incision the texture is found approaching to semicartilaginous firmness, giving great resistance to the knife. The tubular portions are observed to be drawn near to the surface of the kidney: it appears in short like a contraction of every part of the organ, with less interstitial deposit than in the last variety. This form of disease existed in a case from which I had a drawing executed about three years ago, it also existed in Bonham; and a most decidedly marked instance of it may be found in Stewart, where however the kidney was of a lighter colour than in the other cases, which were more of a purplish gray tinge. I believe the case of Smith belonged to the same. In most of these cases the urine has been highly coagulable by heat, at times forming a large curdled deposit, though in one case (Castles) where an approach to this appearance was found on the outside of the kidney, but with marked structural change in the liver, and with confirmed bronchial congestion, only a dense bran-like deposit of a brown colour was produced by the application of heat.

Although I hazard a conjecture as to the existence of these three different forms of disease, I am by no means confident of the correctness of this view. On the contrary it may be that the first form of *degeneracy* to which I refer never goes much beyond the first stage; and that all the other cases, including Sallaway, together with the second series, and the third, are to be considered only as modifications, and more or less advanced states of one and the same disease.

(In the above extract the names of some of the patients forming Bright's clinical cases have been left in, the numerical references to the finely-coloured plates of the volume being omitted.)

Bright's book established his reputation all over Europe and he became the principal medical consultant in the London of his day. He had a substantial clinical unit at Guy's and this contained not only wards but also consulting and examination rooms and a clinical laboratory. This was the first such unit in which pathology could be so intimately linked to the clinical picture of disease. But Bright should not be thought of as having only described glomerular nephritis and providing the differentiation between the cardiac and renal causes of dropsy: in *Cases and observations connected with disease of the pancreas and duodenum* (1832)[1153] he provided original accounts of pancreatic diabetes and pancreatic steatorrhoea. In 1836, in *Observations on jaundice*[1154], he gave the first description of acute yellow atrophy of the liver. In the same year (1836)[1155], in *Guy's Hospital Reports* (as with a number of his publications), he became the first to describe unilateral or 'Jacksonian' epilepsy. In papers of 1836 and 1840 he recorded his fully-developed views on *Cases and observations, illustrative of renal disease accompanied with the secretion of albuminous urine*[1156]. In 1836–39, in joint authorship with Thomas Addison who was teaching at Guy's at the same time, he published part of an *Elements of the practice of medicine*[1157] (which remained incomplete) and, after his death, in 1860, the New Sydenham Society published his *Clinical memoirs on abdominal tumours and intumescence*[1158].

Thomas Addison (1793–1860) – no clinician but a brilliant lecturer and pathologist – was not fond of drugs and, with John Morgan (1797–1847) wrote the first book in English on the effects of poisons on the living body; this work, of 1829[1159], was followed by a paper of 1837[1160] recording the first attempt to use static electricity therapeutically. Addison published in the *London Medical Gazette* of 1849 a historic paper *Anaemia: disease of the supra-renal capsules*[1161] which included the classical description of what has become known as pernicious or Addisonian anaemia; this account was given in the course of his record of the condition due to lesions of the adrenals now known as 'Addison's disease'. Addison's account of the anaemia 'incident to adult males' which 'usually occurs between the ages of twenty and sixty; sometimes proceeding to an extreme degree in a few weeks, but more frequently commencing insidiously...' continues[1161]:

Its approach is first indicated by a certain amount of languor and restlessness, to which presently succeed a manifest paleness of the countenance, loss of muscular strength, general relaxation or feebleness of the whole frame, and indisposition to, or incapacity for, bodily or mental exertion. These symptoms go on increasing with greater or less rapidity: the face, lips, conjunctivae, and external surface of the body, become more and more bloodless; the tongue appears pale and flabby; the heart's action gets exceedingly enfeebled, with a weak, soft, usually large, but always strikingly compressible pulse; the appetite may or may not be lost; the patient experiences a distressing and increasing sense of helplessness and faintness; the heart is excited, or rendered tumultuous in its action, the breathing painfully hurried by the slightest exertion, whilst the whole surface bears some resemblance to a bad wax figure; the patient is no longer able to rise from his bed; slight edema perhaps shows itself about the ankles; the feeling of faintness and weakness becomes extreme, and he dies either from sheer exhaustion, or death is preceded by signs of passive effusion or cerebral oppression. With all this, the emaciation or wasting of the body, though sometimes considerable, is not unfrequently quite disproportionate to the failure of the powers of the circulation – relaxation and flabbiness, rather than wasting of the flesh, being one of the most remarkable features of the disorder.

Addison had been preceded in his account of the anaemia by James Scarth Combe (1796–1883) whose paper was read on May 1st, 1822 and was published (*History of a case of anaemia*)[1162] in 1824. But it was Addison's lucid description which led to the condition becoming widely recognized. Anton Biermer (1827–1892) in 1872[1163] gave a fuller account of pernicious anaemia and became the first to describe retinal haemorrhages in the condition which, in continental Europe, is frequently known as 'Biermer's disease'. Addison's most singular claim to distinction is that he was the first to show the importance of the adrenal glands to clinical medicine, his full account of 'Addison's disease' being given in his monograph *On the constitutional and local effects of disease of the suprarenal capsules*[1164] published in London in 1855. Of this great work Garrison[1165] says: 'This book was regarded merely as a scientific curiosity in Addison's time, but it is now recognized as of epoch-making importance, since, in connection with the physiologic work of Claude Bernard, it inaugurated the study of the diseases of the ductless glands...'

Addison provided a number of other clinical descriptions and these are assembled in *A collection of the published writings*[1166], the tribute of the New Sydenham Society published in 1868.

The third of the great Guy's triumvirate was Thomas Hodgkin (1798–1866), a Quaker always seen in the traditional dress of the Society of Friends. Hodgkin, sensitive and markedly independent of spirit, described aortic insufficiency in 1828–29[1167], 3 years before Corrigan, but is more usually remembered for his paper *On some morbid appearances of the absorbent glands and spleen*[1168] of 1832. This provided the first proper account of the lymphadenoma which Wilks, in 1865, called 'Hodgkin's disease'. Hodgkin, much of whose later life was devoted to travelling, philanthropic works and reforming interests, was also an outstanding pathologist whose *Lectures on the morbid anatomy of the serous and mucous membranes* (1836–40)[1169] did a great deal to provoke interest in England on the tissues and their pathology.

One-third of the way through the nineteenth century the best of English medicine was both rational and based firmly on a sound basic knowledge of pathology. It was, however, bereft of the understanding of the nature of disease which was to come later in the century with the germ and cell theories and was, in the terms of practical therapeutics, markedly ineffective. The excellence of its gross pathology is shown by the *Illustrations of the elementary forms of disease*[1170] – a magnificent work of 1838, still unsurpassed, in which Sir Robert Carswell (1793–1857) provided an atlas containing plates selected from over 2000 water-colours painted and lithographed by his own hand. Carswell was professor of morbid anatomy at University College, London. The standard of illustration in Carswell's book was almost matched by Joseph Hodgson (1788–1869), of Birmingham, whose *A treatise on the diseases of arteries and veins* (1815)[1171] provides what Morton[1172] describes as 'the best illustrations of aneurysms and of aortic valvular endocarditis so far published and the first description of non-sacculated dilatation of the aortic arch (Hodgson's disease)'.

James Hope (1801–1841), an Edinburgh graduate who was later connected with St. George's, London, greatly advanced the knowledge of his generation regarding cardiology, cardiac murmurs, aneurysm and valvular disease. In *A treatise on the diseases of the heart and great vessels* (1832)[1173] he gave an account of what has been called 'Hope's early diastolic murmur' in mitreal stenosis. He provided also classical descriptions of cardiac asthma and cardiac neurosis and, in 1834[1174], published a fine atlas of pathology made from his own drawings.

William Charles Wells, physician to St. Thomas's Hospital, whose observation of coagulable urine has already been noted as preceding Bright's description of chronic nephritis, showed that the red colour of blood was not iron but the complex organic material later identified as haematin. This finding, of 1797[1175], came before the start of the nineteenth century and was followed by the famous *An essay on dew* (1814)[1176] which was a major contribution to physical science and the understanding of relative humidity and the means of artificial ventilation.

But if one wants to examine the medicine of the period just prior to the discovery of anaesthetics it is to the *Lectures on the principles and practice of physic*[1177], published in 1843 by Sir Thomas Watson (1792–1882) that one turns. In its successive editions this beautifully written book remained widely read for a quarter of a century. Watson's lectures were first published in the *Medical Times and Gazette* (1840–42) and are remarkable not only for their scope and style but also for their advocacy of the use of rubber gloves in order to achieve antisepsis. Watson also advised the cleansing of the hands in a solution of chloride of lime before obstetric deliveries were undertaken.

This valuable piece of tuition has its parallel in what is probably the most notable achievement of the so-called 'New Vienna School' of German medicine. Of this school, Josef Skoda (1805–1881) was the leading clinician. His main contribution is the *Abhandlung über Perkussion und Auskultation*[1178], published in Vienna in 1839, classifying the sounds obtained on percussion by their pitch and tone. There is a valuable English translation of 1853 – a work of importance as it is due to Skoda that percussion became widely used in clinical practice and that the usefulness of resonance as a diagnostic sign was understood. Skoda's colleague, also a Bohemian, was the pathologist, Carl Rokitansky (1804–1878). Rokitansky generated theories later dismissed with some force by Virchow but the best of his work is embodied in his *Die Defecte der Scheidewände der Herzens* (1875)[1179] in which, after 14 years devoted to the study of the subject, Rokitansky gave a brilliant account, still important, of defects of the septum of the heart. His other main work is the *Handbuch der pathologischen Anatomie* (1842–46)[1180], based on the vast number of autopsies performed by Rokitansky, and which establishes him as one of the great writers of modern times on gross pathology.

The major achievement of the German school was the insight obtained by Ignaz Philipp Semmelweis (1818–1865) into the nature of puerperal sepsis. Semmelweis, a Hungarian, was a pupil of both Skoda and Rokitansky. In 1846 he became assistant in the first obstetric ward of the Allgemeines Krankenhaus in Vienna. Semmelweis noted that the two obstetric wards differed in mortality rate, the worst being that in which students came straight from the autopsy room to examine the women patients. The cleanliness in the least afflicted of the wards largely resulted from its use for the instruction of midwives. In 1847 one of Rokitansky's assistants died following a minor wound obtained at dissection and Semmelweis noted that the postmortem appearances closely resembled those of the women who died following delivery. He then instituted hygienic procedures which dropped the mortality rate from 9.92 to 3.8% and convinced him that puerperal fever was a septicaemia. These conclusions were published in 1847–49[1181] and in the later *Die Aetiologie, der Begriff und die Prophylaxis des Kindbettfiebers*[1182] of 1861. The latter work, although badly presented, is one of the most important books of medical science and established Semmelweis as the pioneer of antisepsis in obstetrics. Sadly, his sensitive personality was unequal to the controversy provoked by his ideas and teaching and, after leaving Vienna and becoming professor of obstetrics in the University of Budapest, he ultimately died in an asylum on August 13th, 1865.

His first publication had been preceded by some 5 years by the appearance of a paper on *The contagiousness of puerperal fever*[1183] by Oliver Wendell Holmes (1809–1894). Holmes was the first to conclude that puerperal fever is contagious. In a series of views that stirred intense opposition amongst the orthodox obstetricians of Philadelphia, he taught that women in the lying-in period should not be attended by those who had been conducting postmortem examinations or been exposed to other such sources of infection, including other cases of puerperal fever. Holmes also insisted that the hands should be washed in a solution of calcium chloride and that the clothes should be changed after attending a case of the disease. He mentioned the similar precautions being taken by Semmelweis in his *Puerperal fever, as a private pestilence*[1184] published in Boston in 1855. The full development of Holmes's understanding of medicine and its history was written in his splended, widely-known *Medical essays: 1842–1882*[1185] which appeared, again in Boston, in 1883.

Holmes was adverse to the 'slavery of the drugging system' which characterized nineteenth century medicine just as it had formed a main part of the art of medicine throughout its history. In Germany, Christian F. S. Hahnemann (1755–1843), the founder of homeopathy, although developing a highly theoretical and non-objective system embodied in his *Organon der rationellen Heilkunde*[1186] of 1810, advanced views which became of great influence and did at least serve to oppose the polypharmacy and dangerously large drug doses of the day. In America, Jacob Bigelow (1786–1879), professor of materia medica at

Harvard, showed himself to be one of the greatest of medical botanists (*American medical botany*[1187] 1817-20); perhaps from his profound knowledge of the body's ability to restore health given appropriate and undamaging care, he was able to guide his own and later generations with his masterly *A discourse on self-limited diseases*[1188] of 1835. It is from Bigelow's *American medical botany*[1187] (Plate XI) that the illustration of the Hemlock (*Conium maculatum*) forming Figure 120 is taken.

The cell theory and Rudolf Virchow

The development of the cell theory was preceded by a sound nineteenth century knowledge of gross anatomy and an appreciation of the tissues as well as of the organs of the body. The leading British anatomist of the period, now more frequently remembered as a neurologist and physiologist, was Sir Charles Bell (1774-1842). Bell's *A system of dissections* (1799-1801)[1189] was published while he was still a student but it serves to summarize the anatomy of the early part of the century. He published on operative surgery in 1807-09[1190] and in 1811 brought out his *Idea of a new anatomy of the brain*[1191] which contains an initial reference to his early experimental work on the ventral spinal nerve roots. He published again on operative surgery in 1821[1192] the year before Magendie showed that the anterior spinal nerve roots have motor functions, whereas the posterior roots are sensory. Also in 1821, in an essay *On the nerves; giving an account of some experiments on their structure and functions...*[1193], he described the facial paralysis since known as 'Bell's palsy'. The culmination of his work came with the publication in 1830 of *The nervous system of the human body*[1194] which records his demonstration of the mixed sensory-motor function of the fifth cranial nerve.

Charles Bell became professor of surgery at Edinburgh in 1836 – a little before the publication of *The races of men* (1850)[1195] by the famed Edinburgh anatomist, Robert Knox (1791-1862). Knox was one of the best teachers of anatomy of the century and a devoted disciple of the methods of Bichat. He produced *A manual of artistic anatomy*[1196] in 1852 but is somewhat luridly remembered because of his association with the criminals who supplied material for his dissecting room. A landlord called William Hare, in November 1827, sold to Knox the body of an old man who had owed rent. Hare, and his associate Burke, seem after this event to have found the sale of dissecting material a useful means of providing themselves with funds. Knox, in the view of the townspeople, was implicated in these felonies; as a result of the subsequent outcry he fell from popularity and ended his life in obscure circumstances. His memorial, in one sense, is Lord Warburton's Anatomy Act of 1832 which, with suitable safeguards, made provision that unclaimed bodies should be made available to the medical schools.

The development of the cell theory, one of the cornerstones of modern biological science, was almost entirely the work of the botanists and microscopists. As early as 1665[768] Robert Hooke had first used the word 'cell' to describe a unit of histological structure. It was not until 1831 that the botanist, Robert Brown (1773-1858) discovered the cell nucleus; Brown also discovered the function of pollen in the replication of plants – announcing both of his observations in a paper *On the organs and mode of fecundation in Orchideae and Asclepiadeae*[1197] published in the *Transactions of the Linnean Society* 1829–32. Within a short time Rudolph Wagner (1805–1864) described the nucleolus (1835)[1198]

The importance of the cell nucleus was first fully realized by Matthias Jacob Schleiden (1804–1881) who, before becoming professor of botany in three centres in Germany had studied both law and medicine. Schleiden[1119] showed that plant tissues are composed of and developed from groups of cells. He emphasized the importance of the nucleus but failed to understand the process of cell division.

Theodor Schwann (1810–1882), professor of anatomy and physiology at Liège, discovered nucleated cells in animal tissues and, stimulated by contact with Schleiden, demonstrated the nucleus in the cells of many types of tissues of both plant and animal origin – thus establishing the basic similarity of all types of living tissues and going a long way towards the definition of the cell theory. In the same important work (*Mikroskopische Untersuchungen über die Uebereinstimmung in der Struktur und dem Wachsthum der Thiere und Pflanzen*)[1200] of 1839 he described the neurilemma, the 'sheath of Schwann'. There is an English translation of this fundamental text of biology dated 1847 and published by the Sydenham Society.

By the mid-century the cell theory was becoming well understood. Hugo von Mohl (1805–1872), in a work of 1851[1201] of which there is an excellent translation dated the following year, described cell division and provided informative drawings of the process in its simple appearances. In 1852, Robert Remak (1815–1865) became the first to show that the growth of new tissues came about by the division of existing cells[1202]. Remak, the first Jew to be given an academic appointment in a German university, discovered the non-medullated nerve fibres (the fibres of Remak) and published accounts of these structures in 1836[1203] and 1838[1204]. In 1844[1205] he became the first to describe the nerve ganglia of the heart and in 1855[1206] he published an important simplification of von Baer's classification of the embryonic germ-layers.

Perhaps the most inspiring character associated with the development of the cell theory and the modern understanding of the tissues was Jacob Henle (1809–1885). Henle was born near Nuremberg and, although of a Jewish family, became professor of anatomy at Zürich, Heidelberg, and then Göttingen. He was the first to describe the epithelia of the skin and intestines and to define the structure and function of columnar and ciliated epithelium; his classical researches on the epithelia appeared in publications of 1837[1207] and 1838[1208] and established his reputation as the master histologist of the Germany of his day.

The beginnings of the germ theory mingled with the understanding of cells and tissues as structures which could form the seat and cause of disease and Henle, in *Von den Miasmen und Contagien* (1840)[1209] laid down postulates regarding the relationships between micro-organisms and disease which served to prevent much confusion as the possible parasitic, causal and commensal roles of microbes became understood. Henle's fundamental contribution to bacteriology becomes evident from a reading of the English translation (1938) of this work on contagion.

His *Allgemeine Anatomie*[1210] of 1841 records his many histological discoveries of the period and contains his remarkably simple histological classification of the tissues. The tissues are considered from a physiological, functional point of view in addition to their microscopical anatomy and the work is the first major treatise of its kind. Its account of the demonstration of smooth muscle in the walls of arterioles is, of itself, important and provides a basis for the contemporary understanding of the action of many of the drugs which affect the cardiovascular system.

Between 1855 and 1871, Henle published the three volumes of the *Handbuch der systematischen Anatomie des Menschen*[1211] – usually considered one of the finest of the modern systems of anatomy. The work is illustrated diagrammatically by Henle and is of monumental importance.

Many structures of the body are described by Henle's name but none bring it into more frequent use than the 'loop of Henle' describing the functionally vitally important segment of the renal tubules. But to attach his name to one structure and allow the memory of his massive contributions to fade is something to be avoided. So much so, that Garrison provides one of his most notable judgements with the observation that: 'Altogether, the histological discoveries of Henle take rank with the anatomical discoveries of Vesalius.'[1212]

Another pioneer microscopist whose name is still in frequent use but whose contributions were of a breadth that is easily forgotten was Johann Evangelista Purkinje (1787–1869). Purkinje's graduation thesis of 1819[1213] from Prague was on subjective visual phenomena and earned him both the admiration of Goethe and the chair of physiology at Breslau. He was the first (1823)[1214] to classify fingerprints and gave (1825)[1215] the first description of the germinal vesicle in the embryo. In 1835[1216] he provided the classical paper on ciliary epithelial motion and in 1839 one of his students (Bogislaus Palicki)[1217] gave the first description of the 'Purkinje fibres' of the myocardium. Purkinje, the first to use the microtome, was also a pharmacologist of importance responsible for some of the early experiments (1829) on camphor, belladonna, stramonium and a number of other substances. He has an extensive *Opera omnia*[1218] dated 1918–73.

The cell theory can be considered to have reached many aspects of its ultimate expression in the work of Rudolph Albert von Kölliker (1817–1905). Kölliker, a Swiss who graduated from Heidelberg, was Henle's prosector at Zürich in 1843 and became professor of anatomy at Zürich 3 years later. In 1847 he was called to the chair at Würzburg and remained there throughout his remaining active life. He was one of the first to apply the cell theory of Schwann to descriptive embryology and in 1841[1219,1220] demonstrated the cellular origin of the spermatozoa. He provided an important study of smooth muscle (1848)[1221] and in the *Handbuch der Gewebelehre des Menschen*[1222] of 1852 he produced what amounts to the first formal textbook of histology. In 1849, with von Siebold, he founded the *Zeitschrift für wissenschaftliche Zoologie* which he edited for the next 50 years and built into the leading German organ of its science. He has a work of 1856[1223] which is of interest as showing the effects of poisons on muscular contraction and, with Heinrich Müller, he became (1856) the first to measure the action currents generated by contractile cardiac muscle[1224]. His great compass is shown by the appearance from his pen in 1861 of the first formal study of comparative embryology[1225] and – looking beyond the fully established cell theory to the mechanisms involved in cellular gene transmission – he anticipated the future by clearly suggesting (*Die Bedeutung der Zellenkerne für die Vorgänge der Vererbung*, 1885)[1226] that the cell nucleus can act as a transmitter of hereditary characteristics.

The cell theory had profound effects upon the study of embryology, effects which culminated in the work of Wilhelm His; it also provided the foundation upon which Rufolf Virchow built the modern knowledge of cellular pathology – an understanding as important as the germ theory to the practice of modern medicine.

Schwann, who formulated the cell theory, and his immediate successors, concentrated their attention upon the nucleus and cell wall and made little reference to the cell protoplasm. In January, 1839 Purkinje made the first attempt to generalize about the living groundwork or substance of cells; he used the word 'protoplasma', a term which had found a previous place in the religious literature in which it described 'the first created thing'.

By that time it was recognized that a plant cell contained a nucleus set in a viscous substance, now called protoplasm, the whole being usually enclosed in a readily demonstrable cell wall. Largely due to the brilliant work of the botanist, Ferdinand Julius Cohn (1828–1898), of Breslau, it was soon appreciated that the same was true of the animal cell – even if the cell wall was, in animal tissues, much less readily visible. Cohn, in publications of 1850[1227] and 1853[1228], after studying the protococcus, concluded that animal and vegetable protoplasm are analogous, if not identical, substances. In later years (1872, 1876)[1229] Cohn became renowned for his work in bacteriology, providing an influential morphological classification of bacteria. From the time of Cohn's publication of 1850 it was increasingly recognized that protoplasm is the essential living substance.

Attention then turned to the cell wall – so constantly present in plants and so frequently almost absent in animals. The first to suggest that an animal cell need not have a cell wall was Franz Leydig (1821–1908), professor of zoology at Tübingen and the first (1850) to describe the interstitial cells of the testis (Leydig cells)[1230]. Interest in the subject continued and almost at the end of the century, in 1895, Charles Overton (1865–1933), then at Zürich but later professor of pharmacology at Lund, following a careful study of the osmotic properties of living cells, advanced the theory that the cytoplasm was modified at the cell surface to form a cell membrane. Widespread acceptance of this theory and study of the characteristics of the cell membrane has been prolific in results of great importance to contemporary pharmacology. Charles Overton's other major contribution was the publication in 1901 of the lipid theory of narcosis[1231].

At first specimens for microscopical examination were prepared in the fresh state by being held between layers of vegetable pith and sliced with a razor. Effective staining techniques began with Joseph von Gerlach (1820–1896) whose transparent mixture of carmine, ammonia and gelatin (Gerlach's stain)[1232] was the first effective histological stain. Virchow did practically all his work with carmine although living in the era during which differential staining became established. The microtome, first used by Purkinje, was more widely introduced by Wilhelm His in 1866 but it was not perfected for another decade.

The master histologist was Maximilian Schultze (1825–1874), professor of anatomy at Halle and later successor to Helmholtz at Bonn. Schultz produced a new era in histology with three great monographs on the nerve-endings of the sense organs, specifically the internal ear (1858)[1233], the nose (1862, 1863)[1234] and the retina (1866)[1235]. He had a lasting effect on the cell theory with his essay of 1861[1236] in which he defined the cell as a mass of nucleated protoplasm, suggesting that the cell envelope or membrane is a physicochemical event possibly due to the effects of surface tension on the cell contents. The same essay showed the importance of successive divisions of the cell nucleus in the generation of the muscle fibre and settled the controversy regarding the place of the cell in muscle tissue. In his monograph *Das Protoplasma der Rhizopoden und der Pflanzenzellen*[1237] published in Leipzig in 1863 Schultze clearly used the word 'protoplasm' and showed that this is almost identical in all living cells. In a further study of the same year he provided the most accurate account of his time of the segmentation of the frog's egg[1238].

The discovery of the centrosome came in a publication of 1877 by Walther Flemming (1843–1905), professor at Prague and then Kiel[1239]. Flemming's slightly later work provided the classical study, beautifully and accurately illustrated, of cell division and karyokinesis. There is a translation (1965) of a major part of this piece of work of 1879 and 1880 (*Beiträge zur Kenntniss der Zelle und ihrer Lebenserscheinungen*)[1240] which ranks in importance with the contributions to the cellular doctrine of Schwann and Virchow. Flemming drew together and completed the fragmentary earlier observations of others and showed that the protoplasm comprises an active, contractile mesh-work (which he called 'chromatin') and an inert, semi-fluid interstitial material (achromatin). The impressive and precise drawings of cell types and cell division forming part of his great monograph illustrate one of the more important of the nineteenth century's texts in biology.

The expression of the interest in cellular and tissue structures reached, in terms of embryology, one of its highest points of accomplishment in the work of Wilhelm His (1831–1904), of Basel, Switzerland. The great work of His was on the origin and development of tissues (histogenesis) – achievements aided by a distinguished background and by His being able to number Remak, Virchow and Kölliker amongst his teachers. He was professor of anatomy, first at Basel and, from 1872 to 1904, at Leipzig.

In his early work His provided monographs on the histology of the lymphatics (1861)[1241] and lymphatic vessels (1863)[1242], the former of these two publications has illustrations drawn by His and showing his fine draughtsmanship. In 1865 he published a major paper[1243] which established the beginnings of his reputation as the greatest of all embryologists produced by the nineteenth century. In the same year his new classification of the tissues, a study based on histogenesis, appeared as *Die Häute und Höhlen des Körpers* (1865)[1244]; this work, on the tissue layers and spaces of the body, showed that the serous cavities of the organism arise in the mesoderm and are lined by a special membrane which His now called endothelial.

His, more than any other worker, was responsible for the introduction of an effective microtome (*Beschreibung eines Mikrotoms*, 1870)[1245] and from his use of this instrument developed the idea of mounting serial sections from which three-dimensional demonstration models were built. These models, giving an accurate picture of the tissues from one embryo, not only greatly aided the teaching for which His became well known but also eliminated many early errors derived from less systematic and representational studies. He has a work of 1874[1246] in which

ANATOMIE

MENSCHLICHER EMBRYONEN

VON

WILHELM HIS.

I.

EMBRYONEN DES ERSTEN MONATS.

ATLAS.
TAFEL I — VIII.

———————

LEIPZIG
VERLAG VON F. C. W. VOGEL
1880.

Figure 127 Wilhelm His. Title page from: *Anatomie menschlicher Embryonen.*
(1880–85).

the developing tissues and organs were compared to malleable tubes and plates – a concept which led to the subject of developmental mechanics.

In 1880–85 His produced what is possibly his masterpiece, the now famous *Anatomie menschlicher Embryonen*[1247], published in three parts and with a substantial atlas of which Figure 127 represents the title page and Figure 128 a typical plate showing the way in which, for the first time, the human embryo was studied as a whole. The atlas amply demonstrates the unrivalled nature of His's drawings of this period.

His remained distinguished as an anatomist and was one of the founders of

418

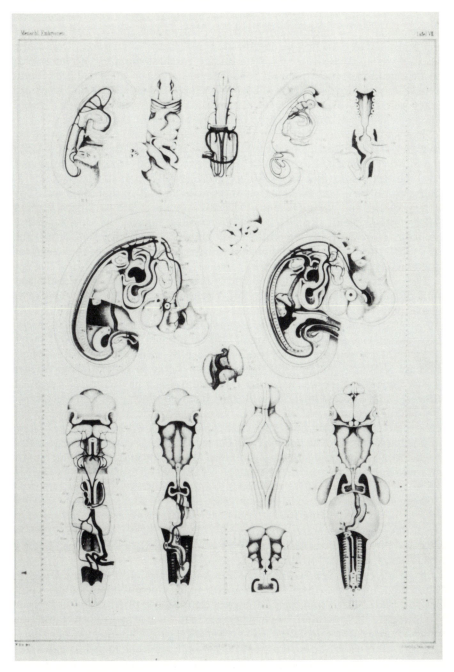

Figure 128   Wilhelm His. Plate from *Anatomie menschlicher Embryonen*. (1880–85).

the Anatomische Gesellschaft; in 1895 he wrote its report (*Die anatomische Nomenclatur*)[1248] so making himself largely responsible for the Basle Nomina Anatomica (BNA), the first standardized nomenclature of anatomy. One of the curiosities of his career arose from his interest in physiognomy. This led him to the identification of the remains of Johann Sebastian Bach which had been found in a coffin in the garden of the old Johanniskirche; His's studies and measurements were used to produce a bust, modelled by the sculptor Seffer, widely acknowledged as an immediately recognizable likeness of the composer.

The whole knowledge of embryology, as the nineteenth century became far advanced, was summarized by the brilliant Francis Maitland Balfour (1851–1882) whose two volume *A treatise on comparative embryology* (1880–81)[1249] appeared only shortly before Balfour, elected professor of animal morphology at Cambridge in 1882, was killed mountaineering in the July of that same year. The century closed and the new century began with the writings of 1892[1250] and 1912[1251] of Wilhelm Roux (1850–1924) whose interest in developmental mechanics (for which he coined the term 'entwicklungsmechanik') formed the basis for the beginnings of experimental embryology – a branch of the science of which he is regarded as the founder.

The greatest of pathologists and one of the towering figures in the establishment of modern medicine was Rudolf Virchow (1821–1902), the founder of cellular pathology. Born in Pomerania, Virchow graduated from Berlin in 1843 and in 1847 began the *Archiv für pathologische Anatomie und Physiologie*, known worldwide as 'Virchow's Archiv'. In 1849, having come into conflict with the governmental authorities, Virchow accepted the chair of pathological anatomy at Würzburg. In 1856, his reputation as an investigator and teacher already established, he was asked back to Berlin where he became professor of pathology and director of the Pathological Institute which had been created for him. He engaged in a wide range of professional activities but was also active in social affairs and was largely responsible for securing a workable sewage system for Berlin (*Ueber die Canalisation von Berlin*, 1868)[1252]; he was also responsible for bringing about the regular inspection of schoolchildren and for many improvements in the hygiene of schools – a subject on which he published in 1869[1253]. He remained active in politics, joining the Prussian Lower House in 1862 and serving in the Reichstag from 1880 to 1893. In advanced age he received many honours, dedicating the Pathological Museum with its vast collection of over 20000 specimens prepared by himself, in 1899. Shortly before his death he witnessed the completion (January, 1902) of the great Berlin municipal hospital which is now named after him.

In 1845, only a few weeks after the first description[1254] of leukaemia by John Hughes Bennett (1812–1875), Virchow independently published his report (*Weisses Blut*, 1845)[1255] on the postmortem examination of a case of leukaemia; Virchow gave this condition its current name and there is an English translation of this historic paper dated 1945. Still in the period before his move to Würzburg, Virchow published three papers (1847)[1256-1258] in the journal he had founded; the first of these (*Zur Entwickelungsgeschichte des Krebses*) provided a fine account of cancer and suggested that one of its exciting causes was local irritation.

Virchow was given, at Würzburg, the first chair of pathological anatomy in Germany. He spent the next few years applying the cell theory to morbid

420

CELLULAR PATHOLOGY

AS BASED UPON

PHYSIOLOGICAL AND PATHOLOGICAL HISTOLOGY.

TWENTY LECTURES

DELIVERED IN THE

PATHOLOGICAL INSTITUTE OF BERLIN

DURING THE

MONTHS OF FEBRUARY, MARCH, AND APRIL, 1858.

BY

RUDOLF VIRCHOW,

PUBLIC PROFESSOR IN ORDINARY OF PATHOLOGICAL ANATOMY, GENERAL PATHOLOGY AND THERAPEUTICS, IN THE UNIVERSITY OF BERLIN; DIRECTOR OF THE PATHOLOGICAL INSTITUTE, AND PHYSICIAN TO THE CHARITÉ HOSPITAL, ETC. ETC.

TRANSLATED FROM THE SECOND EDITION OF THE ORIGINAL,

BY

FRANK CHANCE, B.A., M.B. CANTAB.

LICENTIATE OF THE ROYAL COLLEGE OF PHYSICIANS; PHYSICIAN TO THE BLENHEIM FREE DISPENSARY AND INFIRMARY.

WITH

NOTES AND NUMEROUS EMENDATIONS, PRINCIPALLY FROM MS. NOTES OF THE AUTHOR,

AND

ILLUSTRATED BY 144 ENGRAVINGS ON WOOD.

LONDON:

JOHN CHURCHILL, NEW BURLINGTON STREET.

MDCCCLX.

Figure 129 Rudolf Virchow. Title page from: *Cellular pathology*... translated by Frank Chance (1860).

histology and building up evidence of the importance of the cell in all vital phenomena. Still only 28 years of age when he went to Würzburg, he published the first description of pulmonary aspergillosis in 1856[1259] (the year he returned to Berlin); in this same year he produced his *Gesammelte Abhandlungen zur wissenschaftlichen Medicin*[1260] which includes the paper on Weisses Blut and three later works on leukaemia.

In 1858, Virchow gave the name 'leukocytosis' to the condition first described by William Addison (1802–1881), author in 1843[1261] of a number of the early observations of blood corpuscles and by many accounted the first haematologist. In 1858 Virchow published one of his more important works, *Ueber die Natur der constitutionellsyphilitischen Affectionen* (republished as a book in 1859)[1262], a major study on the pathology of syphilis, in which he re-explored the knowledge that this disease ubiquitously affected all the organs and tissues of the body; Virchow's own study of the disease demonstrated that the causative agent of the disease was spread by the blood to the infected tissues.

The same year (1858) saw the publication of one of the great books of the history of medicine – Virchow's *Die Cellularpathologie in ihrer Begründung auf physiologische und pathologische Gewebelehre*[1263]; it is this work, published in Berlin, which established Virchow as the greatest figure in the history of pathology and the architect, with the exponents of the germ theory, of much of the modern understanding of disease. Of this epoch-making work, there is an English translation of 1860 (*Cellular Pathology as based upon physiological and pathological histology*)[1264] by Frank Chance, the title page of which provides Figure 129. With the knowledge of cell division at his disposal Virchow developed his doctrine *Omnis cellula e cellula* which declared that all cells arise from previously existing cells. This formed the basis for the series of lectures given in the Pathological Institute of Berlin during February, March and April 1858 which provided the substance of Virchow's book. Its Figure 3, early in the first lecture, showing some of the types of cells Virchow had recognized, is reproduced as Figure 130. Here is the passage in which he notes how each advance in medical

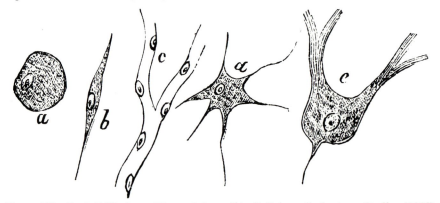

Figure 130   Rudolf Virchow. Figure 3 from *Die Cellularpathologie...* Berlin, (1858).

a. Hepatic cell. *b*. Spindle-shaped cell from connective tissue. *c*. Capillary vessel. *d*. Somewhat large stellate cell from a lymphatic gland. *e*. Ganglion-cell from the cerebellum. The nuclei in every instance similar.

understanding has begun with discoveries concerning the structures of the body – and moves from this to the recognition 'that the cell is really the ultimate morphological element in which there is any manifestation of life' [1265]:

> The present reform in medicine, of which you have all been witnesses, essentially had its rise in new anatomical observations, and the exposition also, which I have to make to you, will therefore principally be based upon anatomical demonstrations. But for me it would not be sufficient to take, as has been the custom during the last ten years, pathological anatomy alone as the groundwork of my views; we must add thereto those facts of general anatomy also, to which the actual state of medical science is due. The history of medicine teaches us, if we will only take a somewhat comprehensive survey of it, that at all times permanent advances have been marked by anatomical innovations, and that every more important epoch has been directly ushered in by a series of important discoveries concerning the structure of the body. So it was in those old times, when the observations of the Alexandrian school, based for the first time upon the anatomy of man, prepared the way for the system of Galen; so it was, too, in the Middle Ages, when Vesalius laid the foundations of anatomy, and therewith began the real reformation of medicine; so, lastly, was it at the commencement of this century, when Bichat developed the principles of general anatomy. What Schwann, however, has done for histology, has as yet been but in a very slight degree built up and developed for pathology, and it may be said that nothing has penetrated less deeply into the minds of all than the cell-theory in its intimate connection with pathology.
>
> If we consider the extraordinary influence which Bichat in his time exercised upon the state of medical opinion, it is indeed astonishing that such a relatively long period should have elapsed since Schwann made his great discoveries, without the real importance of the new facts having been duly appreciated. This has certainly been essentially due to the great incompleteness of our knowledge with regard to the intimate structure of our tissues which has continued to exist until quite recently, and, as we are sorry to be obliged to confess, still even now prevails with regard to many points of histology to such a degree, that we scarcely know in favour of what view to decide.
>
> Especial difficulty has been found in answering the question, from what parts of the body action really proceeds – what parts are active, what passive; and yet it is already quite possible to come to a definitive conclusion upon this point, even in the case of parts the structure of which is still disputed. The chief point in this application of histology to pathology is to obtain a recognition of the fact, that the cell is really the ultimate morphological element in which there is any manifestation of life, and that we must not transfer the seat of real action to any point beyond the cell.

The following is the expression of the doctrine that 'Where a cell arises, there a cell must have previously existed . . .' [1266]:

> Even in pathology we can now go so far as to establish, as a general principle, *that no development of any kind begins* de novo, *and consequently as to reject the theory of equivocal* [spontaneous] *generation just as much in the history of the development of individual parts as we do in that of entire organisms.* Just as little as we can now admit that a tænia can arise out of saburral mucus, or that out of the residue of the decomposition of animal or vegetable matter an infusorial animalcule, a fungus, or an alga, can be formed,

equally little are we disposed to concede either in physiological or pathological histology, that a new cell can build itself up out of any non-cellular substance. Where a cell arises, there a cell must have previously existed (*omnis cellula e cellula*), just as an animal can spring only from an animal, a plant only from a plant. In this manner, although there are still a few spots in the body where absolute demonstration has not yet been afforded, the principle is nevertheless established, that in the whole series of living things, whether they be entire plants or animal organisms, or essential constituents of the same, an eternal law of *continuous development* prevails. There is no discontinuity of development of such a kind that a new generation can of itself give rise to a new series of developmental forms. No developed tissues can be traced back either to any large or small simple element, unless it be unto a cell.

Virchow's book is notable for its mastery of the history of its subject and for its display of the vast increase in the knowledge of cellular and tissue pathology made by its author. *Die Cellularpathologie...* [1263] underlies the structural element of the modern understanding of disease to the degree that the great atlas of Vesalius underlies the modern view of gross anatomy. In a single volume Virchow had produced one of the greatest monuments of the nineteenth century.

Curiously, one of Virchow's mistakes was in relationship to the nature of carcinoma. In his *Die krankhaften Geschwülste* (1863–67) [1267], of which only three volumes were published, he advanced a theory of the connective tissue origin of carcinoma. This was disproved by Carl Thiersch (1822–1895), professor of surgery at Erlangen and inventor of the so-called Thiersch skin graft, who produced, in a publication of 1865 [1268], evidence strongly suggesting the epithelial cell origin of carcinoma. In work which led to the final recognition of Virchow's error, Heinrich Waldeyer-Hartz (1836–1921) demonstrated the epithelial origin of carcinoma (*Die Entwicklung der Carcinome*, 1867 and 1872) [1269].

The most distinguished of Virchow's pupils was Julius Cohnheim (1839–1884) who, despite his short life, became professor of pathology at Kiel, then Breslau, and then Leipzig. In 1863 he published the results of an important series of investigations on the sugar-forming ferments [1270]. His reputation established him as the finest experimental pathologist of the century, his most noted works being on inflammation (in which, in 1873, he showed the passage of leukocytes through the walls of the capillaries resulting in their accumulation at the site of injury [1271]), the bone marrow changes in pernicious anaemia (1876) [1272], and tuberculosis (which he proved to be contagious by successfully inoculating tuberculous material into the anterior chamber of the rabbit eye). The latter finding, ending a long period of controversy, appeared in *Die Tuberkulose vom Standpunkte der Infectionslehre* [1273] published in Leipzig in 1880. Cohnheim, in 1877–80, produced the *Vorlesungen über allgemeine Pathologie* [1274] which, apart from Virchow's *Die Cellularpathologie* [1263], was the most widely influential textbook on pathology of the century – its standing being such that a translation was published by the New Sydenham Society in 1889–90.

The last of the great pathologists and histologists of the century which saw both sciences shaped into their modern form was Carl Weigert (1845–1904) of Silesia. Weigert was the first to stain bacteria and in *Ueber Bakterien in der Pockenhaut* (1871) [1275] he not only demonstrated that carmine will stain cocci but also began investigations in haemorrhagic smallpox. These studies, in 1874–75, revealed the lesion produced by smallpox virus in the skin and showed the resulting 'coagulation necrosis'[1276]. In 1876 Weigert showed that methyl violet will demonstrate the presence of cocci in the tissues[1277]; his later studies much advanced the differential staining techniques used in the examination of the nervous system and led to a widespread appreciation of the usefulness of analine dyes in histopathology. Weigert is also remembered for his having produced the classical study of the morbid anatomy of Bright's disease (1879)[1278], for his provision of the first description of the pathological lesion in myocardial infarction (1880)[1279], and for his having first noted the connection between myasthenia gravis and hypertrophy of the thymus (1901)[1280].

Physiology and Claude Bernard

The pioneer experimental physiologist of the century and its founder experimental pharmacologist was François Magendie (1783–1855), of Bordeaux. A remorseless vivisectionist, Magendie nevertheless produced some of the more fundamental observations of modern times – he also produced the first modern textbook of therapeutics. As early as 1813 he produced what is now regarded as the classical study of the physiology of deglutition and emesis (*Mémoire sur le vomissement*)[1281]. In 1817 this was followed by the *Mémoire sur l'émétine, et sur les trois espèces d'ipecacuanha*[1282] which reported the isolation of emetine; a century later, at a time which coincided with the beginnings of the age of chemotherapy, Edward Bright Vedder (1878–1952), in a study of *Experiments undertaken to test the efficacy of the ipecac treatment of dysentery* (1911)[1283], demonstrated the amoebicidal effect of emetine. Vedder's work led to the widespread use of emetine in amoebic dysentery – a use which looked back at Megendie's isolation of the alkaloid.

In 1821, Magendie showed that the chemical differences between blood and tissue fluid result in osmotic effects at the vessel walls[1284]; he showed also that absorption of fluids and semi-solids is a function of the blood vessels and is not restricted to the lymphatics. In the same year he became the founder of the *Journal de physiologie expérimentale* which became of great influence in the development of its subject. In 1822, in a work which has been judged Magendie's greatest contribution to experimental physiology, he provided experimental proof of Bell's law, showing conclusively that the anterior roots of the spinal nerves are motor in function, whereas the posterior roots are sensory[1285].

To the pharmacologist of today Magendie's most important book was the *Formulaire pour la préparation et l'emploi de plusieurs nouveaux médicamens, tels que la noix vomique, la morphine . . .* of 1822[1286]. Magendie, always factual in his interests and always unable to develop theories or generalizations, was working soon after the original isolation of a number of the alkaloids. In his *'Formulaire . . .'* he gathered together the available information on many of these promising new substances. Thus, by means of this important book, he became the author who introduced morphine, veratrine, brucine, emetine, quinine and strychnine into the practice of medicine. The effect of the work was widespread, an English translation appearing in 1824.

In 1827 he gave the first satisfactory description of the cerebrospinal fluid[1287].

In 1839, in *Lectures on the blood*[1288], a volume published in Philadelphia, he performed the first formal experiments in anaphylaxis, showing that repeated injections of egg albumen killed rabbits which had been able to tolerate the initial injection. Edward Jenner, in 1798, had previously seen anaphylaxis in patients given smallpox variolation but these studies of Magendie represent the beginning of experimental immunology in its allergic aspects.

In his later major publications Magendie (*Phénomènes physiques de la vie*, 1842)[1289] carried his interest in physiology into the practice of clinical medicine, thus beginning a further improvement of the subject. His last substantial work, *Recherches physiologiques et cliniques sur le liquide céphalo-rachidien ou cérébro-spinal* (1842)[1290] represented a return to his old interest in the cerebrospinal fluid; it provided also the description of what has become known as the Foramen of Magendie.

Although Magendie can be regarded as the founder of organized experimental physiology in France, earlier experiments of this type had been undertaken. Julien Legallois (1770–1814), in 1801, the year in which he received his medical degree, produced a work in which he anticipated the idea of the body producing internal secretions[1291]. His subsequent studies, important but marked by brutal vivisection, showed that bilateral division of the vagus can result in fatal bronchopneumonia and that a small, carefully positioned, lesion of the medulla can inhibit breathing. These latter experiments began the understanding of the respiratory centre in the medulla. These findings were reported in the *Expériences sur le principe de la vie* (1812)[1292] by which Legallois is remembered.

The understanding of the *noeud vital* was completed by Marie Jean Flourens (1794–1867) who convincingly showed that asphyxia results from a lesion of the bilateral respiratory centre in the medulla oblongata. This was noted in the second edition (1842) of Flourens' *Recherches expérimentales sur les propriétés et les fonctions du système nerveux, dans les animaux vertébrés* of 1824[1293] – the same work provided experimental proof that vision depends on the intact state of the cerebral cortex. These observations had been preceded by a classical demonstration (1823)[1294] that removal of the cerebrum allowed the maintenance of reflex function but with the loss of cerebration and volition whereas ablation of the cerebellum produced disturbances of balancing and equilibrium. Thus, Flourens, who had conducted these experiments in pigeons, became responsible for the vital demonstration that the cerebrum is the part of the brain concerned with the processes of thought, the cerebellum being the organ maintaining control over the co-ordination of body movements, its lesions resulting in ataxia. In 1830[1295] Flourens showed that damage or destruction of the semicircular canals produces loss of equilibrium with section of an individual semicircular canal producing vertiginous motion around an axis relating to the ablated canal. Flourens thus inferred that both the cerebellum and the semicircular canals must be intact for proper motor co-ordination of movement to be possible. In a mid-century paper which attracted relatively little attention (*Note touchant l'action de l'éther sur les centres nerveux*, 1847)[1296] Flourens showed that chloroform had an anaesthetic effect very like that of ether. This startling observation actually slightly preceded Simpson's demonstration of the usefulness of chloroform.

Much of modern haemodynamics and perhaps more of the contemporary interest in blood viscosity began with the orderly and rather beautiful experiments of Jean Léonard Poiseuille (1799–1869). Poiseuille was the first since the clergyman Stephen Hales to add importantly to the knowledge of the physiology of the heart and circulation. Almost exactly a century after the original blood pressure experiment of Hales (1733), Poiseuille replaced the long glass tube which Hales had used with a mercury manometer connected to the artery by a hollow lead tip filled with potassium carbonate to prevent blood clotting. His graduation thesis (*Recherches sur la force du coeur aortique*, 1828)[1297] describes this 'haemo-dynamometer' with which he showed that the blood pressure varies with respiration. Poiseuille also measured the degree of arterial dilatation produced by the heart beat. There is an English translation of 1828.

Poiseuille's law, relating to the flow of liquids in tubes and fundamental to the modern studies of blood viscosity, arises from his *Recherches expérimentales sur le mouvement des liquides dans les tubes de très petits diamètres* of 1840[1298]. This work not only elaborates and defines the viscosity coefficient but shows Poiseuille as the inventor of the viscosimeter with which the early measurements on the viscosity of fluids were undertaken. In 1860 Poiseuille brought his studies of blood pressure and related subjects to fruition with his *Sur la pression du sang dans le système artériel*[1299].

The real importance of the vagus nerve was shown by the brothers Weber, of Wittenberg. Ernst Heinrich Weber (1795–1878), for a long period professor of anatomy and physiology at Leipzig, discovered the inhibitory effect of the vagus in a series of classical experiments in which he was associated with his brother, Eduard Friedrich Weber (1806–1871). The experiment involved electromagnetic stimulation between electrodes placed in the nostril of the frog and the spinal cord at the level of the fourth vertebra[1300]. Progressive narrowing of the field localized the inhibitory effect leading to the cessation of cardiac action. The vagi were shown to be the communicators of the inhibitory stimulus and, although later workers showed that the vagus contains acceleratory as well as inhibitory fibres, the understanding of the physiological actions of the vagus on the heart – as shown by the Webers – remains one of the classics of physiology. The work represents a beginning of our understanding of the autonomic nervous system – an understanding upon which much of modern therapeutics depends.

Ernst Weber published *Anatomia comparata nervi sympathici*[1301] in 1817 and *De aure et auditu hominis et animalium*[1302] in 1820. Both of these works advanced the application of the experimental method to the problems of physiology. The two brothers then published the famous *Wellenlehre*[1303], on the hydrodynamics of wave motion, for the first time measuring the velocity of the pulse wave, in 1825. This work showed that the pulse wave is slightly delayed in transmission – an understanding which ushered in much precise physical measurement in medicine; it was followed by Ernst Weber's *De pulsu, resorptione, auditu et tactu* (1834)[1304] which contains Weber's still-used hearing test. There has been a recent (1978) English translation – motivated perhaps by the fact that the work embodies Weber's law proposing that the intensity of sensation is not directly proportional to the strength of the stimulus. The findings were augmented by Gustav Fechner (1801–1887) in a way which produced the Weber–Fechner law[1305], approximated by the expression that the intensity of sensation varies with the logarithm of the stimulus: a hint of the insight given by the application of physics to biology, an approach followed by Ervin Ferry (1868–1956) who, in a paper on the *Persistence of vision* (1892)[1306], was able to further modify Weber's law.

The main English exponent of the experimental technique applied to physiology was Marshall Hall (1790–1857) who began his publications of note with a work of 1831[1307], in which he very clearly distinguished arterioles from venules and capillaries, but who is better known for the paper *On the reflex function of the medulla oblongata and medulla spinalis* (1833)[1308] in which he showed the difference between unconscious reflexes and volitional action. He used the term 'reflex action' – and this has found its own lasting place in the nomenclature of medicine. Hall also has an important work of 1851 on the neuro-muscular transmission of epilepsy[1309] and in 1856 he gave a description of one of the earlier methods of artificial respiration[1310].

The first English medical school fully to recognize the importance of physiology to medicine was University College, London, where William Sharpey (1802–1880) became the first incumbent of the newly-created chair in anatomy and physiology. Sharpey has an interestingly illustrated paper *On a peculiar motion excited in fluids by the surfaces of certain animals* (1830)[1311] – a work of importance in the early understanding of cilia and ciliary motion. He is perhaps more famous for his having been the first to devote his whole career to physiology – and for the excellence of his teaching which produced graduates of the calibre of Michael Foster, Burdon-Sanderson and Schäfer.

England's other distinguished physiologist was Sir William Bowman (1816–1892) whose two part essay *On the minute structure and movements of voluntary muscle* (1840, 1841)[1312] provided the classical description of striated muscle. 'Bowman's capsule', as part of the glomerulus of the kidney, was described, in relationship to the uriniferous tubule, in the essay *On the structure and use of the Malpighian bodies of the kidney*[1313] published in the *Philosophical Transactions* in 1842. The other anatomical structure which carries Bowman's name is the ciliary muscle (Bowman's muscle) – for he was the first to make major improvements to ophthalmic surgery in England. His splendid *Lectures on the parts concerned in the operations on the eye, and on the structure of the retina*[1314], of 1849, gave the first good description of the microscopical anatomy of the eye. This was followed by a work of 1852 describing further advances in its subject[1315] and an attempt to make an artificial pupil. He provided also the first scientific attempt at treating lachrymal obstructions and disorders (1857–59)[1316].

In Germany some aspects of the progress of the first part of the nineteenth century, the period of 30 or so years which saw the beginnings of modern scientific medicine and great intellectual strides made in physiology and medicinal chemistry, were represented by the work of Justus von Liebig (1803–1873) who, in 1831, discovered both chloroform and chloral. The publication of these discoveries came in 1832[1317]. Chloroform was independently discovered by Liebig, Guthrie and Soubeiran. Samuel Guthrie (1782–1848) produced a paper announcing a *New mode of preparing a spirituous solution of chloric ether*[1318] in 1832. This involved the production of chloroform by distilling alcohol with chlorinated lime; it also gave the drug the name 'chloric ether'. The *Recherches sur quelques combinaisons du chlore*[1319] of Eugène Soubeiran (1793–1858) appeared in 1831, but it is difficult to determine who actually first discovered chloroform.

Liebig, in 1842, published a work on the processes of nutrition – a book which greatly increased understanding of the importance of metabolic studies in scientific physiology[1320]. Somewhat sadly, Liebig's preoccupation with the chemical and material aspects of physiology led him to miss the living, organic aspect of the processes of fermentation and putrefaction – processes which he believed to be only catalytic and chemical. He has a well-known publication[1321], dating from 1853, 20 years before his death, in which he gives a fine account of what is now known as Liebig's method of estimating urea.

Friedrich Wöhler (1800–1882), an associate of Liebig, crowned the achievement of the early German chemists by both synthesizing urea and demonstrating that benzoic acid, after ingestion, appears as hippuric acid in the urine. Both of these findings are of fundamental importance. The synthesis of urea by heating ammonium cyanate was reported in *Ueber künstliche Bildung des Harnstoffs* (1828)[1322] and was the first time that an organic compound had been made from inorganic starting materials. As such it showed that there is no essential chemical difference between the components of living and inanimate things. The discovery thereby provided the basis for the splendid successes of Emil Fischer and the later synthetic chemists. The second great discovery began in 1824 and was confirmed in 1842 (*Umwandlung der Benzoësäure in Hippursäure im lebenden Organismus*)[1323]. It was this work that Wöhler demonstrated that benzoic acid, taken in the diet, is excreted in the urine as hippuric acid. This observation showed that animals can synthesize complex organic materials and do not have to take these into the body preformed by plants or other animals. Other examples of chemical synthesis by animal tissues soon came to light, Wöhler's observation providing an entry to the modern understanding of animal metabolism.

The beginnings of the modern knowledge of the physiology of digestion came from the work of two American and one English investigators. John Richardson Young (1782–1804) showed that the gastric juice flowed at the same time as the saliva. He also showed the essential principle of the gastric juice to be an acid, but incorrectly thought it to be phosphoric acid. This work, *An experimental inquiry into the principles of nutrition, and the digestive process*[1324], was published in Philadelphia in 1803. Young's error was corrected by William Prout (1785–1850) who proved that the acid of the gastric juice is free hydrochloric acid. Prout's now well-known study *On the nature of the acid and saline matters usually existing in the stomachs of animals*[1325] appeared in *Philosophical Transactions* in 1824. It was followed by one of medicine's more remarkable small books – the *Experiments and observations on the gastric juice, and the physiology of digestion*[1326], published in 1833 by William Beaumont (1785–1853), a surgeon in the United States Army. Beaumont, whose studies began in a remote field outpost in the forests of Michigan, describes an incident in which part of the anterior upper abdominal wall and diaphragm of a Canadian half-breed, Alexis St. Martin, was blown away by the discharge of a musket. He then gives an account of the surgical care over several months of this patient who survived, despite initial prolapse of part of the left lung into the wound, but was left with a gastric fistula. By means of a long series of careful experiments Beaumont showed that gastric juice flows, not continuously, but in response to food and that mechanical stimulation of the stomach and its mucous membrane produces only congestion. Beaumont at one stage had to bring Alexis St. Martin back almost 2000 miles from one of his travels so that the studies could continue – but he used his opportunities to such good effect that he was able to determine the action of gastric juice on various types of foodstuffs, thereby beginning much of the modern knowledge of dietetics. His studies of the chemistry of the juice convinced him that it contained hydrochloric acid and another substance active in the process of digestion. Theodor Schwann (1810–1882) showed the latter agent to be pepsin (*Ueber das Wesen des Verdauungsprocesses*, 1836)[1327].

Physiology, in the first half of the nineteenth century, began the process which, in the last half of the century, produced the successes of Helmholtz, Claude Bernard, and Carl Ludwig. Hermann von Helmholtz (1821–1894), born in Potsdam, ultimately became professor of physiology and pathology at Königsberg and then holder of the chairs of anatomy and physiology at Bonn, physiology at Heidelberg, and physics at Berlin. He was to some extent preceded by the resonance theory of Albrecht von Haller (1747)[897] and the theory of hearing of Guichard Joseph Du Verney (1648–1730) whose publication on the subject was dated 1683[1328].

From these beginnings, Helmholtz, already trained as a physician, became the master mathematical physicist of the age. Early in life he published his important essay *Ueber die Erhaltung der Kraft, eine physikalische Abhandlung* (1847)[1329] which gave universal application to the fundamental doctrine of physics concerned with the conservation of energy. This essay established the first law of thermodynamics that all modes of energy are capable of transformation between one another but are otherwise both indestructible and impossible of creation. In a publication of 1848 Helmholtz, using isolated preparations, showed that the muscles are the principal source of animal heat[1330]. In 1850 he reported measurements of the velocity of the nervous impulse[1331]. In 1851 he announced the invention of the ophthalmoscope[1332] – an event which began a new era in ophthalmology. In 1852 he published his theory of colour vision[1333] and in 1854–55 wrote an account of the mechanism of accommodation[1334], the latter subject being studied with the ophthalmometer which he had devised in 1852. In 1863 he published one of his masterpieces, *Die Lehre von der Tonempfindungen als physiologische Grundlage für die Theorie der Musik*[1335] – this provided Helmholtz's theory of hearing, a proposal upon which the modern theories of resonance are based; there is an English translation (1875) of the third edition of this work – and it shows him as both a physicist of enormous capability and as a cultured and sensitive musician. There is also an English translation (1874) of his later work of 1869[1336] which includes a description of what has come to be called 'Helmholtz's ligament' of the malleus; the book gives a fine account of his studies on the working of the middle ear and the processes of hearing.

The first to found a physiological laboratory in the United States (1871) was Henry Pickering Bowditch (1840–1911), whose laboratory was at Harvard. Bowditch was also the first to establish the 'all-or-nothing' principle[1337] of the contraction of cardiac muscle; in *Note on the nature of nerve-force* (1885)[1338] and a later paper of 1890[1339] he reported the indefatigability of nerve – a point contested[1340] by Julius Bernstein (1839–1917).

The beginnings of the neuron theory lie in the experimental studies of Augustus Volney Waller (1816–1870) of Elverton Farm, Kent. These works were reported in *Experiments on the section of the glossopharyngeal and hypoglossal nerves of the frog, and observations of the alterations produced thereby in the structure of their primitive fibres* (1850)[1341]. Waller showed that if a nerve was cut the axis-cylinders in the distal stump would soon degenerate, while the nerve fibres in the proximal segment would survive much longer. He inferred that the nerve cells nourish the nerve fibres. Waller also demonstrated that section of the anterior spinal nerve root caused degenerative changes showing that the parent cells of the motor fibres lie in the spinal cord; division of the sensory, posterior spinal root showed that the parent cells of the cut axons lay in the posterior root ganglia.

The gross functioning of some of these nervous pathways was then shown by Friedrich Leopold Goltz (1834–1902), a pupil of Helmholtz and professor of physiology at Halle then Strassburg. Goltz did important work on shock, vagal inhibition, and the functioning of the semicircular canals but his most informative work was on the effects of sectioning major central nervous system pathways. In 1869 he studied the frog following excision of either the brain or spinal cord[1342]. Garrison[1343] gives this account of the findings:

> He showed how the decerebrated or "spinal" frog will hop, swim, jump out of boiling water, croak like the frogs in Aristophanes, and adjust itself mechanically to every stimulation, but will otherwise sit like a mummy and, though surrounded with food, die of starvation, because it is a spinal machine, devoid of volition, memory, or intelligence. If the optic thalami remain intact, the animal will show some intelligence in regard to its own nutrition and sexual instinct; but ablation of the cerebral hemispheres in the dog is followed by restless movements, unintelligent response to stimuli, and inability to feed itself or to swallow.

The higher in the evolutionary scale the animal, the greater were the effects of decerebration: the most profound effect resulting from amentia in man. Goltz reported his work on dogs in 1874[1344] and 1892[1345]. He managed to keep a dog alive for about 8 months after subtotal decerebration and showed such animals incapable of purposive movement but capable of fairly satisfactory locomotion and co-ordination. With Ernst Ewald (1855–1921) he showed, in 1896[1346], that impregnation of the bitch was possible after severance of the spinal cord. Garrison summarized the meaning of these studies with the following[1347]:

> Goltz's exposition of the "spinal" animal as a brainless mechanism which, in Bernard Shaw's phrase, "blunders into death," and of the animal deprived of its spinal cord as a conscious intelligence with lessened power of coördination and adaptation, initiated much of the work of recent times upon the complex reflexes of the body.

The understanding of the more detailed functioning of the nervous system was sketched in by a number of workers. These included Ludwig Türck (1810–1868) who, in 1851, showed that degeneration in an axon shows the direction in which it conducts impulses, ascending tracts degenerating above the site of section and descending tracts below it[1348]. Türck then provided (1868) the results of his vitally important investigations into the cutaneous distribution of the successive pairs of spinal nerves[1349]. Charles Edouard Brown-Séquard (1817–1894), in a set of elegant studies published in 1863[1350], described the pathways of conduction in the spinal cord; the stimuli he examined included touch, vibration, pain, temperature and the like. The British investigator, Sir Charles Scott Sherrington (1857–1952) showed the association of the lateral horn cells with the sympathetic outflow (1892)[1351] and the features of the proprioceptive system (1906)[1352]. Sherrington did much to advance understanding of the reflex arc but he also studied re-enforcement and antagonism in both simple and compound reflexes; his unusual and subtle understanding of the nervous system emphasized its linking and integrating function, uniting the reflex and voluntary capabilities of the whole organism.

The greatest of all figures of nineteenth century physiology was Claude Bernard (1813–1878; Figure 131). He was born in Saint Julien in the Rhône, the son of a winemaker of the region. In Paris he became an associate of Magendie; he was one of the most brilliant and gifted of experimental physiologists and was the originator of the technique of producing disease by chemical or physical manipulation: thus, he is virtually the founder of those branches of experimental pathology and medicine which have been indispensible to the later progress of science. He discovered (1848) the glycogenic function of the liver[1353] and, in 1849, the digestive action of the pancreatic juice[1354]. In the next year he published *Chiens rendus diabétiques*[1355], reporting that experimental puncture of the fourth ventricle produced glycosuria. In 1852 he announced the discovery of the vaso-motor nerves[1356]. He continued his work on the sympathetic system with a further report of 1854[1357] and then, in 1855, produced *Leçons de physiologie expérimentale appliquée à la médecine*[1358] which, amongst many experiments, noted his catheterization of a dog's heart. His work on the glycogenic function of the liver and the essential part played by this organ in the processes of digestion led, in 1855, to the concept of the 'internal secretions' and the understanding that the body can synthesize as well as break down complex organic substances during metabolism[1359].

The famous work of Claude Bernard on motor nerve endings paralysed with curare appeared in 1856[1360] and proved the excitability of muscle functionally separated from its nerve; it provided the classical demonstration of the correctness of von Haller's doctrine of irritability; it offered also the beginnings of knowledge on the structure and function of the motor end-plate and the actions of the neuromuscular blocking agents, such as curare. Bernard's demonstration of the action of curare in stopping the transmission of the impulse from the motor nerve to the voluntary muscle that it serves is given in a paper on the *Analyse physiologique des propriétés des systèmes musculaires et nerveux au moyen du curare*[1361] published in 1856. He continued to work on pharmacological subjects and many aspects of physiology for much of his life and in 1857 published an extensive study of the effects of poisonous substances and drugs[1362].

In 1858[1363] he reported one of his major achievements – the discovery of glycogen – and in the same year produced the two volume *Leçons sur la physiologie et la pathologie du système nerveux*[1364]. The latter work contained his description of the lesion of the cervical sympathetic which is now known as 'Horner's syndrome'. The modern name for the condition traces its origin to the report *Ueber eine Form von Ptosis* (1869)[1365] of Johann Horner (1831–1886).

1858 also saw the publication of Bernard's discovery of the separate vasodilator and vasoconstrictor elements of the vasomotor system and the

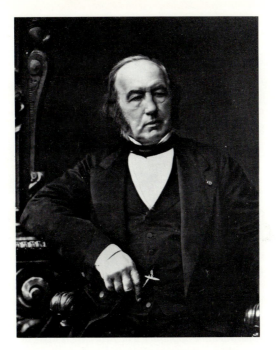

Figure 131   Claude Bernard (1813–1878).

explanation of the way in which these nerves regulate the supply of blood to the structures of the body[1366]. Keenly aware of the importance of the vasomotor system in the functioning of the digestive tract, Bernard, in 1864, reported the results (the 'paralytic secretions') brought about by sectioning the glandular nerves[1367].

Rewards for his achievements came somewhat later than might have been expected. Eventually, during the lifetime of Magendie, a chair in physiology was created for Bernard at the Sorbonne. In 1855 he succeeded Magendie as professor of physiology at the Collège de France. Napoleon III admired him so greatly that he created two special laboratories for him and, in 1869, made him a Senator. The publications of his later life included the finely-written *Leçons de pathologie expérimentale*[1368] of 1872; the *Leçons sur le diabète et la glycogenèse animale* (1877)[1369], showing that in diabetes mellitus glycaemia is followed by glycosuria; the *Leçons sur les anesthésiques et sur l'asphyxie* (1875)[1370], following much earlier work showing that chloroform anaesthesia could be both prolonged and deepened by the administration of morphine; and then, in 1878, the year in which he died, *La fermentation alcoolique*[1371], in which Bernard showed that he disputed Pasteur's belief that a ferment was a living thing or process deriving from a micro-organism. There is also a famous posthumous work, the *Leçons de physiologie opératoire*[1372] of 1879 which, in countless examples, exhibits Bernard's operative technique and command of the experimental method. The

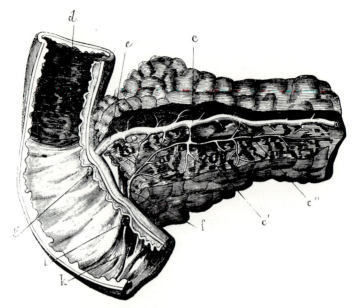

Figure 132 Claude Bernard. The human pancreas and duodenum. From: *Leçons de physiologie expérimentale appliquée à la médecine.* Paris (1855–56). Vol. II.

book is difficult reading for the modern student due to the then unaltered attitudes to vivisection.

Following Claude Bernard's great publications through almost chronologically emphasizes that early in his career he discovered certain isolated physiological facts – and then developed these, seeking an increasing understanding of each by deliberate, beautifully executed experiments. These were pieced together by a power of thinking in physiological terms which amounted to a unique insight. Perhaps his greatest achievement was to understand the glycogenic function of the liver and thereby unravel much regarding the place of hepatic function in general metabolism. Almost equally important was his understanding of pancreatic function in relation to digestion. Figure 132 shows his drawing of the human pancreas and duodenum – structures of the greatest importance in his studies for he showed how digestion in the stomach was only a beginning, the pancreatic juice splitting fats after their emulsification and converting starch to sugar whilst also acting on some of the proteins still in their native state. The third great achievement was the unravelling of the vasomotor system and the setting upon sound lines the understanding of its vasodilator and vasoconstrictor elements. To today's anaesthetist his experiments with curare and neuromuscular blockade are fundamental to daily practice – and to the physician Bernard's work on carbon dioxide and his showing that it displaces oxygen from the erythrocytes remains conspicuous as the basis of many later developments.

The work of Claude Bernard led to rapid progress in understanding the internal biochemical environment of the body, its processes of digestion and metabolism, and the place of the ductless glands in these processes.

Much of the present knowledge of the circulation and its physiology stems from the work of Carl Ludwig (1816–1895) who eventually became professor of physiology at Leipzig. Ludwig was a brilliant teacher responsible for the early training of many of the next generation who attained eminence. He wrote *Beiträge zur Lehre vom Mechanismus der Harnsecretion* (1843)[1373] – the classical study on renal secretion – and (1847) changed the haemodynamometer of Poiseuille into a kymograph by the simple means of adding a float to the top of the mercury column, and causing this float, equipped with a stylus, to write on a rotating drum[1374]. He later published on osmosis (1849)[1375], experimental ventricular fibrillation (1850)[1376], the nerve supply to the salivary glands (1851)[1377], the maintenance of isolated organs by perfusion or the provision of an artificial circulation (1865)[1378] and, from Leipzig, announced the discovery of the vasomotor reflexes (1867)[1379].

Knowledge of the circulation was then advanced by Sir Michael Foster (1836–1907), who made an extensive visit to the German laboratories of physiology accompanied by Sharpey, and became the first professor of physiology at Cambridge in 1883. Foster became second only to Ludwig as a teacher and from his Cambridge school of physiology stems much of the later achievement of the English-speaking physiologists and physicians of the late Victorian and the Edwardian eras. Foster published a well-known textbook in 1877[1380] and a volume, *Lectures on the history of physiology* (1901)[1381]. The latter work remained of interest for so long that it was reprinted in 1924 and in 1970. It contains Foster's own work, virtually all on the heart, and showing that all parts of the cardiac tissue exhibit the heartbeat, for any part of the heart, divided from the rest of the organ, will continue to beat rhythmically until its death supervenes.

Studies which involved keeping tissues alive for a while following their removal from the body were greatly facilitated by the work of Carl Ludwig and further advanced by Sydney Ringer (1834–1910) whose paper *Regarding the action of hydrate of soda, hydrate of ammonia, and hydrate of potash on the ventricle of the frog's heart* (1880–82)[1382] appeared just over 100 years ago. 'Ringer's solution', which was shown later to be capable of supporting the beating of the mammalian heart, demonstrated the importance of calcium salts to physiological tissues.

One of Sir Michael Foster's most brilliant pupils at Cambridge, Walter Holbrook Gaskell (1847–1914) then laid the histological foundations for the contemporary understanding of the autonomic nervous system. Gaskell's classical report *On the rhythm of the heart of the frog, and on the nature of the action of the vagus nerve* (1882)[1383] disclosed the acceleratory nerves of the heart and established that the motor impulses from the ganglia in the sinus venosus control the rate and force of the action of the heart but do not initiate the actual heartbeat: the latter was shown to be due to the intrinsic contractile capability of heart muscle itself and to the contraction wave which, passing from one cardiac muscle fibre to the next, spreads across the auricular wall. In his *On the innervation of the heart* (1883–84)[1384], Gaskell demonstrated that the efferent vasoconstrictor fibres of the system originated in the lateral horn of the spinal cord. In 1886 he wrote *On the structure, distribution, and function of the nerves which innervate the visceral and vascular system*[1385]; in this he traced the path of the preganglionic neurons and showed that the sympathetic fibres originate only in the thoracic and lumbar outflow. In 1908 he published on *The origin of vertebrates*[1386] and, at the end of his life, wrote *The involuntary nervous system*[1387] – a book which summarized his life's work and appeared, in 1916, 2 years following his death.

Foster's successor as professor of physiology at Cambridge was John Newport Langley (1852–1925). Almost at the end of the nineteenth century, in association with William Lee Dickinson (1862–1904), Langley published *On the local paralysis of peripheral ganglia, and on the connexion of different classes of nerve fibres with them* (1889)[1388]. This paper added yet another item to the nomenclature in which the autonomic nervous system is still discussed, for Langley and Dickinson showed that if Foster's synapse (the ganglion of a sympathetic nerve) was painted with nicotine then the transmission of the nerve impulse across it would be blocked. These findings preceded a brilliant series of studies, reported in *On reflex action from sympathetic ganglia*[1389] with Sir Hugh Kerr Anderson (1865–1928), a paper of 1894, and *On the reaction of cells and of nerve-endings to certain poisons, chiefly as regards the reaction of striated muscle to nicotine and to curari*[1390], of 1905. These publications, both in the *Journal of Physiology*, introduced the concept of a receptor site or substance with which a drug must interact in order to exert its biological effect. They were followed by Langley's splendid monograph, *The autonomic nervous system* (1921)[1391], in which he defined the efferent function of the autonomic nervous system and divided it into its orthosympathetic and parasympathetic divisions.

The turn of the century also saw the scientific development of the concept of the vitamin deficiency diseases. Sir Frederick Gowland Hopkins (1861–1947), professor of biochemistry at Cambridge, in 1892–93 published what is now a well-known method of estimating uric acid in urine[1392] and, with Sydney Cole (1877–1952), in 1901 reported the isolation of tryptophan[1393]. He then found that while mice soon died on a diet of zein (which is free of tryptophan), carbohydrates and fat, they survived if tryptophan was added. With Edith Gertrude Willcock he wrote *The importance of individual amino-acids in metabolism*[1394]. This was published in 1906, the year in which he produced *The analyst and the medical man*[1395] predicting the existence of the vitamins. The concept of the 'accessory factors' became fully developed in his *Feeding experiments illustrating the importance of accessory factors in normal dietaries* (1912)[1396]. His later work explained the production of lactic acid during the contraction of muscle (1907)[1397] and reported the isolation of glutathione (1921)[1398]. In 1929 he shared the Nobel Prize in Physiology for his discovery of the growth-promoting vitamins.

Several of the more significant advances of the period in respiratory physiology were produced by John Scott Haldane (1860–1936), one-time director of the Mining Research Laboratory at Birmingham and a major contributor to the developing subject of industrial hygiene. His name is more frequently used by the pharmacologist in connection with his *A new form of apparatus for measuring the respiratory exchange of animals* (1892)[1399] – the paper which recorded the development of the Haldane apparatus for the analysis of respiratory gases. In 1898 he reported his potassium ferricyanide method for measuring oxygen combined with haemoglobin[1400] and in 1901 described his means of determining haemoglobin – the Haldane haemoglobinometer[1401]. In 1905, writing with John Gillies Priestley (1880–1941), he gave the final proof of the place of carbon dioxide excess in controlling and stimulating respiration[1402]. In the 1913 publication on *Physiological observations made on Pike's Peak, Colorado, with special reference to adaptation to low barometric pressures*[1403], working with Claude Gordon Douglas (1882–1963) and others, he provided the best work to that date on the processes of adaptation to high altitudes. At the outbreak of World War I, in a now famous paper whose first author was Johanne Christiansen – *The absorption and dissociation of carbon dioxide by human blood* (1914)[1404] – he provided the CO_2 dissociation curves which have been so important in understanding the mechanisms of gaseous exchange. Late in the war, in an essay on *The therapeutic administration of oxygen* (1917)[1405], he began the modern use of oxygen therapy and, in 1922, produced one of the modern classics – his book on *Respiration*[1406]. He survived long enough to produce a second edition, written with J. G. Priestley, in 1935.

The haemoglobinometer which Haldane devised in 1901 was actually a modification of the instrument originally invented by Sir William Gowers (1845–1915) and reported in the *Practitioner* in 1878[1407]. The work on gaseous exchange which he had undertaken was augmented by Sir Joseph Barcroft (1872–1947), professor of physiology at Cambridge from 1925 to 1937, whose *The respiratory function of the blood*[1408] appeared in 1925–28. Barcroft's studies on the oxygen-carrying capacity of the blood bring the nineteenth century progress in physiology close to the present day. It was a notable progress, and one which made physiology become the pulse of medicine.

Surgery and Joseph Lister

The surgery of the nineteenth century continued that of the previous century, except that the centre of influence swung from Paris to London as a result of the teaching and practice of John Hunter. American surgery came into separate existence during this period but, for all practical purposes, surgical intervention in the skull, chest, abdomen, joints and eyes remained impossible until almost two-thirds of the century had passed.

There are no finer examples of the state of both operative surgery and the ethics of surgery at the beginning of the century than the writings of John Bell (1763–1820) of Edinburgh. John Bell, regarded as the founder of modern surgical anatomy, was the first to ligate the gluteal artery; he also ligated both the internal iliac and the common carotid arteries at a time when inhalational anaesthesia had not yet begun. His three volume *The principles of surgery* (1801–08)[1409], finely illustrated with his own drawings, epitomizes the surgical knowledge of the period. His *Letters on professional character and manners* (1810)[1410] serve the same function for the medical ethics of the day.

Possibly the most colourful of the early nineteenth century surgeons was Sir Astley Paston Cooper (1768–1841). Born in Norfolk and a pupil of John Hunter's, Cooper is remembered for having become demonstrator in anatomy at St. Thomas's Hospital at the early age of twenty-one and for having, in later life, become one of the chief embellishments of the tradition of Guy's. He was appointed surgeon to Guy's in 1800 and thereafter occupied himself with incessant dissecting and in the development of a rapid but unhasty operative technique. His publications on relieving deafness by myringotomy (1801)[1411] earned him the Copley medal. His study of *The anatomy and surgical treatment of abdominal hernia* (1804–07)[1412] is one of the great classics of surgical literature – it records his observations on femoral hernia and is the source of the eponyms 'Cooper's ligament' and 'Cooper's hernia'. In 1805 he ligated the common carotid artery; the patient died but a second case, ligated in 1808, survived. This was reported in *A case of aneurism of the carotid artery* (1809)[1413]; the eventual autopsy findings were noted in an *Account of the first successful operation, performed on the carotid artery, for aneurism, in the year 1808; with the post-mortem examination in 1821*[1414] – a paper in *Guy's Hospital Reports* of 1836.

In 1817 Cooper performed the quite remarkable feat of ligating the abdominal aorta. The patient died the following day but dissection suggested that with a lesser degree of aortic disease he might well have survived. The feat was recorded in the *Surgical essays*[1415] which, in 1818–19, Cooper published in joint authorship with Benjamin Travers (1783–1858), the noted vascular and ophthalmic surgeon of St. Thomas's Hospital. Cooper then published on diseases of the breast (1829)[1416], in which he noted cystic changes, and the thymus gland (1832)[1417], of which he gave an excellent account of the anatomy. He wrote on the ligation of arteries and nerves in 1836[1418] and in the same year published a *Case of a femoral aneurism, for which the external iliac artery was tied, with an account of the preparation of the limb, dissected at the expiration of eighteen years* (1836)[1419]. The latter account records what must be one of the more striking surgical cases of Regency times, for the artery was tied in 1808 and the patient's life was thereby prolonged until 1826. The very first successful ligation of the carotid seems to have taken place a few months before Cooper's case of 1808 and was reported by Amos Twitchell (1781–1850) in an essay on *Gun-shot wound of the face and neck; ligature of the carotid artery* (1842–43)[1420], the title of which shows one indication for these heroic procedures. The lengths to which, under the conditions of the time, such heroism could be driven is illustrated by the fact that in 1824 Cooper amputated at the hip joint.

Most of the great names of the period were excellent anatomists whose knowledge, derived from frequent dissection, permitted rapid operative technique. This was true of Abraham Colles (1773–1843), professor of surgery at Dublin, whose article *On the fracture of the carpal extremity of the radius* (1814)[1421] describes what is now known as 'Colles' fracture' and who ligated the subclavian artery in 1811 and in 1813. His accounts of these operations were included in a publication of 1815[1422]. In an important work (*Practical observations on the venereal disease, and on the use of mercury*, 1837)[1423] Colles began the use of small doses of mercury in the treatment of syphilis.

The same knowledge of anatomy characterized the work of Robert Liston (1794–1847), a man of great stature and strength who became professor of clinical surgery at University College, London. His most important book is that on *Practical Surgery* (1837)[1424]; it records his suggestion that a mirror might be used for viewing the larynx. He introduced a method of flap amputation, a device for crushing urinary stones, and is said[1425] to have been 'possessed of such Herculean strength that he could amputate a thigh with the aid of only one assistant, while compressing the artery with his left hand and doing all the sawing and cutting with his right'. If this indicates something of the surgery of the time, the fact that on December 21st, 1846, Liston became the first surgeon in Britain to perform a major operation with the aid of an anaesthetic shows the changes in the art of surgery that began late in his lifetime.

James Syme (1799–1870), one of the finest of Scottish surgeons and for a short period Liston's successor at University College, bore a special relationship to many of these temporal changes. He is remembered for 'Syme's amputation' – the amputation which he first successfully performed on September 8th, 1842. His early works catalogue substantial contributions to the characteristic ablational surgery of the nineteenth century. They include his account of 1828 of excision of the lower jaw for osteosarcoma[1426], his *Three cases in which the elbow-joint was successfully excised* (1829)[1427], his *Treatise on the excision of diseased joints* (1831)[1428] and his famous commentary of 1843 on *Amputation at the ankle-joint*[1429]. But he was quick to adopt the improved practices of the new era which began in the mid-century: he wrote *On the use of ether in the performance of surgical operations* (1847–48)[1430] and was one of the very first in Europe to use ether on such occasions and adopt the practice of anaesthesia. Syme was also the teacher and father-in-law of Joseph Lister and was one of the earliest surgeons to adopt Lister's antiseptic methods. His later writings included his *Contributions to the pathology and practice of surgery* (1848)[1431] and a *Case of iliac aneurism* (1862)[1432] – a case in which he opened the aneurysmal sac and ligated the common iliac and internal and external iliac arteries.

Sir William Fergusson (1808–1877), a pupil of Robert Knox in Edinburgh, became professor of surgery at King's College Hospital, London – a chair in which he was succeeded by Lord Lister. Fergusson was the real creator of conservative surgery, developing Syme's idea that excision was to be preferred to amputation whenever possible to its logical conclusion. Especially noted for a long and successful series of operations on harelip and cleft-palate, he wrote *A system of practical surgery* (1842)[1433]. The fourth edition of this work (1857) described Fergusson's vaginal speculum[1434]. In 1867 he published a fine study, *Lectures on the progress of anatomy and surgery during the present century*[1435], which gives an account, still of great use, of the history of the first half of the nineteenth century.

Sir Benjamin Brodie (1783–1862), ultimately surgeon to St. George's Hospital, began his career as a physiologist, much influenced by Bichat. He has an important work of 1814 on the nervous control of gastric secretion[1436]. He was the first to operate on varicose veins and published on this subject in 1816[1437]. His most important work is on *Pathological and surgical observations on the diseases of the joints* (1818)[1438], a volume which provides the first account of the clinical features of anklyosing spondylitis. He described what is now called 'Brodie's abscess' in 1828[1439] and, in 1846, gave the first description of intermittent claudication in man[1440]; in the same work he provided the first account of his test for valvular insufficiency in varicose veins (a test now usually attributed to Trendelenburg).

Brodie became the most illustrious medical man of his age, President of the Royal Society, Sergeant Surgeon to William IV and to Queen Victoria, and President of the Royal College of Surgeons. With the passing of the first Medical Act of 1858, a statute born out of great controversy and the subject of no less than 17 earlier attempts at legislation, the General Medical Council came into being –

almost exactly 125 years ago. Brodie, although then 75 years of age, was elected President of the General Council of Medical Education and Registration, as what we now know as the GMC was then called.

Many of the surgeons of this vintage left their names attached to clinical conditions in a way which makes them frequently remembered. One such was Guillaume Dupuytren (1777–1835), whose many publications include one of 1826 giving the first clear account of the pathology of congenital dislocation of the hip[1441], another of 1831 describing 'Dupuytren's contracture' of the palmar aponeurosis[1442], and a notable work (*Leçons orales de clinique chirurgicale*, 1832–34)[1443] in which he shows the excellence of his knowledge of physiology and pathology and describes an operation of 1812 in which he became the first to excise the lower jaw successfully.

Paul Pierre Broca (1824–1880), later famous as an anthropologist, in 1861 described 'Broca's area'[1444], claiming that the third left frontal convolution of the brain is the centre of articulate speech. He became the first to trephine in order to drain a cerebral abscess, the position of which had been diagnosed by functional localization. Thus his work greatly advanced the early attempts at neurosurgery, even though Pierre Marie (1853–1940), in 1906[1445], disputed Broca's claim to have identified the speech centre and proposed that aphasia is of one of three types: anarthria, when the defect is of articulation; motor aphasia, involving Broca's centre; or Wernicke's, sensory, aphasia.

Of the German school, Carl Ferdinand von Graefe (1787–1840), of Warsaw, but later professor of surgery at Berlin, is remembered for his *Rhinoplastik* of 1818[1446] and for a work of 1820 describing an operation for congenital cleft palate[1447]; these publications and his practice made him the founder of modern plastic surgery.

American surgery began its independent growth in the nineteenth century – its special contributions being the virtual founding of the operative gynaecological surgery of the modern age, and the epoch-making introduction of surgical anaesthesia. Representatives include Philip Syng Physick (1768–1837) – often called 'the Father of American Surgery' – an Edinburgh graduate and pupil of John Hunter's, who became professor of surgery at the University of Pennsylvania. His writings had less impact than his teaching but he has publications of 1812–13[1448], showing him to have been the first to have used a stomach tube in cases of poisoning; 1816, showing his use of absorbable kid and buckskin ligatures[1449]; 1822, describing his introduction of the use of a seton in cases of un-united fracture[1450]; 1826, giving an account of his operation for the making of an artificial anus[1451]; and 1828, recording his invention of the 'forceps, employed to facilitate the extirpation of the tonsil'[1452].

The pioneer ovariotomist, hardly believed in his first accounts of the operation and its circumstances, was Ephraim McDowell (1771–1830), a pupil of John Bell of Edinburgh. In 1795 he began to practice in the small community of Danville, Kentucky, at that time on the frontier of civilization. In 1809 he removed a massive ovarian cyst from a Mrs Crawford, aged 47, who survived for over 30 years. This, and two later cases were reported, somewhat obscurely (*Three cases of extirpation of diseased ovaria*)[1453], in 1817 before attracting the interest of other pupils of John Bell at Edinburgh. McDowell's original account of his three cases was reprinted in 1938.

The somewhat miserable state of the obstetric science of the time is shown by the degree to which vesicovaginal fistula was then recognized as a problem. It was solved by James Marion Sims (1813–1883), a graduate of Jefferson Medical College, Philadelphia, who invented the lateral posture (Sims' position) for examining or operating on the female patient, and who devised the duck-bill, or Sims', speculum. To these improvements Sims added the use of a silver wire suture, which avoided the sepsis that had previously broken down most attempts at repair of such fistulae, and the use of a catheter, which kept the bladder empty while the fistula healed. He published his brilliant results in *On the treatment of vesico-vaginal fistula*[1454] in 1852 and gave an account of *Silver sutures in surgery*[1455] in 1858. Sims went to New York and established the State Hospital for Women in 1855. He subsequently visited Europe and performed his operation in many of the great surgical centres of the day. In 1861 he wrote on *Amputation of the cervix uteri*[1456] and in 1862 *On vaginismus*[1457]. His *Clinical notes on uterine surgery* (1866)[1458] had a widespread impact on the developing science of gynaecological surgery and, in the *British Medical Journal* of 1878, he showed the breadth of his operative skills with an important paper, *Remarks on cholecystotomy in dropsy of the gall-bladder*[1459]. Despite his several achievements, Sims will always be remembered for his work on vesicovaginal fistula; his paper of 1852 on this subject was reprinted in *Medical Classics* in 1938.

of intense controversy – some of it, involving the participants in the discoveries, bitter and unedifying. Of the attempts of antiquity, the nepenthe of Homer – nepenthe being supposed to be a drug that brings forgetfulness of grief – is thought to have been Indian hemp. The use of the soporific sponge of the Salernitans is not recorded in the writings of Paré and seems to have died out in the seventeenth century. The surgeons of the eighteenth and early nineteenth centuries are said to have intoxicated patients undergoing amputation, arterial ligation, and operations such as repair of large hernias with alcohol or opium. In 1800, Sir Humphry Davy (1778–1829), of Penzance, experimented on himself with nitrous oxide and suggested that it might be used in surgical operations when there is no great loss of blood[1460]. This aroused the interest of William Paul Barton (1786–1856) who, in 1808, wrote *A dissertation on the chymical properties and exhilerating effects of nitrous-oxide gas* – a thesis presented to the University of Pennsylvania and cited by Chauncey D. Leake (1975)[1461]. Barton, who was interested in the effects of nitrous oxide on behaviour, later became professor of botany at Philadelphia and wrote a useful *Vegetable materia medica of the United States* (1817–18)[1462]. Thoughts of using nitrous oxide in a manner suggested by Humphry Davy seem to have disappeared, the gas being used only in itinerant medicine shows where it had an entertainment value.

The early medical history of ether seems to have been comparable. There is an anonymous note, often ascribed to Michael Faraday (1791–1867), the founder of electrochemistry, in the *Quarterly Journal of the Arts*[1463] for 1818, which suggests that inhalation of ether would produce much the same effects as nitrous oxide:

V. *Effects of Inhaling the Vapour of sulphuric Ether.*

When the vapour of ether mixed with common air is inhaled, it produces effects very similar to those occasioned by nitrous oxide. A convenient mode of ascertaining the effect is obtained by introducing a tube into the upper part of a bottle containing ether, and breathing through it; a stimulating effect is at first perceived at the epiglottis, but soon becomes very much diminished, a sensation of fulness is then generally felt in the head, and a succession of effects similar to those produced by nitrous oxide. By lowering the tube into the bottle, more of the ether is inhaled at each inspiration, the effect takes place more rapidly, and the sensations are more perfect in their resemblance to those of the gas.

In trying the effects of the ethereal vapour on persons who are peculiarly affected by nitrous oxide, the similarity of sensation produced was very unexpectedly found to have place. One person who always feels a depression of spirits on inhaling the gas, had sensation of a similar kind produced by inhaling the vapour.

It is necessary to use caution in making experiments of this kind. By the imprudent inspiration of ether, a gentleman was thrown into a very lethargic state, which continued with occasional periods of intermission for more than 30 hours, and a great depression of spirits; for many days the pulse was so much lowered that considerable fears were entertained for his life.

Ether frolics became popular in the United States and Crawford Williamson Long (1815-1878), a graduate of the University of Pennsylvania, is said to have noted that a participant in such a frolic fell heavily but with no indication of pain. On March 30th, 1842, Crawford Long, at Jefferson, Georgia, removed a small cystic tumour from the back of the neck of a patient under the influence of ether. He thereby became the first to use ether vapour as an anaesthetic successfully but did not publish his results until others (including Morton) had independently made the same discovery. Eventually, in the *Southern Medical and Surgical Journal* of 1849, Crawford Long published *An account of the first use of sulphuric ether by inhalation as an anaesthetic in surgical operations*[1464]. There is no doubt that Long was the first to make professional use of ether as an anaesthetic. This fact is clearly established in *Long, the discoverer of anaesthesia. A presentation of his original documents*[1465] – a work published in 1897 by Hugh Hampton Young (1870-1945).

Long's failure to publish robbed his work of the effect it would have had in introducing ether anaesthesia into everyday practice.

Events then returned to nitrous oxide, for in Hartford, Connecticut, late in 1844, a young dentist, Horace Wells (1815-1848) witnessed an exhibition of the social use of the gas and noted that the subject fell but without pain. Wells soon began to use nitrous oxide successfully in dental extractions. He communicated his results to his friend and former partner, William Thomas Green Morton (1819-1868) and, through Morton, a student at Harvard Medical School, arranged to demonstrate the technique before John Collins Warren (1778-1856). The demonstration, in January 1845, was a disaster and although Wells survived to write *A history of the discovery of the application of nitrous oxide gas, ether, and other vapours, to surgical operations*[1466] – a work published in 1847 – he ended his life, by inhaling ether and causing bleeding by venesection, the following year.

Morton, in the meantime, remained interested in the possibilities of anaesthesia. Dissatisfied with nitrous oxide and looking for a more potent agent, he noted a comment of his preceptor, Charles T. Jackson (1805-1880), a chemist of some considerable standing, on the anaesthetic effects of chloric ether. From Jackson, Morton learnt that sulphuric ether is also an anaesthetic. Morton used this agent to extract a bicuspid tooth and then returned to John Collins Warren, persuading him to give this further anaesthetic a trial. Without the nature of the agent being disclosed this trial took place on October 16th, 1846, Warren excising a vascular tumour from below the jaw on the left side of the neck of a patient who clearly felt no pain.

Morton, who had independently discovered the anaesthetic use of ether, tried to patent the discovery and published an item entitled *Circular. Morton's Letheon* (1846)[1467]. Fortunately, Henry Jacob Bigelow (1818–1890) recognized the true nature of Morton's 'Letheon' and announced it to the world in a paper read before the Boston Society of Medical Improvement on November 9th, 1846. The announcement was repeated in Bigelow's excellent paper, *Insensibility during surgical operations produced by inhalation*[1468], published in the *Boston Medical and Surgical Journal* (1846).

Warren and Bigelow were largely responsible for ether anaesthesia being rapidly and widely adopted in the practice of surgery. Bigelow remained generous to Morton's reputation and claim of discovery in his *Ether and chloroform: a compendium of their history and discovery* (1848)[1469]. He has a publication of 1852 showing him to have undertaken the first excision of the hip joint in America[1470] and a further publication of 1869 in which he gives the first proper account of the iliofemoral (Bigelow's) ligament[1471]. He was a participant in the fine historical study, *A century of American medicine 1776–1876*[1472] written by Edward H. Clarke, Bigelow and others, and published in 1876.

The terms 'anaesthetic' and 'anaesthesia' were initially proposed by Oliver Wendell Holmes. On January 19th, 1847, Sir James Young Simpson (1811–1870), professor of obstetrics at Edinburgh, became the first to use ether in midwifery in Great Britain. Although this use was successful, Simpson set about finding a less irritating and more rapidly acting alternative. His deliberate experiments, using a number of volatile liquids, led him to become the first (November 4th, 1847) to use chloroform. Impressed with his results, he published them a week later (*London Medical Gazette*, 1847) and followed this announcement with his historic publication, *Discovery of a new anaesthetic agent, more efficient than sulphuric ether*[1473] – a paper contributed to the *Lancet* in the notable year, 1847, that saw the widespread practice of effective anaesthesia begin the transformation of surgery.

For all practical purposes, surgery, until 1847, had been limited to life-saving procedures, usually destructive, in which speed was of the essence. For the patient the experience was horrendous. With the advent of ether and chloroform anaesthesia the surgeon was given time for the performance of skilled, conservative techniques – and was freed of some of the apprehension and all of the operative agony of the patient. The surgery of the first half of the nineteenth century was a continuation of that of the previous 100 or even 200 years. The surgical skills of the last half of the century begin today's operative capability. It does perhaps cause one to pause for a moment to realize how recent has been the change.

Sir Thomas Spencer Wells (1818–1897), of St. Albans, was a pupil of Stokes and Graves in Dublin, and was a surgeon in the Royal Navy (1841–48) at the time anaesthetics became widely used. He performed his first ovariotomy in 1858 and achieved a great reputation as a pioneer gynaecological surgeon. His *Diseases of the ovaries*[1474] was published in 1865–72 and his paper giving *Remarks of forci-pressure and the use of pressure-forceps in surgery*[1475] appeared in the *British Medical Journal* in 1879. The latter paper is the source of the 'Spencer Wells forceps', ubiquitous amongst the items of modern surgical equipment. Spencer Wells was one of those who saw their practice changed by anaesthesia, just as many contemporary doctors watched their practice transformed by penicillin.

A gynaecologist of the generation that never saw pre-anaesthetic surgery was Robert Lawson Tait (1845–1899), of Edinburgh. Tait's eventual success in gynae-cological surgery made his unit at Birmingham, where he settled in 1871, famous. By 1879 he was able to write on *Removal of normal ovaries*[1476] – a subject which showed how elective surgery could grow in the presence of anaesthesia. In 1881 he described oöphorectomy[1477] and, following John S. Parry (1843–1876) and his publication on *Extra-uterine pregnancy*[1478] of 1876, Lawson Tait, in 1884, described *Five cases of extra-uterine pregnancy operated upon at the time of rupture*[1479]. Tait's first successful operation on a ruptured ectopic was performed on March 1st, 1883 – an advance of which the present time is the centenary. Although Tait lived well into the period of Listerian principles he refused to acknowledge Lister's ideas, deriding them because he did not see sepsis due to scrupulous cleanliness and the use of warm or boiled water to flush out the abdomen or pelvis. The statistics of his success appear in his *General summary of conclusions from one thousand cases of abdominal section*[1480] – a fine work, published in Birmingham in 1884 and suggesting that his technique approached that of asepsis. He wrote again on ectopic pregnancy in 1888 and, in 1890 described the *Surgical treatment of typhilitis*[1481]; this historic work, which appeared in the *Birmingham Medical Review*, deserves its own special place in the traditions, for Tait was the first (May, 1880) British surgeon to diagnose acute appendicitis and treat it by excision of the appendix. His later works describe his method of Caesarean section in cases of placenta praevia (1890)[1482] and his paper *On the method of flap-splitting in certain plastic operations* (1887–88)[1483] describes the operation which he had devised for the repair of a rectocele. Part of Tait's success seems to have been due to a gentle, sensitive skill which left little tissue in a state vulnerable to infection. The gentleness contrasts with a somewhat savage style of controversy and a characteristically pungent pattern of argument. Another factor contributing to his fine results seems to have arisen from his adoption of deliberate cleanliness. It is certain that no such full measure of success could have preceded surgical anaesthesia.

The description of 'McBurney's point', and the associated sign indicating the need for surgical intervention in acute appendicitis, came in the year of Tait's death, 1899. In that year, Charles McBurney (1845–1913), of Massachusetts, in his paper *Experience with early operative interference in cases of disease of the vermiform appendix* (1889, reprinted 1938)[1484] described his sign and stated that it was to be 'determined by the pressure of one finger' applied at a point $1\frac{1}{2}$–2 inches from the anterior superior iliac spine and on a straight line drawn from the spinous process itself to the umbilicus.

Apart from the discovery of anaesthesia, the second great influence which transformed surgery and made it part of the rapid growth of scientific medicine in

444

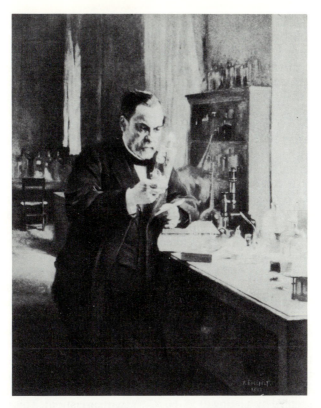

Figure 133 Louis Pasteur (1822–1895). [*From: William Osler. The evolution of modern medicine . . . New Haven, Yale Univ. Press (1921).*]

the latter half of the nineteenth century, was the establishment of the germ theory, associated with the growth of bacteriology in the hands of Pasteur and Robert Koch, and the immediate application of the theory by Lister.

Early in the rapid sequence of events which led to the cell theory, Theodor Schwann (1810–1882), in 1837, confirmed observations made 1 year earlier by Baron Charles Cagniard-Latour (1777–1859) who had noted that yeasts, examined microscopically, appeared as globules which seemed to be of a living and vegetable nature. Cagniard-Latour (*Mémoire sur la fermentation vineuse*, 1838)[1485] provided the earliest demonstration of the true nature of yeasts. Schwann discovered the yeast cell independently and extended the earlier observations by showing that yeasts caused fermentation which could be prevented by heating. Schwann, by virtue of his paper of 1837 reporting these findings[1486], became the founder of the germ theory of putrefaction and fermentation.

Twenty years later (1857)[1487], Louis Pasteur (Figure 133; 1822–1895), then dean and professor of chemistry in the Faculty of Sciences at Lille, investigated lactic acid fermentation of milk, alcoholic fermentation of beers and wine, and other fermentation processes (1859, 1860)[1488, 1489]. He found that the conversion

445

of sugar to lactic acid during fermentation is due to small corpuscles, acting in isolation or in groups. Pasteur thus found that each process depended on a specific ferment which, especially in the fermentation or souring of milk, seemed capable of reproduction, as if living. He then showed that if he heated the fluid and sealed the containing vessel the milk would remain unfermented for long periods.

At this time putrefaction, fermentation, souring and infection were all thought to be due to miasma or foul air. Pasteur, knowing already that yeasts, as micro-organisms, were capable of multiplication by division, doubted this theory and thought that specific ferments carried by the air, rather than the air itself, were responsible for some of these processes. His epoch-making paper is the *Mémoire sur les corpuscles organisés qui existent dans l'atmosphère. Examen de la doctrine des générations spontanées*[1490] of 1861. In this work he put blood, milk or urine in glass tubes, drew the ends of the tubes into a capillary bent at an angle, and then heated the tubes to destroy the ferment or fermenting agent already present. The contents of the tubes remained unfermented – although they were in contact with air through the open capillary. This finding marked the downfall of the theory of spontaneous generation and provided the basis for the germ theory. It was merely a step from the demonstration that a specific agent must be present to cause fermentation to the germ theory of disease – and from this to modern bacteriology and immunology.

In 1863 Pasteur confirmed that putrefaction or fermentation was a biological process due to 'animalcules' which could be carried by the air[1491]; in the same year he became the first to differentiate between aerobic and anaerobic organisms[1492, 1493]. He then turned his attention to studying the fermentation of wine (1866)[1494] and, in 1868 showed that the spoiling of wine by the growth of micro-organisms could be prevented by heating to 55–60 °C[1495] (pasteurization). This discovery was of enormous commercial value and was followed by Pasteur's application of the germ theory to unravelling the cause of the disease *pébrine* which was then ruining the vitally important French silkworm industry. Discovery of the cause of this silkworm disease failed to solve the problem and revealed a second disease, *flâcherie*. This period of investigation, lasting some 5 years and associated with certain personal tragedies, was recorded by Pasteur in his *Études sur la maladie des vers à soie*[1496], published in two volumes in 1870.

He resumed his studies on fermentation in 1876, this time studying the spoiling of beer by micro-organisms[1497], and again showing the value of pasteurization. At this stage Pasteur was defining a ferment as a living form originating from a germ – a view contested in a posthumous essay written by Claude Bernard – but the definition, and the avenues of investigation that it opened, carried Pasteur into areas that were more and more those of the medical man concerned with the causes of infectious disease.

The anthrax bacillus had already been discovered and shown to be non-filterable and Koch (1876) had cultivated the organism in pure culture and shown its relationship to the disease[1498]. Without knowing of Koch's work, Pasteur studied anthrax in 1877[1499]. He seeded 50 ml of urine with one drop of blood from an infected animal, having previously sterilized the urine by heating. After allowing the culture to grow, he seeded a second 50 ml sample of sterile urine with one drop of the culture. By such serial dilutions he produced a final dilution of the original drop of blood of about 1 in 1000 million. The final culture was clearly supporting a huge growth of bacilli, indicating that these had multiplied in the subcultures. Pasteur then showed that one drop of the final culture injected into a healthy animal caused death from anthrax just as certainly as did a drop of blood freshly taken from an infected beast. It seemed clear that anthrax was caused by the bacillus and that was capable of replication. Pasteur, in this and similar experiments, convincingly showed that micro-organisms could be the cause of disease – and not merely the consequence of infection or present co-incidentally with the disease.

At the same time, in 1877, working with Jules François Joubert, Pasteur discovered the *Vibrion septique*, the first anaerobic pathogen to be detected[1500]. Interestingly, these two workers also noticed the antagonism between the growth of *Bacillus anthracis*, the anthrax bacillus, and other bacteria growing in the cultures; thus, they recorded one of the earliest observations on antibiosis.

In 1879 (*Sépticémie puerpérale*)[1501] Pasteur described the streptococcus of puerperal sepsis. The following year, after noting that fowls inoculated with an attenuated variant of the chicken cholera organism became immune to subsequent challenge with the bacterium, and developing the idea of protective inoculation by the use of cultures of the living organism in an attenuated form, Pasteur published the vitally important paper, *Sur les maladies virulentes, et en particulier sur la maladie appelée vulgairement choléra des poules* (1880)[1502], which can now be seen as one of the foundation stones of the modern science of immunology. The paper marked the beginning of Pasteur's work on the prophylaxis of disease by the use of attenuated organisms; it was accompanied, in the same year, by a paper (*Sur l'étiologie du charbon*)[1503] in which Pasteur was associated with two of his most brilliant pupils, Charles Chamberland (1851–1908) and Pierre Émile Roux (1853–1933), and in which he gave an account of the first use of an attentuated bacterial vaccine employed for therapeutic purposes.

In 1881, again in co-authorship with some of his students, Pasteur published the paper, *Sur la rage*[1504], which recorded the beginnings of his studies on rabies. It was his work on this subject which brought Pasteur his greatest acclaim. In 1884, with Chamberland and Roux, he demonstrated the rabies virus in the blood[1505]. In 1885 he reported the development of his specific vaccine for the treatment of rabies[1506]. His first patient was an Alsatian boy, Joseph Meister, badly savaged by a rabid dog, who was successfully treated in July, 1885. In 1885 and 1886 Pasteur produced his papers, *Méthode pour prévenir la rage après morsure*[1507], in which he gave a full account of his rabies vaccine and the results he had obtained in using it. These papers established the value of preventive inoculation with an attenuated organism. By this discovery, reflecting what Pasteur realized may be part of the natural history in which the great diseases wax and wane in historical time, perhaps as their causative organisms augment or attenuate, Pasteur ushered in one of the most notable achievements of therapeutics. In response to his triumph the French public subscribed the sum of two-and-a-half million francs which made possible the building of the Institut Pasteur, Paris, which Pasteur himself directed from 1889 to 1895.

Arising from his work on rabies Pasteur provided what seems to be the first record of the pneumococcus. This appears in a paper (*L'organisme micro-*

scopique trouvé par M. Pasteur dans la maladie nouvelle provoquée par la salive d'un enfant mort de la rage[1508] published by Joseph Parrot (1829–1883) in 1881. Independently of Pasteur, the pneumococcus was discovered by George Miller Sternberg (1838–1915), one of the earliest of the bacteriologists, a pioneer of the subject in America, and the first to photograph the tubercule bacillus in that country. Sternberg, author of *A manual of bacteriology* (1893)[1509], became US Surgeon General from 1893 to 1902.

Pasteur's total contribution to medicine and therapeutics was so vast that it has been equalled few times in the history of medicine. A founder of bacteriology, the discoverer of the real nature of the processes of putrefaction and fermentation, he not only destroyed the theory of spontaneous generation but also developed and established the practice of preventive vaccination and immunization using deliberately attenuated micro-organisms. Figure 133, the portrait of Pasteur in his laboratory, is taken from the fine, seven volume, *Oeuvres de Pasteur, réunies par Pasteur Vallery-Radot*[1510] and published in Paris in 1922–39.

There was an element of serendipity, like that involved in Fleming's discovery of penicillin, in what is to the physician Pasteur's most important discovery. Fielding Garrison[1511] notes that Pasteur's 'discovery of preventive inoculation was due to the accidental fact that virulent cultures of chicken cholera virus, during a vacation from the laboratory, became sterile or inactive, and, when injected, were found to act as preventive vaccines against a subsequent injection of a virulent character.' A less acute mind might have discarded these unexpected observations, rather than exploring them. Horace Walpole's word (coined upon the title of the fairytale *The Three Princes of Serendip*, the heroes of which 'were always making discoveries, by accidents and sagacity, of things they were not in quest of') may not be the right one. There is more to it than making happy discoveries by accident – there is also a perseverance in exploring the ramifications of the unexpected and trivial. Pasteur's curiosity seems to have been such that a very lean and unpromising fact that was novel would trigger systematic experiment – and the thing that makes his writings instructive is each experimental design and the logic that provides them with sequence.

The great problem of the germ theory – were the micro-organisms the cause or the consequence of the diseases in which they seemed to be involved – was clearly expressed, on August 3rd, 1864, by Thomas Spencer Wells in speaking to the annual meeting, at Cambridge, of the British Medical Association.

The central problem – cause or consequence – was tackled by Robert Koch (Figure 134; 1843–1910). Koch, of Klausthal, Hannover, a medical graduate (1866) of Göttingen, had been greatly influenced by Jacob Henle and his theory of contagion. After serving in the Franco-Prussian War, Koch became Kreis-physicus (a district physician or type of general practitioner) at Wollstein; there he had time to indulge his private interest in microscopy.

The anthrax bacillus had already been described and Koch began his studies by attempts to explore its life cycle. By April, 1876 he was able to report to the eminent botanist, Ferdinand Cohn, of Breslau that he had not only produced a pure culture of *Bacillus anthracis* but had also worked out its complete life cycle including the spore-forming capability. A few days later, at Cohn's invitation, he demonstrated his culture methods and the findings of his study at the Botanical

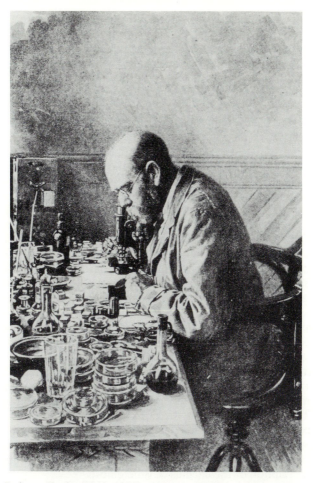

Figure 134 Robert Koch (1843–1910). [*From: William Osler. The evolution of modern medicine . . . New Haven, Yale Univ. Press (1921).*]

Institute at Breslau. Cohn immediately published Koch's results (*Die Aetiologie der Milzbrand-Krankheit, begründet auf die Entwicklungsgeschichte des Bacillus anthracis*)[1498] in a historic paper (1876) which has been reprinted with an English translation in *Medical Classics*, 1938. The work demonstrated that the organism, cultured for several generations under artificial laboratory conditions could produce the disease in a number of varieties of animals. It was clear that the organism was the cause of the disease – and Koch's finding was declared the most important bacteriological discovery then made.

In 1877 Koch wrote a paper describing his method of making smears of bacteria on cover slips, fixing them by gentle heat, staining them with Weigert's aniline dyes, and photographing them so that they could be classified and compared[1512]. This work laid the foundation for many of the technical methods of today.

Koch then used these methods to inoculate organisms obtained from various sources into animals, these studies being accompanied by parallel culture and sub-culture of the organisms *in vitro*. He showed that, in respect of the bacteria from six different kinds of surgical infection, the organism bred true through several generations, both in animals and on laboratory culture. This work was recorded in his great study of the aetiology of bacterial infectious disease (*Untersuchungen über die Aetiologie der Wundinfectionskrankheiten*[1513], published in 1878. This established the specificity of wound infection for the first time. It appears in an English translation, dated 1880, and published by the New Sydenham Society.

The rapidity of translation itself suggests the importance of the findings. This recognition led to Koch's preferment to a position in the Imperial Health Department (1880). There he produced an important report on methods of disinfection (1881)[1514] and introduced solid culture media – a great technical innovation – by spreading liquid gelatin with meat infusion broth on glass plates; once the coagulum had set it permitted the culture of organisms in pure growth without resorting to the cumbersome liquid media previously employed.

On March 24th, 1882, Koch announced the discovery of the tubercule bacillus. The work concerned is remarkable for its dependence upon the staining techniques and means of culture which Koch had devised. It was reported in *Die Aetiologie der Tuberculose*[1515] – a paper of 1882 notable not only for the discovery of the causative organism of tuberculosis but also for its provision of the first statement of 'Koch's postulates'. The paper was published in an English translation (*The Etiology of Tuberculosis*) in 1938.

Koch wrote at a time when '$\frac{1}{7}$ of all people die of tuberculosis' and, 'if only the productive middle aged class is considered, tuberculosis carries away a third and often more of these.' He stained his material with an alcoholic solution of methylene blue and potassium hydroxide, then removed the cover slips into a concentrated solution of vesuvin; following this treatment the tubercule bacilli contrasted with other cellular materials and were stained 'a beautiful blue'. Koch noted that only lepra bacilli stained in this way, apart from the tubercule bacilli. This is his description of the bacillus of tuberculosis[1516]:

> The bacteria made visible by this method show a behavior which, in many respects, is characteristic. They have a rod shaped form and thus belong to the group of bacilli. They are very thin and are from a quarter to one-half of the diameter of a red blood corpuscle in length; however, at times they attain greater length, up to the full diameter of a red blood cell. In shape and size they bear a striking similarity to the lepra bacilli; yet they differ from the latter in that they appear a little slimmer and pointed at the ends. Also with Weigert's nuclear staining method, the lepra bacilli take up the stain, which the tubercle bacilli do not do. The bacilli are present in large numbers in all situations where the tuberculous process is early in origin and making rapid progress; they then usually form little groups which are pressed closely together and at times are arranged in bundles. Many times these lie within cells and present a picture like that of lepra bacilli heaped within the cells. On the other hand, many free bacilli are found. Particularly on the borders of large caseous foci, crowds of bacilli which are not inclosed in cells are found.
>
> As soon as the height of the tuberculous process is passed the bacilli become

more rare, are found only in small groups or entirely alone on the edges of tuberculous foci, along with weakly stained and at times scarcely recognizable bacilli, which are dying or already dead. Finally, they may disappear completely, yet they are rarely entirely absent and then only in those cases in which the tuberculous process is arrested.

Koch devised a method whereby 'serum of cattle or sheep blood, which is obtained as purely as possible, is poured into cotton stoppered test tubes and daily, for six consecutive days, is heated to a temperature of 58 °C for an hour at a time. By this means it is possible to sterilize the serum completely in most instances, although not always, when everything else may fail. Then it is heated to 65 °C for several hours, indeed, until it has become coagulated and firm.' It is not difficult to imagine the numbers of experiments that must have gone into settling upon these technical details. Using slopes or other preparations of such media, Koch observes that [1517]:

> The cultures resulting from the growth of tubercle bacilli first appear to the naked eye in the second week after inoculation, usually not until after the tenth day, as very tiny points and dry scales, which, according to whether the tuberculous material is more or less broken up during inoculation and brought into contact with a larger surface of the culture medium by means of rubbing motions, lie about the fragments of the tubercles in tiny or wide areas.

He then has a series of most satisfying passages in which he has quite characterized the cultural features of the organism on his medium [1518]:

> The colony of bacilli, furthermore, forms such a compact mass that the little scale can be raised easily from the solidified blood serum with a platinum wire and can broken up only by the exertion of a certain amount of pressure. The markedly slow growth which is attained only at incubator temperature, the peculiarly dry and scale like condition of these bacillary colonies occur in no other known type of bacteria, so that confusion of the cultures of tubercle bacilli with those of other bacteria is impossible; and after only a small amount of practice nothing is easier to detect at once than accidental contamination of the cultures. The growth of the colonies ceases after several weeks, as has been said already, and further enlargement probably does not occur because the bacilli are lacking in motility and are forced out on the culture medium only through the growth process itself, which, because of the slow proliferation of the bacilli, naturally can proceed only in very short dimensions. In order to keep such a culture going, it must be transplanted to new culture material at some time after the first inoculation, approximately after 10 to 14 days.

In this work, of 100 years ago, Koch, in his animal experiments, had identified appropriate species and was writing of 'four to six guinea pigs' being inoculated each time with the material to be tested for virulence; he also has animals which remained 'uninjected for controls'.

'Koch's postulates', which became vital in the face of a rapid influx of knowledge regarding bacteriology – an influx which could have produced much confusion – were rooted in Koch's early attraction to the teachings of Henle. The latter has a famous essay (*Von den Miasmen und Contagien*)[1519] in his *Patho-*

logische Untersuchungen of 1840 in which he sets down clear postulates regarding the aetiological relationships of micro-organisms to disease. It was these postulates of Henle which Koch later developed. This subject has been well discussed by Charles Singer and E. Ashworth Underwood (1962) who give the following as being Koch's postulates, in their finally developed form:

In order to prove that an organism is the inseparable cause of a disease it is necessary to demonstrate[1520]:

(1) The constant presence of the organism in every case of the disease.
(2) The preparation of a pure culture, which must be maintained for repeated generations.
(3) The reproduction of the disease in animals by means of a pure culture removed by several generations from the organisms first isolated.

Just before his discovery of the tubercule bacillus, Koch, in 1881, introduced steam sterilization as being more efficient than the chemical methods advocated by Lister. In 1883, when he was still only 40, he visited Egypt and India as head of the German Cholera Commission. There he discovered the cholera vibrio and the route of its transmission by drinking water, food and fomites. He published this further important discovery in a paper *Ueber die Cholerabakterien* (1844)[1521] which appeared the year after the announcement of the discovery of the Koch-Weeks bacillus[1522]. For the latter contribution, the detection of the bacillus of infectious conjunctivitis, Koch received 100000 marks from the Prussian State.

When he was 42 years of age Koch was appointed professor of hygiene and bacteriology at the University of Berlin. In 1890–1891 he introduced tuberculin in the treatment of tuberculosis[1523] and, although he brought out new tuberculin (Tuberculin R) in 1897[1524], this proved to be his one major mistake. Even though Koch limited the claims for tuberculin to the suggestion that it might prove curative in early phthisis, Koch's reputation and the worldwide fear of the disease led to inflated expectations. Koch was at this time Director of the Institute for Infectious Diseases in Berlin – an appointment made on the founding of the Institute in 1891. His reputation survived the disappointment of tuberculin, this being aided by the recognition that the substance provided the most reliable means of diagnosing the existence of present or past infection with the tubercule bacillus. Work on the immunological aspects of the disease continued, sporadic studies being pursued until the advent of effective multiple chemotherapy overwhelmed their interest in the years immediately after 1950.

Koch's later studies included Rinderpest in South Africa, Texas fever, blackwater fever, tropical malaria, plague, malaria in Italy, Rhodesian red-water fever, trypanosomiasis and recurrent fever in German East Africa and, again, sleeping sickness in Africa. He published on several of these subjects in 1898[1525] and, in 1903, introduced his prophylactic measures, almost universally adopted since, for the control of typhoid[1526]. His second error came at the London Tuberculosis Congress of 1900 when he expressed the view that there was little danger of transmission of the bovine tubercule bacillus to man, the bovine and human tubercule bacilli having been separated and studied by Theobald Smith (1859–1934) in 1898[1527].

Koch, aged 62, received the Nobel Prize in 1905, the award being given for his work on tuberculosis. Without doubt the greatest and most influential bacteriologist of his day, his fundamental importance may lie in his having been the first to show a specific organism (anthrax) to be the cause of a definite disease, and in his having developed the postulates which made a science rather than a source of confusion of the vast increase in the knowledge of microbiology which characterized the late nineteenth century. To the contemporary scientist much of Koch's attraction must lie in his genius for developing new and practical technical methods. These, in their original and modified forms, permitted the vast discoveries of his contemporaries and successors. One example of the practical things that came from his laboratory is the Petri dish, today in universal use, which was a modification of Koch's solid media on glass plates and was designed (others produced a similar invention in 1885) by Richard Julius Petri (1852–1921), one of Koch's assistants and author of the paper, *Eine kleine Modification des Koch'schen Plattenverfahrens*[1528] of 1887. Koch died in 1910, his ashes being placed, as he wished, in the Berlin Institute for Infectious Diseases. There is a *Gesammelte Werke*[1529], of two volumes (in three) published in Leipzig in 1912.

With the methodology largely available the massive increase in the knowledge of medical bacteriology was, in the last 20 years of the nineteenth century, almost without precedent. Gerhard Henrik Hansen (1841–1912) discovered the leprosy bacillus in 1871 and published his findings in 1874[1530]. Albert Ludwig Neisser (1855–1916) recorded the discovery of the gonococcus in 1879[1531]. The causative organism of typhoid, *Salmonella typhi*, was discovered by Carl Joseph Eberth (1835–1926) and reported in 1880[1532]. Friedrich Fehleisen (1854–1924) produced his paper *Ueber Erysipel*[1533] announcing the identification of the *Streptococcus pyogenes* in 1882. Theodor Albrecht Klebs (1834–1913) gave the first account of *Corynebacterium diphtheriae*, the Klebs–Loeffler bacillus, the causal pathogen of diphtheria, in 1883[1534]. The following year Friedrich Loeffler (1852–1915) described the cultivation of the diphtheria organism and the production of the characteristic membrane by pure cultures of the germ swabbed on the mucous membranes of animals[1535]. Also in 1884 Arthur Nicolaier (1862–1900), in *Ueber infectiösen Tetanus*[1536], discovered, but could not isolate, the causative organism of tetanus. In 1886, Theodor Escherich (1857–1911) gave an account of *Escherichia coli*, causing the whole genus *Escherichia* to be named after him[1537]. Sir David Bruce (1855–1931) in a *Note on the discovery of a micro-organism in Malta fever* (1887)[1538] showed the causative pathogen to be *Brucella (Micrococcus) melitensis*. This same year saw the discovery of *Neisseria meningitidis*, the causative agent in cerebrospinal meningitis, by Anton Weichselbaum (1845–1920)[1539]. Angusto Ducrey (1860–1940), in *Il virus dell' ulcera venera*[1540], of 1889, closed the extraordinary decade which had also seen the discovery of the tubercule bacillus by showing *Haemophilus ducreyi* (Ducrey's bacillus) to be the causal organism of the venereal infection, chancroid.

Among the notable reports of the next decade, the discovery of *Haemophilus influenzae* in 1892[1541] stands out, not only for the importance of the organism in bronchitis and respiratory tract infections but also because Richard Friedrich Pfeiffer (1858–1945) wrongly thought it to be the causative organism of the viral illness, influenza. In America, William Henry Welch (1850–1934) and George Nuttall (1862–1937), in 1892, announced the discovery of the gas gangrene bacillus, *Clostridium Welchii* or *Cl. perfringens*[1542]. In 1894, in a paper on *La peste bubonique à Hong-Kong*[1543], published in the *Annals of the Pasteur Institute*, Alexandre Emile Yersin (1863–1943) gave the first account of the plague bacillus, *Pasteurella (Yersinia) pestis*, which he had isolated from excised buboes. In 1898 the dysentery bacillus was discovered by Kiyoshi Shiga (1870–1957), after whom the *Shigellae* are named[1544]. And then, soon after the opening of the present century, Jules Jean Bordet (1870–1961) and Octave Gengou (1875–1957), in *Le microbe de la coqueluche*[1545], again in the *Annals of the Pasteur Institute*, reported the discovery of the 'Bordet–Gengou bacillus', *Haemophilus (Bordetella) pertussis*, the causative agent of whooping cough.

At the beginning of the last decade of the century, Pasteur's idea of the prophylactic use of attenuated organisms was extended to the use of toxins and antitoxins – a prime mover in this new development being Emil Adolf von Behring (1854–1917), a Prussian army surgeon who became professor of hygiene at Halle and then Marburg. Pasteur and his pupils knew that the clear filtrate of some organisms could exert pathological effects. In 1889, in another observation the potential of which may not be, even today, fully exhausted, Hans Buchner (1850–1902) had shown that the bactericidal power of defibrinated blood was possessed by the blood serum, even when this was free from cells, and was lost if the serum was heated to 55 °C for 1 hour. There was, therefore, a heat-labile property that could kill bacteria in the cell-free serum[1546].

In effect, von Behring, while working in Koch's Institute with Baron Shibasaburo Kitasato (1856–1931), extended Pasteur's observations to a second generation and showed that the serum of animals immunized by means of attenuated diphtheria toxins could be used as either a preventive or therapeutic inoculation against virulent diphtheria in other animals. The protective agent was clearly an antitoxin, capable of neutralizing the toxin of the disease, and the discovery of the antitoxins to tetanus and diphtheria was announced in von Behring and Kitasato's joint paper *Ueber das Zustandekommen der Diphtherie-Immunität und der Tetanus-Immunität bei Thieren*[1547] of 1890. It is this notable paper which began the prophylactic and therapeutic use of antitoxins. Emil von Behring has a later paper of 1894 dealing more fully with the clinical potential of diphtheria antitoxin[1548] and a still later work of 1913–1914 extending the knowledge of the subject[1549]. In 1900, von Behring became the first recipient of the Nobel Prize for Medicine.

Studies on the cellular expression of immunity and resistance to infection rest upon the work with *Daphnia* of the great Russian biologist, Elie Metchnikoff (1845–1916). In 1884, Metchnikoff showed how amoeboid cells in the interstitial fluid and blood engulf organisms or microscopical foreign particles, so destroying the ingested bacteria in the phenomenon of phagocytosis[1550]. Metchnikoff produced a classical set of lectures on the pathology of inflammation in 1892[1551] and this was immediately translated into French; it appeared in an important English version in 1893. In 1903, Metchnikoff, who was awarded a Nobel Prize in 1908, published a joint work with Pierre Roux annoucing the successful transmission of syphilis from man to higher apes[1552].

At the turn of the century Sir Almroth Wright (1861–1947) devised an agglutination test permitting the diagnosis of undulant fever (1897)[1553] and then went on to make typhoid vaccination practicable. Writing with Sir William

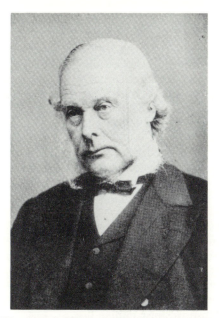

Figure 135   Joseph Lister, 1st Baron Lister (1827–1912).

Leishman (1865–1926), he recorded his *Remarks on the results which have been obtained by the antityphoid inoculations*[1554] in 1900. In 1903 and 1904, with Stewart Douglas (1871–1936), in two important papers called *An experimental investigation of the rôle of the blood fluids in connection with phagocytosis*[1555], Almroth Wright showed the existence of the thermolabile opsonins in both normal and immune serum.

There is a curiously interesting paper, *On some properties in achromatic object-glasses applicable to the improvement of the microscope*[1556] which appears in the *Philosophical Transactions of the Royal Society* for 1830 and which antedates much that has been recounted regarding the developments from Pasteur's work onwards. It was contributed by Joseph Jackson Lister (1786–1869), the father of Lord Lister, and represents the working out of the basic idea of the modern microscope with its achromatic lenses. Chromatic aberration was due to the reflected light rays from the mirror of the microscope being divided into the spectrum. Joseph Jackson Lister's innovation was to design a doublet lens – a plano-concave lens of flint glass to which a convex lens of crown glass was cemented – which permitted the making of the achromatic microscope.

Joseph Lister, ultimately 1st Baron Lister (Figure 135; 1827–1912), graduated from the University of London in 1852 and then, in 1854, after moving to Edinburgh, became house-surgeon to Syme. The eldest daughter of Syme later became Lister's wife. In 1858 Lister produced one of his most valuable papers, *On the early stages of inflammation*[1557]. In 1862, having already become professor of surgery in the University of Glasgow, Lister produced his essay *On the coagulation of the blood*[1558]; this was a Croonian Lecture which was published in 1863 and showed that, in contradistinction to previous theories, blood clotting within blood vessels depended upon their injury. By this time Lister had shown that blood, protected from contamination, could be kept free from putrefaction indefinitely. This led him towards Pasteur's ideas and away from the concept of spontaneous generation. In 1865 he made his reputation as a surgeon with his classical paper *On excision of the wrist for caries*[1559].

At this stage Lister seems to have been impressed with the fact that the mortality in amputation, despite his adoption of the clean techniques of Syme, was of the order of 45%. The threshold of his understanding seems to have come with his observation that excellence of healing, healing by first intention, was usually achieved without purulence, in disregard to the then current doctrine of 'laudable pus'. Perhaps influenced by his father's interest in microscopy, he proved receptive to Pasteur's ideas on the significance of micro-organisms as a cause of infection.

Aware that heat sterilization was of little application to work on living tissues, he turned his attention to chemical antiseptics, or means of germ killing. In the *Lancet* of 1867 he produced his first work on the antiseptic principle in surgery. This was the essay *On a new method of treating compound fracture, abscess, ... with observations on the conditions of suppuration*[1560]. Looking for something which could be used during operations to kill germs, although these had not yet been shown to cause human disease, Lister settled upon the use of carbolic acid. Once he had fully realized the significance of Pasteur's discoveries regarding fermentation, Lister produced, again in 1867 and in the *Lancet*, his paper *On the antiseptic principle in the practice of surgery*[1561] which represents an epoch-making contribution to surgical science.

Seemingly undeterred by criticism, Lister developed a carbolized catgut ligature (1869)[1562] which let him close operative wounds completely, and in 1870 he wrote *On the effects of the antiseptic system of treatment upon the salubrity of a surgical hospital*[1563]. In the same year he brought the most simple possible method of using carbolic sterilization to field conditions with his paper, *A method of antiseptic treatment applicable to wounded soldiers in the present war* (1870)[1564]. He reported the isolation of *Bacillus lactis* in 1873[1565], wrote again on the subject in 1877–78[1566], and was, within a few years, able to operate on joints and extend the anatomical territory potentially available to surgical intervention more vigorously than any previous surgeon.

In 1869 Lister became Syme's successor at Edinburgh. In 1877 he accepted the chair in surgery at King's College, London. He was president of the Royal Society from 1895 to 1900 and, in 1897, became the first man of medicine to be raised to the peerage.

Both Oliver Wendall Holmes and Ignaz Semmelweis had, before Lister, striven to obtain antisepsis in obstetrics. Lister recognized the contributions of both, but was the first to understand the implications to surgery of the discoveries of Pasteur. Listerism allowed surgery to extend into the hollow cavities of the body and, even after the idea of asepsis rather than antisepsis had been developed, it still allowed the surgeon to produce greatly improved results under battlefield conditions. Although he did not himself invade the closed spaces of the body, the cranial cavity and the chest and abdomen, Lister's work fluently applied the nineteenth century progress in microbiology to a new age.

There is a fine, two volume, *Collected Papers*[1567], published in 1909, 3 years before his death. Of Lister, it has been written that when he 'was laid at rest in West Hampstead Cemetery, England had buried her greatest surgeon'[1568]. His principle of antisepsis, and his methods against bacteria and their invasion, was of the same effect as today's asepsis, the prevention of microbial access to the wound. It is clear that he left a considerate tradition of surgery, respectful of the need to prevent invasion by pathogens once the defences of the body had been breached. He ends his paper of 1867 on the antiseptic principle with the following passage commenting on the change which the method has brought about in his surgical wards at Glasgow[1561]:

> There is, however, one point more that I cannot but advert to – namely, the influence of this mode of treatment upon the general healthiness of a hospital. Previously to its introduction, the two large wards in which most of my cases of accident and of operation are treated were amongst the unhealthiest in the whole surgical division of the Glasgow Royal Infirmary, in consequence, apparently, of those wards being unfavourably placed with reference to the supply of fresh air; and I have felt ashamed, when recording the results of my practice, to have so often to allude to hospital gangrene or pyaemia. It was interesting, though melancholy, to observe that, whenever all, or nearly all, the beds contained cases with open sores, these grievous complications were pretty sure to show themselves; so that I came to welcome simple fractures, though in themselves of little interest either for myself or the students, because their presence diminished the proportion of open sores among the patients. But since the antiseptic treatment has been brought into full operation, and wounds and abscesses no longer poison the atmosphere with putrid exhalations, my wards, though in other respects under precisely the same circumstances as before, have completely changed their character; so that during the last nine months not a single instance of pyaemia, hospital gangrene, or erysipelas has occurred in them.
>
> As there appears to be no doubt regarding the cause of this change, the importance of the fact can hardly be exaggerated.

The pioneer of visceral surgery was Christian Albert Billroth (1829–1894), professor of surgery at Zürich and then Vienna. His major works include an excellent set of lectures on surgical pathology and therapeutics (1863)[1569], a description of the first resection of the oesophagus (1872)[1570], a report of the first successful resection of the pylorus for neoplasia, the Billroth I operation (1881)[1571], and a study (written by Ernst Hauer) of Billroth's long series of intestinal resections and anastomotic operations (1884)[1572]; the Billroth II gastro-enterostomy was recorded by Viktor von Hacker (1852–1933) in a paper published in 1885[1573].

Carl Thiersch (1822–1895), professor of surgery at Erlangen and then Leipzig, a great pioneer of Listerism, produced a number of works including the classical description (1867) of phosphoric necrosis of the jaw[1574] and a paper of 1874 which gives his first account of transplantation of the skin – the skin graft for which his name has become famous[1575].

Lister's antiseptic methods gradually merged into the present-day idea of asepsis. The great pioneer in the change was Ernst von Bergmann (1836–1907), a

Russian who ultimately held the surgical chair at Würzburg and then Berlin. He used corrosive sublimate as an antiseptic and then evolved methods of steam sterilization and, finally, the modern aseptic ritual. He has publications of 1887[1576] and 1888[1577] which show how much he was able to advance the surgical treatment of intracranial disease.

Sir James Paget (1814–1899), whose name is associated with Paget's disease of the nipple (eczema of the nipple with cancerous changes; 1874)[1578] and with Paget's disease (osteitis deformans; 1877, 1882)[1579], whilst still a first year medical student at St. Bartholomew's, discovered trichina in a muscle during dissection. His tutor, Sir Richard Owen (1804–1892) named the parasite *Trichina spiralis* and published an account of the condition in 1835[1580].

The late phases of the nineteenth century ended not only enriched by the knowledge of pathology derived from the cell theory, the practical advantages of antisepsis with their theoretical basis in the germ theory, and with the boon of inhalational anaesthesia – they ended also with a wealth of new clinical observation, some of these observations expressing themselves in the modern specialties.

Modern ophthalmology derives largely from the work of Friedrich von Graefe (1828–1870). In 1857 he described an operation for strabismus[1581]. In 1857 and the following few years he introduced iridectomy for the treatment of glaucoma[1582]. In 1859 he showed that central retinal artery thrombosis can be a cause of sudden blindness[1583]. In 1860 and in later publications he showed the importance of optic neuritis in the pathogenesis of several kinds of vision impairments[1584]. In 1864 he wrote an account[1585] of the failure of the upper eyelid to follow the eyeball as the latter is rolled downwards in exophthalmic goitre (von Graefe's sign of the current textbooks) and in 1867, amongst his several later works, he provided a monograph which forms the basis of contemporary knowledge of the diagnostic symptomology of the ocular paralyses[1586].

In obstetrics the great change was the lessened mortality from infection – but features of present practice also appeared. In 1860 Credé's method of delivering the placenta by gentle external manual expression was described[1587]. It had been anticipated by a century in the writing (*Practical directions, shewing a method of preserving the perinaeum in birth, and delivering the placenta without violence*, 1767)[1588] of John Harvie, Smellie's successor, but the eighteenth century idea had been ignored. Carl Siegmund Credé (1819–1892) not only brought in his method of placental expression but also, in works of 1884 and in his influential teaching, introduced the use of silver nitrate drops instilled into the eyes of new-born infants to prevent ophthalmia neonatorum[1589].

The modern concept of paediatrics was virtually begun by Eduard Henoch (1820–1910), of Berlin. He described what is now known as 'Henoch's purpura' in a paper of 1868[1590]; he also gave the first account *Ueber Purpura fulminans* in 1887[1591], and brought out the book, *Vorlesungen über Kinderkrankheiten*[1592], which so much affected contemporary and later attitudes to the care of children, in 1881.

Modern neurology derives from the French school of medicine and found its formative nineteenth century expression in the works of Jean Martin Charcot (1825–1893). In 1862, Charcot became physician to the hospital of the Salpêtrière – an institute with which his name has ever since been associated. He produced one of the earliest reports of intermittent claudication in man (1859)[1593], gave the first description of the lightning pains in tabes dorsalis (1866)[1594], began the formal study of geriatrics in the same year[1595], gave a brilliant account of tabetic arthropathy (Charcot's joints) in 1868[1596] and, again in 1868, in a paper on the *Histologie de la sclérose en plaques*[1597] gave an account of the appearances in multiple sclerosis.

Charcot's contributions to the morbid anatomy of neurological disease are of lasting importance. He described the histological lesions of the spinal cord in muscular atrophy (1869)[1598] and provided the first demonstration of the atrophy of the anterior horns of the spinal cord in poliomyelitis (1870)[1599]. He wrote the splendid *Leçons sur les maladies du système nerveux faites à La Salpêtrière*[1600] of 1872-1887 and, in their three volumes, these lectures remain informative. There is an English translation of 1877-1889. Charcot wrote also the *Leçons sur les localisations dans les maladies du cerveau* (1876-1880)[1601] which is an intellectual giant of a work adding vastly to the knowledge of the localization of functions and lesions in diseases of the brain. The illustrations, and studies working out the central nervous system pathways involved in some of these lesions, in themselves make these works memorable. Charcot made many other contributions to the literature. These include (with Jean Albert Pitres, 1848-1928) the three papers on *Les centres moteurs corticaux chez l'homme* of 1877, 1878 and 1883 (published as a book in 1895)[1602] which eliminated all doubt about the existence of cortical motor centres in man and, finally, Charcot's *Oeuvres complètes*[1603] – a nine volume masterpiece, published in 1888-1894, which forms a fitting memorial to the teaching and discoveries of a clinic now considered to have been the finest neurological centre of modern times.

The principal British neurologists of the transition of the centuries were John Hughlings Jackson (1834-1911), Sir William Richard Gowers (1845-1915), and Sir Victor Horsley (1857-1916). Hughlings Jackson wrote much that was ahead of time and appreciated only more recently. In 1863 he published a paper on *Unilateral epileptiform seizures, attended by temporary defect of sight*[1604]. What is now called 'Jacksonian epilepsy' had, as a unilateral seizure, been previously recorded but Jackson gave such an excellent account of the condition that it has since always been associated with his name. He is largely responsible for the widespread recognition of the importance of the ophthalmoscope in neurological diagnosis and he wrote on this subject between 1863 and 1866[1605]. He studied aphasia for 30 years, wrote on this subject in 1864[1606], and is substantially responsible for the present understanding of this condition, of which, in a manner like that of Charcot, he was keenly aware of the psychological elements in the clinical presentation. His *Notes on the physiology and pathology of language* (1866)[1607] form a fascinating entry to subjects still being explored. He gave the first notable account (1867)[1608] of syringomyelia (in a paper in association with Jacob Augustus Clarke; 1817-1880) and he predicted, from clinical observations, the existence of motor areas in the frontal lobes of the cerebrum. Later the same year (1870) Gustav Fritsch (1838-1891) and Eduard Hitzig (1838-1907) showed that electrical stimulation of the frontal cortex did indeed cause movements of the peripheral elements of the opposite side of the body[1609]. His other publications include his *Remarks on the relations of different divisions of the central nervous system to one another and to parts of the body*[1610] – an important paper of 1898 which began the concept of functional 'levels' in the nervous system.

The first haemocytometer was produced by Louis Malassez (1842–1909) and reported in 1874[1611]; the instrument was modified and named by Sir William Gowers, later professor of clinical medicine at University College, London. Gowers gave an important account of the changes in the retinal arteries in Bright's disease (1876)[1612]; his *The diagnosis of diseases of the spinal cord* (1880)[1613] described 'Gowers's tract', and in 1881 he published a classical account of epilepsy[1614]. The latter book remains one of the most important on its subject. A fine teacher, Gowers produced his *Lectures on the diagnosis of diseases of the brain*[1615] in 1885 and his finest work, *A manual of diseases of the nervous system*[1616], in 1886–1888. His later studies include a paper *On myopathy and a distal form* (1902)[1617] which describes the form of progressive muscular dystrophy known as 'the distal myopathy of Gowers'. His work on muscular dystrophy preserves his name in the form of 'Gowers' sign' – the condition in which, with the hands, the patient climbs up the legs on rising from the floor; the sign is characteristic but not specific for muscular dystrophy as it occurs in any disorder in which the pelvic girdle muscles are weakened.

Sir Victor Horsley was the founder of neurosurgery in England. Gowers and Horsley together wrote a paper, *A case of tumour of the spinal cord. Removal; recovery*[1618], in 1888, which records the first successful excision of an extra-medullary tumour of the spinal cord. Horsley did important work on the physiology of the nervous system. In 1884 he reported the effects of excision of the thyroid in the monkey[1619]. The picture he described is now considered to be the mixed syndrome resulting from myxoedema and parathyroid excision. In 1886 he wrote on *Functional nervous disorders due to loss of thyroid gland and pituitary body*[1620]. This work provided the first successful attempts at hypophy-sectomy in animals – two dogs surviving for 5 months or longer after pituitary excision.

Horsley then became interested in the localization of central nervous system functions and, with Charles Edward Beevor (1854–1907) of the National Hospital, Queen Square, published *A minute analysis (experimental) of the various movements produced by stimulating in the monkey different regions of the cortical centre for the upper limb . . .*[1621]. This important paper, of 1887, was followed by *A record of experiments upon the functions of the cerebral cortex* (1889)[1622]. Then, in a joint publication with Francis Gotch (1853–1913) (*On the mammalian nervous system, its functions, and their localisation determined by an electrical method*)[1623]. Horsley showed that minute electrical currents are produced by the functioning brain. By recording these currents with the string galvanometer, Horsley and his colleagues laid the foundation for the later development of electroencephalography.

With the present century only just started, Horsley, with Robert Clarke (1850–1926), using an apparatus which allowed the accurate localization of electrodes placed experimentally in the brain, undertook the work which led to their paper on *The structure and functions of the cerebellum examined by a new method* (1908)[1624]. This study led the way to modern stereotactic neurological surgery. It appeared one year before Horsley's *The Linacre Lecture on the function of the so-called motor area of the brain* (1909)[1625] which showed that ablation of the precentral gyrus or cortex in man abolished athetosis.

Cholera in England

Asiatic cholera broke out in Sunderland in October, 1831, the following being the record of the first few cases [1626]:

Allison, aged fifty, a painter of earthenware residing in a low situation on the bank of the Wear two miles above the town, was attacked at 4 a.m. on the 5th August with vomiting and purging of a watery whitish fluid, like oatmeal and water. His hands and feet were cold, his skin covered with clammy sweat, his face livid and the expression anxious, his eyes sunken, his lips blue, thirst excessive, his breath cold, his voice weak and husky, and his pulse almost imperceptible. He passed into a stage of reactive fever and got well. Arnott, a farm-labourer on the opposite bank of the Wear from the man Allison, was seized at 2 a.m. on the 8th August with precisely the same symptoms, and died in twelve hours. Neither he nor Allison had any intercourse or relation with seamen or the shipping of Sunderland. Another case on the 8th August came to light afterwards. A woman in the village of West Bolden, four miles from Sunderland, on the Newcastle road, was found by a surgeon from the town to be suffering from choleraic sickness, of which she died twelve hours from its onset.

A week after these cases in the country not far from Sunderland, there occurred the death, on 14th August, of one of the Wear pilots named Henry. He had been troubled with diarrhoea for some time before, but not so as to keep him from his occupation. Having gone down in the direction of Flamborough Head to look for ships, he picked up a vessel between that and the Wear, piloted her in, and, a few days after, piloted her out again. The identity of the vessel was never traced, but it was alleged that she had come from an infected port abroad. The last time Henry was in his boat he was seized with violent vomiting and purging, and died at his house after an illness of twenty hours. A brother pilot, who looked in at the house on the day of his death, fell into a similar choleraic disorder, but recovered. On the 28th August a shipwright died of the same; also about the end of August two persons at a distance of four or five miles from Sunderland. In September, it is said, there were other cases and fatalities. Early in October the authentic particulars of cholera in Sunderland begin. Dixon attended one case, which was fatal on the 9th October. Another case, which came to light three months after, was that of a girl of twelve, named Hazard, residing on the Fish Quay, who was well enough on Sunday the 16th October to have been twice at church. She was seized in the middle of the night following with the sudden and appalling symptoms of choleraic disease and died on the Monday afternoon. A few doors off on the same quay lived a keelman named Sproat, aged sixty; he occupied a large, clean, well-ventilated room on the first-floor of a house in the most open part of the quay, opposite to a crowded part of the anchorage. He was in failing health, and had been troubled with diarrhoea for a week or ten days previous to the 19th October, on which day he had to give up work. Next day, Thursday, the 20th, a surgeon who had been sent for found him vomiting and purging, but not at all collapsed, with no thirst, and in good spirits. He improved so much that on Friday he had toasted cheese for supper and on Saturday a mutton chop for dinner, after which he went out to his keel on the river for a few minutes. On his return he was seized with rigor, cramps, vomiting and purging. Medical aid was not sent for until seven on Sunday morning, when he was found in a sinking state, pulseless, speaking in a husky whisper, his face livid and pinched, his limbs cramped, the purgings like "meal washings." He continued like that for three days, and died on Wednesday, the 26th October, at noon.

This came to be reckoned the first death from Asiatic cholera in England.

His grandchild, a girl of eleven, while moving about the room an hour after the death, was suddenly seized with faintness, pains in the stomach-region, vomiting and purging of watery matters; she was taken to the Infirmary and soon got well. The day after his father's death, Thursday, the 27th October, William Sproat, junior, a fine athletic young keelman, who had attended on his parent during his illness, was found lying in a low damp cellar near to the Fish Quay, suffering from choleraic symptoms; he had been ill only a few hours, and was removed (with his daughter as above) to the Infirmary the same evening. He became gradually worse: on the 30th he was continually throwing himself about, moaning and biting the bedclothes; on the 31st he was lying on his back comatose, his eyes open, the pupils wide and insensible, and the breathing stertorous, in which state he died the same day. An old nurse at the Infirmary (Turnbull) helped to place the body in the coffin, went to bed in a state of considerable fear, and was seized at one in the morning with symptoms of cholera, of which she died after a few hours.

Meanwhile there had been two other fatal cases unconnected with the Sproats or the Fish Quay. On the quay of Monk Wearmouth, across the river, lived a shoemaker named Rodenburg, aged thirty-five. He occupied a poor hovel and had a large family, but he was in good work and wages. On Sunday, the 30th October, he had pork for dinner, and what was left of it for supper. In the middle of the night he was seized with vomiting, and with purging of a fluid like water-gruel in vast quantities; when visited by the medical men, he spoke in a husky whisper, his nails were blue, his skin livid, covered by cold sweat, his limbs cramped. The spasms ceased about nine o'clock on Monday morning; about noon he asked to be raised in bed, and died as they were raising him. On the very same night, between Sunday and Monday, a keelman named Wilson, who lived with his wife in a decent room in the High Street, and had attended the Methodist chapel on Sunday, was seized with cholera at 4 a.m. on Monday, and died the same afternoon at three.

The account, displaying many of the features of cholera, is that preserved by Charles Creighton (1847–1927), who also prepared an English translation of August Hirsch's (1817–1894) *Handbuch der historisch-geographischen Pathologie*[1627]; the latter study is possibly the best book on its subject and was published, in its translation, by the New Sydenham Society in 1883–1886.

The outbreak of Asiatic Cholera in Sunderland in 1831 was part of the spread of this illness, not previously endemic in Britain, from its ancient sites in India to China, Japan, Asiatic Russia and Eastern Europe early in the nineteenth century. Virtually the whole of Britain and Europe was involved by the winter of 1832. Unlike plague, the disease travelled slowly – a little slower than people, by the means of transport then available – moved or migrated. This rate of spread allowed for some measure of action by the authorities of the time.

In June, 1831 a Central Board of Health was established under the authority of the Privy Council. From the beginning it was clear that if the Board was to accomplish anything useful in the face of the advancing disease, then it must work through organizations which already existed. Essentially, these organizations comprised the Parish Officers and Justices of the Peace, whose real functions were to implement the provisions of the Poor Law. Thus, when the Board met at the end of June and made its recommendations to the Privy Council these, historically, became the first such set of proposals of modern times to influence the public health by means of local government.

The background of the beginnings of public hygiene lay in reports by Sir James Phillips Kay-Shuttleworth (1804–1877) on the fate of cotton operatives in Manchester (1832), the investigations leading up to this report, and the later reports on the training of pauper children (1841) and public education (1852–62). Thomas Southwood Smith (1788–1861) had produced his book *A treatise on fever*[1628] in 1830 and, as physician to the London Fever Hospital, was to produce a report to the Poor Law Commissioners on the physical causes of preventable mortality and morbidity amongst the poor (1838).

Cholera, taking some advantage of the conditions these reports set out to change, moved fast enough to excite great anxiety. Although none of the members of the Central Board of Health set up to deal with the problem had ever seen a case of cholera and nothing was known of the cause or method of transmission of the disease, the recommendations of the Board were extreme. Each town or village was to appoint a local Board of Health, the medical member of this body was to correspond with the Board of Health in London, and in each town or neighbourhood one or more places was to be 'immediately pointed out as places to which every case of the disease as soon as detected might be removed in conveyances appropriated exclusively for the purpose'. The Board proposed that 'expurgators' should remove the sick to the appointed places – just as contacts were to be sent to isolation hospitals; help, if needed, was to be provided by the military, the police, and a system of fines. When these proposals, shorn of the 'expurgators' and the provisions for fines, were made public both the scheme and its originators were quickly attacked by Thomas Wakley, editor of the *Lancet*. Wakley's other attacks included that on John Elliotson (1791–1868)[1629], a friend of Dickens and Thackeray and among the first to operate with the aid of hypnotism, and Sir William Wilde (1815–1876), who in 1853 wrote the first British book to place the treatment of middle ear disease on a sound footing and provide diseases of the ear with a firm basis in pathology[1630].

Despite publication and implementation of a final set of regulations, the epidemic which followed the first cases of cholera at Sunderland caused about 22 000 deaths by early June, 1832. The epidemic waned by December, and the Central Board of Health was then dissolved. The measures taken late in the epidemic had been assisted by the sensible provisions of the Cholera Prevention Act of February, 1832 – this permitted direction by Orders in Council and these provided for the nursing of the sick poor in their own homes, the cleansing of infected houses, the covering of drains and cesspools, and the destruction of clothing and bedding which had belonged to the dead. The useful effect of these provisions was limited by the lack of resources.

The second great cholera epidemic in Britain produced cases in Edinburgh late in 1848. The disease spread to involve London by the December and the whole of the country by June, 1849. The epidemic was worse than that of 1831–32 and it is reckoned that some 54 000 persons died of the infection in England and Wales.

During and prior to the period of the second epidemic, a great deal of attention was focused on the care of the poor and the need for improvements in hygiene. In this movement Sir Edwin Chadwick (1800–1890), then secretary to the Poor Law Commission but previously a lawyer, became of commanding influence. He provided reports on poor law reform (1834–42) and cemeteries (1843–55) but it was his *Report . . . from the Poor Law Commissioners on an enquiry into the sanitary conditions of the labouring population of Great Britain*[1631] of 1842 which highlighted the abject results of the Industrial Revolution and vividly displayed the insanitary conditions under which much of the working section of the population was then living. The value of the report lay in its reliance on a careful analysis of the causes of death in 1838 and 1839. As a result of this and earlier reports the Public Health Act of 1848 ('The Chadwick Act') passed onto the statute book and the General Board of Health was instituted. Chadwick became a salaried member of the General Board and played a conspicuous part in the process of reform – until his dictatorial manner and demanding tone so greatly antagonized both the medical profession and the local authorities that, in July, 1854, the motion in Parliament to extend the Public Health Act for a further term was defeated. The demise of Chadwick roughly coincided with the later stages of the third great cholera epidemic, that of 1853–54, and there is little doubt that the failure of the General Board to arrest cholera contributed to the outcome. Chadwick has often been said to have begun the modern era of public health. A fitting tribute to his benefaction was produced by Sir Benjamin Ward Richardson (1828–1896) whose two volume work, *The health of nations. A review of the works of Edwin Chadwick*[1632] was published in London in 1887.

The person who solved the problem of the transmission of cholera was John Snow (1813–1858), of Westminster Hospital, London. Snow is often thought of as the first specialist anaesthetist. In 1847 he gave an account of an ether inhaler which was the first to regulate the amount of ether vapour received by the patient[1633]. In 1848 he described his invention of a chloroform inhaler[1634]. In 1850 he produced a work showing that he had attempted to devise a means of carbon dioxide absorption during anaesthesia[1635]. In 1858, after delivering Queen Victoria by means of chloroform in 1853 and again in 1857, he wrote a classical study, *On chloroform and other anaesthetics: their action and administration*[1636]. These contributions put the administration of anaesthetic vapours on a scientific basis and displayed an approach to obscure problems which became relevant to cholera.

In the first cholera outbreak, early in 1832, Snow, then an apprentice in Newcastle-on-Tyne, helped to deal with the cholera epidemic at Killingworth colliery. This experience left him believing that the infection might be spread by foods, fluids, or hands, if contaminated with the bodily discharges. In 1849, in the second epidemic, when 140 deaths occurred in an orphan asylum at Tooting, he confirmed his impression and seems to have discarded the old ideas that the illness was spread by 'miasma' or foul air. The children he recognized might spread infection by contagion and by contaminating one another with gastro-intestinal discharges.

Later in 1849, Snow investigated a cholera outbreak which caused over 600 deaths in the area of Golden Square, London. Snow showed that all but ten of the 69 people who had died in Broad Street drew their water from the pump in that same street. Contact with the pump in Broad Street existed in several of the ten patients in the group. Snow also traced the pipelines of the different water companies supplying the streets in the area and found that some supplies were associated with gross outbreaks of the disease, while others were almost clear. Putting his several observations together he concluded that faecal material from the cholera cases contaminated the water supplies, either by draining through the soil to the wells from the cesspits or by direct involvement of the rivers and sources of supplies. In 1849 he published *On the mode of communication of cholera* (of which the second edition gives the story of the Broad Street well) and his paper *On the pathology and mode of communication of the cholera*[1637].

In 1849, the year of Snow's publication, William Budd (1811–1880), of Bristol, reached the same conclusion. Both Snow and Budd therefore came close to anticipating the germ theory of Pasteur. Budd later strengthened the theory of water-borne infection and in 1873 published on *Typhoid fever; its nature, mode of spreading, and prevention*[1638]. Snow's results were also confirmed when the General Board of Health itself investigated cholera death rates in the areas supplied by the various water companies in nine London parishes.

These results were presented to the General Board by Sir John Simon (1816–1904) who became the first medical officer for the City of London. Simon, next to Chadwick the most important reformer of the public health and hygiene of the nineteenth century, published his famous *Public health reports*[1639] in 1887. His later work, *English sanitary institutions, reviewed in their course of development, and in some of their political and social relations*[1640], of 1890, dissects the public health problem of the day, discusses the growth and purposes of the public health improvement, and has been of lasting influence. Simon's skill and natural diplomacy, supported by the factual analyses in his reports, initiated the Sanitary Act of 1866 and the modern era of public health management. By means of this Act and the associated legislation of the period, the local authorities of the day obtained improved powers to clean up towns and reduce the cause of illness within them. Implementation of these powers became possible with the passing of the Local Government Board Act of 1871 – and, with the passing of the old poor law provisions, these Boards took over the care of the poor and the public health, so bringing together two needs which are frequently manifestations of one problem.

The last of the great epidemics of cholera in Britain, that of 1866, was contemporaneous with the passing into law of the Sanitary Act. Its effects destroyed public complacency and lent force to the movement to provide clean drinking water and the means of the hygienic disposal of waste and sewage. Thus, before any drug active against the *Vibrio cholerae* had been described, the methods of prevention of the disease had been provided by sanitary reform. The most important English treatise on hygiene was *A manual of practical hygiene*[1641] written by Edmund Alexander Parkes (1819–1876). In this work, the first major English study of its kind, Parkes was aided by Lord Sidney Herbert (1810–1861), who was Secretary for War at the time of the outbreak of the Crimean War in 1854. Those early involved in bringing forward proposals for public health organization in the United States were Lemuel Shattuck (1793–1859) and his

465

colleagues N. P. Banks and J. Abbott who put forward their *Report of a general plan for the promotion of public and personal health, devised, prepared, and recommended by the commissioners appointed under a resolve of the legislature of Massachusetts relating to a sanitary survey of the State*[1642]. Although this historic item was published in Boston in 1850 – and led to Shattuck being called 'the Chadwick of America' – a Board of Health was not established until 1869. There is a facsimile of the Report dated 1948.

Chadwick's other great gift to his nation was to convince William Farr (1807–1883) to leave clinical practice and enter the office of the Registrar General. Farr's *Vital statistics*[1643], which ranks with Graunt's 'Observations' as a fundamental contribution to its subject, appeared in 1837; it was reprinted in 1974. He devised what is known as 'Farr's law', that the graphical expression of an epidemic shows a first rapid ascent, then slopes slowly to a maximum, only to fall more rapidly than it mounted. He has an important later study on life expectation (1875)[1644] and this appeared in the same year that Henry Wyldbore Rumsey (1809–1876) published his finely critical *Essays and papers on some fallacies of statistics concerning life and death, health and disease* (1875)[1645].

The Medical Reform

The nineteenth century saw the established earlier practices of the profession of medicine radically changed in response to a demand for reform. Much of this demand arose from the new Middle Class, made rich by the Industrial Revolution and equipped to demand better medical attention than could be provided by the few Edinburgh graduates then available and the rest of the profession with its widely varying standards. A similar demand arose within the profession itself: the younger graduates, especially those of Edinburgh, could envisage the dangers to the whole profession from its obvious inadequacies – and the great mass of surgeons and apothecaries wanted to advance themselves by better training and separate themselves from the totally unqualified.

The professional ambitions of the apothecaries gradually increased from the date of the Rose case which, in 1704, gave them a legal right to practise medicine. It is from this date that the general practitioner or family doctor began to emerge. The momentum of the change increased when, in 1748, Parliament refused to pass a Bill granting the apothecaries the monopoly of pharmaceutical retail trade. More and more apothecaries then practised medicine, fewer kept retail shops, and in 1774 the Court of the Society of Apothecaries decided to restrict their Livery to those members who practised medicine.

In the early part of the nineteenth century, Sir Joseph Banks, President of the Royal Society, undertook an enquiry on the best method of improving medical education. Banks had been much concerned with the Apothecaries' Physic Garden at Chelsea and, in 1815, the Society of Apothecaries secured an Act whereby all apothecaries in England and Wales, other than those already in practice, were required to be examined and licensed by the Society after serving a five-year apprenticeship. This momentous Apothecaries' Act of 1815 attained the objective of providing a medical qualification effective anywhere in the Kingdom but, intentionally or not, it put the control of virtually the whole of general medical practice into the hands of the Society by making it possible for it to prosecute anyone who set up as a doctor without the Apothecaries' licence. There followed a period of controversial and constructive effort by the Society and the subsequent shape of medicine in Britain owes much to the wisdom with which these great powers were exercised. Certificates were demanded showing that courses in anatomy and physiology and in the theory and practice of medicine had been pursued, in addition to the period of apprenticeship. Most usefully of all, the Society demanded evidence that the candidates for its licence had walked the wards of a recognized hospital for at least 6 months.

The old Company of Surgeons had become the Royal College of Surgeons in 1800 and, so that its members could achieve a status which ranked at least equal to that of the apothecaries, the Surgeons increased the requirements for their diploma. The demands of both bodies could then be met by the additional hospital experience and an additional course of lectures in surgery. Many candidates then began to seek the double qualification of 'College and Hall' – so beginning the practical tradition of the properly qualified general practitioner who could claim a basic level of competence as both physician and surgeon.

The extent of the success of the 1815 Act, despite its imperfections, can be judged by from figures given by Frederick F. Cartwright[1646] who notes that: 'In the years 1842–4 only sixteen licences were granted by the universities and thirty-seven by the Royal College of Physicians. The remaining English licences, 953 in number, were granted by 'college and hall', that is by the Royal College of Surgeons and the Society of Apothecaries.'

Nevertheless, in 1840, the status of the majority of country doctors remained little more than that of a skilled tradesman whose essential qualifying body was not a university with its several faculties but was instead a Livery Company of the City of London and with a background rooted in commerce. Additionally, the apothecary, if only that licence had been obtained, was still obligated to provide some sort of potion – he could still not legally charge for advice without medicine.

Much of the further call for reform arose from within the ranks of these compulsory vendors of medicines who, even when a statuatory fee of 2 shillings and sixpence per visit was authorized, remained unable, for financial reasons, to relinquish their interest in the retail dispensing trade and leave this to the chemists and druggists – themselves becoming more prosperous and organized since a dissident fraction of the membership of the Society of Apothecaries, led by the quaker Jacob Bell, in 1841, joined with the better of the chemists and druggists to establish the present-day Pharmaceutical Society of Great Britain.

It is now quite difficult to realize how late was the development of any real English university education for the great majority of students of medicine. Charing Cross Hospital was founded by Benjamin Golding in 1821 with the specific intention of providing such an education. Seven years later, University College was founded in Gower Street and in 1831 King's College was established in the Strand, London. Both of these latter institutes had medical departments from the beginning and both acquired or founded hospital teaching facilities within a few years. Even so, teaching was still related to the requirements of the Society of Apothecaries when the University of London was incorporated by its Charter of 1836. It offered degrees in medicine 2 years later but these were not accepted as licences for the practice of medicine until 1854. Thus, the Penny

Black, the first adhesive postage stamp of such interest to philatelists, issued in 1840, is of the same date as the first medical degrees conferred on university-educated medical graduates in London. And when the first London medical degrees were accepted as a licence to practice in 1854, ether anaesthesia was already well known, and chloroform had been introduced by James Young Simpson in Edinburgh some 7 years before; Rudolf Virchow's '*Cellular Pathologie*' of 1858 and Louis Pasteur's presentation of his germ theory to the Sorbonne University in 1864 both came early in the professional lives of this particular group of graduates from London.

In London, university medical education to an organized curriculum barely preceded the great discoveries and ideas which form the scientific basis of medicine. Subsequently, the great advances in scientific knowledge meant that although the licence of the Society of Apothecaries held its place for many years and was the most popular medical qualification, educating the practitioner of medicine outside a university was less and less practicable – and apprenticeship gave way to university and science-based training.

This transition underlay the final call for medical reform and produced a movement which aimed at an integrated, educated medical profession with one recognized qualification that would ensure a competent standard of practice throughout the country and mark off its registered practitioners from the un-qualified.

Slowly the practitioner of family medicine had emerged from the Elizabethan grocer who also dealt in medicinal herbs and compounded pills and potions. With modern medical science beginning, important figures in the final reform movement included Thomas Wakley, who founded the *Lancet* in 1823, and Charles Hastings, who in 1816 either founded or revived the Worcester Medical and Surgical Society, the forerunner of the British Medical Association established in 1855. As the reform movement gathered strength the Society of Apothecaries continued to be of great standing and importance – almost all of the new provincial universities established in England during the nineteenth century started as a medical school organized to satisfy the requirements of the Apothe-caries' examiners. In 1851 St. Mary's Hospital opened in Paddington with a dis-tinguished medical and surgical staff – but as no resident Apothecary had been appointed the institution was refused recognition until this had been accomplished.

In 1858, with the passing into law of the historic Medical Act of October that year, the reform movement reached its fruition, bringing into being what was then known as 'the General Council of Medical Education and Registration of the United Kingdom'. Not only did this Act, even though it bore the marks of compromise and the 17 previous attempts at such legislation, establish a formal Medical Register – it also instructed the Council to publish for the first time a national pharmacopoeia, and gave it powers to rationalize medical education. The General Medical Council later became widely known for its work, based on a quite modest and inconspicuous section of the Medical Act, which gave it powers to erase from the Register the names of doctors convicted of a criminal offence or judged guilty of infamous conduct in a professional respect.

The potential to rationalize medical education and the pharmacopoeia of practical medicine must seem of equal or greater importance than the Register

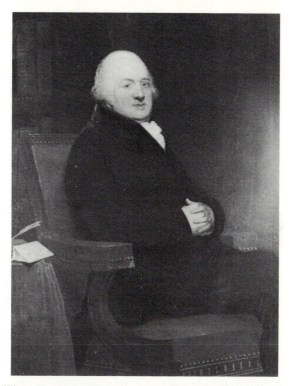

Figure 136   William Saunders. First President of the Medical and Chirurgical Society, London. [*Portrait in the possession of the Royal Society of Medicine.*]

and the power to delete from it – but, of the names added in 1865, that of Elizabeth Garrett (1836–1917) is one of the more historic: after satisfying the requirements for the licence of the Society of Apothecaries, this candidate, later Dr Elizabeth Garrett-Anderson, became the first woman to obtain an English registrable medical qualification. This accomplishment, possible only because the regulations of the Society did not exclude female candidates (the possibility of a woman applying having not been envisaged), led to the founding of the Royal Free Medical School and Hospital for Women, in which Garrett-Anderson was associated with her friend, Sophia Jex-Blake, who qualified from Edinburgh.

Outstanding amongst the eclectic and honourable associations which have been important in the growth of the profession, is the Royal Society of Medicine which had its beginnings in the Medical Society of London, itself founded in 1773..The Medical Society of London flourishes today but from its troubled early years sprang the Medical and Chirurgical Society of London, founded in May 1805. This was to be 'a Society comprehending the several branches of the medical profession' and was to 'be established in London for the purpose of conversation on professional subjects, for the reception of communications, and for the formation of a Library...'[1647]. The first President was William Saunders (Figure 136) and in August 1834 the growing Society received its Charter and became 'The Royal Medical and Chirurgical Society' whose members were then designated Fellows.

The original objectives of the Society were preserved but, as the nineteenth century advanced, it became clear that there would be many advantages from a joining together of the several, sometimes quite small, medical fraternities that had arisen in London. After numerous attempts this was achieved, the necessary Supplemental Charter being received by the Council of the old Society at its house at 20, Hanover Square on June 5th, 1907. The new by-laws of the united societies – now the Royal Society of Medicine – were adopted from June 14th, 1907. There is a pleasing account, by Maurice Davidson (1955)[1647], which describes the founding and growth of the Royal Society of Medicine, the building and opening of its present-day premises at 1, Wimpole Street, London, and the development and activities of the Society's vastly important Library.

The drugs of the nineteenth century

The investigation of the alkaloids began with the nineteenth century. Considering that man has from the very earliest times made use of natural plant drugs for medicinal or spiritual purposes, it must be surprising that knowledge of the active principles of such botanical drugs does not antedate the first decade of the nineteenth century. It is perhaps equally startling that it still remains difficult to present a definition of an alkaloid – a class of drug principles of which over 900 examples are now known – to which there are no exceptions. Among these examples we must number morphine, quinine, nicotine, strychnine and reserpine. An alkaloid is usually understood to be of plant origin; to have a basic, salt-forming, ammonia-like character (the property from which the group derives its name, alkaloid meaning alkali-like); to contain nitrogen, and to produce physiological effects in animals and man. Perhaps oddly, the 900 or more examples come from a comparatively restricted range of plants. They occur mainly in Rubiaceae, Papaveraceae, Fumariaceae, Solanaceae, Leguminosae and Apocynaceae. To a much less extent they are found in the Rosaceae, Graminaceae, Labiatae and Compositae. Although there are exceptions, the same genus, in some cases related genera, yield the same or structurally-related alkaloids. An example is that seven distinct genera of Solanaceae produce the important alkaloid hyoscyamine, the optically active form of the atropine which remains in everyday use.

This class of drugs remains important in medicine and their first representative in the literature is the paper of 1802, *Mémoire sur l'opium*[1648], by Charles Louis Derosne (1780–1846) 'pharmacien de Paris'. Derosne observed that a syrupy extract of opium, when diluted with water, gave a crystalline deposit. He separated this crystalline matter and tried to purify it; by his efforts he prepared the first alkaloid, probably impure narcotine. When he added alkali to the diluted opium syrup he obtained a different substance – this must have contained the alkaloid, morphine. However, it seems clear that Derosne failed to realize that he was dealing with the active physiological principle of the vitally important drug, opium.

This was first grasped by the German, Friedrich Wilhelm Sertürner

(1783–1841) who was born in Neuhaus, near Paderborn in Westphalia. When he was 16 years of age Sertürner became an apprentice in the pharmacy of Paderborn and from 1809 he had his own pharmacy. While he was still an apprentice, in 1805, he published his first paper on opium[1649], giving an account of the discovery of meconic acid in the drug substance. In 1806 he published a second, epoch-making paper in which he announced the isolation of morphine, a new organic base that was apparently related to ammonia. He prepared a number of salts and showed that the new substance was characterized by its solubility in acid water and its precipitation from such solution by ammonia. Thus, it had the character of a weak base. Testing its physiological effects he found it produced sleep in a dog – he therefore supposed that he had identified *der eigentliche betäubende Grundstoff* of opium, the specific narcotic principle of opium, and he called the new substance morphine, after the god of sleep, Morpheus. He has a classic paper of 1817 in which he explores the physiological effects of morphine on himself and three young men[1650]. The credit for successfully applying the simple methods of chemical analysis developed late in the eighteenth century to pharmacological problems connected with plant drugs must, therefore, be given to Sertürner who not only first isolated a typical alkaloid in a pure state but also described its chemical and physiological properties in unmistakable terms. Despite its obvious importance now, this work attracted little notice until attention was drawn to it by the French chemist, Joseph Gay-Lussac (1778–1850) in 1817. The result, no doubt influenced by Sertürner's paper of that year, was the concentration of a great deal of scientific effort on the alkaloids.

The term 'alkaloid' was given to these fascinating substances by K. F. W. Meissner (1792–1853) of Halle who coined the term to describe those alkali-like weak bases obtained from crude drug sources by Sertürner's method. The method soon produced useful results in other hands. In 1810 Bernardino Gomes (1769–1823) treated an alcoholic extract of cinchona bark with alkali and obtained a crystalline precipitate which he called *cinchonino*[1651]. This provides one of the earlier papers on the subject available in English for there is a translation of the paper by Gomes in the *Edinburgh Medical and Surgical Journal* of 1811. Subsequent work by Pierre Pelletier and J. B. Caventou on the material Gomes had isolated showed that it was a mixture of two alkaloids and these, when separated, were called quinine and cinchonine.

The man who had possibly the greatest influence on this early search for the active principles of drugs was François Magendie (1783–1855), the great French physiologist who became the teacher of Claude Bernard. As early as 1809 Magendie was studying the Javanese arrow poison, *Upas tiente*, a powerful convulsant later shown to be strychnine. In 1817 Pierre Joseph Pelletier (1788–1842) and Magendie published their paper *Recherches chimiques et physiologiques sur l'ipécacuanha*[1652] in which they reported experiments with different species of ipecacuanha[1282] and showed that the emetic properties of this drug were due to an alkaloid which they named emetine. They were unable to isolate the drug in pure form and it was later shown to be a mixture of at least three alkaloids.

Pelletier then became associated with Joseph Bienaimé Caventou (1795–1877). Following their successful isolation of quinine and cinchonine from cinchona these two workers, in 1819, reported the preparation of the alkaloids strychnine and brucine from nux vomica (*Mémoire sur un nouvel alcali végétal (la strychnine) trouvé dans la fève de Saint-Ignace, la noix vomique, etc*)[1653]. Between 1820 and 1840 a considerable number of alkaloids were isolated and purified and descriptions of their properties entered the literature; in addition to those mentioned the alkaloids of this period included aconitine, atropine, berberine, codeine, colchicine, coniine, curarine, hyoscyamine, piperine, quinidine, thebaine, and varatrine. Of these, the isolation of codeine may be noted, having been reported in the paper *Nouvelles observations sur les principaux produits de l'opium* (1832)[1654] by Pierre Jean Robiquet (1780–1840).

At the beginning of this very fertile period the reaction of François Magendie to the early discoveries of Pelletier and Caventou was of great importance. In 1821, seeing the potential clinical use of these new, isolated drugs, Magendie published his famous pocket formulary, *Formulaire pour la préparation et l'emploi de plusieurs nouveaux médicamens, tels que la noix vomique, la morphine, l'acide prussique, la strychnine, la vératrine, les alcalis des quinquinas, l'emetine, l'iode*[1286]. Magendie seems to have been the first to use the pure alkaloids in the treatment of disease – and he carried many of these new drugs into clinical medicine, thereby beginning the modern age of therapeutics. Across the Atlantic, Magendie's book was almost exactly contemporaneous with *The pharmacopoeia of the United States of America*[1655]; this, the first official US pharmacopoeia, was published in Boston in December 1820. Its text is in both Latin and English but the book is remarkable for the brevity of its descriptions and for the way that much that was traditional but pointless had been cleared away.

The moderately wide variety of drugs entering therapeutics in the third decade of the century is shown by the reports of Johann Schenk, whose experience with cod-liver oil was noted in 1822[1656] and 1826 and led to the extensive use of the substance in Europe. At the same time, Georges Serulas (1774–1832) reported, in 1822, the discovery of iodoform[1657] and in 1829 Jean Lugol (1786–1851) wrote on the effects of iodine in scrofulous diseases[1658] (a paper which began the use of Lugol's solution).

However, the great interest of the period lies in the history of the glycosides, whose discovery and investigation proceeded in parallel with that of the alkaloids. The glycosides are an ill-defined and numerous group of substances, found mainly in plants, which have in common the property of yielding a sugar-like substance, often glucose itself, as a result of certain chemical processes. The real biological function of the plant glycosides has not been established but it is probable that they provide the plant with a means of storing, in a harmless form, poisonous and physiologically active substances which can be broken down by enzymes, often from adjacent cells, when this is required. They are generally crystalline solids which are at least sparingly soluble in water and, as only soluble substances can be transported in a plant by movements of the sap, this leads to the hypothesis that plants convert into glycosides either harmful or useless substances (which can be deposited in the barks, fruit rinds, or seed coats where they can do no harm and will eventually be shed) or decorative and attractive materials, such as the floral pigments (which can be formed in the leaves and, in the proper season, transported to the flowers or fruits to attract, for example, the insect agents of pollination). At all events, whatever the function of these substances, their solutions have the property of rotating the plane of polarized light, usually to the left, and under the influence of aqueous solutions of acids they can be split (hydrolysed) into one or more sugars and a non-sugar portion, named the aglycone. This hydrolysis can also be effected by the naturally occurring enzymes in neighbouring cells, the enzymes being curiously specific and effective only for one glycoside or for a group of closely related glycosides.

The first glycoside to be isolated was salicin which was obtained from willows in an impure state in 1825 and in a pure form in 1829. Salicin is the active constituent of willow (*Salix spp.*) bark and was for centuries used as a remedy against fever and eventually against acute rheumatism; its medicinal use dates at least to the days of classical Greek antiquity. Its hydrolytic products are D-glucose and saligenin (salicyl alcohol, *ortho*-hydroxybenzyl alcohol. One of the early works of note on the substance and its derivatives is the *Recherches sur la salicine et les produits qui en dérivent*[1659] published by Raffaele Piria (1815–1865) in 1839; Piria made salicylic acid from salicin. Salicylic acid (*ortho*-hydroxybenzoic acid) was then synthesized by H. Gerland who, in 1852, reported[1660] that 'If nitrous acid (prepared by acting on arsenious acid with nitric acid) is passed through a dilute warm aqueous solution of anthranilic acid, till no more nitrogen is evolved, it remains clear, and yields, on evaporation, fine long needles of an acid free from nitrogen, and possessing the composition and properties of salicylic acid.' Thus, from salicin, the active principle of the ancient remedy, oil of wintergreen, we get to the beginnings of the synthetic chemistry that has had such a profound effect upon medicine.

Of all the glycoside-yielding plants, perhaps one of the medically most important is the foxglove, *Digitalis purpurea*, the subject of William Withering's beautiful study of 200 years ago (1785)[1053]. The isolation of an active principle in digitalis, amorphous digitalin, was reported in 1845 (*Mémoire sur la digitale pourprée*)[1661] by Augustin Homolle (1808–1875). Digitalin (Digitalinum Purum Germanicum) is still noted in our contemporary pharmacopoeias as 'a standardized mixture of glycosides from the seeds of *Digitalis purpurea*, containing 100 units of activity in 1 g'[1662]. It has to be carefully distinguished from digitoxin (which is completely and readily absorbed when given by mouth and is the most potent of the digitalis glycosides and the most cumulative in action) and from the now universally-used digoxin (the crystalline glycoside obtained from the leaves of *Digitalis lanata*).

Other events of the period included the making of methyl alcohol in 1834, the year in which aniline and pyrrole were found in coal tar. Carbolic acid was first prepared from coal tar by Friedlieb Runge (1795–1867) and this was reported in 1834[1663] 2 years after Samuel Guthrie (1782–1848) had announced his discovery of the modern method of making chloroform by distilling alcohol with chlorinated lime[1318]. The whole of the first third or so of the century can be summarized in the splendid *The elements of materia medica; comprehending the natural history, preparation, properties, composition, effects, and uses of medicines* published by Jonathan Pereira (1804–1853) in 1839–40[1108]. This was the first outstanding English work on the subject, Pereira being a lecturer in the medical school of the London Hospital and becoming Professor of Materia Medica at the School of Pharmacy established by the Pharmaceutical Society of Great Britain. Part one of his work deals with the general action and classification of medicines and the mineral materia medica. Some of his definitions now reflect the early stages of the present-day branches of the science[1664]:

PHARMACOLOGY (*Pharmacology*, from Φάρμακον, *a medicine*, and Λόγος, *a discourse*), or *Materia Medica*, is a branch of acology devoted to the consideration of medicines. It is subdivided into *Pharmacognosia*, which treats of simples, or unprepared medicines; *Pharmacy*, which teaches the modes of collecting, preparing, and preserving medicines; and lastly, *Pharmacodynamics*, which is devoted to the consideration of the effects and uses of medicines.

The work is a rich source of information on the history and natural history of the drugs known at the time. It is one of the most readily available synopses of this type of information, an example being Pereira's note beginning his account of mercury and its compounds[1665]:

Hydrar'gyrum.—Mer'cury or Quick'silver.

HISTORY.—No mention is made of quicksilver in the Old Testament; nor does Herodotus allude to it. From this we might infer that both the ancient Hebrews and Egyptians were unacquainted with it. But we are told on the authority of an Oriental writer, that the Egyptian magicians, in their attempts to imitate the miracles of Moses, employed wands and cords containing mercury, which under the influence of the solar heat, imitated the motion of serpents (D'Herbelot, *Bibliothèque Orient.* art. *Moussa*). Both Aristotle and Theophrastus (*De Lapidibus*) mention αργυρος χυτὸς, (*argentum liquidum*): and the first of these naturalists says that Dædalus (who is supposed to have lived about 1300 years before Christ) communicated a power of motion to a wooden Venus by pouring quicksilver into it. We are also told that Dædalus was taught this art by the priests of Memphis. Pliny (*Hist. Nat.* lib. xxxiii.) and Dioscorides (lib. v. cap. cx.) also speak of mercury, and the latter writer describes the method of obtaining it from cinnabar.

Mercury was first employed medicinally by the Arabian physicians Avicenna and Rhazes; but they only ventured to use it externally against vermin and cutaneous diseases. We are indebted to that renowned empiric Paracelsus for its administration internally.

SYNONYMES.—The names by which this metal has been distinguished are numerous. Some have reference to its silvery appearance and liquid form; as υδράργυρος, *hydrargyrus* and *hydrargyrum*, (from ύδωρ, *aqua* and αργυρος, *silver*); others to its mobility and liquidity, as well as its similarity to silver, such as *argentum vivum, aqua argentea, aqua metallorum*, and *quicksilver*. It has been called *Mercury*, after the messenger of the gods, on account of its volatility.

NATURAL HISTORY.—Mercury is comparatively a rare substance. It is found in the metallic state, either pure (*native* or *virgin mercury*), in the form of globules, in the cavities of the other ores of this metal, or combined with silver (*native amalgam*). Bisulphuret of mercury (*native cinnabar*) is the most important of the quicksilver ores, since the metal of commerce is chiefly obtained from it. The principal mines of it are those of Idria in Carniola, and Almaden in Spain. The latter yielded 10,000 lbs. of cinnabar annually to Rome in the time of Pliny (*Hist. Nat.* xxxiii.) Protochloride of mercury (*mercurial horn ore* or *corneous mercury*) is another of the ores of mercury. Traces of this metal have also been met with in common salt, during its distillation with sulphuric acid, by Rouelle, Proust, Westrumb, and Wurzer (Gmelin, *Handb. d. Chemie,* i. 1282).

Part II (the volume of 1840) is concerned with the vegetable and animal materia medica and is a detailed source of information on scientifically-orientated medical botany. On this subject, on which learning was then in many respects at its height, Pereira's book serves to revise and augment William Woodville's finely-illustrated *Medical botany: containing systematic and general descriptions, with plates of all the medicinal plants, indigenous and exotic, comprehended in the catalogues of the materia medica, as published by the Royal Colleges of Physicians of London and Edinburgh...* [129] Second edition of 1810 (four volumes).

The knowledge of medical botany was important, for most of the drugs used in medicine until very recent times were of vegetable origin. For the most part, their active principles, once these were isolated, were found to be alkaloids, with a few glycosides. The introduction of these active principles and an increasing number of synthetic chemicals gradually changed the situation. The change was aided by the activities of an alert pharmaceutical industry, which could better produce and market such drugs, and by the interests of physicians, who soon came to value the availability of uniform and stable purified plant principles or pure chemicals with which predictable results could be obtained.

The degree of predictability was perhaps less than the pioneers might have hoped. Few of the extracted alkaloids were ideal for their desired use; many proved toxic and associated with narrow margins (the therapeutic ratio) between the effective dose and the toxic dose level. Few of the plant-derived substances had a broad therapeutic ratio. An example of such a plant drug, still of importance, is digitalis: the therapeutic ratio is so narrow that William Withering titrated the dose to the level which produced the first symptoms of toxicity, and then dropped back slightly from this to determine the therapeutically optimal dose. The ratio was so narrow that the dose needed to be determined, and adjusted separately, for each individual patient.

In order to overcome some of these difficulties and to advance knowledge, chemists tried to characterize the complex chemical alkaloids and glycosides in a rational manner. In some cases the effort, in respect of organic compounds, was aided by the concept of a carbon ring structure visualized by F. A. Kekule (1829–1896). The attempt proved surprisingly difficult and little real progress was made during the nineteenth century. Only after the theory and technique of organic chemistry had developed to a sufficiently advanced level could the problem of understanding the molecular structure of these complex entities be attempted successfully. It was, in fact, not until the decade beginning with 1960 that the structure of almost all of the important alkaloids had been established. Similarly, it was not until this time that it was possible to claim that the majority of these structures had been synthesized.

Modern pharmacology could begin at a much earlier stage – as soon as chemically pure compounds with unvarying physicochemical characteristics could be compared and evaluated in a systematic manner in appropriate biological models and systems. Before the mid-nineteenth century simple but useful additions to the drugs available continued to be made. An example is embodied in the *Treatise on the oleum jecoris aselli, or cod-liver oil, as a therapeutic agent in certain forms of gout, rheumatism, and scrofula; with cases*[1666] – a work published in Edinburgh by John Hughes Bennett (1812–1875) in 1841. Bennett had visited continental Europe and his book served to introduce cod-liver oil into English medical use. If his indications, as specific illnesses, were overly hopeful, the value of the vitamins so provided to the general nutrition of those with serious diseases is not hard to imagine.

Of the mid-nineteenth century chemical drugs and alkaloids, the discovery of amyl nitrite by Antoine Balard (1802–1876) in 1844[1667]; the isolation of papaverine from opium by Georg Merck (1825–1873) in 1848[1668]; the disclosure of the antiseptic properties of carbolic acid by François Lemaire (born 1814) in 1860[1669]; and the isolation of cocaine, from the coca leaf brought from Peru, by Albert Niemann (1834–1861), and reported in 1860[1670], will serve as examples. Georg Merck's isolation of papaverine from opium led him to develop his family's seventeenth century Angel Apothecary in Darmstadt. He built this into a major commercial concern supplying alkaloids and this later led to the expansion of Merck and Company in Rahway, New Jersey.

Pharmacology, as a separate science, can be said to have been founded shortly before the mid-century. Its real originator was Rudolf Buchheim (1820–1879) whose *Lehrbuch der Arzneimittellehre*[1671] was published in Leipzig, dated 1853–1856, and who is considered the most important of the early instructors in pharmacology. His work was almost contemporaneous with that of Claude Bernard, whose *Leçons sur les effets des substances toxiques et médicamenteuses*[1362], of 1857, is especially notable within the context of the development of medicines.

The year 1864 saw the appearance of the *British Pharmacopoeia published under the direction of the General Council of Medical Education and Registration of the United Kingdom pursuant to the Medical Act, 1858*[1672]. This was the first official British pharmacopoeia and was to replace the earlier pharmacopoeias of the Colleges of Physicians of London, Edinburgh, and Dublin. It comprised two parts and an appendix: the first part was the materia medica; the second part gave the preparations and compounds, and the appendix listed the reagents for chemical analysis and the chemical processes involved in making the Part II items. There was also a revision of the pharmaceutical weights and measures of the Kingdom and this is of some importance to those reading earlier medical and related texts.

The materia medica of 1864 is possibly more interesting than the preparations – it being in some ways more informative to know what was available to be used in therapy, rather than to know what medicines were made of these materials. The materia medica of the first British Pharmacopoeia includes, as shown in Table 3, a total of 311 separate substances. It is still largely herbal in nature for 187 (60.1%) of all of these substances are of vegetable origin.

Most of the vegetable materials are of a quite straightforward 'botanical' nature characteristic of the earlier pharmacopoeias. Excluding items which would now be considered foodstuffs, perfumes, condiments, flavourings, and excipients, the 169 botanical substances include beer yeast, lemon juice, cod liver

Table 3   *The British Pharmacopoeia (1864); Part I – the contents of the materia medica*

Vegetable	Botanical	169	
	Alkaloids	7	
	Other active		
	plant principles	2	
	Miscellaneous	9	
	Total	187	
Mineral	Chemical	103	
	Miscellaneous	6	
	Total	109	
Animal	Mammal	9	
	Insect	6	
	Total	15	
Total		311	

oil, and hips (which might be the most valuable as providing a range of vitamins); colchicum corm, digitalis, ergot, fig, fern root, ipecacuan, opium, squill, and senna (from which, in a difficult situation, useful or essential medicines might be made); camphor, hemlock, and nux vomica (among the plant poisons) and sassafras and leaf tobacco (among the known plant carcinogens). There is also the interesting dandelion root (*Taraxacum Dens Leonis*, 'the fresh Roots; gathered between September and February, from meadows and pastures in Britain') which for ages has had a reputation as a herbal diuretic. This reputation has been examined in recent studies. P. P. Rutherford and A. C. Deacon (1972) have reported on *The mode of action of dandelion root β-fructofuranosidases on inulin*[1673] and Elizabeth Rácz-Kotilla, G. Rácz and Ana Solomon (1974) have advised positive findings in a study on *The action of Taraxacum Officinale extracts on the body weight and diuresis of laboratory animals*[1674].

The seven alkaloids and two other active plant principles in the 1864 materia medica are the following:

Aconitia, 'An Alkaloid ... obtained from Aconite Root',

Atropia, 'An Alkaloid ... obtained from Belladonna Root',

Sulphate of Beberia, 'The Sulphate of an Alkaloid ... prepared from Bebeeru Bark',

Digitalin, 'The active principle obtained from Digitalis',

Hydrochlorate of Morphia, 'The Hydrochlorate of an Alkaloid ... prepared from Opium',

Sulphate of Quinia, 'The Sulphate of an Alkaloid ... prepared from Yellow-Cinchona Bark, and from the bark of Cinchona lancifolia *Mutis*',

Santonin, 'A crystalline neutral principle obtained from Santonica'

Strychnia, 'An Alkaloid . . . obtained from Nux Vomica', and

Veratria, 'An Alkaloid . . . obtained from Cevadilla; not quite pure'.

Of these substances, the atropine, digitalin, morphine salt, quinine salt and, in difficult circumstances, perhaps also the santonin, could have essential uses. The product of the aconite root, and the strychnine, are lethal poisons with no place in therapeutics.

The 'miscellaneous' group of nine substances among the items of vegetable origin include rectified spirit and sherry, which are difficult to classify.

The 103 chemical substances, most of them inorganic, in the analysis represented in Table 3, include ether, chloroform, prepared chalk, sulphate of iron, iodine, iodide of potassium, bicarbonate of soda, and salt – all items of present-day use or of use if the better drugs which have replaced them were swept away. Among the toxic substances there is arsenious acid, a whole range of antimony salts, white bismuth, calomel and many derivatives of mercury, and several lead salts.

The small number of substances of animal origin include prepared lard, castor (from the beaver – 'The Preputial Follicles and their Secretion . . . from the Hudson's Bay Territory'), spermaceti (from 'The Sperm Whale, inhibiting the Pacific and Indian Oceans. Nearly pure Cetine, separated by cooling and purification from the oil contained in the head'), musk (from Moschus moschiferus *Linn.* – 'Native of Thibet and other parts of Central Asia. The inspissated Secretion from the preputial follicles, dried; imported from China'), and prepared suet. The handful of items of insect origin include cantharides ('The Beetle, dried; collected in Russia, Sicily, and Hungary'), cochineal ('The female Insect, dried; reared in Mexico and Teneriffe') and the leech ('1. Sanguisuga officinalis *Savigny,* The Speckled Leech; and 2. S. medicinalis *Sav.,* The Green Leech, imported chiefly from Hamburg').

The British Pharmacopoeia for 1864 contains a list of books to which reference has been made in its text – these books contain the plates of the official plants. These sources therefore provide illustrations to the different botanical items when these are needed. Due to the vagaries of botanical nomenclature over time, especially when authorities are not quoted and names have changed more than once, this listing can be helpful. One of the source books is Stephenson and Churchill's *Medical botany* . . . [1675] of 1831; following its index this provides a 'Tabular Index of the Latin Names' – this shows the early nineteenth century uses for these plant medicines. Adjunctive information, for late in the century, is provided by the very fine 'Materia Medica Table of the Organic Kingdom' which is provided in the *Companion to the latest edition of the British Pharmacopoeia . . . by Peter Squire* [1676], 12th edition (1880).

Developments late in the century involved both the methods of pharmacology and the introduction of new drugs, some of them synthetic. Alexander Crum Brown (1838–1922) and Sir Thomas Fraser (1841–1919), at Edinburgh, became the first to investigate the relationship between the chemical composition of drugs and their physiological effects (1868–69) [1677]. Fraser, in important papers of 1890 and 1892 (*Strophanthus hispidus: its natural history, chemistry, and pharmacology*) [1678] gave an account of the ordeal poison, *Physostigma venenosum*, the calabar bean of parts of Africa; from this source he extracted the alkaloid physostigmine and showed that this constricts the pupil, slows the heart, promotes lachrymal and salivary secretion, and greatly increases intestinal activity. He also showed that atropine prevents or reverses these effects – thereby demonstrating a basic antagonism of action between atropine and physostigmine and adding to the knowledge which led to an understanding of the balanced pharmacological mechanisms of the autonomic nervous system. Fraser became Professor of Materia Medica at Edinburgh and, working again with Brown, who was a chemist, showed that with many alkaloids changing the nitrogen in the compound from a tertiary form to a quarternary ammonium base produced a chemical which had curare-like activity in mammals, regardless of the original and characteristic physiological effect of the starting alkaloid. This was one of the early generalizations relating chemical structure in highly active substances to their pharmacology.

The drugs introduced at this period included digitoxin, which was isolated from digitalis by Johann Schmiedeberg (1838–1921) in 1875[1679]; hyoscine (scopolamine), isolated by Albert Ladenburg (1842–1911) and reported in 1881[1680]; paraldehyde, which was introduced as a narcotic by Vincenzo Cervello (1854–1919) in 1884[1681]; and antipyrine, the antipyretic agent synthesized by Wilhelm Filehne (1844–1927) in 1884[1682]. Antipyrine (phenazone) is dimethyl phenyl pyrazoline and Filehne went on to make the dimethyl amino derivative[1683] of antipyrine, so producing amidopyrine (Pyramidon; aminophenazone). Both of these substances were early noted to have anti-inflammatory as well as anti-pyretic activity. They also possibly cause fatal agranulocytosis and blood dyscrasias; they do cause skin eruptions and so have declined in use, but the 4-butyl, 2-phenyl derivative of antipyrine was later introduced as phenylbutazone (4-butyl-1,2-diphenyl-pyrazolidine-3,5-dione). This has perhaps been a difficult series of drugs. There is no doubt that amidopyrine causes agranulocytosis and the risk is sufficiently great to make the drug unsuitable for use. Martindale, for example, notes that the 'Onset of agranulocytosis may be sudden and unpredictable.'[1684] In respect of phenylbutazone, the same source notes that the 'More severe reactions include reactivation of gastric and duodenal ulcers with perforation, haematemesis and melaena, hepatitis, hypertension, and, more rarely, agranulocytosis, thrombocytopenia, and aplastic anaemia.'[1685]

Starting points in the search for new, patentable drugs tended to start with known substances with a modest degree of activity, and – by adjustments to molecular structure – improve that activity. At the time when a search for effective sedatives and hypnotics began, alcohol, chloral hydrate, and paraldehyde were already known and the mild anticonvulsant effect of potassium bromide had been noted in epileptics. Eugen Baumann (1846–1896) then discovered sulphonal[1686], or 2,2di(ethyl sulphonyl) propane, which was (1888) introduced by Alfred Kast[1687] as a safe soporific. This substance is now seldom, if ever, used as it has a very slow onset of action and successive doses tend to have a cumulative effect. However, its preparation in 1886[1686] underlies part of the later development of the important barbiturate series of drugs. Substances related to urea had been shown to have a mild narcotic action and, impressed with sulphonal, Joseph von Mering (1849–1908), assisted by the biochemist Emil Fischer (1852–1919), now sought a series of compounds similar to the sulphonals but containing a urea moiety. An example was found in diethyl acetyl urea, and this was shown to be a soporific comparable to sulphonal. By doubling the urea moiety and closing the ring, Fischer and von Mering obtained diethyl malonyl urea, a compound which had already been synthesized but its significance over-looked. The biological studies showed the compound to be safer and more rapid in action and to be more effective. It is said that Fischer was in Verona, Italy when von Mering telegraphed the successful results of the studies. The drug was there-fore trademarked Veronal, after the quiet and restful place where the news of success was received; Fischer and von Mering published their historic paper *Ueber eine neue Klasse von Schlafmitteln*[1688] announcing its synthesis, that of barbitone (Diethylmalonylurea) in 1903. From this discovery stemmed the whole range of the widely used barbiturate series of drugs.

It can now be seen that the barbiturates have many disadvantages, despite which they are frequently used as hypnotics. Although they differ widely in dosage, duration of action, and therapeutic ratio, they all depress the central nervous system, produce tolerance, lead to dependence, enhance the effects of alcohol, and have an abuse potential associated with gross toxic effects if taken in overdose. They also interfere with the metabolism of other drugs and cause enzyme induction. The non-barbiturate hypnotics, some of which have a far wider margin of safety between the therapeutic and toxic dose levels, are now rapidly replacing the barbiturates. The modern benzodiazepines, nitrazepam and flurazepam, are to be preferred because of their relatively low incidence of toxic effects, abuse usage, and drug interactions. Even so, Fischer and von Mering's achievement was real, the derivatives of barbitone formed an important part of therapeutics until the middle of the present century, and these same drugs retain their special uses.

The late nineteenth century search for drugs to relieve pain and fever coincided with the search which produced the anti-inflammatory, analgesic agents already mentioned. Some of its roots lay in the attempts to find substitutes for quinine, which was popular in fevers and the molecule of which was found to contain benzene rings; other roots lay in what seem to have been empirical suggestions that aniline, already isolated from coal tar by William Perkin (1838–1907), appeared to lessen fever in those exposed to it. Additionally, Friedlieb Runge (1795–1867) had prepared carbolic acid, or phenol, from coal tar. The antiseptic properties of phenol had been appreciated by Lister and put to surgical use – but the substance was also reputed to reduce fevers, although, like aniline, it was far too toxic to be used in this way. Most importantly, salicin and salicylic acid had been prepared – and the latter is the *ortho*-carboxyl substituted derivative of phenol. Salicyclic acid (*ortho*-hydroxybenzoic) has definite bacterio-static and fungicidal properties but is too irritant for continuous application to the skin. Phenol, carbolic acid (hydroxybenzene) is caustic to the skin; taken by mouth it causes extensive local corrosion and profound depression of the central nervous system with circulatory and respiratory failure; aqueous solutions of Liquified Phenol of 0.2–1% are bacteriostatic, stronger solutions are bactericidal – the action depending on the sensitivity of the organism and the temperature and being markedly slow against spores or acid-fast bacteria.

The toxicity of aniline, phenol, and salicyclic acid was found to be controlled by simple acetylation. This has been one of the more fertile observations.

In 1887 Oscar Hinsberg and Alfred Kast (1856–1903), in their paper *Ueber die*

Wirkung des Acetphenetidins[1689], introduced phenacetin. This drug, enormously widely used, can be regarded as the ethyl ester of *para*-acetylamino phenol. The compound (1-acetamido-4-ethoxybenzene) effectively masked the amino group by acetylation and the phenolic hydroxyl group by ethylation. It was hoped that the properties of both aniline and phenol were combined in the parent compound, *para*-amino phenol, and the toxicity reduced by the manipulations. It is said that the large scale manufacture of phenacetin was achieved when Carl Duisburg (1861–1935), director of research at the dye factory of Friedrich Bayer, seeking to use a supply of crude *para*-amino phenol, proposed acetylating the amino group and blocking the hydroxyl with a methyl or ethyl configuration. At all events, phenacetin received wide usage as an analgesic and antipyretic. Adverse effects, at doses of 1 g or more daily, have included methaemoglobinaemia, sulphaemoglobinaemia and occasionally haemolytic anaemia, skin rashes and jaundice. Prolonged administration of large doses has been shown to be associated with renal papillary necrosis and this has led to regulatory action against the drug in the United Kingdom.

Another antipyretic analgesic of the same vintage and arising from the same concepts in early medicinal chemistry was acetanilide or antifebrin. This compound (*N*-phenylacetamide) was introduced by Arnold Cahn and Paul Hepp in 1887 after studies of its usefulness in typhoid fever[1690]. It has been replaced by safer substances.

Of these safer medicaments the most remarkable is acetyl salicylic acid. This seems to have excited no interest when it was first produced in 1853 by Charles Gerhardt (1816–1856), professor of chemistry at Strassburg. Discussing the sodium salt of salicylic acid, Chauncey Leake (1975) makes the medically interesting comment that 'It seems to have been the histologist, Solomon Stricker (1834–1898) who noted its beneficial effect in acute rheumatic disorders . . . and noted that sodium salicylate appears to be able to arrest acute rheumatic fever.'[1691] The reference which Leake cites in this passage is dated 1876[1692] and it is perhaps curious that Garrison (1927) notes these important observations only in an Appendix where he lists '1877 – Stricker treats articular rheumatism with salicylic acid.'[1693]

It is said that the pharmaceutical company of Friedrich Bayer & Co., at Elberfeld, where Heinrich Dreser (1860–1924) was director of research, wished to introduce a non-irritating derivative of salicylic acid. Dreser had been professor of pharmacology at Göttingen and, as Leake recounts, 'One of his chemists brought him a sample of acetyl salicylic acid hoping it would be less irritating to the stomach of his father than sodium salicylate necessary to control arthritic pain. Dreser demonstrated relative lack of local irritation from acetyl salicylic acid by using gills of live goldfish.'[1691] Aspirin was the trade name selected by the Company and under this name Dreser introduced this drug into medicine in a paper in *Pflüger's Archiv*, dated 1899, and entitled *Pharmakologisches über Aspirin (Acetylsalicylsäure)*[1694]. Of this paper, the initial page forms Figure 137.

As the nineteenth century drew to its close Wilhelm Röntgen (1845–1923), in *Ueber eine neue Art von Strahlen*[1695] of 1895 announced the discovery of the X-rays which Kölliker named 'Roentgen rays' and for which the inventor received the Nobel Prize for Physics in 1901. Röntgen's paper appeared in an English translation in *Nature* in 1896 – and the discovery was immediately applied to

(Aus dem pharm. Laboratorium der Farbenfabriken vorm. Friedr. Bayer & Co., Elberfeld.)

Pharmakologisches über Aspirin (Acetylsalicylsäure).[1]

Von

Professor Dr. med. **H. Dreser.**

Bei vielen auf „Erkältung" zurückgeführten Krankheitszuständen wäre der Gebrauch des salicylsauren Natrons sicher viel populärer, wenn es nicht durch seinen widerlich süsslichen Geschmack, der sich nur schlecht corrigiren lässt, solche Abneigung hervorriefe. Hier vermag die pharmaceutische Chemie auf synthetischem Wege ein Präparat vielleicht herzustellen, das die unliebsamen Erscheinungen in den „ersten Wegen" vermeidet, wozu ausser dem widerlichen Geschmack auch die Belästigung des Magens zählt. Nach der Resorption müsste sich die wirksame Salicylsäure möglichst rasch aus dem neuen Producte abspalten.

Vergleicht man den Geschmack der Lösungen von benzoësaurem, salicylsaurem, orthomethoxybenzoësaurem Natron, so ergibt sich, dass der widerlich süssliche Geschmack durch das freie Phenolhydroxyl der Salicylsäure bedingt ist. Die medicinisch werthvolle Wirkung der Salicylsäure ist aber in Folge der Substitution des Phenolwasserstoffatoms durch Methyl ganz verloren gegangen, denn das orthomethoxybenzoësaure Natron entbehrt jeglicher desinficirenden Wirkung. Die Bindung derartiger Methoxylgruppen ist chemisch so fest, dass innerhalb des Organismus eine Spaltung und Regeneration von Sali-

---

1) Nachdem die Herren Dr. C. Witthauer (Aspirin, ein neues Salicylpräparat. Die Heilkunde, Aprilheft 1899) und Dr. Jul. Wolgemuth (Ueber Aspirin [Acetylsalicylsäure], Therapeut. Monatshefte 1899, Maiheft) ihre günstigen klinischen Erfahrungen über Aspirin berichtet haben, sollen der Vollständigkeit halber auch die Ergebnisse der pharmakologischen Vorprüfung hier mitgetheilt werden, welche bereits in ihren Grundzügen ausgeführt war, bevor das Aspirin zur klinischen Prüfung angeboten wurde.

Figure 137 Heinrich Dreser. *Pharmakologisches über Aspirin (Acetylsalicylsäure),* (1899).

medicine. Within 2 years, in 1897, Leopold Freund (1868–1944) published an account of the first use of X-rays in irradiation therapy[1696]. Before the century closed, in 1898, in their account *Sur une substance nouvelle radio-active, contenue dans la pechblende*[1697], Pierre Curie (1859–1906) and Marie Curie (1867–1934) announced the isolation of radium from pitchblende and demonstrated its remarkable degree of radioactivity. For this discovery they shared with Becquerel (the discoverer, in 1896, of radioactivity) the Nobel Prize for Physics in 1903; Marie Curie, in 1911, also received the Nobel Prize for Chemistry.

The drugs of the late part of the century included the isolation of ephedrine (1887)[1698], the extraction of pure emetine from ipecacuanha (1894–95)[1699], the first suggestion that cocaine might be used as a local anaesthetic (1868)[1700], a later very clear proposal for such use in 1880[1701], and the introduction (1885) of the use of amyl nitrite in the treatment of anginal pain and angina pectoris by Sir Thomas Lauder Brunton (1844–1916). Thomas Brunton produced an excellent work called *A text-book of pharmacology, therapeutics and materia medica*[1702] in 1885. This summarized his experience as a physician at St. Bartholomew's where he undertook formal and well-organized studies on the effects of a number of drugs on the cardiovascular system. By the late segment of the century the leading German pharmacologist of the day had become Johann Schmiedeberg (1838–1921), professor at Dorpat and Strassburg, who made extensive studies of the effects of the new drugs being discovered on the circulation and produced the very systematic *Grundriss der Arzneimittellehre*[1703] of 1883. The German schools of the time showed an early interest in the pharmacology of drugs and their effects on living tissues, as distinct from the pharmaceutical concerns related to the preparation, identification and standardization of drugs. The pioneer in this almost physiological approach to the subject was Rudolf Buchheim of Dorpat. Schmiedeberg was Buchheim's most illustrious pupil. He succeeded Buchheim at Dorpat in 1866 but in 1872 moved to Strassburg where the first real pharmacological institute had been created.

Schmiedeberg showed that muscarine, the alkaloid which he and his pupils isolated from the poisonous mushroom *Amanita muscaria*, and electrical stimulation of the vagus nerve slowed the heart's movement, both effects being antagonized by atropine. These effects were shown to occur at the nerve endings and not in the cardiac muscle tissue itself. These observations laid part of the foundation for the later understanding of the autonomic nervous system and were important in first showing a similarity between the effects of a drug at its site of action and stimulation of the relevant autonomic nerve. Schmiedeberg is also remembered for important studies on the cardiac glycosides and for his very early interest in the mechanisms of drug absorption, distribution and excretion from the body.

The drugs of the nineteenth century are, in a sense, less than the intellectual achievement that accompanied and produced them. At their best these achievements were those of experimental pharmacology – and the first laboratory that can be said to have been devoted exclusively to that subject was Rudolf Buchheim's at Dorpat (Tartu). This was about 1846. Buchheim insisted that the effects of drugs on the body should be explained and understood, as well as measured and described. His book, *Lehrbuch der Arzneimittellehre*[1671], published in Leipzig and dated 1853–1856, is one of the fundamentals of the subject.

Pharmacology, as an independent experimental science, was firmly established by Buchheim's pupil, Johann Oswald Schmiedeberg, who defined its purpose as being the study of the damage and change wrought in a living organism by chemical substances, other than foods. In 1875, in one of his more important specific contributions[1679], he reported the isolation of digitoxin from digitalis. In 1883, when he was professor of pharmacology and director of the pharmacological institute in the University of Strassburg, he published his brilliant *Grundriss der Arzneimittellehre*[1703] – a work which was of considerable influence. Schmiedeberg attracted scores of students to his institute at Strassburg – and it is from this nucleus that independent departments of pharmacology were established in a great number of universities.

Discussion

The nineteenth century opened with the Industrial Revolution, even in Britain, far from complete – and with the attitudes of modern medicine at hardly more than a formative stage. Those attitudes were substantially influenced by the French school and up to the mid-century, if not beyond it, the advances made in medicine were largely French. From the mid-century, German medicine, chemistry, and pharmacology became ascendant. The striking achievements of the British and American schools were the provision of classic descriptions of disease, the discoveries of inhalational anaesthesia, and the establishment of antiseptic surgery.

From the English school the most distinguished publication marking the beginning of the nineteenth century was Heberden's *Commentarii de morborum historia et curatione*[945] of 1802. The doctor who has time to read nothing more than the English edition of Heberden, Withering's *An account of the foxglove...* (1785)[1053] and Jenner's *An inquiry...* (1798)[1038] has at least found the time needed to study those items of closest practical relevance to medicine before it assumed modern dress.

1819 saw the publication of the first edition of Laennec's *De l'auscultation médiate...*[1130] and it is this book, if only one were to be chosen, which might stand for the great French achievement of integrating the clinical manifestations of disease in the living with the excellence of pathology that typified the followers of Bichat at the time; it is also the beginning of practical instrumental auscultation – the first technique to reveal the morbid anatomy of the lesion in the living patient. If one were to date modern medicine from any one event, it might well be from the 1819 date of the appearance of Laennec's book. The preparation of modern medicines (apart from Withering's herbal remedy of digitalis, and Jenner's smallpox vaccine) might be said to date from a little earlier – from 1805, when Sertürner isolated morphine[1649].

In 1827–31 Richard Bright published his very fine *Reports of medical cases...*[1151], and this work, providing the original description of essential nephritis (Bright's disease) and differentiating cardiac from renal dropsy, typifies the splendid clinical descriptions provided by the British school in the period about one-third of the way through the century.

In 1839 Theodor Schwann (following slightly earlier work by Schleiden) published his *Mikroskopische Untersuchungen*...[1200], and this treatise gave what was, in effect, a definition of the cell theory – a theory forming one of the cornerstones of nineteenth century biological progress.

In 1846 Morton introduced ether anaesthesia (previously used in 1842 by Long) and the great invention of anaesthesia by the American school was announced, in Boston, and in Bigelow's paper *Insensibility during surgical operations produced by inhalation*[1468]. The following year (1847) Sir James Young Simpson of Edinburgh introduced chloroform anaesthesia in obstetrics[1473].

In 1858 Virchow's *Die Cellularpathologie*...[1263] was published, making Virchow, with the exponents of the germ theory, the architect of much of the modern understanding of disease. In the same year Claude Bernard discovered the vasoconstrictor and vasodilator nerves, and these observations (following his slightly earlier work on vasomotor function) serve as examples of the great contributions made to medicine by the French physiologist and teacher.

In 1861 Pasteur published his epoch-making *Mémoire sur les corpuscles organisés qui existent dans l'atmosphère*...[1490] – thereby providing one of the most fundamental observations of the germ theory. In 1867 Lister introduced antiseptic surgery[1561]. We have, therefore, a tradition of a little less than 125 years of surgery which, from Lister's day to the present, could use both inhalational anaesthesia and the techniques of antisepsis or asepsis.

In 1882 Koch discovered the tubercule bacillus (this was 4 years after Edison, in 1878, had invented the platinum wire, incandescent lamp).

In 1895 Röntgen discovered X-rays (in the same year that Marconi invented wireless).

Against this nineteenth century cascade of achievement we must place the drugs available. The best of the first British Pharmacopoeia of 1864 must seem to be (apart from sources of vitamins, not then described) digitalis, opium, atropine, a salt of morphine, quinine sulphate, ether, chloroform, ferrous sulphate, iodine, sodium bicarbonate, salt and a few other household remedies. To set against these items, there are some substantially toxic plant and mineral substances. Jenner's vaccine must be added to the list of things which would be considered highly useful.

The conclusion cannot be escaped that after many, many centuries, knowledge and understanding had suddenly vastly increased – but, in the face of serious illness, the means of effective medical intervention must have seemed few and far between.

References

1118.   Heberden, William, Snr. (1745). As ref. 935 but pp. 14–15
1119.   Heberden, William, Snr. (1745). As ref. 935 but p. 16
1120.   Heberden, William, Snr. (1745). As ref. 935 but pp. 16–17
1121.   Withering, William (1785). As ref. 1053 but p. 186
1122.   Withering, William (1785). As ref. 1053, but p. 186
1123.   Garrison, Fielding H. (1929). As ref. 179 but p. 408
1124.   Louis, Pierre Charles Alexandre. Recherches anatomico-pathologiques sur la phthisie. Paris, *Gabon & Cie.*, 1825

1125. Louis, Pierre Charles Alexandre. Recherches anatomiques, pathologiques et thérapeutiques sur la maladie connue sous les noms de gastro-entérite; fièvre putride, adynamique, ataxique, typhoïde, etc. 2 vols. Paris, *J. B. Baillière*, 1829

1126. Louis, Pierre Charles Alexandre. Recherches sur les effets de la saignée dans quelques maladies inflammatoires, et sur l'action de l'émétique et des vésicatoires dans la pneumonie. Paris, *J. B. Baillière*, 1835

1127. Bichat, Marie François Xavier. Traité des membranes en général et diverses membranes en particulier. Paris, *Richard, Caille & Ravier*, an VIII, (1800)

1128. Bichat, Marie François Xavier. Recherches physiologiques sur la vie et la mort. Paris, *Brosson, Gabon et Cie.*, an VIII, (1800)

1129. Bichat, Marie François Xavier. Traité d'anatomie descriptive. 5 vols. Paris, *Gabon & Cie.*, an X-XII, (1801-03)

1130. Laennec, René Théophile Hyacinthe. De l'auscultation médiate, ou traité du diagnostic des maladies des poumons et du coeur. 2 vols. Paris, *J. A. Brosson & J. S. Chaudé*, 1819

1131. Laennec, René Théophile H. As ref. 1130 but 2nd (1826) edn.

1132. (Laennec, René). A treatise on the diseases of the chest, in which they are described according to their anatomical characters, and their diagnosis established on a new principle by means of acoustick instruments. Translated from the French of R. T. H. Laennec, MD with a preface and notes by John Forbes, MD London, *Underwood*, 1821

1133. Laennec, René (1821). As ref. 1132 but pp. 1-16

1134. Laennec, René (1821). As ref. 1132 but pp. 284-285

1135. Garrison, Fielding H. (1929). As ref. 179 but p. 412

1136. Cheyne, John. An essay on hydrocephalus acutus, or dropsy in the brain. Edinburgh, *Mundell, Doig & Stevenson*, 1808

1137. Cheyne, John. The pathology of the membranes of the larynx and bronchia. Edinburgh, *Mundell, Doig & Stevenson*, 1809

1138. Cheyne, John. A case of apoplexy in which the fleshy part of the heart was converted into fat. *Dublin Hosp. Rep.*, 1818, **2**, 216-23

1139. Adams, Robert. Cases of diseases of the heart, accompanied with pathological observations. *Dublin Hosp. Rep.*, 1827, **4**, 353-453

1140. Spens, Thomas. History of a case in which there took place a remarkable slowness of the pulse. *Med. Commentaries*, (1792), Edinburgh, 1793, **7**, 458-65

1141. Adams, Robert. A treatise on rheumatic gout, or chronic rheumatic arthritis, of all the joints. London, *J. Churchill*, 1857

1142. Graves, Robert James. (Palpitation of the heart with enlargement of the thyroid gland). *Lond. Med. Surg. J. (Renshaw)*, 1835, **7**, 516-17

1143. Graves, Robert James. A system of clinical medicine. Dublin, *Fannin & Co.*, 1843

1144. Stokes, William. An introduction to the use of the stethoscope. Edinburgh, *Maclachlan & Stewart*, 1825

1145. Stokes, William. A treatise on the diagnosis and treatment of diseases of the chest. Dublin, *Hodges & Smith*, 1837

1146. Stokes, William. Observations on some cases of permanently slow pulse. *Dublin Q. J. Med. Sci.*, 1846, **2**, 73-85

1147. Stokes, William. The diseases of the heart and aorta. Dublin, *Hodges & Smith*, 1854

1148. Corrigan, Sir Dominic John. On permanent patency of the mouth of the aorta, or inadequacy of the aortic valves. *Edinb. Med. Surg. J.*, 1832, **37**, 225-45

1149. Wells, William Charles. On the presence of the red matter and serum of blood in the urine of dropsy, which has not originated from scarlet fever. *Trans. Soc. Improve. Med. Chir. Knowl.*, 1812, **3**, 194-240

1150. Blackall, John. Observations on the nature and cure of dropsies. London, *Longman*, 1813

1151. Bright, Richard. Reports of medical cases selected with a view of illustrating the symptoms and cure of diseases by a reference to morbid anatomy. 2 vols. London, *Longman*, 1827-31

1152. Bright, Richard (1827-31). As ref. 1151 but pp. 67-69

1153. Bright, Richard. Cases and observations connected with disease of the pancreas and duodenum. *Med.-Chir. Trans.*, 1832, **18**, 1-56

1154. Bright, Richard. Observations on jaundice. *Guy's Hosp. Rep.*, 1836, **1**, 6

1155. Bright, Richard. Fatal epilepsy, from suppuration between the dura mater and arachnoid, in consequence of blood having been effused in that situation. *Guy's Hosp. Rep.,* 1836, **1,** 36–40

1156. Bright, Richard. Cases and observations, illustrative of renal disease accompanied with the secretion of albuminous urine. *Guy's Hosp. Rep.,* 1836, **1,** 338–400; 1840, **5,** 101–161

1157. Bright, Richard and Addison, Thomas. Elements of the practice of medicine. Vol. 1, pts. 1–3. London, *Longmans,* (1836)–39

1158. Bright, Richard. Clinical memoirs on abdominal tumours and intumescence. London, *New Sydenham Soc.,* 1860

1159. Addison, Thomas and Morgan, John. An essay on the operation of poisonous agents upon the living body. London, *Longman, Rees,* 1829

1160. Addison, Thomas. On the influence of electricity, as a remedy in certain convulsive and spasmodic diseases. *Guy's Hosp. Rep.,* 1837, **2,** 493–507

1161. Addison, Thomas. Anaemia; disease of the supra-renal capsules. *Lond. Med. Gaz.,* 1849, **43,** 517–18

1162. Combe, James Scarth. History of a case of anaemia. *Trans. Med-Chir. Soc. Edinb.,* 1824, **1,** 194–204

1163. Biermer, Anton. Eine eigenthumliche Form von progressiver perniciöser Anämie. *Korresp Bl. Schweiz. Ärz.,* 1872, **2,** 15–18

1164. Addison, Thomas. On the constitutional and local effects of disease of the supra-renal capsules. London, *S. Highley,* 1855

1165. Garrison, Fielding H. (1929). As ref. 179 but p. 423

1166. Addison, Thomas. A collection of the published writings. London, *New Sydenham Soc.,* 1868

1167. Hodgkin, Thomas. On the retroversion of the valves of the aorta. *Lond. Med. Gaz.,* 1828–29, **3,** 433–43

1168. Hodgkin, Thomas. On some morbid appearances of the absorbent glands and spleen. *Med-Chir. Trans.,* 1832, **17,** 68–114

1169. Hodgkin, Thomas. Lectures on the morbid anatomy of the serous and mucous membranes. 2 vols. London, *Simpkin, Marshall & Co.,* 1836–40

1170. Carswell, Sir Robert. Illustrations of the elementary forms of disease. London, *Longman, etc.,* 1838

1171. Hodgson, Joseph. A treatise on the diseases of arteries and veins. London, *T. Underwood,* 1815

1172. Morton, Leslie T. As ref. 1853, p. 368

1173. Hope, James. A treatise on the diseases of the heart and great vessels. London, *W. Kidd,* 1832

1174. Hope, James. Principles and illustrations of morbid anatomy. London, *Whittaker & Co.,* 1834

1175. Wells, William Charles. Observations and experiments on the colour of blood. *Phil. Trans.,* 1797, **87,** 416–31

1176. Wells, William Charles. An essay on dew. London, *Taylor & Hessay,* 1814

1177. Watson, Sir Thomas, Bart. Lectures on the principles and practice of physic. 2 vols. London, *J. W. Parker,* 1843

1178. Skoda, Josef. Abhandlung über Perkussion und Auskultation. Wien, 1839

1179. Rokitansky, Carl, Friherr von. Die Defecte der Scheidewände der Herzens. Wien, *W. Braumüller,* 1875

1180. Rokitansky, Carl, Freiherr von. Die Defecte der Scheidewände der Herzens. Wien, *W. Braumüller u. Seidel,* 1842–46

1181. Semmelweis, Ignaz Philipp. Höchst wichtige Erfahrungen über die Aetiologie der in Gebäranstalten epidemischen Puerperalfieber. *Z. k. k. Ges. Aerzte Wien,* 1847–48, **4,** pt. 2, 242–44; 1849, **5,** 64–65

1182. Semmelweis, Ignaz Philipp. Die Aetiologie, der Begriff und die Prophylaxis des Kindbettfiebers. Pest, Wien & Leipzig, *C. A. Hartleben,* 1861

1183. Holmes, Oliver Wendell. The contagiousness of puerperal fever. *N. Engl. Q. J. Med. Surg.,* 1842–43, **1,** 503–30

1184. Holmes, Oliver Wendell. Puerperal fever, as a private pestilence. Boston, *Ticknor & Fields,* 1855

1185. Holmes, Oliver Wendell. Medical essays: 1842–1882. Boston, *Houghton Mifflin & Co.,* 1883

1186. Hahnemann, Christian Friedrich Samuel. Organon der rationellen Heilkunde. Dresden, *Arnold,* 1810

1187. Bigelow, Jacob. American medical botany. 3 vols. Boston, *Cummings & Hilliard,* 1817–20

1188. Bigelow, Jacob. A discourse on self-limited diseases. Boston, *N. Hale,* 1835

1189. Bell, Sir Charles. A system of dissections. 2 vols. Edinburgh, *Mundell & Son,* 1799–1801

1190. Bell, Sir Charles. A system of operative surgery. 2 vols. London, *Longham,* 1807–09

1191. Bell, Sir Charles. Idea of a new anatomy of the brain. London, *Strahan & Preston,* (1811)

1192. Bell, Sir Charles. Illustrations of the great operations of surgery. London, *Longman,* 1821

1193. Bell, Sir Charles. On the nerves; giving an account of some experiments on their structure and functions, which lead to a new arrangement of the system. *Phil. Trans.,* 1821, **111,** 398–424

1194. Bell, Sir Charles. The nervous system of the human body. 2nd edn., London, *Longmans,* 1830

1195. Knox, Robert. The races of men. London, *H. Renshaw,* 1850

1196. Knox, Robert. A manual of artistic anatomy. London, *H. Renshaw,* 1852

1197. Brown, Robert. On the organs and mode of fecundation in Orchideae and Asclepiadeae. *Trans. Linn. Soc.,* 1829–32, **16,** 685–746

1198. Wagner, Rudolph. Einige Bemerkungen und Fragen über das Keimbläschen (vesicula germinativa). *Arch. Anat. Physiol. Wiss. Med.,* 1835, 373–7

1199. Schleiden, Matthias Jakob. Beiträge zur Phytogenesis. *Arch. Anat. Physiol. Wiss. Med.,* 1838, 137–76

1200. Schwann, Theodor. Mikroskopische Untersuchungen über die Uebereinstimmung in der Struktur und dem Wachsthum der Thiere und Pflanzen. Berlin, *Sander,* 1839

1201. Mohl, Hugo von. Grundzüge der Anatomie und Physiologie der vegetabilischen Zelle. Braunschweig, *F. Vieweg und Sohn,* 1851

1202. Remak, Robert. Ueber extracelluläre Entstenhung thierischer Zellen und über die Vermehrung derselben durch Theilung. *Arch. Anat. Physiol. Wiss. Med.,* 1852, 47–57

1203. Remak, Robert. Vorläufige Mittheilungen microscopischer Beobachtungen über den innern Bau der Cerebrospinalnerven und über die Entwickelung ihrer Formelemente. *Arch. Anat. Physiol. Wiss. Med.,* 1836, 145–61

1204. Remak, Robert, Observationes anatomicae et microscopicae de systematis nervosi structura. Berolini, *sumtibus et formis Reimerianis,* 1838

1205. Remak, Robert. Neurologische Erläuterungen, *Arch. Anat. Physiol. (Lpz.),* 1844, 463–72

1206. Remak, Robert. Untersuchungen über die Entwickelung der Wirbelthiere. Berlin, *G. Reimer,* 1855

1207. Henle, Friedrich Gustav Jacob. Symbolae ad anatomiam villorum intestinalium, imprimis eorum epithelii et vasorum lacteorum. Berolini, *A. Hirschwald,* 1837

1208. Henle, Friedrich Gustav Jacob. Ueber die Ausbreitung des Epithelium im menschlichen Körper. *Arch. Anat. Physiol. Wiss. Med.,* 1838, 103–28

1209. Henle, Friedrich Gustav Jacob. Von den Miasmen und Contagien. In his *Pathologische Untersuchungen,* Berlin, 1840, pp. 1–82

1210. Henle, Friedrich Gustav Jacob. Allgemeine Anatomie. Leipzig, *L. Voss,* 1841

1211. Henle, Friedrich Gustav Jakob. Handbuch der systematischen Anatomie des Menschen. 3 vols. Braunschweig, *F. Vieweg u. Sohn,* 1855–71

1212. Garrison, Fielding H. (1929). As ref. 179 but p. 458

1213. Purkinje, Johann Evangelista (Purkyně). Beiträge zur Kenntniss des Sehens in subjectiver Hinsicht. Prag, *Fr. Vetterl von Wildenkron,* 1819

1214. Purkinje, Johann Evangelista (Purkyně). Commentatio de examine physiologico organi visus et systematis cutanei. Vratislaviae, *typis Universitatis,* (1823)

1215. Purkinje, Johann Evangelista (Purkyně). Symbolae ad ovi ovium historiam ante incubationem. Vratislaviae, *typ. Universitatis,* 1825

1216. Purkinje, Johann Evangelista and Valentin, Gabriel Gustav. De phaenomeno generali et fundamentali motus vibratorii continui in membranis. Wratislaviae, *sumpt. A. Schulz et soc.,* 1835

1217. Palicki, Bogislaus. De musculari cordis structura, (Breslau), 1839

1218. Purkinje, Johann Evangelista (Purkyně). Sebrané sipsy. Opera omnia. Tom. 1–12. v. Praze, *Purkyňova Spolestnost,* 1918–73

1219. Kölliker, Rudolph Albert von. Beiträge zur Kenntniss der Geschlechtsverhältnisse und der Samenflüssigkeit wirbelloser Thiere. Berlin, *W. Logier,* 1841

1220. Kölliker, Rudolph Albert von. Ueber das Wesen der sogenannten Saamenthiere. *N. Notiz. a.d. Geb. d. Natur-und Heilk.,* Weimar, 1841, **19**, 4–8

1221. Kölliker, Rudolph Albert von. Beiträge zur Kenntniss der glatten Muskeln. *Z. Wiss. Zool.,* 1848, **1**, 48–87

1222. Kölliker, Rudolph Albert von. Handbuch der Gewebelehre des Menschen. Leipzig, *W. Engelmann,* 1852

1223. Kölliker, Rudolph Albert von. Physiologische Untersuchungen über die Wirkung einiger Gifte. *Virchows Arch. Pathol. Anat.,* 1856, **10**, 3–77, 235–96

1224. Kölliker, Rudolph Albert von and Müller, Heinrich. Nachweis der negativen Schwankung des Muskelstroms am natürlich sich contrahirenden Muskel. *Verh. Phys.-Med. Ges. Würzburg,* 1856, **6**, 528–33

1225. Kölliker, Rudolph Albert von. Entwicklungsgeschichte des Menschen und der höheren Thiere. Leipzig, *W. Engelmann,* 1861

1226. Kölliker, Rudolph Albert von. Die Bedeutung der Zellenkerne für die Vorgänge der Vererbung. *Z. Wiss. Zool.,* 1885, **42**, 1–46

1227. Cohn, Ferdinand Julius. Zur Naturgeschichte des Protococcus pluvialis, Breslau, 1850

1228. Cohn, Ferdinand Julius. Untersuchungen über die Entwicklungsgeschichte der mikroskopischen Algen und Pilzen, Bonn, 1853

1229. Cohn, Ferdinand Julius. Untersuchungen über Bacterien. *Beitr. Biol. Pflanzen,* 1872, **1**, Heft 2, 127–224; Heft 3, 141–207; 1876, 2, Heft 2, 249–276

1230. Leydig, Franz. Zur Anatomie der männlichen Geschlechtsorgane und Analdrüsen der Säugethiere. *Z. Wiss. Zool.,* 1850, **2**, 1–57

1231. Overton, Charles Ernest. Studien über die Narkose. Jena, *G. Fischer,* 1901

1232. Gerlach, Joseph von. Mikroskopische Studien aus dem Gebiete der menschlichen Morphologie. Erlangen, *F. Enke,* 1858

1233. Schultze, Maximilian Johann Sigismund. Ueber die Endigungsweise des Hörnerven im Labyrinth, *Arch. Anat. Physiol. Wiss. Med.,* 1858, 343–81

1234. Schultze, Maximilian Johann Sigismund. Untersuchungen über den Bau der Nasenschleimhaut, namentlich die Structur und Endigungsweise der Geruchsnerven bei dem Menschen und den Wirbelthieren. *Abh. Naturf. Ges. Halle,* 1862, **7**, 1–100

1235. Schultze, Maximilian Johann Sigismund. Zur Anatomie und Physiologie der Retina. Bonn, *M. Cohen u. Sohn,* 1866

1236. Schultze, Maximilian Johann Sigismund. Ueber Muskelkörperchen und das, was man eine Zelle zu nennen habe. *Arch. Anat. Physiol. Wiss. Med.,* 1861, 1–27

1237. Schultze, Maximilian Johann Sigismund. Das Protoplasma der Rhizopoden und der Pflanzenzellen. Leipzig, *Engelmann,* 1863

1238. Schultze, Maximilian Johann Sigismund. Observationes nonnulae de ovorum ranarum segmentatione, quae "Furchungsprocess" dicitur. Bonnae, *Formis C. Georgi,* 1863

1239. Flemming, Walther. Beobachtungen über die Beschaffenheit des Zellkerns. *Arch. Mikr. Anat.,* 1877, **13**, 693–717

1240. Flemming, Walther. Beiträge zur Kenntniss der Zelle und ihrer Lebenserscheinungen. *Arch. Mikr. Anat.,* 1879, **16**, 302–436; 1880, **18**, 151–259

1241. His, Wilhelm, Snr. Untersuchungen über den Bau der Lymphdrüsen. Leipzig, *W. Engelmann,* 1861

1242. His, Wilhelm, Snr. Ueber das Epithel der Lymphgefässwurzeln und über die von Recklinghausen'schen Saftcanälchen. *Z. Wiss. Zool.,* 1863, **13**, 455–73

1243. His, Wilhelm, Snr. Beobachtungen über den Bau des Säugethier-Eierstockes. *Arch. Mikr. Anat.,* 1865, **1**, 151–202

1244. His, Wilhelm, Snr. Die Häute und Höhlen des Köpers. Basel, *Schweighauser,* 1865

1245. His, Wilhelm, Snr. Beschreibung eines Mikrotoms. *Arch. Mikr. Anat.,* 1870, **6**, 229–32

1246. His, Wilhelm, Snr. Unsere Körperform und das physiologische Problem ihrer Entstehung. Leipzig, *F. C. W. Vogel,* 1874

1247. His, Wilhelm, Snr. Anatomie menschlicher Embryonen. 3 pts. and atlas. Leipzig, *F. C. W. Vogel,* 1880–85

1248. His, Wilhelm, Snr. Die anatomische Nomenclatur. Leipzig. *Veit & Co.,* 1895. English translation by L. F. Barker, 1907

1249. Balfour, Francis Maitland. A treatise on comparative embryology. 2 vols. London, *Macmillan & Co.,* 1880–81

1250. Roux, Wilhelm. Beiträge zur Entwickelungsmechanik des Embryo. Ueber die künstliche Hervorbringung halber Embryonen durch Zerstörung einer der beiden ersten Furchungs-kugeln, sowie über die Nachentwickelung (Postgeneration) der fehlenden Körperhälfte. *Virchows Arch. Pathol. Anat.,* 1888, **114,** 113–53, 246–91

1251. Roux, Wilhelm. Terminologie der Entwicklungsmechanik. Leipzig, *W. Engelmann,* 1912

1252. Virchow, Rudolf Ludwig Karl. Ueber die Canalisation von Berlin. *Vjschr. Gerichtl. Öff. Med.,* 1868, n.F. **9,** 1–43

1253. Virchow, Rudolf Ludwig Karl. Ueber gewisse, die Gesundheit benachtheiligende Einflüsse der Schulen. *Virchows Arch. Pathol. Anat.,* 1869, **46,** 447–70

1254. Bennett, John Hughes. Case of hypertrophy of the spleen and liver, in which death took place from suppuration of the blood. *Edinb. Med. Surg. J.,* 1845, **64,** 413–23

1255. Virchow, Rudolf Ludwig Karl. Weisses Blut. *N. Notiz. Geb. Natur- u. Heilk.,* 1845, **36,** 151–56

1256. Virchow, Rudolf Ludwig Carl. Zur Entwickelungsgeschichte des Krebses. *Virchows Arch. Pathol. Anat.,* 1847, **1,** 94–201

1257. Virchow, Rudolf Ludwig Karl. Ueber die acute Entzündung der Arterien. *Virchows Arch. Pathol. Anat.,* 1847, **1,** 272–378

1258. Virchow, Rudolf Ludwig Karl. Die pathologischen Pigmente. *Virchows Arch. Pathol. Anat.,* 1847, **1,** 379–404, 407–86

1259. Virchow, Rudolf Ludwig Karl. Beiträge zur Lehre von den beim Menschen vorkommenden pflanzlichen Parasiten. *Virchows Arch. Pathol. Anat.,* 1856, **9,** 557–93

1260. Virchow, Rudolf Ludwig Karl. Ueber farblose Blutkörperchen und Leukämie. In his *Gesammelte Abhandlungen zur wissenschaftlichen Medicin,* Frankfort a.M., *Meidinger,* 1856, pp. 147–218

1261. Addison, William. Experimental and practical researches on inflammation and on the origin and nature of tubercles of the lungs. London, *J. Churchill,* 1843

1262. Virchow, Rudolph Ludwig Karl. Ueber die Natur der constitutionell-syphilitischen Affectionen. *Virchows Arch. Pathol. Anat.,* 1858, **15,** 217–336

1263. Virchow, Rudolph Ludwig Karl. Die Cellularpathologie in ihrer Begründung auf physiologische und pathologische Gewebelehre. Berlin, *A. Hirschwald,* 1858

1264. (Virchow, Rudolf). Cellular pathology as based upon physiological and pathological histology. Twenty lectures delivered in the Pathological Institute of Berlin during the months of February, March, and April, 1858, by Rudolf Virchow, translated from the second edition of the original by Frank Chance. London, *J. Churchill,* 1860

1265. Virchow, Rudolf (1860 trans.). As ref. 1264 but pp. 2, 3

1266. Virchow, Rudolf (1860 trans.). As ref. 1264 but pp. 27, 28

1267. Virchow, Rudolf Ludwig Karl. Die krankhaften Geschwülste. Vol. 1–3, Heft 1. Berlin, *A. Hirschwald,* 1863–67

1268. Thiersch, Carl. Der Epithelialkrebs namentlich der Haut. 1 vol. and atlas. Leipzig, *W. Engelmann,* 1865

1269. Waldeyer-Hartz, Heinrich Wilhelm Gottfried. Die Entwicklung der Carcinome. *Virchows Arch. Pathol. Anat.,* 1867, **41,** 470–523; 1872, **55,** 67–159

1270. Cohnheim, Julius Friedrich. Zur Kenntnis der zuckerbildenden Fermente. *Virchows Arch. Pathol. Anat.,* 1863, **28,** 241–53

1271. Cohnheim, Julius Friedrich. Neue Untersuchungen über die Entzündung. Berlin, *A. Hirschwald,* 1873

1272. Cohnheim, Julius Friedrich. Erkrankung des Knochenmarkes bei perniciöser Anämie. *Virchows Arch. Pathol. Anat.,* 1876, **68,** 291–93

1273. Cohnheim, Julius Friedrich. Die Tuberkulose vom Standpunkte der Infectionslehre. Leipzig, *A. Edelmann,* 1880

1274. Cohnheim, Julius Friedrich. Vorlesungen über allgemeine Pathologie. 2 vols. Berlin, *A. Hirschwald,* 1877–80

1275. Weigert, Carl. Ueber Bakterien in der Pockenhaut. *Zbl. Med. Wiss.,* 1871, **9,** 609–11

1276. Weigert, Carl. Anatomische Beiträge zur Lehre von den Pocken. 2 pts. Breslau, *M. Cohn u. Weigert,* 1874–75

1277. Weigert, Carl. Ueber eine Mykose bei einem neugeborenen Kinde (Bakterienfärbung mit Anilinfarben). *Jber. Schles. Ges. Vaterl. Cultur,* (1875), 1876, **53**, 229

1278. Weigert, Carl. Die Bright'sche Nierenerkrankung vom pathologisch-anatomischen Standpunkte. *Samml. Klin. Vortr.,* 1879, Nr. 162–63 (Inn. Med., Nr. 55), 1411–60

1279. Weigert, Carl. Ueber die pathologische Gerinnungs-Vorgänge. *Virchows Arch. Pathol. Anat.,* 1880, **79**, 87–123

1280. Weigert, Carl. Pathologisch-anatomischer Beitrag zur Erb'schen Krankheit (Myasthenia gravis). *Neurol. Zbl.,* 1901, **20**, 597–601

1281. Magendie, François. Mémoire sur le vomissement. Paris, *Crochard,* 1813. A translation of the above is in *Ann. Phil.,* London, 1813, **1**, 429–38

1282. Magendie, François and Pelletier, Pierre Joseph. Mémoire sur l'émétine, et sur les trois espèces d'ipecacuanha. *J. Gén. Méd. Chir. Pharm.,* 1817, **59**, 223–31

1283. Vedder, Edward Bright. Experiments undertaken to test the efficacy of the ipecac treatment of dysentery. *Bull. Manila Med. Soc.,* 1911, **3**, 48–53

1284. Magendie, François. Mémoires sur le mécanisme de l'absorption chez les animaux à sang rouge et chaud. *J. Physiol. Esp. Pathol.,* 1821, **1**, 1–17, 18–31

1285. Magendie, François. Expériences sur les fonctions des racines des nerfs rachidiens. *J. Physiol. Exp. Pathol.,* 1822, **2**, 276–79; 366–71. See J. F. Fulton, *Selected readings in the history of physiology,* 2nd edn., 1966, pp. 280–85

1286. Magendie, François. Formulaire pour la préparation et l'emploi de plusieurs nouveaux médicamens, tels que la noix vomique, la morphine, *etc.* Paris, *Méquignon-Marvis,* 1822

1287. Magendie, François. Mémoire sur un liquide qui se trouve dans le crâne et le canal vertébral de l'homme et des animaux mammifères. *J. Physiol. Exp. Pathol.,* 1825, **5**, 27–37; 1827, **7**, 1–29, 66–82

1288. Magendie, François. Lectures on the blood. Philadelphia, *Harrington, Barrington & Haswell,* 1839

1289. Magendie, François. Leçons sur les phénomènes physiques de la vie. 4 vols. Paris, *J. B. Baillière,* 1836–38

1290. Magendie, François. Recherches physiologiques et cliniques sur le liquide céphalorachidien ou cérébro-spinal. 1 vol. and atlas. Paris, *Méquignon-Marvis,* 1842

1291. Legallois, Julien Jean César. Le sang, est-il identique dans tous les vaisseaux qu'il parcourt? Paris, *Thèse,* (1801)

1292. Legallois, Julien Jean César. Expériences sur le principe de la vie. Paris, *D'Hautel,* 1812. English translation, Philadelphia, 1813

1293. Flourens, Marie Jean Pierre. Recherches expérimentales sur les propriétés et les fonctions du système nerveux, dans les animaux vertébrés. Paris, *Crevot,* 1824

1294. Flourens, Marie Jean Pierre. Recherches sur les propriétés et les fonctions du système nerveux dans les animaux vertébrés. *Arch. Gén. Méd.,* 1823, **2**, 321–70

1295. Flourens, Marie Jean Pierre. Expériences sur les canaux semi-circulaires de l'oreille. *Mém. Acad. R. d. Sci. (Paris),* 1830, **9**, 455–77

1296. Flourens, Marie Jean Pierre. Note touchant l'action de l'éther sur les centres nerveux. *C. R. Acad. Sci. (Paris),* 1847, **24**, 340–44

1297. Poiseuille, Jean Léonard Marie. Recherches sur la force du coeur aortique. Paris, *Thèse No. 166,* 1828. English translation in *Edinb. Med. Surg. J.,* 1829, **32**, 28–38

1298. Poiseuille, Jean Léonard Marie. Recherches expérimentales sur le mouvement des liquides dans les tubes de très petits diamètres. *C. R. Acad. Sci. (Paris),* 1840, **11**, 961–67, 1041–48; 1841, **12**, 112–15

1299. Poiseuille, Jean Léonard Marie. Sur la pression du sang dans le système artériel. *C. R. Acad. Sci. (Paris),* 1860, **51**, 238–42

1300. Weber, Eduard Friedrich Wilhelm and Weber, Ernst Heinrich. Experimenta, quibus probatur nervos vagos rotatione machinae galvanomagneticae irritatos, motum cordis retardare et adeo intercipare. *Ann. Univ. Med. (Milano),* 1845, 3 ser., **20**, 227–33

1301. Weber, Ernst Heinrich. Anatomia comparata nervi sympathici. Lipsiae, *C. H. Reclam,* 1817

1302. Weber, Ernst Heinrich. De aure et auditu hominis et animalium. Lipsiae, *apud G. Fleischerum,* 1820

1303. Weber, Ernst Heinrich and Weber, Eduard Friedrich Wilhelm. Wellenlehre. Leipzig, *W. Engelmann,* 1825

1304. Weber, Ernst Heinrich. De pulsu, resorptione, auditu et tactu. Annotationes anatomicae et physiologicae. Lipsiae, *C. F. Koehler,* 1834

1305. Fechner, Gustav Theodor. Ueber ein wichtiges psychophysisches Grundgesetz und dessen Beziehung zue Schätzung der Sterngrössen. *Abh. k. sächs. Ges. Wiss. (Lpz.), Maths.-Phys. Cl.,* (1858), 1859, **4,** 455–532

1306. Ferry, Ervin Sidney. Persistence of vision. *Am. J. Sci.,* 1892, 3 ser. **44,** 192–207

1307. Hall, Marshall. A critical and experimental essay on the circulation of the blood. London, *R. B. Seeley & W. Burnside,* 1831

1308. Hall, Marshall. On the reflex function of the medulla oblongata and medulla spinalis. *Phil. Trans.,* 1833, **123,** 635–65

1309. Hall, Marshall. Synopsis of cerebral and spinal seizures of inorganic origin and of paroxysmal form as a class; and of their pathology as involved in the structures and actions of the neck. London, *J. Mallett,* 1851

1310. Hall, Marshall. On a new mode of effecting artificial respiration. *Lancet,* 1856, **1,** 229

1311. Sharpey, William. On a peculiar motion excited in fluids by the surfaces of certain animals. *Edinb. Med. Surg. J.,* 1830, **34,** 113–22

1312. Bowman, Sir William. On the minute structure and movements of voluntary muscle. *Phil. Trans.,* 1840, **130,** 457–501; 1841, **131,** 69–72

1313. Bowman, Sir William. On the structure and use of the Malpighian bodies of the kidney. *Phil. Trans.,* 1842, **132,** 57–80

1314. Bowman, Sir William. Lectures on the parts concerned in the operations on the eye, and on the structure of the retina. London, *Longmans,* 1849

1315. Bowman, Sir William. Observations on artificial pupil, with a description of a new method of operating in certain cases. *Med. Times Gaz.,* 1852, n.s., **4,** 11–14, 33–35

1316. Bowman, Sir William. On the treatment of lacrymal obstructions. *Ophthal. Hosp. Rep.,* 1857–59, **1,** 10–20, 88

1317. Liebig, Justus von. Ueber die Verbindungen, welche durch die Einwirkung des Chlors auf Alkohol, Aether, ölbildendes Gas und Essiggeist entstehen. *Ann. Pharm. (Heidelberg),* 1832, **1,** 182–230

1318. Guthrie, Samuel. New mode of preparing a spirituous solution of chloric ether. *Am. J. Sci. Arts,* 1832, **21,** 64–65; **22,** 105–06

1319. Soubeiran, Eugène. Recherches sur quelques combinaisons du chlore. *Ann. Chim. (Paris),* 1831, 2 sér., **48,** 113–57

1320. Liebig, Justus von. Die organische Chemie in ihrer Anwendung auf Physiologie und Pathologie. Braunschweig, *F. Vieweg,* 1842

1321. Liebig, Justus von. Ueber einige Harnstoffverbindungen und eine neue Methode zur Bestimmung von Kochsalz und Harnstoff im Harn. *Ann. Pharm. (Heidelberg),* 1853, **85,** 289–328

1322. Wöhler, Friedrich. Ueber künstliche Bildung des Harnstoffs. *Ann. Phys. Chem. (Leipzig),* 1828, **12,** 253–6

1323. Wöhler, Friedrich. Umwandlung der Benzoësäure in Hippursäure im lebenden Organismus. *Ann. Phys. Chem. (Leipzig),* 1842, **56,** 638–41

1324. Young, John Richardson. An experimental inquiry into the principles of nutrition, and the digestive process. Philadelphia, *Eaken & Mecum,* 1803

1325. Prout, William. On the nature of the acid and saline matters usually existing in the stomachs of animals. *Phil. Trans.,* 1824, **114,** 45–49

1326. Beaumont, William. Experiments and observations on the gastric juice, and the physiology of digestion. Plattsburgh, *F. P. Allen,* 1833. Facsimile reprint, Cambridge, *Harvard Univ. Press,* 1929

1327. Schwann, Theodor. Ueber das Wesen des Verdauungsprocesses. *Arch. Anat. Physiol. Wiss. Med.,* 1836, 90–138

1328. Duverney, Guichard Joseph. Traité de l'organe de l'ouie; contenant la structure, les usages et les maladies de toutes les parties de l'oreille. Paris, *E. Michallet,* 1683. English translation, 1737

1329. Helmholtz, Hermann Ludwig Ferdinand von. Ueber die Erhaltung der Kraft, eine physikalische Abhandlung. Berlin, *G. Reimer,* 1847

492

1330. Helmholtz, Hermann Ludwig Ferdinand von. Ueber die Wärmeentwickelung bei der Muskelaction. *Arch. Anat. Physiol. Wiss. Med.*, 1848, 144–64

1331. Helmholtz, Hermann Ludwig Ferdinand von. Vorläufiger Bericht über die Fortpflanzungsgeschwindigkeit der Nervenreizung. *Arch. Anat. Physiol. Wiss. Med.*, 1850, 71–73

1332. Helmholtz, Hermann Ludwig Ferdinand von. Beschreibung eines Augen-Spiegels zur Untersuchung der Netzhaut im lebenden Auge. Berlin, *A. Förstner,* 1851. English translation by T. H. Shastid, 1916

1333. Helmholtz, Hermann Ludwig Ferdinand von. Ueber die Theorie der zusammengesetzten Farben. *Arch. Anat. Physiol. Wiss. Med.,* 1852, 461–82; *Ann. Phys. Chem.,* 1852, **87,** 45–66

1334. Helmholtz, Hermann Ludwig Ferdinand von. Ueber die Accommodation des Auges. *v. Graefes Arch. Ophthal.,* 1854–55, **1,** 2 Abt., 1–74

1335. Helmholtz, Hermann Ludwig Ferdinand von. Die Lehre von der Tonempfindungen als physiologische Grundlage für die Theorie der Musik. Braunschweig, *F. Vieweg u. Sohn.* 1863. English translation of 3rd edn., London, 1875

1336. Helmholtz, Hermann Ludwig Ferdinand von. Die Mechanik der Gehörknöchelchen und des Trommelfells. Bonn, *M. Cohen & Sohn,* 1869. English translation, 1874

1337. Bowditch, Henry Pickering. Ueber die Eigenthümlichkeiten der Reizbarkeit, welche die Muskelfasern des Herzens zeigen. *Arb. Physiol. Anst. Leipzig,* (1871), 1872, **6,** 139–76

1338. Bowditch, Henry Pickering. Note on the nature of nerve-force. *J. Physiol. (Lond.),* 1885, **6,** 133–35

1339. Bowditch, Henry Pickering. Ueber den Nachweis der Unermüdlichkeit des Säugethiernerven. *Arch. Anat. Physiol., Physiol. Abt.,* 1890, 505–08

1340. Bernstein, Julius. Ueber die Ermüdung und Erholung der Nerven. *Pflüg. Arch. Ges. Physiol.,* 1877, **15,** 289–327

1341. Waller, Augustus Volney. Experiments on the section of the glossopharyngeal and hypoglossal nerves of the frog, and observations of the alterations produced thereby in the structure of their primitive fibres. *Phil. Trans.,* 1850, **140,** 423–429

1342. Goltz, Friedrich Leopold. Beiträge zur Lehre von den Functionen der Nervencentren des Frosches. Berlin, *A. Hirschwald,* 1869

1343. Garrison, Fielding H. (1929). As ref. 179 but p. 540

1344. Goltz, Friedrich Leopold. Ueber die Functionen des Lendenmarks des Hundes. *Pflüg. Arch. Ges. Physiol.,* 1874, **8,** 460–98

1345. Goltz, Friedrich Leopold. Der Hund ohne Grosshirn. *Pflüg. Arch. Ges. Physiol.,* 1892, **51,** 570–614

1346. Goltz, Friedrich L. and Ewald, Ernst Julius R. Der Hund mit verkürztem Rückenmark. *Pflüg. Arch. Ges. Physiol.,* 1896, **63,** 362–400

1347. Garrison, Fielding H. (1929). As ref. 179 but p. 541

1348. Türck, Ludwig. Ueber den Zustand der Sensibilität nach theilweiser Trennung des Rückenmarkes. *Z. k. k. Ges. Aerzte Wien,* Abt. I, 1851, **7,** 189–201

1349. Türck, Ludwig. Ueber die Haut-Sensibilitätsbezirke der einzelnen Rückenmarksnervenpaare. *Denkschr. k. Akad. Wiss. (Wien), Math.-Nat. Cl.,* 1868, **29,** 299–326

1350. Brown-Séquard, Charles Edouard. Recherches sur la transmission des impressions de tact, de chatouillement, de douleur, de température et de contraction (sens musculaire) dans la moëlle épinière. *J. Physiol. (Paris),* 1863, **6,** 124–45, 232–48, 581–646

1351. Sherrington, Sir Charles Scott. Notes on the arrangement of some motor fibres in the lumbo-sacral plexus. *J. Physiol. (Lond.),* 1892, **13,** 621–772

1352. Sherrington, Sir Charles Scott. On the proprio-ceptive system, especially in its reflex aspect. *Brain,* 1906, **29,** 467–82

1353. Bernard, Claude. De l'origine du sucre dans l'économie animale. *Arch. Gén. Méd.,* 1848, 4 sér., **18,** 303–19. Reprinted, with translation, in *Med. Classics,* 1939, **3,** 552–80

1354. Bernard, Claude. Du suc pancréatique et de son rôle dans les phénomènes de la digestion. *C. R. Soc. Biol. (Mémoires),* (1849) 1850, **1,** 99–115. Reprinted, with translation, in *Med. Classics,* 1939, **3,** 581–617

1355. Bernard, Claude. Chiens rendus diabétiques. *C. R. Soc. Biol. (Paris),* (1849), 1850, **1,** 60

1356. Bernard, Claude. Influence du grand sympathique sur la sensibilité et sur la calorification. *C. R. Soc. Biol. (Paris),* (1851), 1852, **3,** 163–64

493

1357. Bernard, Claude. Recherches expérimentals sur le grand sympathique et spécialement sur l'influence que la section de ce nerf exerce sur la chaleur animal. *C. R. Soc. Biol. (Paris), (Mémoires),* (1853), 1854, **5**, 77–107

1358. Bernard, Claude. Leçons de physiologie expérimentale appliquée à la médecine. Vols. 1 and 2. Paris. *J. B. Baillière,* 1855–56

1359. Bernard, Claude. Sur le mécanisme de la formation du sucre dans le foie. *C. R. Acad. Sci. (Paris),* 1855, **41**, 461–69

1360. Bernard, Claude. Analyse physiologique des propriétés des systèmes musculaire et nerveux au moyen du curare. *C. R. Acad. Sci. (Paris),* 1856, **43**, 825–29

1361. Bernard, Claude (1856). As ref. 821

1362. Bernard, Claude. Leçons sur les effets des substances toxiques et médicamenteuses. Paris, *J. B. Baillière,* 1857

1363. Bernard, Claude. Nouvelles recherches expérimentales sur les phénomènes glycogéniques du foie. *C. R. Soc. Biol. (Mémoires),* (1857) 1858, 2 sér., **4**, 1–7

1364. Bernard, Claude. Leçons sur la physiologie et la pathologie du système nerveux. 2 vols. Paris, *J. B. Baillière,* 1858

1365. Horner, Johann Friedrich. Ueber eine Form von Ptosis. *Klin. Mbl. Augenheilk.,* 1869, **7**, 193–98

1366. Bernard, Claude. De l'influence de deux ordres de nerfs qui déterminent les variations de couleur du sang veineux dans les organes glandulaires. *C. R. Acad. Sci. (Paris),* 1858, **47**, 245–53, 393–400

1367. Bernard, Claude. Du rôle des actions réflexes paralysantes dans le phénomène des sécrétions. *J. Anat. Physiol. (Paris),* 1864, **1**, 507–13

1368. Bernard, Claude. Leçons de pathologie expérimentale. Paris, *J. B. Baillière,* 1872

1369. Bernard, Claude. Leçons sur le diabète et la glycogenèse animale. Paris, *J. B. Baillière,* 1877

1370. Bernard, Claude. Leçons sur les anesthésiques et sur l'asphyxie. Paris, *J. B. Baillière,* 1875

1371. Bernard, Claude. La fermentation alcoolique. *Rev. Sci. (Paris),* 1878, **16**, 49–56

1372. Bernard, Claude. Leçons de physiologie opératoire. Paris, *J. B. Baillière,* 1879

1373. Ludwig, Carl Friedrich Wilhelm. Beiträge zur Lehre vom Mechanismus der Harnsecretion. Marburg, *N. G. Elwert,* 1843

1374. Ludwig, Carl Friedrich Wilhelm. Beiträge zur Kenntniss des Einflusses der Respirationsbewegungen auf den Blutlauf im Aortensystem. *Arch. Anat. Physiol. Wiss. Med.,* 1847, 242–302

1375. Ludwig, Carl Friedrich Wilhelm. Ueber die endosmotischen Aequivalente und die endosmotische Theorie. *Z. Rat. Med.,* 1849, **8**, 1–52

1376. Hoffa, Moritz and Ludwig, Carl Friedrich Wilhelm. Einige neue Versuche über Herzbewegung. *Z. Rat. Med.,* 1850, **9**, 107–44

1377. Ludwig, Carl Friedrich Wilhelm. Neue Versuche über die Beihilfe der Nerven zur Speichelabsonderung. *Z. Rat. Med.,* 1851, n.F. **1**, 254–77

1378. Ludwig, Carl Friedrich Wilhelm. Die physiologischen Leistungen des Blutdrucks. Leipzig, *S. Hirzel,* 1865

1379. Cyon, Elie de and Ludwig, Carl Friedrich Wilhelm. Die Reflexe eines der sensiblen Nerven des Herzens auf die motorischen der Blutgefässe. *Arb. Physiol. Anst. Leipzig,* (1866), 1867, **1**, 128–49

1380. Foster, Sir Michael. A text-book of physiology. London, *Macmillan,* 1877

1381. Foster, Sir Michael. Lectures on the history of physiology. Cambridge, *Univ. Press,* 1901

1382. Ringer, Sidney. Regarding the action of hydrate of soda, hydrate of ammonia, and hydrate of potash on the ventricle of the frog's heart. *J. Physiol. (Lond.),* 1880–82, **3**, 195–202

1383. Gaskell, Walter Holbrook. On the rhythm of the heart of the frog, and on the nature of the action of the vagus nerve. *Phil. Trans.,* 1882, **173**, 993–1033

1384. Gaskell, Walter Holbrook. On the innervation of the heart. *J. Physiol. (Lond.),* 1883–84, **4**, 43–127

1385. Gaskell, Walter Holbrook. On the structure, distribution, and function of the nerves which innervate the visceral and vascular system. *J. Physiol. (Lond.),* 1886, **7**, 1–80

1386. Gaskell, Walter Holbrook. The origin of vertebrates. London, *Longmans, Green,* 1908

1387. Gaskell, Walter Holbrook. The involuntary nervous system. Part 1. London, *Longmans, Green & Co.,* 1916

1388. Langley, John Newport and Dickinson, William Lee. On the local paralysis of peripheral ganglia, and on the connexion of different classes of nerve fibres with them. *Proc. R. Soc.,* 1889, **46**, 423–31

1389. Langley, John Newport and Anderson, Sir Hugh Kerr. On reflex action from sympathetic ganglia. *J. Physiol. (Lond.),* 1894, **16**, 410–40

1390. Langley, John Newport. On the reaction of cells and of nerve-endings to certain poisons, chiefly as regards the reaction of striated muscle to nicotine and to curari. *J. Physiol. (Lond.),* 1905, **33**, 374–413

1391. Langley, John Newport. The autonomic nervous system. Cambridge, *W. Heffer,* 1921

1392. Hopkins, Sir Frederick Gowland. On the estimation of uric acid in the urine. *J. Pathol. Bact.,* 1892–93, **1**, 451–59

1393. Hopkins, Sir Frederick Gowland and Cole, Sydney William. A contribution to the chemistry of proteids. I. A preliminary study of a hitherto undescribed product of tryptic digestion. *J. Physiol. (Lond.),* 1901, **27**, 418–28

1394. Willcock, Edith Gertrude and Hopkins, Sir Frederick Gowland. The importance of individual amino-acids in metabolism. *J. Physiol. (Lond.),* 1906, **35**, 88–102

1395. Hopkins, Sir Frederick Gowland. The analyst and the medical man. *Analyst,* 1906, **31**, 385–404

1396. Hopkins, Sir Frederick Gowland. Feeding experiments illustrating the importance of accessory factors in normal dietaries. *J. Physiol. (Lond.),* 1912, **44**, 425–60

1397. Fletcher, Sir Walter Morley and Hopkins, Sir Frederick Gowland. Lactic acid in amphibian muscle. *J. Physiol. (Lond.),* 1907, **35**, 247–309

1398. Hopkins, Sir Frederick Gowland. On an autoxidisable constituent of the cell. *Biochem. J.,* 1921, **15**, 286–305

1399. Haldane, John Scott. A new form of apparatus for measuring the respiratory exchange of animals. *J. Physiol. (Lond.),* 1892, **13**, 419–30

1400. Haldane, John Scott. A contribution to the chemistry of haemoglobin and its immediate derivatives. *J. Physiol. (Lond.),*1898, **22**, 298–306

1401. Haldane, John Scott. The colorimetric determination of haemoglobin. *J. Physiol. (Lond.),* 1901, **26**, 497–504

1402. Haldane, John Scott and Priestley, John Gillies. The regulation of the lung-ventilation. *J. Physiol. (Lond.),* 1905, **32**, 225–66

1403. Douglas, Claude Gordon *et al.* Physiological observations made on Pike's Peak, Colorado, with special reference to adaptation to low barometric pressures. *Phil. Trans. B,* 1913, **203**, 185–318

1404. Christiansen, Johanne Ostenfeld *et al.* The absorption and dissociation of carbon dioxide by human blood. *J. Physiol. (Lond.),* 1914, **48**, 244–71

1405. Haldane, John Scott. The therapeutic administration of oxygen. *Br. Med. J.,* 1917, **1**, 181–83

1406. Haldane, John Scott. Respiration. New Haven, *Yale Univ. Press,* 1922

1407. Gowers, Sir William Richard. The numeration of blood corpuscles and the effect of iron and phosphorus on the blood. *Practitioner,* 1878, **21**, 1–17

1408. Barcroft, Sir Joseph. The respiratory function of the blood. 2 pts. Cambridge, *Univ. Press,* 1925–28

1409. Bell, John. The principles of surgery. 3 vols. (in 4). Edinburgh, London, *T. Cadell & W. Davies,* 1801–08

1410. Bell, John. Letters on professional character and manners. Edinburgh, *J. Moir,* 1810

1411. Cooper, Sir Astley Paston, Bart. Further observations on the effects which take place from the destruction of the membrana tympani of the ear; with an account of an operation for the removal of a particular species of deafness. *Phil. Trans.,* 1801, **91**, 435–50

1412. Cooper, Sir Astley Paston, Bart. (1804–07). As ref. 1011

1413. Cooper, Sir Astley Paston, Bart. A case of aneurism of the carotid artery. *Med.-Chir. Trans.,* 1809, **1**, 1–12, 222–33

1414. Cooper, Sir Astley Paston, Bart. Account of the first successful operation, performed on the carotid artery, for aneurism, in the year 1808; with the post-mortem examination, in 1821. *Guy's Hosp. Rep.,* 1836, **1**, 53–58

1415. Cooper, Sir Astley Paston, Bart. and Travers, Benjamin. Surgical essays. 2 vols. London, *Cox & Son,* 1818–19

1416. Cooper, Sir Astley Paston, Bart. Illustrations of the diseases of the breast. London, *Longman, Rees & Co.,* 1829

1417. Cooper, Sir Astley Paston, Bart. The anatomy of the thymus gland. London, *Longman,* 1832

1418. Cooper, Sir Astley Paston, Bart. Some experiments and observations on tying the carotid and vertebral arteries, and the pneumo-gastric, phrenic, and sympathetic nerves. *Guy's Hosp. Rep.,* 1836, **1,** 457–75, 654

1419. Cooper, Sir Astley Paston, Bart. Case of a femoral aneurism, for which the external iliac artery was tied, with an account of the preparation of the limb, dissected at the expiration of eighteen years. *Guy's Hosp. Rep.,* 1836, **1,** 43–52

1420. Twitchell, Amos. Gun-shot wound of the face and neck; ligature of the carotid artery. *N. Engl. Q. J. Med. Surg.,* 1842–43, **1,** 188–93

1421. Colles, Abraham. On the fracture of the carpal extremity of the radius. *Edinb. Med. Surg. J.,* 1814, **10,** 182–86

1422. Colles, Abraham. On the operation of tying the subclavian artery. *Edinb. Med. Surg. J.,* 1815, **11,** 1–25

1423. Colles, Abraham. Practical observations on the venereal disease, and on the use of mercury. London, *Sherwood, Gilbert & Piper,* 1837

1424. Liston, Robert. Practical surgery. London, *J. Churchill,* 1837

1425. Garrison, Fielding H. (1929). As ref. 179 but p. 482

1426. Syme, James. Case of osteo-sarcoma of the lower jaw. *Edinb. Med. Surg. J.,* 1828, **30,** 286–90

1427. Syme, James. Three cases in which the elbow-joint was successfully excised. *Edinb. Med. Surg. J.,* 1829, **31,** 256–66

1428. Syme, James. Treatise on the excision of diseased joints. Edinburgh, *A. Black,* 1831

1429. Syme, James. Amputation at the ankle-joint. *Lond. Edinb. Mon. J. Med. Sci.,* 1843, **3,** 93–96

1430. Syme, James. On the use of ether in the performance of surgical operations. (*Lond. Edinb.*) *Month. J. Med. Sci.,* 1847–48, **8,** 73–76

1431. Syme, James. Contributions to the pathology and practice of surgery. Edinburgh, *Sutherland & Knox,* 1848

1432. Syme, James. Case of iliac aneurism. *Med.-Chir. Trans.,* 1862, **45,** 381–87

1433. Fergusson, Sir William. A system of practical surgery. London, *J. Churchill,* 1842

1434. Fergusson, Sir William. System of practical surgery. 4th edn. London. *J. Churchill,* 1857

1435. Fergusson, Sir William. Lectures on the progress of anatomy and surgery during the present century. London, *J. Churchill & Sons,* 1867

1436. Brodie, Sir Benjamin Collins, Bart. Experiments and observations on the influence of the nerves of the eighth pair on the secretions of the stomach. *Phil. Trans.,* 1814, **104,** 102–06

1437. Brodie, Sir Benjamin Collins, Bart. Observations on the treatment of varicose veins of the legs. *Med.-Chir. Trans.,* 1816, **7,** 195–210

1438. Brodie, Sir Benjamin Collins, Bart. Pathological and surgical observations on the diseases of the joints. London, *Longman,* 1818

1439. Brodie, Sir Benjamin Collins, Bart. On trephining the tibia. *Lond. Med. Gaz.,* 1828, **2,** 70–74

1440. Brodie, Sir Benjamin Collins, Bart. Lectures illustrative of various subjects in pathology and surgery. London, *Longman,* 1846

1441. Dupuytren, Guillaume, le baron. Mémoire sur un déplacement originel ou congénital de la tête des fémurs. *Répert. Gén. Anat. Physiol. Pathol.,* 1826, **2,** 82–93

1442. Dupuytren, Guillaume, le baron. De la rétraction des doigts par suite d'une affection de l'aponévrose palmaire, opération chirurgicale qui convient dans ce cas. *J. Univ. Hebd. Méd. Chir. Prat.,* 1831, 2 sér., **5,** 352–65. Reprinted, with translation, in *Med. Classics,* 1939, **4,** 127–50

1443. Dupuytren, Guillaume, le baron. Leçons orales de clinique chirurgicale. 4 vols. Paris, *Germer-Baillière,* 1832–34

1444. Broca, Pierre Paul. Remarques sur le siège de la faculté du langage articulé, suivie d'une observation d'aphémie (perte de la parole). *Bull. Soc. Anat. Paris,* 1861, **36,** 330–57

1445. Marie, Pierre. Revision de la question de l'aphasie; la troisième circonvolution frontale gauche ne joue aucun rôle spécial dans la fonction du langage. *Sem. Méd. (Paris),* 1906, **26,** 241–47

1446. Graefe, Carl Ferdinand von. Rhinoplastick, oder die Kunst den Verlust der Nase organisch zu ersetzen. Berlin, *Reimer,* 1818

1447. Graefe, Carl Ferdinand von. Die Gaumennath, ein neuentdecktes Mittel gegen angeborene Fehler der Sprache. *J. Chir. Augenheilk.,* 1820, **1,** 1–54

1448. Physick, Philip Syng. Account of a new mode of extracting poisonous substances from the stomach. *Eclectic Repert.,* 1812–13, **3,** 111, 381

1449. Physick, Philip Syng. (Buck-skin and kid ligatures). *Eclect. Repert.,* 1816, **6,** 389

1450. Physick, Philip Syng. A case of fracture of the bone of the under jaw, successfully treated with a seton. *Philad. J. Med. Phys. Sci.,* 1822, **5,** 116–18

1451. Physick, Philip Syng. Extracts from an account of a case in which a new and peculiar operation for artificial anus was performed. *Philad. J. Med. Phys. Sci.,* 1826, **13,** 199–202

1452. Physick, Philip Syng. Description of a forceps, employed to facilitate the extirpation of the tonsil. *Am. J. Med. Sci.,* 1828, **2,** 116–17

1453. McDowell, Ephraim. Three cases of extirpation of diseased ovaria. *Eclect. Repert. Analyt. Rev.,* 1817, **7,** 242–44

1454. Sims, James Marion. On the treatment of vesico-vaginal fistula. *Am. J. Med. Sci.,* 1852, n.s., **23,** 59–82. Reprinted in *Med. Classics,* 1938, **2,** 677–712

1455. Sims, James Marion. Silver sutures in surgery. New York, *S. S. & S. W. Wood,* 1858

1456. Sims, James Marion. Amputation of the cervix uteri. *Trans. N.Y. Med. Soc.,* 1861, 367–71

1457. Sims, James Marion. On vaginismus. *Trans. Obstet. Soc. Lond.,* (1861), 1862, **3,** 356–67

1458. Sims, James Marion. Clinical notes on uterine surgery. London, *R. Hardwicke,* 1866

1459. Sims, James Marion. Remarks on cholecystotomy in dropsy of the gall-bladder. *Br. Med. J.,* 1878, **1,** 811–15

1460. Davy, Sir Humphry. Researches, chemical and philosophical, chiefly concerning nitrous oxide. London, *J. Johnson,* 1800. Reprinted, London, Butterworths, 1972

1461. Leake, Chauncey Depew. An historical account of pharmacology to the twentieth century. Springfield, Illinois, *Charles C. Thomas,* 1975, p. 132

1462. Barton, William Paul Crillon. Vegetable materia medica of the United States. 2 vols. Philadelphia, *M. Carey & Son,* 1817–18

1463. Anonymous. Effects of inhaling the vapour of sulphuric ether. *Q. J. Arts,* 1818, **4,** 158–159

1464. Long, Crawford Williamson. An account of the first use of sulphuric ether by inhalation as an anaesthetic in surgical operations. *South. Med. Surg. J.,* 1849, **5,** 705–713

1465. Young, Hugh Hampton. Long, the discoverer of anaesthesia. A presentation of his original documents. *Johns Hopk. Hosp. Bull.,* 1897, **8,** 174–84

1466. Wells, Horace. A history of the discovery of the application of nitrous oxide gas, ether, and other vapours, to surgical operations. Hartford, *J. G. Wells,* 1847

1467. Morton, William Thomas Green. Circular. Morton's Letheon. Boston, *Dutton & Wentworth,* (1846)

1468. Bigelow, Henry Jacob. Insensibility during surgical operations produced by inhalation. *Boston Med. Surg. J.,* 1846, **35,** 309–17, 379–82

1469. Bigelow, Henry Jacob. Ether and chloroform: a compendium of their history and discovery. Boston, *D. Clapp.* 1848

1470. Bigelow, Henry Jacob. Resection of the head of the femur. *Am. J. Med. Sci.,* 1852, **24,** 90

1471. Bigelow, Henry Jacob. The mechanism of dislocation and fracture of the hip. With the reduction of the dislocations by the flexion method. Philadelphia, *H. C. Lea,* 1869

1472. Clarke, Edward Hammond *et al.* A century of American medicine 1776–1876. By Edward H. Clarke, H. J. Bigelow, S. D. Gross, T. Gaillard Thomas and J. S. Billings, Philadelphia, *H. C. Lea,* 1876

1473. Simpson, Sir James Young. Discovery of a new anaesthetic agent, more efficient than sulphuric ether. *Lond. Med. Gaz.,* 1847, n.s., **5,** 934–37; *Lancet,* 1847, **2,** 549

1474. Wells, Sir Thomas Spencer. Diseases of the ovaries. 2 vols. London, *J. Churchill,* 1865–72

1475. Wells, Sir Thomas Spencer. Remarks on forcipressure and the use of pressure-forceps in surgery. *Br. Med. J.,* 1879, **1,** 926–28; **2,** 3–4

1476. Tait, Robert Lawson. Removal of normal ovaries. *Br. Med. J.,* 1879, **1**, 813–14

1477. Tait, Robert Lawson. A case of removal of the uterine appendages. *Br. Med. J.,* 1881, **1**, 766–67

1478. Parry, John S. Extra-uterine pregnancy. Philadelphia. *H. C. Lea,* 1876

1479. Tait, Robert Lawson. Five cases of extra-uterine pregnancy operated upon at the time of rupture. *Br. Med. J.,* 1884, **1**, 1250–51

1480. Tait, Robert Lawson. General summary of conclusions from one thousand cases of abdominal section. Birmingham, *R. Birbeck,* 1884

1481. Tait, Robert Lawson. Surgical treatment of typhilitis. *Bgham Med. Rev.,* 1890, **27**, 26–34, 76–89

1482. Tait, Robert Lawson. An address on the surgical aspect of impacted labour. *Br. Med. J.,* 1890, **1**, 657–61

1483. Tait, Robert Lawson. On the method of flap-splitting in certain plastic operations. *Br. Gynaec. J.,* 1887–88, **3**, 367–76; 1891–92, **7**, 195–214

1484. McBurney, Charles. Experience with early operative interference in cases of disease of the vermiform appendix. *N. Y. Med. J.,* 1889, **50**, 676–84. Reprinted in *Med. Classics,* 1938, **2**, 506–31

1485. Cagniard-Latour, Charles, Baron. Mémoire sur la fermentation vineuse. *Ann. Chim. Phys.,* 1838, **68**, 206–22

1486. Schwann, Theodor. Vorläufige Mittheilung betreffend Versuche über die Weingährung und Fäulniss. *Ann. Phys. Chem. (Leipzig),* 1837, **41**, 184–93

1487. Pasteur, Louis. Mémoire sur la fermentation appelée lactique. *C. R. Acad. Sci. (Paris),* 1857, **45**, 913–16

1488. Pasteur, Louis. Nouveaux faits pour servir à l'histoire de la levure lactique. *C. R. Acad. Sci. (Paris),* 1859, **48**, 337–38

1489. Pasteur, Louis. Expériences relatives aux générations dites spontanées. *C. R. Acad. Sci. (Paris),* 1860, **50**, 303–07, 849–54; **51**, 348–52, 675–78

1490. Pasteur, Louis. Mémoire sur les corpuscles organisés existent dans l'atmosphère. Examen de la doctrine des générations spontanées. *Ann. Sci. Nat. (Zool.),* 1861, **16**, 5–98

1491. Pasteur, Louis. Nouvel exemple de fermentation determinée par des animalcules infusoires pouvant vivre sans gaz oxygène libre, et en dehors de tout contact avec l'air de l'atmosphere. *C. R. Acad. Sci. (Paris),* 1863, **56**, 416–21

1492. Pasteur, Louis. Recherches sur la putréfaction. *C. R. Acad. Sci. (Paris),* 1863, **56**, 1189–94

1493. Pasteur, Louis. Examen du rôle attribué au gaz oxygène atmosphérique dans la destruction des matières animales et végétales après la mort. *C. R. Acad. Sci. (Paris),* 1863, **56**, 734–40

1494. Pasteur, Louis. Études sur le vin. Paris, *Imp. impériale,* 1866

1495. Pasteur, Louis. Études sur le vinaigre. Paris, *Gauthier-Villars,* 1868

1496. Pasteur, Louis. Études sur la maladie des vers à soie. 2 vols. Paris, *Gauthier-Villars,* 1870

1497. Pasteur, Louis. Études sur la bière, . . . avec une théorie nouvelle de la fermentation. Paris, *Gauthier-Villars,* 1876

1498. Koch, Robert. Die Aetiologie der Milzbrand-Krankheit, begründet auf die Entwicklungsgeschichte des Bacillus anthracis. *Beitr. Biol. Pflanzen,* 1876, **2**, 277–310. Reproduced with translation in *Med. Classics,* 1938, **2**, 745–820

1499. Pasteur, Louis and Joubert, Jules François. Etude sur la maladie charbonneuse. *C. R. Acad. Sci. (Paris),* 1877, **84**, 900–06

1500. Pasteur, Louis and Joubert, Jules François. Charbon et septicémie. *C. R. Acad. Sci. (Paris),* 1877, **85**, 101–15

1501. Pasteur, Louis. Septicémie puerpérale. *Bull. Acad. Méd. (Paris),* 1879, 2 sér., **8**, 505–508

1502. Pasteur, Louis. Sur les maladies virulentes, et en particulier sur la maladie appelée vulgairement choléra des poules. *C. R. Acad. Sci. (Paris),* 1880, **90**, 239–48

1503. Pasteur, Louis, Chamberland, Charles and Roux, Pierre Paul Emile. Sur l'etiologie du charbon. *C. R. Acad. Sci. (Paris),* 1880, **91**, 86–94

1504. Pasteur, Louis *et al.* Sur la rage. *C. R. Acad. Sci. (Paris),* 1881, **92**, 1259–60

1505. Pasteur, Louis. Nouvelle communication sur la rage. *C. R. Acad. Sci. (Paris),* 1884, **98**, 457–63, 1229–31

1506. Pasteur, Louis. Méthode pour prévenir la rage après morsure. *C. R. Acad. Sci. (Paris),* 1885, **101**, 765–74

1507. Pasteur, Louis. Méthode pour prévenir la rage après morsure. *C. R. Acad. Sci. (Paris),* 1885, **101**, 765–74; 1886, **102**, 459–69; 835–8; **103**, 777–85

1508. Parrot, Joseph. L'organisme microscopique trouvé par M. Pasteur dans la maladie nouvelle provoquée par la salive d'un enfant mort de la rage. *Bull. Acad. Méd. Paris,* 1881, 2 sér., **10**, 379

1509. Sternberg, George Miller. A manual of bacteriology. New York, *W. Wood & Co.,* 1893

1510. Pasteur, Louis. Œuvres de Pasteur, réunies par Pasteur Vallery-Radot. 7 vols. Paris, *Masson,* 1922–39

1511. Garrison, Fielding H. (1929). As ref. 179 but p. 577

1512. Koch, Robert. Verfahrungen zur Untersuchung, zum Conserviren und Photographiren der Bacterien. *Beitr. Biol. Pflanzen,* 1877, **2**, 399–434

1513. Koch, Robert. Untersuchungen über die Aetiologie der Wundinfectionskrankheiten. Leipzig, *F. C. W. Vogel,* 1878. English translation, New Sydenham Society, 1880

1514. Koch, Robert. Ueber Desinfection. *Mitt. k. GesundhAmte,* 1881, **1**, 234–82

1515. Koch, Robert. Die Aetiologie der Tuberkulose. *Berl. Klin. Wschr.,* 1882, **19**, 221–30. Reprinted with translation in *Med. Classics,* 1938, **2**, 821–80

1516. Koch, Robert (1882, in 1938 translation). As ref. 1515 but p. 856

1517. Koch, Robert (1882, in 1938 translation). As ref. 1515 but p. 863

1518. Koch, Robert (1882 in 1938 translation). As ref. 1515 but p. 864

1519. Henle, Friedrich Gustav Jacob (1840). As ref. 1209

1520. Singer, Charles and Underwood, E. Ashworth. A short history of medicine. Oxford, *Clarendon Press.* 2nd edn. 1962, pp. 379–380

1521. Koch, Robert. Ueber die Cholerabakterien. *Dtsch. Med. Wschr.,* 1884, **10**, 725–28

1522. Koch, Robert. Bericht über die Thätigkeit der deutschen Cholerakommission in Aegypten und Ostindien. *Wien. Med. Wschr.,* 1883, **33**, 1548–51

1523. Koch, Robert. Weitere Mittheilungen über ein Heilmittel gegen Tuberkulose. *Dtsch. Med. Wschr.,* 1890, **16**, 1029–32; **17**, 101–02, 1189–92

1524. Koch, Robert. Ueber neue Tuberkulinpräparate. *Deutsch. Med. Wschr.,* 1897, **23**, 209–13

1525. Koch, Robert. Reise-Bericht über Rinderpest, Bubonenpest in Indien und Afrika, Tsetse- oder Surrakrankheit, Texasfieber, tropische Malaria, Schwarzwasserfieber. Berlin, *J. Springer,* 1898

1526. Koch, Robert. Die Bekämpfung des Typhus. Berlin, *A. Hirschwald,* 1903

1527. Smith, Theobold. A comparative study of bovine tubercle bacilli and of human bacilli from sputum. *J. Exp. Med.,* 1898, **3**, 451–511

1528. Petri, Richard Julius. Eine kleine Modification des Koch'schen Plattenverfahrens. *Zbl. Bakt.,* 1887, **1**, 279–80

1529. Koch, Robert. Gesammelte Werke. 2 vols (in 3). Leipzig, *G. Thieme,* 1912

1530. Hansen, Gerhard Henrik Armauer. Indberetning til det Norske mediciniske Selskab i Christiania om en med understøttelse af selskabet foretagen reise for at anstille undersøgelser angående spedalskhedens årsager, tildels udførte sammen med forstander Hartwig. *Norsk. Mag. f. Laegevidensk.,* 1847, 3 R., **4**, 9 Heft, 1–88; Case reports, i–liii. For an English translation of the paper, see *Br. For. Med.-Chir. Rev.,* 1875, **55**, 459–89

1531. Neisser, Albert Ludwig Siegmund. Ueber eine der Gonorrhoe eigentümliche Micrococcus-form. *Zbl. Med. Wiss.,* 1879, **17**, 497–500

1532. Eberth, Carl Joseph. Die Organismen in den Organen bei Typhus abdominalis. *Virchows Arch. Pathol. Anat.,* 1880, **81**, 58–74

1533. Fehleisen, Friederich. Ueber Erysipel. *Dtsch. Z. Chir.,* 1882, **16**, 391–97. English translation, 1886

1534. Klebs, Theodor Albrecht Edwin. Ueber Diphtherie. *Verh. Congr. Inn. Med.,* 1883, **2**, 139–54

1535. Loeffler, Friedrich. Untersuchungen über die Bedeutung der Mikroorganismen für die Entstehung der Diphtherie biem Menschen, bei der Taube und beim Kalbe. *Mitt. k. GesundhAmte,* 1884, **2**, 421–99

1536. Nicolaier, Arthur. Ueber infectiösen Tetanus. *Dtsch. Med. Wschr.,* 1884, **10**, 842–44

1537. Escherich, Theodor. Die Darmbakterien des Säuglings und ihre Beziehungen zur Physiologie der Verdauung. Stuttgart, *F. Enke,* 1886

1538. Bruce, Sir David. Note on the discovery of a micro-organism in Malta fever. *Practitioner,* 1887, **39**, 161–70

1539. Weichselbaum, Anton. Ueber die Aetiologie der akuten Meningitis cerebro-spinalis. *Fortschr. Med.,* 1887, **5,** 573–83, 620–26

1540. Ducrey, Augusto. Il virus dell' ulcera venerea. *Gazz. Int. Sci. Med.,* 1889, **11,** 44

1541. Pfeiffer, Richard Friedrich Johannes. Vorläufige Mittheilungen über die Erreger der Influenza. *Dtsch. Med. Wschr.,* 1892, **18,** 28

1542. Welch, William Henry and Nuttall, George Henry Falkiner. A gas-producing bacillus (Bacillus aërogenes capsulatus nov. spec.) capable of rapid development in the blood-vessels after death. *Johns Hopk. Hosp. Bull.,* 1892, **3,** 81–91. Reprinted in *Med. Classics,* 1941, **5,** 852–85

1543. Yersin, Alexandre Emile Jean. La peste bubonique à Hong-Kong. *Ann. Inst. Pasteur,* 1894, **8,** 662–667

1544. Shiga, Kiyoshi. Ueber den Dysenteriebacillus (Bacillus dysenteriae). *Zbl. Bakt.,* 1898. 1 Abt., **24,** 817–28, 870–74

1545. Bordet, Jules Jean Baptiste Vincent and Gengou, Octave. Le microbe de la coqueluche. *Ann. Inst. Pasteur,* 1906, **20,** 731–41; 1907, **21,** 720–26

1546. Buchner, Hans. Ueber die bakterientödtende Wirkung des zellenfreien Blutserums. *Zbl. Bakt.,* 1889, **5,** 817–23; **6,** 1–11

1547. Behring, Emil Adolf von and Kitasato, Shibasaburo. Ueber das Zustandekommen der Diphtherie-Immunität und der Tetanus-Immunität bei Thieren. *Dtsch. Med. Wschr.,* 1890, **16,** 1113–1114

1548. Behring, Emil Adolf von. Die Behandlung der Diphtherie mit Diphtherieheilserum. *Dtsch. Med. Wschr.,* 1893, **19,** 543–47; 1894, **20,** 645–46

1549. Behring, Emil Adolf von. Ueber ein neues Diphtherieschutzmittel. *Dtsch. Med. Wschr.,* 1913, **39,** 873–76; 1914, **40,** 1139

1550. Metchnikoff, Elie. Über eine Sprosspilzkrankheit der Daphnien. Beitrag zur Lehre über den Kampf der Phagocyten gegen Krankheitserreger. *Virchows Arch. Pathol. Anat.,* 1884, **96,** 177–95

1551. Metchnikoff, Elie (Mechnikov, Ilya Ilyich). Lektsii o sravnitelnoi pathologii vospaleniy. St. Petersburg, *K. L. Rikker,* 1892

1552. Metchnikoff, Elie and Roux, Pierre Paul Emile. Etudes expérimentales sur la syphilis. *Ann. Inst. Pasteur,* 1903, **17,** 809–21; 1904, **18,** 1–6

1553. Wright, Sir Almroth Edward and Smith, Frederick. On the application of the serum test to the differential diagnosis of typhoid and Malta fever. *Lancet,* 1897, **1,** 656–59

1554. Wright, Sir Almroth Edward and Leishman, Sir William Boog. Remarks on the results which have been obtained by the antityphoid inoculations. *Br. Med. J.,* 1900, **1,** 122–29

1555. Wright, Sir Almroth Edward and Douglas, Stewart Ranken. An experimental investigation of the rôle of the blood fluids in connection with phagocytosis. *Proc. R. Soc. (Lond.),* 1903–04, **72,** 357–370; 1904, **73,** 128–42

1556. Lister, Joseph Jackson. On some properties in achromatic object-glasses applicable to the improvement of the microscope. *Phil. Trans.,* 1830, **120,** 187–200

1557. Lister, Joseph, 1st Baron Lister. On the early stages of inflammation. *Phil. Trans.,* 1858, **148,** 645–702

1558. Lister, Joseph, 1st Baron Lister. On the coagulation of the blood. *Proc. R. Soc. (Lond.),* (1862), 1863, **12,** 580–611

1559. Lister, Joseph, 1st Baron Lister. On excision of the wrist for caries. *Lancet,* 1865, **1,** 308–12, 335–38, 362–64

1560. Lister, Joseph, 1st Baron Lister. On a new method of treating compound fracture, abscess, etc., with observations on the conditions of suppuration. *Lancet,* 1867, **1,** 326–29, 357–59, 387–89, 507–09; **2,** 95–96. Reprinted in *Med. Classics,* 1937, **2,** 28–71

1561. Lister, Joseph, 1st Baron Lister. On the antiseptic principle in the practice of surgery. *Lancet,* 1867, **2,** 353–56, 668–69. Reprinted in *Med. Classics,* 1937, **2,** 72–83

1562. Lister, Joseph, 1st Baron Lister. Observations on ligature of arteries on the antiseptic system. *Lancet,* 1869, **1,** 451–55

1563. Lister, Joseph, 1st Baron Lister. On the effects of the antiseptic system of treatment upon the salubrity of a surgical hospital. *Lancet,* 1870, **1,** 4–6, 40–2. Reprinted in *Med. Classics,* 1937, **2,** 84–101

1564. Lister, Joseph, 1st Baron Lister. A method of antiseptic treatment applicable to wounded soldiers in the present war. *Br. Med. J.,* 1870, **2,** 243–44

1565. Lister, Joseph, 1st Baron Lister. A further contribution to the natural history of bacteria and the germ theory of fermentative changes. *Q. J. Micr. Sci.,* 1873, n.s. **13**, 380–408

1566. Lister, Joseph, 1st Baron Lister. On the lactic fermentation and its bearings on pathology. *Trans. Pathol., Soc. Lond.,* 1877–78, **29**, 425–67

1567. Lister, Joseph, 1st Baron Lister. Collected papers. 2 vols. Oxford, *Clarendon Press,* 1909

1568. Garrison, Fielding H. (1929). As ref. 179 but p. 591

1569. Billroth, Christian Albert Theodor. Die allgemeine chirurgische Pathologie und Therapie. Berlin, *G. Reimer,* 1863

1570. Billroth, Christian Albert Theodor. Ueber die Resection des Oesophagus. *Arch. Klin. Chir.,* 1872, **13**, 65–69

1571. Billroth, Christian Albert Theodor. Offenes Schreiben an Herrn Dr. L. Wittelshöfer. *Wien. Med. Wschr.,* 1881, **31**, 161–65, 1427

1572. Hauer, Ernst. Darmresektion und Enterorhaphieen, 1878–83. *Z. Heilk,* 1884, **5**, 83–108

1573. Hacker, Viktor von. Zur Casuistik und Statistik der Magenresectionen und Gastro-enterostomieen. *Verh. Dtsch. Ges. Chir.,* 1885, **14**, Pt. II, 62–71

1574. Thiersch, Carl. De maxillarum necrosi phosphorica. Lipsiae, *apud A. Edelmannum,* 1867

1575. Thiersch, Carl. Ueber die feineren anatomischen Veränderungen bei Aufheilung von Haut auf Granulationen. *Verh. Dtsch. Ges. Chir.,* 1874, **3**, 69–75

1576. Bergmann, Ernst von. Zur Sublimatfrage. *Therap. Mh.,* 1887, **1**, 41–44

1577. Bergmann, Ernst von. Die chirurgische Behandlung von Hirnkrankheiten. Berlin, *A. Hirschwald,* 1888

1578. Paget, Sir James, Bart. On disease of the mammary areola preceding cancer of the mammary gland. *St. Barth. Hosp. Rep.,* 1874, **10**, 87–89. Reprinted in *Med. Classics,* 1936, **1**, 75–78

1579. Paget, Sir James, Bart. On a form of chronic inflammation of bones (osteitis deformans). *Med.-Chir. Trans.,* 1877, **60**, 37–64; 1882, **65**, 225–36. Reprinted in *Med. Classics,* 1936, **1**, 29–71

1580. Owen, Sir Richard. Description of a microscopic entozoon (Trichina spiralis) infesting the muscles of the human body. *Lond. Med. Gaz.,* 1835, **16**, 125–127; *Trans. Zool Soc. Lond.,* 1835, **1**, 315–24

1581. Graefe, Friedrich Wilhelm Ernst Albrecht von. Beiträge zur Lehre vom Schielen und von der Schiel-Operation. *v. Graefes Arch. Ophthal.,* 1857, **3**, 1 Abt., 177–286

1582. Graefe, Friedrich W. E. A. von. Ueber die Iridectomie bei Glaucom und über den glaucomatösen Process. *v. Graefes Arch. Ophthal.,* 1857, **3**, 2 Abt., 456–560; 1858, **4**, 2 Abt., 127–61; 1862, **8**, 2 Abt., 242–313

1583. Graefe, Friedrich W. E. A. von. Ueber Embolie der Arteria centralis retinae als Ursache plötzlicher Erblindung. *v. Graefes Arch. Ophthal.,* 1859, **5**, 1 Abt., 136–57

1584. Graefe, Friedrich Wilhelm Ernst Albrecht von. Ueber Complication von Sehnervenentzündung mit Gehirnkrankheiten. *v. Graefes Arch. Ophthal.,* 1860, **7**, 2 Abt., 58–71

1585. Graefe, Friedrich Wilhelm Ernst Albrecht von. Ueber Basedow'sche Krankheit. *Dtsch. Klinik,* 1864, **16**, 158–59

1586. Graefe, Friedrich W. E. A. von. Symptomenlchre der Augenmuskellähmungen. Berlin, *H. Peters,* 1867

1587. Credé, Carl Siegmund Franz. De optima in partu naturali placentum amovendi ratione. Lipsiae, *A. Edelmannum,* (1860)

1588. Harvie, John (1767). As ref. 975

1589. Credé, Carl Sigmund Franz. Die Verhütung der Augenentzündung der Neugeborenen. Berlin, *A. Hirschwald,* 1884

1590. Henoch, Eduard Heinrich. Über den Zusammenhang von Purpura und Intestinalstörungen. *Berl. Klin. Wschr.* 1868, **5**, 517–19

1591. Henoch, Eduard Heinrich. Ueber Purpura fulminans. *Berl. Klin. Wschr.,* 1887, **24**, 8–10

1592. Henoch, Eduard. Vorlesungen über Kinderkrankheiten. Berlin, *A. Hirschwald,* 1881. English translation, New York, 1882

1593. Charcot, Jean Martin. Sur la claudication intermittente. *C. R. Soc. Biol. (Paris),* (1858), *Mémoires,* 1859, 2 sér., **5**, 225–38

1594. Charcot, Jean Martin and Bouchard, Abel. Douleurs fulgurantes de l'ataxie sans incoordination des mouvements; sclérose commençante des cordons postérieurs de la moelle épinière. *Gaz. Méd. Paris,* 1866, 3 sér., **21**, 122–24

1595. Charcot, Jean Martin. Leçons sur les maladies des vieillards et les maladies chroniques. Paris, *A. Delahaye,* 1867

1596. Charcot, Jean Martin. Sur quelques arthropathies qui paraissent dépendre d'une lésion du cerveau ou de la moëlle épinière. *Arch. Physiol. Norm. Pathol.,* 1868, **1,** 161–78

1597. Charcot, Jean Martin. Histologie de la sclérose en plaques. *Gaz. Hôp. (Paris),* 1868, **41,** 554–55, 557–58, 566

1598. Charcot, Jean Martin and Joffroy, Alex. Deux cas d'atrophie musculaire progressive avec lésions de la substance grise et des faisceaux antéro-latéraux de la moelle épinière. *Arch. Physiol. Norm. Pathol.,* 1869, **2,** 744–60

1599. Charcot, Jean Martin and Joffroy, Alex. Une observation de paralysie infantile s'accompagnant d'une altération des cornes antérieures de la substance grise de la moelle. *C. R. Soc. Biol. (Paris),* (1869), 1870, 5 sér., **1,** 312–15

1600. Charcot, Jean Martin. Leçons sur les maladies du système nerveux faites à La Salpêtrière. 3 vols. Paris, *A. Delahaye,* 1872–87. English translation, 1877–89

1601. Charcot, Jean Martin. Leçons sur les localisations dans les maladies du cerveau. Paris, *V. A. Delaye,* 1876–80. English translation (New Sydenham Society), 1883

1602. Charcot, Jean Martin and Pitres, Jean Albert. Les centres moteurs corticaux chez l'homme. Paris, *Rueff & Cie.,* 1895

1603. Charcot, Jean Martin. Œuvres complètes. 9 vols. Paris, 1888–94

1604. Jackson, John Hughlings. Unilateral epileptiform seizures, attended by temporary defect of sight. *Med. Times Gaz.,* 1863, **1,** 588–89

1605. Jackson, John Hughlings. Observations on defects of sight in brain disease. *Ophthal. Hosp. Rep.,* 1863–65, **4,** 10–19, 389–446; 1865–66, **5,** 51–78, 251–306. Reprinted in *Med. Classics,* 1939, **3,** 918–26

1606. Jackson, John Hughlings. Loss of speech: its association with valvular disease of the heart, and with hemiplegia on the right side. Defects of smell. Defects of speech in chorea. Arterial regions in epilepsy. *Clin. Lect. Rep. Lond. Hosp.,* 1864, **1,** 388–471

1607. Jackson, John Hughlings. Notes on the physiology and pathology of language. *Med. Times Gaz.,* 1866, **1,** 659–62

1608. Clarke, Jacob Augustus Lockhart and Jackson, John Hughlings. On a case of muscular atrophy, with disease of the spinal cord and medulla oblongata. *Med.-Chir. Trans.,* 1867, **50,** 489–96

1609. Fritsch, Gustav Theodor and Hitzig, Eduard. Ueber die elektrische Erregbarkeit des Grosshirns. *Arch. Anat. Physiol. Wiss. Med.,* 1870, 300–32. Translation in *J. Neurosurg.,* 1963, **20,** 905–16. Reprinted, with translation, in R. H. Wilkins, *Neurosurgical classics,* New York, 1965

1610. Jackson, John Hughlings. Remarks on the relations of different divisions of the central nervous system to one another and to parts of the body. *Br. Med. J.,* 1898, **1,** 65–69

1611. Malassez, Louis Charles. Nouvelle méthode de numération des globules rouges et des globules blancs du sang. *Arch. Physiol. Norm. Pathol.,* 1874, 2 sér., **1,** 32–52

1612. Gowers, Sir William Richard. The state of the arteries in Bright's disease. *Br. Med. J.,* 1876, **2,** 743–45

1613. Gowers, Sir William Richard. The diagnosis of disease of the spinal cord. London, *J. & A. Churchill,* 1880

1614. Gowers, Sir William Richard. Epilepsy and other chronic convulsive diseases. London, *J. & A. Churchill,* 1881

1615. Gowers, Sir William Richard. Lectures on the diagnosis of diseases of the brain. London, *J. & A. Churchill,* 1885

1616. Gowers, Sir William Richard. A manual of diseases of the nervous system. Vol. 1. London, *J. & A. Churchill,* 1886

1617. Gowers, Sir William Richard. On myopathy and a distal form. *Br. Med. J.,* 1902, **2,** 89–92

1618. Gowers, Sir William Richard and Horsley, Sir Victor Alexander Haden. A case of tumour of the spinal cord. Removal; recovery. *Med.-Chir. Trans.,* 1888, **71,** 377–430

1619. Horsley, Sir Victor Alexander Haden. A recent specimen of artificial myxoedema in a monkey. *Lancet,* 1884, **2,** 827

1620. Horsley, Sir Victor Alexander Haden. Functional nervous disorders due to loss of thyroid gland and pituitary body. *Lancet,* 1886, **1,** 5

1621. Beevor, Charles Edward and Horsley, Sir Victor Alexander Haden. A minute analysis (experimental) of the various movements produced by stimulating in the monkey different regions of the cortical centre for the upper limb, as defined by Professor Ferrier. *Phil. Trans. B.,* 1887, **178**, 153–68

1622. Horsley, Sir Victor Alexander Haden and Sharpey-Schaffer, Sir Edward Albert. A record of experiments upon the functions of the cerebral cortex. *Phil. Trans. B.,* (1888), 1889, **179**, 1–45

1623. Gotch, Francis and Horsley, Sir Victor Alexander Haden. On the mammalian nervous system, its functions, and their localisation determined by an electrical method. *Phil. Trans. B.,* 1891, **182**, 267–526

1624. Horsley, Sir Victor Alexander Haden and Clarke, Robert Henry. The structure and functions of the cerebellum examined by a new method. *Brain,* 1908, **31**, 45–124

1625. Horsley, Sir Victor Alexander Haden. The Linacre Lecture on the function of the so-called motor area of the brain. *Br. Med. J.,* 1909, **2**, 125–32

1626. Creighton, Charles (1891–94; reprint 1965). As ref. 586 but Vol. II pp. 796–97

1627. Hirsch, August. Handbuch der historisch-geographischen Pathologie. 2 vols. Erlangen, *F. Enke,* 1860–64. An English translation by Charles Creighton in 3 vols. was published by the New Sydenham Society in 1883–86

1628. Smith, Thomas Southwood. A treatise on fever. London, *Longman, etc.,* 1830

1629. Elliotson, John. Numerous cases of surgical operations without pain in the mesmeric state. London, *H. Baillière,* 1843

1630. Wilde, Sir William Robert Wills. Practical observations on aural surgery and the nature and treatment of diseases of the ear. London, *J. Churchill,* 1853

1631. Chadwick, Sir Edwin. Report . . . from the Poor Law Commissioners on an enquiry into the sanitary conditions of the labouring population of Great Britain. London, *W. Clowes & Sons,* 1842

1632. Richardson, Sir Benjamin Ward. The health of nations. A review of the works of Edwin Chadwick. 2 vols. London, *Longmans, Green & Co.,* 1887

1633. Snow, John. On the inhalation of the vapour of ether in surgical operations. London, *J. Churchill,* 1847

1634. Snow, John. On the inhalation of chloroform and ether. With description of an apparatus. *Lancet,* 1848, **1**, 177–80

1635. Snow, John. On narcotism by the inhalation of vapours. *Lond. Med. Gaz.,* 1850, n.s., **11**, 749–54; 1851, n.s., **12**, 622–27

1636. Snow, John. On chloroform and other anaesthetics: their action and administration. London, *J. Churchill,* 1858; facsimile, 1950

1637. Snow, John. On the pathology and mode of communication of the cholera. *Lond. Med. Gaz.,* 1849, **44**, 730–32, 745–52, 923–29

1638. Budd, William. Typhoid fever; its nature, mode of spreading, and prevention. London, *Longmans, Green & Co.,* 1873

1639. Simon, Sir John. Public health reports. 2 vols. London, *J. & A. Churchill,* 1887

1640. Simon, Sir John. English sanitary institutions, reviewed in their course of development, and in some of their political and social relations. London, *Cassell & Co.,* 1890

1641. Parkes, Edmund Alexander. A manual of practical hygiene. London, *John Churchill & Sons,* 1864

1642. Report of a general plan for the promotion of public and personal health, devised, prepared, and recommended by the commissioners appointed under a resolve of the legislature of Massachusetts relating to a sanitary survey of the State. Boston, *Dutton & Wentworth,* 1850; facsimile, 1948

1643. Farr, William. Vital statistics. In McCulloch, J. R., A statistical account of the British Empire, 2nd edn., London, 1839, **2**, 521–90. Vital statistics. London, *E. Stanford,* 1885

1644. Farr, William. Supplement to the thirty-fifth annual report of the Registrar-General of Births and Marriages in England. London, *Eyre & Spottiswoode,* 1875

1645. Rumsey, Henry Wyldbore. Essays and papers on some fallacies of statistics concerning life and death, health and disease. London, *Smith, Elder & Co.,* 1875

1646. Cartwright, Frederick F. (1977). As ref. 178 but pp. 53, 54

1647. Davidson, Maurice. The Royal Society of Medicine: the realization of an ideal (1805–1955). London, *Royal Society of Medicine,* 1955

1648. Derosne, Charles Louis. Mémoire sur l'opium. *Ann. Chim.,* 1802, **45**, 257–85

1649. Sertürner, Friedrich Wilhelm Adam. Darstellung der reinen Mohnsäure (Opiumsäure); nebst einer chemischen Untersuchung des Opiums, mit vorzüglicher Hinsicht auf einen darin neu entdeckten Stoff. *J. Pharm. (Lpz.),* 1805, **14,** 47–93

1650. Sertürner, F. W. A. Ueber das Morphium, eine neue salzfähige Grundlage, und die Mekonsäure, als Hauptbestandtheile des Opiums. *Gilbert's Ann. d. Physik. Leipzig,* 1817, **25,** 56–89

1651. Gomes, Bernardino Antonio. Ensaio sobre o cinchonino, e sobre sua influencia em a virtude da quina, e de outras cascas. *Mem. Acad. Reale Sci. Lisboa,* 1810, **3,** 202–217. English translation of the paper, see *Edinb. Med. Surg. J.,* 1811, **7,** 420–31

1652. Pelletier, Pierre Joseph and Magendie, Francois (1817). As ref. 836

1653. Pelletier, Pierre Joseph and Caventou, Joseph Bienaimé. Mémoire sur un nouvel alcali végétal (la strychnine) trouvé dans la fève de Saint-Ignace, la noix vomique, *etc. J. Pharm. (Paris),* 1819, **5,** 145–174

1654. Robiquet, Pierre Jean. Nouvelles observations sur les principaux produits de l'opium. *Ann. Chim. (Paris),* 1832, 2 sér., **51,** 225–67

1655. Pharmacopoeia of the United States of America. Boston, *C. Ewer,* 1820

1656. Schenk, Johann Heinrich. Erfahrungen über die grossen Heilkräfte des Leberthrans gegen chronische Rheumatismen und besonders gegen das Hüft- und Lendenweh. *J. Pract. Heilk.,* 1822, **55,** 6 St., 31–58; 1826, **62,** 3 St., 3–40

1657. Sérullas, Georges Simon. Mémoire sur l'iodure de potassium, l'acide hydriodique et sur un composé nouveau de carbone, d'iode et d'hydrogène. *Ann. Chim. Phys.,* 1822, 2 sér., **20,** 163–68

1658. Lugol, Jean Guillaume August. Mémoire sur l'emploi de l'iode dans les maladies scrofuleuses. Paris, *Baillière,* 1829

1659. Piria, Raffaele. Recherches sur la salicine et les produits qui en dérivent. *C. R. Acad. Sci. (Paris),* 1839, **8,** 479–85

1660. Gerland, H. New formation of salicylic acid. *J. Chem. Soc.,* 1852, **5,** 133–35

1661. Homolle, Augustin Eugene. Mémoire sur la digitale pourprée. *J. Pharm. Chim.,* 1845, 3me. sér., **7,** 57–83

1662. Martindale, 27th edn. (1977). As ref. 1 but p. 490

1663. Runge, Friedlieb Ferdinand. Ueber einige Producte der Steinkohledestillation. *Ann. Phys. Chem. (Lpz.),* 1834, **31,** 65–77, 513–24; **32,** 308–32

1664. Pereira, Jonathan (1839–40). As ref. 1108 but part 1, p. 1

1665. Pereira, Jonathan (1839–40). As ref. 1108 but part 1, p. 436

1666. Bennett, John Hughes. Treatise on the oleum jecoris aselli, or cod liver oil. Edinburgh, *Maclachlan, Stewart & Co.,* 1841

1667. Balard, Antoine Jérome. Mémoire sur l'alcool amylique. *C. R. Acad. Sci. (Paris),* 1844, **19,** 634–41

1668. Merck, Georg Franz. Vorläufige Notiz über eine neue organische Base im Opium. *Ann. Phys. Chem. (Lpz.),* 1848, **66,** 125–28

1669. Lemaire, François Jules. Du coaltar saponiné, désinfectant énergique. Paris, *Germer-Baillière,* 1860

1670. Niemann, Albert. Ueber eine neue organische Base in den Cocablättern. Göttingen, *E. A. Huth,* 1860

1671. Buchheim, Rudolf. Lehrbuch der Arzneimittellehre. Leipzig, *L. Voss,* 1856

1672. British Pharmacopoeia, published pursuant to the Medical Act, 1858. London, *General Medical Council,* 1864

1673. Rutherford, P. P. and Deacon, A. C. The mode of action of dandelion root β-fructofuranosidases on inulin. *Biochem. J.,* 1972, **129,** 511–512

1674. Rácz-Kotilla, Elizabeth, Rácz, G. and Solomon, Ana. The action of *Taraxacum officinale* extracts on the body weight and diuresis of laboratory animals. *Planta medica,* 1974, **26,** 212–217

1675. Stephenson, J. and Churchill, J. M. Medical botany... London, *John Churchill,* 4 vols., 1831, **IV,** (following index)

1676. Companion to the latest edition of the British Pharmacopoeia... by Peter Squire... London, *J. & A. Churchill,* 12th edn., 1880, pp. xxiv–xxxiii

1677. Brown, Alexander Crum and Fraser, Sir Thomas Richard. On the connection between chemical constitution and physiological action. *Trans. R. Soc. Edinb.*, 1868–69, **25**, 151–203, 693–739

1678. Fraser, Sir Thomas Richard. Strophanthus hispidus; its natural history, chemistry, and pharmacology. *Trans. R. Soc. Edinb.*, 1890, **35**, 955–1027; 1892, **36**, 343–457

1679. Schmiedeberg, Johann Ernst Oswald. Untersuchungen über die pharmakologisch wirksamen Bestandtheile der Digitalis purpurea *L. Arch. Exp. Pathol. Pharmak.*, 1875, **3**, 16–43

1680. Ladenburg, Albert. Die natürlich vorkommenden mydriatisch wirkenden Alkaloïde. *Ann. Chem. Pharm.*, 1881, **206**, 274–307

1681. Cervello, Vincenzo. Recherches cliniques et physiologiques sur la paraldéhyde. *Arch. Ital. Biol.*, 1884, **6**, 113–34

1682. Filehne, Wilhelm. Ueber das Antipyrin, ein neues Antipyreticum. *Z. Klin. Med.*, 1884, **7**, 641–42

1683. Filehne, Wilhelm. Ueber das Pyramidon, ein Antipyrinderivat. *Berl. Klin. Wschr.*, 1896, **33**, 1061–63

1684. Martindale, 27th edn. (1977). As ref. 1 but p. 187

1685. Martindale, 27th edn. (1977). As ref. 1 but p. 208

1686. Baumann, Eugen. Ueber Disulfone. *Berl. Dtsch. Chem. Ges.*, 1886, **19**, 2806–14

1687. Kast, Alfred. Sulfonal, ein neues Schlafmittel. *Berl. Klin. Wschr.*, 1888, **25**, 309–14

1688. Fischer, Emil and Mering, Joseph von. Ueber eine neue Klasse von Schlafmitteln. *Therap. Gegenw.*, 1903, **44**, 97–101

1689. Hinsberg, Oscar Heinrich Daniel and Kast, Alfred. Ueber die Wirkung des Acetphenetidins. *Zbl. Med. Wiss.*, 1887, **25**, 145–8

1690. Cahn, Arnold and Hepp, Paul. Sur l'action de l'antifébrine (acétanilide) et de quelques corps analogues. *Progrès Méd.*, 1887, **5**, 43–46

1691. Leake, Chauncey Depew (1975). As ref. 1461 but p. 161

1692. Stricker, Solomon. Ueber die Resultate der Behandlung der Polyarthritis rheumatica mit Salicylsäure. *Berl. Klin. Wschr.*, 1876, **13**, 1–2; 99–103

1693. Garrison, Fielding H. (1929). As ref. 179 but p. 856

1694. Dreser, Heinrich. Pharmakologisches über Aspirin (Acetylsalicylsäure). *Pflüg. Arch. Ges. Physiol.*, 1899, **76**, 306–18

1695. Röntgen, Wilhelm Conrad. Ueber eine neue Art von Strahlen. *S. B. Phys.-Med. Ges. Würzburg*, 1895, 132–41. English translation in *Nature*, 1896, **53**, 274 and 377

1696. Freund, Leopold. Demonstration eines mit Röntgenstrahlen behandelten Falles von Naevus pigmentosus pilosus. *Wien. Klin. Wschr.*, 1897, **10**, 73–74

1697. Curie, Pierre and Curie, Marie Skodowska. Sur une substance nouvelle radio-active, contenue dans la pechblende. *C. R. Acad. Sci. (Paris)*, 1898, **127**, 175–78, 1215–17

1698. Nagai, Nagajosi. Ephedrin. *Pharm. Ztg*, 1887, **32**, 700

1699. Paul, Benjamin Horatio and Cownley, Alfred John. The chemistry of ipecacuanha. *Pharm. J.*, 1894–95, **54**, 111–15, 373–374, 690–92

1700. Moréno y Maïz, Thomas. Recherches chimiques et physiologiques sur l'Erythroxylum coca du Pérou et la cocaïne. Paris, *L. Leclerc*, 1868

1701. Anrep, Vasili Konstantinovich. Ueber die physiologische Wirkung des Cocaïn. *Pflüg. Arch. Ges. Physiol.*, 1880, **21**, 38–77

1702. Brunton, Sir Thomas Lauder, Bart. A text-book of pharmacology, therapeutics and materia medica. London, *Macmillan & Co.*, 1885

1703. Schmiedeberg, Johann Ernst Oswald. Grundriss der Arzneimittellehre. Leipzig, *F. C. W. Vogel*, 1883

7

The Present Century. The Beginnings of Preventive Medicine

Experimental medicine

In the nineteenth century the advancement of science was largely due to an organized, descriptive effort associated with a number of important discoveries. It rested on a freeing of the intellect in a way that permitted scientific empiricism; it was aided by meaningful advances in chemistry and by the use of such essential aids as microscopy. The main interest of twentieth century medicine has been in its social implications and its development of many effective means of therapy.

The biology underlying much modern medical progress rests, to no small extent, on the experiments conducted by Gregor Johann Mendel (1822–1884), an Augustinian monk and abbot of Brünn, who in 1866 had expressed the results of his study on the hybridization of peas in a paper (*Versuche über Pflanzen-Hybriden*)[1704] which appeared in an English translation in Bateson's book *Mendel's principles of heredity*[1705]; this was published in 1909 but Mendel's classic paper, in its translation, was republished, with a valuable introduction by R. A. Fisher, in 1965. The most simple formulation of the Mendelian laws of inheritance, which envisage dominant or unchangeable characteristics ('*a*') and recessive or latent characteristics ('*b*') in the parents of the hybrid, makes Mendel's law identical with Newton's binomial theorem: $(a + b)^2 = a^2 + 2ab + b^2$. Thus, one-half of the hybrids ($2ab$) will breed true to the parental characteristics and the rest will be divided equally between progeny with only the dominant (a) or the recessive (b) characteristic. In the later generations the mixed hybrids will breed according to Mendel's law and the pure dominant or pure recessive progeny will breed true to their kinds. The law seems to be typical of those generalizations which are most unlikely to be observed except as a result of systematic experiment but that can be verified as often as is wanted by repeated experiment.

Mendel's work, largely done in 1865 and the immediately preceding years, had no effect upon the nineteenth century. It had been published in an obscure journal and was not noticed until Hugo Marie de Vries (1848–1935), and his colleagues, repeated and confirmed the work, and de Vries not only advanced the mutation theory but gave an account of the rediscovery of Mendel's findings in a book (*Die Mutationstheorie*)[1706] of 1901–3. (There is an English translation of 1909.) Shortly before this, Sir Francis Galton (1822–1911), who was interested in the pedigrees of Basset hounds, used a brilliant series of statistical methods to develop a 'law of filial regression'; this was expressed in his study *Natural inheritance*[1707] published in 1889. An observer of this time who was convinced that Darwin's theory of natural selection would need to be modified was William Bateson (1861–1926) whose *Materials for the study of variation treated with especial regard to discontinuity in the origin of species*[1708] appeared in 1894. The book gathered together many of the points of discussion of the time and showed that Bateson considered discontinuity to be of more importance than continuous variation and adaptation in the natural world; it shortly preceded de Vries and his full-blown theory of mutation – the latter suggesting the abrupt or spontaneous origin of species.

These concepts have gradually been augmented and modified. Wilhelm Johannsen (1857–1927), the Danish botanist, in 1903, provided support for the Mendelian ideas by showing that in the self-fertilizing plants chosen for study a pure line of progeny could be maintained, seemingly indefinitely, in a way which depended only on the genetic variability[1709]. Johannsen, in 1911, introduced the word 'gene'. Walter Sutton (1877–1916) had already suggested (1903) that the hereditary units (whatever they were) were carried by the cell chromosomes[1710] and in 1910 Thomas Morgan (1866–1945) demonstrated sex-linked inheritance in *Drosophila*[1711]. In 1913 Alfred Sturtevant (1891–1970) published his important paper, *The linear arrangement of six sex-linked factors in Drosophila, as shown by their mode of association*[1712], which showed that the genes are arranged in a linear sequence on the chromosome.

Morgan continued his work with the fruit fly, *Drosophila melanogaster* and, by 1915, was able to map the position of many of the Mendelian factors along the chromosomes of the convenient species he had chosen to study[1713]. By 1927, when ideas of 'emergent evolution' were being advanced to suggest that violent mutations may have little to do with the biological success of species in evolution, Hermann Muller (1890–1967), who studied the genetic effects of radiation, could report the induction of genetic mutations (*Artificial transmutation of the gene*)[1714]. In 1935, in a paper which is fundamental to many recent developments in genetic engineering[1715], Nikolai Timoféeff-Ressovsky and his co-workers reported X-ray mutagenesis in *Drosophila*; in 1944 it became known that deoxyribonucleic acid (DNA) is the basic material for genetic transformation[1716].

The post-1945 developments have included the discovery of the sexual processes in the reproduction of bacteria (1946)[1717], the demonstration that the genetic sex of an individual can be determined by studying the sex chromatin on the inner surface of the nuclear membrane of cells (1949)[1718], and the further demonstration (1952) that DNA is the carrier of genetic information in virus reproduction[1719]. It is interesting, as some of these facts rapidly become widely known, that the normal chromosome number in man (46) was not finally established until 1956[1720]. The view at that time, as if to look back on the story of the development of the understanding of the cell since the early descriptions by Schwann, is given in the helpful summary, *The cell-theory: a restatement, history, and critique*[1721] by John Baker – a three-part communication of 1948, 1949 and 1952.

The complexities of the antigen–antibody reaction and the modern ramifications of the concepts of immunity and the host-defence mechanism have part of their beginnings in the demonstration of the bactericidal power of the defibrinated blood of certain animals. This demonstration was achieved by George Nuttall (1862-1937) and reported in 1888[1722]. Several other workers made similar observations over a short period of time. Following Nuttall's work, Hans Buchner (1850-1902) showed that this ability of the blood, when freed of its fibrin, to lyse or kill bacteria was possessed by the cell-free serum – but was lost if the serum was heated to 55 °C for 1 hour[1723]. That phenomena of this kind were not restricted to the effects of serum on bacteria was demonstrated, in 1892, by George Sternberg (1838-1915) who showed that the serum of an animal which had recovered from vaccinia can neutralize the activity of the causative virus[1724]. This finding was later adapted to provide a number of tests intended to determine whether or not a host had been infected with a specific virus.

Jules Jean Bordet (1870-1961) then provided a classic paper, *Contribution à l'étude du sérum chez les animaux vaccinés* (1895)[1725], showing that the sera of immunized animals contain two different substances which are involved in the process of bacteriolysis. In 1909, Bordet and others published this paper in English in *Studies in immunity*; the two substances later came to be known as sensitizing antibody and complement. The involvement of bacterial agglutinins in these processes was investigated by a number of workers, including Bordet, who published his paper *Sur l'agglutination et la dissolution des globules rouges par le sérum d'animaux injectés de sang défibriné*[1726] in 1898, and the knowledge of such agglutinins was applied to the diagnosis of typhoid by Georges Widal (1862-1929) in 1896[1727]. Bordet's slightly later work, in association with Octave Gengou (1875-1957) concerned complement and the joint paper of these two workers of 1901 established the Bordet–Gengou complement–fixation reaction[1728]. This reaction provided the basis for several of the later tests for infection, including the Wasserman test for the diagnosis of syphilis.

Possibly one of the broadest of the early studies on specific antibacterial immunity and its mechanisms was the classic *L'immunité dans les maladies infectieuses*[1729] published in Paris in 1901 by Elie Metchnikoff (1845-1916). Metchnikoff received a Nobel Prize in 1908, Bordet receiving a similar honour in 1919.

Some of the main events then move forward a little – the template theory of antibody formation being of 1930[1730]; the notable *Die Spezifizität der serologischen Reaktionen*[1731] of Karl Landsteiner (1868-1943) being of 1933, and the demonstration of the fact that antibodies are gamma globulins being of 1939[1732]. Freund's adjuvant dates from 1942[1733] and the important paper, *Experiments on transfer of cutaneous sensitivity to simple compounds*[1734], by Landsteiner and Merrill Chase, is of the same year. This paper began the understanding of the cellular transfer of delayed hypersensitivity. Of the great investigative techniques, with the advances in knowledge represented by their mechanisms, the fluorescent antibody technique of Albert Coons and Melvin Kaplan dates from 1950[1735], the method of immunoelectrophoresis of Pierre Grabar and C. A. Williams from 1953[1736]; the *Kinetic studies on immune hemolysis*[1737] (on complement fixation) by Manfred Mayer and Lawrence Levine dates from 1954 – and the radioimmunoassay of Rosalyn Yalow and Solomon Berson dates from their paper reporting an *Immunoassay of endogenous plasma insulin in man* in 1960[1737a].

The gradual accumulation of understanding on the bodily defences associated with the immune mechanism was accompanied, in 1915, by the first isolation of a filterable virus. This was achieved by Frederick Twort (1877–1950) and reported in a paper in the *Lancet* (*An investigation on the nature of ultra-microscopic viruses*)[1738]. The work demonstrated the transmissible lysis of bacteria by the virus particles. In 1917, Félix d'Herelle (1873–1949) discovered a filterable agent capable of bacteriolysis[1739]; he considered this ultramicroscopic, filter-passing agent to be the same or very similar to that which had been mentioned by Twort. In 1921, d'Herelle described the agent in a book entitled, *Le bactériophage* – from which bacteriophage gets its name.

The previously clear distinction between that which was living, and that which was not, ended with a report by Alfred Gierer and Gerhard Schramm on *Infectivity of ribonucleic acid from tobacco mosaic virus*[1740] published in 1956. This report proved that nucleic acid, and not just the complete virus, possessed infectivity. The realization that no external infectious agent was necessary to prompt the immune mechanism and that the body could produce autoantibodies with pathological consequences came with the paper, of 1956, by Ivan Roitt and his colleagues on *Autoantibodies in Hasimoto's disease* (*lymphadenoid goitre*)[1741]. A year later there appeared the historic demonstration of a new host-defence mechanism: interferon – a protein which appeared in the blood following the interaction of virus with cells and which could interfere with the multiplication of the virus. The discovery, by Alick Isaacs (1921–1967) and Jean Lindenmann was announced in their joint paper *Virus interference. I. the interferon*[1742].

An aspect of the work on the immune system which seems of ever-increasing relevance is that part concerned with graft rejection and the success, or otherwise, of organ transplantation techniques. The subject has proved to be complex and exacting and it is perhaps difficult to remember that as early as 1903, in the great *Festschrift zur sechzigsten Geburtstage von Robert Koch*[1743] published that year, tissue-specific antigens were described by Paul Uhlenhuth (1870–1957). The start of the study of histocompatibility antigens was marked by the appearance in 1916 of the paper on *Further experimental studies on the inheritance of susceptibility to a transplantable tumour, carcinoma (J.W.A.) of the Japanese waltzing mouse*[1744] by Clarence Little (1888–1971) and Ernest Tyzzer (1875–1966). By 1924, Clarence Little had shown that homograft rejection was due to genetic differences between the donor of the graft and its recipient[1745].

The initial discoveries underlying the modern ideas on transplantation genetics and its immune expression are to be credited to Peter Gorer (1907–1961) whose fundamental paper, *The genetic and antigenic basis of tumour transplantation*[1746], appeared in 1937 and 1938. Understanding of the so-called 'laws of transplantation' was placed on a firm scientific basis by the two leading figures, Thomas Gibson and Sir Peter Medawar whose joint paper on *The fate of skin homografts in man*[1747] appeared in 1943. The following year Medawar's continuing studies showed the immunological nature of the mechanism by which transplanted tissues are rejected.

The great 'self-marker' theory of immunological tolerance arose from the work of Sir Frank Macfarlane Burnet and Frank Fenner. In essence, the work attempted to determine why the body does not reject its own tissues and asked how the body marks off 'self' from 'non-self'. Burnet and Fenner's theory of immunity appeared in the 1949 edition of their *The production of antibodies*[1748]. It suggested that tolerance of the body to its normal constituents depends upon their being present and immunologically recognizable at a critical stage of embryonic development. Medawar and his colleagues were able to offer proof of Burnet and Fenner's theory in 1953[1749] and, in 1960, for his work on immunological tolerance, Burnet shared a Nobel Prize with Medawar. The year after the proof of the theory, in 1954, in two important papers reporting *Quantitative studies on tissue transplantation immunity*[1750], Medawar and his colleagues announced the experimental production of immunological tolerance.

Sir Frank Burnet's book, *The clonal selection theory of acquired immunity*[1751] appeared in 1959 – so introducing to a wide audience a concept which is still of discussion. It was of the year following Sir Peter Medawar's paper *The homograft reaction*[1752], of 1958, which showed that a graft would be rejected even if the donor and recipient animals were of the same litter unless they were genetically identical.

Leukocyte typing dates from the 1957 contribution of Rose Marise Payne[1753]. It appears again, with other aspects of histocompatibility, in a paper of 1958 by J. J. van Rood and his co-workers[1754]. The same year Jean Dausset, in a paper entitled *Iso-leuco-anticorps*[1755], announced the discovery of the first histocompatibility antigen. Also in 1958, George Davis Snell, in a notable paper on *Histocompatibility genes of the mouse*[1756], settled the convention whereby the genes determining the outcome of transplantation are called 'histocompatibility genes'. It was not until 1972 that Baruj Benacerraf and Hugh McDevitt were able to produce their study *Histocompatibility-linked immune response genes*[1757] which shows that the ability to produce certain of the immune responses is genetically determined. These groups of workers have made important advances, recognized by the Nobel Prize shared by Dausset, Snell and Benacerraf in 1980.

Related aspects of the overall immune mechanism can be represented by Jacques Miller's 1961 demonstration of the immunological function of the thymus[1758]; the 1962 paper on the *Initiation of immune responses by small lymphocytes*[1759] – the work of James Gowans and colleagues which identified the immunologically competent cell – and the beautiful demonstration of the complete sequence of the first immunoglobulin molecule to be understood in this way. The latter demonstration was reported in the paper *The covalent structure of an entire γG immunoglobulin molecule*[1760] published by Gerald Edelman and his associates in 1969.

Allergic phenomena have come to be of considerable importance in modern drug therapy. In essence, their description and understanding, which is still only partial, is of the present century. The first adequate account of anaphylaxis was given by Paul Portier (1866–1962) and Charles Richet (1850–1935) in their paper *De l'action anaphylactique de certains venins*[1761] of 1902. It was, in fact, Richet who devised the name of the condition. Almost immediately, in 1903, Nicolas Arthus (1862–1945), in *Injections répétées de sérum de cheval chez le lapin*[1762], described the manifestation of anaphylaxis which has become known as the 'Arthus phenomenon'; the title of the paper makes plain the key point regarding repeated exposure to the foreign protein. It was 1910 before John Auer (1875–1948) and Paul Lewis (1879–1929) gave an adequate account of the physiological changes involved in the fatal anaphylactic reaction[1763].

Serum sickness, now a well-known adverse drug effect, was first described in 1903 [1764]. A fine description of the condition and its biological significance was given in *Die Serumkrankheit* (1905, English translation 1951) [1765] published by Clemens Pirquet Von Cesenatico (1874–1929) and Bela Schick (1877–1967) – both famous names, Pirquet having first suggested the name 'allergy' and using it in the title of his important, *Klinische Studien über Vakzination und vakzinale Allergie* [1766], published in Leipzig in 1907.

The period between the two World Wars saw the research work of Sir Thomas Lewis (1881–1945) embodied in the important paper, *Vascular reactions of the skin to injury. II. The liberation of a histamine-like substance in injured skin . . .* [1767], of 1924. This paper, published jointly with Ronald Thomson Grant, suggested that a histamine-like substance (for a while called the 'H-substance') was responsible for the events of anaphylaxis. Sir Thomas then advanced his hypothesis further in his book on *The blood-vessels of the human skin and their responses* (1927) [1768]. In 1932 Carl Dragstedt and his colleagues showed that anaphylaxis was associated with the release of histamine into the circulation [1769]; Lewis's H-substance was thereafter identified with histamine.

The same period produced the valuable study, *Allergic diseases; diagnosis and treatment of bronchial asthma, hay-fever, and other allergic diseases* (1925) [1770], in which Willem Storm Van Leeuwen (1882–1933) showed that allergens are the cause of asthma in many sufferers from the condition, mould spores being a common such allergen, and many patients being relieved by enclosure in an allergen-proof chamber or exposure to high altitudes where such spores are rare or absent. The finding is reminiscent of William Withering's advice regarding long sea voyages as a means of relieving asthma.

Most of the advances in genetics, immunology, and the knowledge of allergic phenomena have arisen from deliberate experiment – the experimental designs exploring from the frontiers of the available information. There is, therefore, in retrospect, a rather logical, coherent picture – even if only a few of the milestones are considered. In some instances there have been important advances in technology – an example is in microscopy: *Das Fluoreszenzmikroskop* [1771], by Oskar Heimstädt, described fluorescence microscopy in 1911; the great advance of electron microscopy was brought forward by Max Knoll and Ernst Ruska in their *Beitrag zur geometrischen Elektronenoptik* [1772] in 1932; phase contrast microscopy was invented by Frits Zernike (1888–1966) and reported in 1935 [1773], but X-ray microscopy was a mid-century invention discussed by Werner Ehrenberg and W. E. Spear in their paper *An electrostatic focussing system and its application to a fine focus X-ray tube* [1774] in 1951.

Modern embryology has been marked by the discovery of 'organizers' by Hans Spemann (1869–1941) and Hilde Mangold in 1924 [1775] and by the demonstration of the place of tissue affinity in the differentiation and morphogenesis of the embryo by Johannes Holtfreter who wrote on this subject in 1939 [1776]. Spemann received the Nobel Prize in 1935 for his discovery of the place of organizers in animal development – and the subject would seem to retain potential, just as a knowledge of any truly specific enzyme involved in the penetration of the oocyte would offer potential for the first specific contraceptive.

Histological science has led from important early contributions by Paul Ehrlich (1854–1915) to quite new techniques, such as tissue culture, which have already become routine laboratory methods. Ehrlich's work is, in its range and variety, remarkable, and eclipsed by his reputation as the founder of chemo-therapy. In its fullness it is to be read in the excellent *Collected papers of Paul Ehrlich. Compiled and edited by F. Himmelweit*[1777] and published in London in three volumes between 1956 and 1960. Two of the things added to histology by Ehrlich are his description of the mast cells in 1879[1778] and the introduction, in 1886, of his method of intravital staining. The latter method, described in his paper *Ueber die Methylenblaureaction der lebenden Nervensubstanz*[1779], provided some of the ideas that led to his discoveries in developing drugs that could enter cells but with a differential toxicity unfavourable to the pathogen.

Ross Granville Harrison (1870–1959), in the *Journal of Experimental Zoology* of 1910, provided an observation fundamental to the development of tissue culture techniques by showing that the outgrowth of nerve fibres from ganglion cells occurs as a mode of protoplasmic movement[1780]. This was soon followed by the paper by Alexis Carrel (1873–1944) on *Rejuvenation of cultures of tissues*[1781] of 1911. Alexis Carrel was given the Nobel Prize in 1912 for this critically important finding that the extra-vital cultivation of tissues was possible and that under such conditions cells could survive and multiply.

One aspect of the work led on to the fine, two volume study on *Degeneration and regeneration of the nervous system*[1782] published in London by Santiago Ramón y Cajal (1852–1934) in 1928. Despite its date, this work remains of current value and was reprinted in 1959. Ramon y Cajal, recipient of a Nobel Prize in 1906, was one of the finest of the neurohistologists of this century and for a long period directed the Institute that bears his name in Madrid. The other aspect of the work led to modern tissue culture to which the groundwork was laid by the historic paper, *The growth, development and phosphatase activity of embryonic avian femora in limb-buds cultivated in vitro*[1783], published by Dame Honor Fell and Robert Robison (1883–1941) in the *Biochemical Journal* of 1929. The first successful cloning of single isolated tissue cells grown *in vitro* was reported by Katherine Sanford and her colleagues in 1948[1784] and the first full account of the lysosomes was given by Kurt Aterman, from a study on the restoration of the rat's liver, published in 1952[1785].

Laboratory medicine

A characteristic of twentieth century medicine is the reliance placed upon the analyses of the laboratory – analyses usually made by experts who have little or no contact with the patient. Examples of such laboratory sciences, now rightly and properly essential, are clinical biochemistry and haematology. The difficulty is in the interpretation of the biological significance of the tests, an area in which the knowledge of the most highly specialized laboratory scientists and the responsi-bilities of the clinician must somehow meet.

The problem has been present since antiquity for the earliest attempts at biochemistry lie in the application of the hypothesis of the four humours – phlegm, blood, yellow bile and black bile – to the examination of urine, to uroscopy. The urine was thought of as having contact with all parts of the patient's body and its examination for colour, consistency, smell, taste, and other characteristics, provided the only kind of direct laboratory test then available. Uroscopy was the diagnostic province of the physician and apothecary; uromancy was the fraudulent practice of the imposter. The difference was that between astronomy and astrology.

The doctor, asked to diagnose the illness of a patient that he had often not seen, from the urine brought by a messenger, had to become an imposter gathering information from the messenger and other circumstances. One of those who, at an early date, saw through the problem and regarded the demand of the patient for such a diagnosis as destructive to the interests of all concerned was Thomas Brian, who entered Cambridge in 1622, achieved his bachelor of arts in 1624–1625 and his mastership in 1629, and was licensed to practice medicine in the same year. He practised first in London and then moved to Colchester in Essex. In 1637, doing for uroscopy what Heberden was to do for theriac, he published *The pisse-prophet or certaine pissepot lectures*[1786]. This rare book is the source of the epigram, *Urina est meretrix, vel mendax* – the *Urine is an harlot, or a lier*, which forms the title of the 1969 study of Brian's book by Ronnie Beth Bush[1787]. Mrs Bush ends her interesting paper with the comment that:

> If *The Pisse-Prophet* were only a description of a 17th-century uroscopist, insecure, disillusioned, indulging in the absolution of honesty, it would be of transient interest. Its appeal lies in its universality. Its author was constantly aware of the inherent conflicts and compromises that form part of the physician–patient relationship. Thomas Brian exemplified a trend of thought. Though his book went through multiple editions, he was rarely quoted and never eulogized. His truths were simply too harsh for public approval. Today, with the softening quality of time, they can be read and acknowledged as unsolved problems of the medical profession.

The discovery of urea in 1773[1788] and that of uric acid in 1776[1789] comprise two of the more notable events in the biochemistry of the eighteenth century – and both discoveries are something like 140 years after Thomas Brian's book of 1637. Progress in the nineteenth century was far more considerable and included the preparation of the first amino acid (cystine) to be isolated (1810)[1790]; the characterization of cholesterol (1815)[1791]; the isolation of both glycine and leucine (1820)[1792]; the demonstration that fats are composed of fatty acids and glycerol (1823)[1793]; the first synthesis of an organic compound (urea) from inorganic materials (1828)[1322]; the isolation of creatine from muscle tissue (1832)[1794]; the elaboration of Pettenkofer's test for bile salts (1844)[1795] and Fehling's test for sugar in the urine (1848)[1796]; Liebig's method of estimating the concentration of urea (1853)[1321]; the demonstration of the first identified excretory product of bile metabolism (coprosterol) in 1857[1797]; the discovery of urobilin in the urine (1868)[1798]; the introduction of the term 'enzyme' in 1878[1799]; the publication of Kjeldahl's method of estimating the quantity of nitrogen in an organic compound (1883)[1800]; the design of Hay's test for the determination of bile acids in urine (1886)[1801]; Max Jaffé's test for creatinine (1886)[1802]; the report of Sir Frederick Gowland Hopkins' method of estimating uric acid in urine (1892–93)[1803], and then the discovery, by Eduard Buchner (1860–1907) of cell-free fermentation[1804]. Buchner had the Nobel Prize in 1907 for this work which began the modern phase in the study of enzymes. The century also saw the classical studies, from 1827 to

1835, of Réné Dutrochet (1776–1847) on the osmotic phenomena involving a semipermeable membrane[1805]; the beginnings of the study of metabolism with the discovery of Friedrich Wöhler (1800–1882) that ingested benzoic acid is excreted in the urine as hippuric acid[1323], and the discovery of nuclein (nucleoprotein) by Johann Miescher (1844–1895) who was the first, in 1871, to propose that there exists a genetic code involved in the transmission of hereditary characteristics[1806]. The late segment of the nineteenth century saw the studies on the chemistry of the cell constituents and cell nucleus by Albrecht Kossel (1853–1927)[1807]; the brilliant electrolyte dissociation theory of Svante Arrhenius (1859–1927) in 1887[1808], and the prediction, in 1898 by Albrecht Kossel, of the polypeptide nature of the protein molecule[1809].

The ascendancy of German chemistry in the nineteenth century is reflected in the fact that, of the 25 publications cited in the catalogue just given, 15 were in German, five in French, four in English, and one in another language.

At the beginning of the twentieth century Phoebus Levene (1869–1940), in 1903, distinguished chemically between DNA and RNA[1810] and the brilliant German biochemist, Emil Fischer (1852–1919) showed (*Untersuchungen über Aminosäuren, Polypeptide und Proteine*, 1906)[1811] that animal and vegetable proteins comprise a series of amino acids united by elimination of the elements of water. *The importance of individual amino-acids in metabolism*[1812] – a publication of 1906 by Edith Willcock and Sir Frederick Gowland Hopkins – led, in the end, to the discovery of the vitamins by showing the importance of tryptophan in the diet. In association with Sir Walter Morley Fletcher (1873–1933), Hopkins then (1907) showed the importance of lactic acid production during striated muscle contraction[1813] and, in a way which further advanced the understanding of the 'interior environment' first appreciated by Claude Bernard, Karl Hasselbalch (1874–1962), with Christen Lundsgaard, in 1912, put forward the Hasselbalch equation regarding the determination of the pH concentration in the blood[1814].

Parts of the understanding of energy kinetics and the mechanisms of cellular respiration came with the discovery of adenosine-5'-triphosphate (ATP) in 1929[1815], the discovery of cytochrome in the same year[1816], the isolation of carbonic anhydrase in 1933[1817], and the appearance, in 1937, of the brilliant study on *Citric acid in intermediate metabolism in animal tissues*[1818] by Sir Hans Krebs (1900–1981) and William Johnson. For the understanding of the citric acid cycle of aerobic carbohydrate metabolism, Krebs shared a Nobel Prize in 1953.

The great achievement of the mid-century relates to the nucleic acids. Erwin Chargaff published work in 1950 that had a profound effect in increasing the understanding of what he termed the *Chemical specificity of nucleic acids and the mechanism of their enzymatic degradation*[1819]. James Dewey Watson and Francis Harry Crick then (1953) produced their epoch-making paper on the *Molecular structure of nucleic acids. A structure for deoxyribose nucleic acid*[1820]. In the same year Maurice Hugh Wilkins and his colleagues produced (again in *Nature*, London) their paper on the *Helical structure of crystalline deoxypentose nucleic acid*[1821]. In 1962, Watson, Crick and Wilkins shared the Nobel Prize for the discovery of the molecular structure of DNA – Wilkins having discovered the double helical structure of this critically important molecule. In *Genetical implications of the structure of deoxyribonucleic acid* (1953)[1822] Watson and Crick went on to explain the chemical mechanism by which cells could, based on the structure of DNA, accurately transmit hereditary characters. Thus, the mid-century saw a vastly increased understanding of genetics in terms of the enormously complicated molecule of the nucleic acids involved. In 1955 Marianne Grunberg-Manago and Severo Ochoa de Albornoz produced their report on the *Enzymatic synthesis and breakdown of polynucleotides; polynucleotide phosphorylase*[1823] showing the discovery of an enzyme which could catalyse the ablation of a terminal phosphate group from ribonucleoside diphosphates. Arthur Kornberg and his colleagues, in 1956, published on the *Enzymatic synthesis of deoxyribonucleic acid*[1824] and in 1959 Ochoa and Kornberg shared the Nobel Prize for their artificial synthesis of nucleic acids by enzymatic means.

The nature and mode of action of oxidation enzymes. Nobel Lecture, December 12, 1955[1825] summarizes the work on oxidizing enzymes of Axel Theorell (1903–1982). Peter Thomas Gilham and Har Khorana published on the synthesis of polynucleotides in 1958[1826] and in 1968 Khorana shared a Nobel Prize for his contribution to this work. In 1961, Sydney Brenner and his associates published their paper on *An unstable intermediate carrying information from genes to ribosomes for protein synthesis*[1827] – so showing the existence of 'messenger' RNA. In the same year J. Heinrich Matthaei and Marshall Nirenberg showed that messenger RNA is needed for protein synthesis and synthetic messenger RNA can be used to unravel certain aspects of the genetic code[1828]. Nirenberg was one of those who, with Khorana, shared the Nobel award in 1968; the third participant of the same Nobel Prize was Robert William Holley who, with colleagues, in 1965, announced the determination of the complete sequence of an alanine transfer RNA[1829].

Recent advances have included those concerned with cyclic adenosine monophosphate, the oncogenes, and the very complex prostaglandins. George Robson, Reginald Butcher and Earl Sutherland published on *Cyclic AMP*[1830] in 1968; Sutherland demonstrated the mediatory effect of this second messenger in a substantial range of hormonal effects and energy transfer systems and received a Nobel Prize in 1971.

An increasing weight of evidence has shown the importance of genetic changes in neoplasia and it has, in 1982, been shown by Clifford J. Tabin and colleagues[1831] from the Massachusetts Institute of Technology and other centres, and by E. Premkumar Reddy and associates at the National Cancer Institute at Bethesda[1832] that a cell line of human bladder carcinoma differed from normal cells only in that one gene exhibited a point mutation which resulted in a glycine residue being replaced by a valine residue in the protein coded for by the affected gene. This would appear to be the first occasion on which the underlying cause of a cancer has been identified in such detail – offering, in terms of the oncogene and of molecular genetics, a possible explanation for the changes responsible for some types of neoplasia.

The term 'prostaglandin' was first used by U.S. von Euler in 1934 to describe the active agent present in human semen and the accessory genital glands[1833]. This material was shown to have both vasodepressor and smooth-muscle stimulating activities. It was later shown that the prostaglandins are synthesized in the body from polyunsaturated fatty acids, arachidonic acid being the main precursor of prostaglandins in man. Work in the last 10 years or so has added to the account of the early prostaglandins, the prostaglandin endoperoxides, thromboxane[1834], and prostacyclin. The latter substance is a potent vasodilator and is the most potent endogenous inhibitor of platelet aggregation yet discovered. It appears possible that a number of diseases are related to an imbalance of the prostacyclin–thromboxane system and studies are presently in progress to explore this hypothesis as it relates to vascular homeostasis in conditions such as occlusive peripheral vascular disease. Studies will obviously explore the place of these agents in diseases associated with thrombotic events in both the arterial and venous systems and in diabetes. The present state of the subject has been reviewed by John R. Vane (1982, 1983)[1835] whose fundamental contribution to the work has been recognized by the recent Nobel Prize.

Haematology and the knowledge of the diseases of the blood is, just as much as biochemistry, a subject of the late nineteenth and the present century. Sir William Osler (1849-1919) gave one of the best of the early descriptions of the blood platelets, reporting in *An account of certain organisms occurring in the liquor sanguinis* (1874)[1836] that white thrombi were composed almost entirely of these structures which have caused so much interest in recent years. It is said that Giulio Bizzozero (1846-1901) gave the blood platelets their name whilst showing, in 1882, their important part in the processes of thrombosis and blood clotting[1837]. In America, in 1906, James Homer Wright (1871-1928) made the initial observations on the megakaryocytes as the parent cells of the blood platelets[1838].

Early observations on the mechanism of blood coagulation were provided by Olof Hammarsten (1841-1932), who showed[1839] that soluble fibrinogen was split into insoluble fibrin with the extrusion of other substances during clotting, and Nicolas Arthus (1862-1945) who, with his associates, showed in 1890 that calcium plays an essential part in the clotting process[1840]. The beginnings of knowledge of some of the first of the clotting factors to be recognized came with the paper on *The preparation and properties of thrombin, together with observations on antithrombin and prothrombin*[1841] published in 1910 by William Howell (1860-1945). Howell's paper of the following year, *The role of antithrombin and thromboplastin (thromboplastic substance) in the coagulation of blood*[1842] added the thromboplastins to the factors which had been described; it preceded the report on *The thromboplastic action of cephalin*[1843] published by Jay McLean (1890-1957) in 1916. Just after World War I, in 1918-19, Howell, with Luther Holt (1855-1924) reported the critically important isolation of heparin[1844].

Some of the methods of measuring events concerned with the formed elements of the blood commemorate the great names of the turn of the century. Paul Ehrlich, in 1879-80, laid the foundation for the differential white cell counting technique[1845]. John Scott Haldane (1860-1936) brought in his haemoglobinometer with his paper of 1901 on *The colorimetric determination of haemoglobin*[1846] – and Victor Vaughan (1851-1929), with his report *On the appearance and significance of certain granules in the erythrocytes of man*[1847], published in 1903, provided the first description of the reticulocytes – an observation which soon led to an understanding of the way in which these cells show recent haematopoiesis. Two measurements of great physiological importance came a decade or so later with the paper on *The variation on the sizes of red blood cells*[1848] by Cecil Price-Jones (1863-1943) and that describing *A method for the determination of plasma and blood volume*[1849] by Norman Keith and his associates; of these two papers, the first, which established the 'Price-Jones curve', was dated 1910; the second, reporting a dye dilution technique for measuring blood volume, was of 1915.

Knowledge of the blood groups and the means of compatible blood transfusion is, essentially, a twentieth century phenomenon. Karl Landsteiner (1868–1943), in 1900, anounced the discovery that human blood contains iso-agglutinins which will agglutinate the erythrocytes of other subjects[1850]. On the basis of his findings he divided human subjects into three blood groups. For this and his continuing work he was given the Nobel Prize in medicine in 1930. In 1906–07, Jan Janský (1873–1921) showed that there are, in fact, four blood groups – which he named A, B, AB, and O[1851]. This work was not noticed until William Moss (1876–1957) published, in 1910, his now well-known paper *Studies on isoagglutinins and isohemolysins*[1852] which came to the same conclusions. Morton gives the sources of French and German summaries of Janský's paper and comments that the work of Moss was complete before he read of it[1853]. In 1927, Landsteiner, with Philip Levine, reported the discovery of the M and N agglutinogens[1854] and then, in 1939, Levine, with Rufus Stetson, announced the discovery of the Rh antigen (*An unusual case of intra-group agglutination*)[1855]. Levine's discovery was published in the *Journal of the American Medical Association* in the year of the outbreak of World War II in Europe. Quite independently, isolated by the German occupation of Belgium, Paul Moureau discovered the Rh factor, reporting his findings (*Recherches sur un nouvel hémo-agglutinogène du sang humain*)[1856] in 1941. Three years before his death, Karl Landsteiner, after making great contributions to the knowledge of blood groups, published with Alexander Wiener the paper *An agglutinable factor in human blood recognized by immune sera for Rhesus blood*[1857] which, in 1940, reported the recognition of the Rh antigen. In 1944 Edwin Cohn (1892–1953) brought in some of the modern techniques of protein fractionation with his work on the *Chemical, clinical, and immunological studies on the products of human plasma fractionation*[1858].

Knowledge of the clinical disorders of blood and the haematopoietic system developed alongside the growth of the cell theory and was aided by the nineteenth century improvements in archromatic microscopy. Acute leukaemia was first described by Nikolaus Friedreich (1825–1882) in 1857[1859]. Eduard Henoch (1820–1910) first described purpura with abdominal pain ('Henoch's purpura')[1860] in 1868 (but Heberden had previously commented on the association). Paul Ehrlich, by means of his cell-staining techniques, differentiated myelogenous from lymphatic leukaemia in 1891[1861]. A fatal pharyngitis associated with gross leukopenia was first reported in 1901[1862] and the first recorded instance of frank agranulocytosis was recorded by Wilhelm Türk (1871–1916) in 1907[1863]. Despite these publications, the term 'agranulocytosis' was not introduced into the literature until it was used by Werner Schultz (1878–1947) who, in 1922, reported four cases with necrotic ulceration of the throat associated with complete or nearly complete disappearance of the poly-morphonuclear leukocytes[1864]. In modern times agranulocytosis, always uncommon as an idiopathic event, has become one of the more conspicuous lesions in the lists of fatal adverse drug reactions.

Earlier confusion in the literature regarding haemophilia was eliminated by William Bulloch (1868–1941) and Sir Paul Fildes (1882–1971) who, in 1911, published a detailed study of the condition and established that females are immune from the clinical consequences of the disease[1865]. Earlier authors had sometimes reported haemophilic episodes in women and a possible explanation arose with the description in 1926, by Erik von Willebrand (1870–1949), of the type of pseudo-haemophilia which, as an inherited bleeding disorder affecting both sexes in its clinical manifestations, has become known as 'von Willebrand's disease'[1866]. The great advance in the treatment of haemophilia, the isolation of Factor VIII, the antihaemophilic globulin, came with the publication in 1937 of the paper on *Hemophilia. II. Some properties of a substance obtained from normal human plasma effective in accelerating the coagulation of hemophilic blood*[1867] – a work by Arthur Patek and Francis Taylor (1900–1959) which began the era of being able to treat the disease usefully. Christmas disease, due to lack of Factor IX, was named after the patient who was the first example to be recorded; the condition was described in a paper of 1952, *Christmas disease, a condition previously mistaken for haemophilia*[1868], by Dr Rosemary Biggs whose contributions to British haematology have been so considerable.

The first description of the monocytic form of leukaemia was given in 1913[1869] but it was not until 1941 that erythroblastosis fetalis was clearly described and shown to be due to rhesus incompatibility between the mother and child. This notable description came in the paper *The rôle of iso-immunization in the pathogenesis of erythroblastosis fetalis*[1870] published by Philip Levine and his colleagues – it led to urgent attempts to find a means of treating and preventing this cause of fetal wastage. Successful exchange transfusion had already (1925) been described by Alfred Hart (1887–1954) and reported in his article, *Familial icterus gravis of the new-born and its treatment*[1871], in the *Canadian Medical Association Journal*. Knowledge of the technique was improved by the publication of Louis Diamond on *Replacement transfusion as a treatment for erythroblastosis fetalis*[1872] in 1948. Fifteen years later, in 1963, this was followed by the work of Albert Liley on *Intrauterine transfusion of foetus in haemolytic disease*[1873] and then, in 1964, Vincent Freda, J. G. Gorman and W. Pollack began the modern means of care with their report of the *Successful prevention of experimental Rh sensitization in man with an anti-Rh gamma$_2$-globulin antibody preparation*[1874].

Of the haematological tests which are now very familiar to the clinician, the title of the paper by Alf Vilhelm Westergren, describing his method of measuring the erythrocyte sedimentation rate (ESR), reminds us of the disease in which, in its acute forms, a markedly raised ESR was a principal feature: Westergren wrote on *Studies of the suspension stability of the blood in pulmonary tuberculosis*[1875]. Wintrobe's paper, *A standardized technique for the blood sedimentation test*[1876], appeared in 1935. Armand James Quick (1894–1977) published his work on *The prothrombin in hemophilia and in obstructive jaundice*[1877] in 1935 and this provided Quick's test for measuring the prothrombin clotting time, and thereby controlling some forms of anticoagulant therapy. The Coombs's test was reported in a *Lancet* article, *Detection of weak and 'incomplete' Rh agglutinins: a new test*[1878], published by Robin Royston Coombs and his associates in 1945.

The last 100 years have built on a knowledge of anaemia which began in antiquity but has advanced at a rate which makes its chronology interesting. William Gardner and Sir William Osler, in *A case of progressive pernicious anaemia, (idiopathic of Addison)*[1879], published in the *Canada Medical and Surgical Journal* in 1877, gave the first full account of pernicious anaemia. Paul Ehrlich described the blood cells in anaemia in papers of 1881[1880]. Guido Banti (1852–1925), in *Dell' anemia splenica*[1881] of 1882, described 'Banti's disease' of splenic anaemia and 12 years later gave an account of the consequential hepatic cirrhosis – 'Banti's syndrome'. In 1884 Otto Leichtenstern (1845–1900) gave one of the first descriptions of subacute combined degeneration of the spinal cord – but he called it 'progressive perniciöse Anämie bei Tabeskranken'[1882], thinking it was a condition of tabetics. Paul Ehrlich first differentiated aplastic anaemia in 1888[1883] and Gustav von Bunge (1844–1920) began the real understanding of the concept of iron-deficiency anaemia in 1895[1884].

With these types of anaemia identified, it was 1910 before James Herrick (1861–1954) published his paper on *Peculiar elongated and sickle-shaped red blood corpuscles in a case of severe anemia*[1885], so first describing sickle cell anaemia, and it was 1913 before Knud Faber (1862–1956) first wrote on simple, achlorhydric anaemia and 'achylia gastrica'[1886]. Osler's classical account of the pregnancy anaemias appeared in his *British Medical Journal* paper, *Observations on the severe anaemias of pregnancy and the post-partum state*[1887], which appeared in the year of his death, 1919.

The American report *Sickle cell anemia*[1888], of 1922, by Verne Mason gave the disease its present name. Then in 1925, Frieda Robscheit-Robbins and George Whipple (1878–1976) published on *Blood regeneration in severe anaemia. II. Favourable influence of liver, heart and skeletal muscle in diet*[1889]. This work led the way for one of the most substantial advances in therapy of the century – the raw liver diet reported by George Minot (1885–1950) and William Murphy in their paper, *Treatment of pernicious anemia by a special diet* (1926)[1890]. For providing this understanding of the means to treat some cases of pernicious anaemia, Whipple, Minot and Murphy shared the Nobel Prize in 1934.

Haematology has perhaps retained the names of those who have done it great service more frequently than some of the modern specialties. Cooley's erythroblastic anaemia, thalassaemia, was described in 1925, and again in 1927 (*Anemia in children, with splenomegaly and peculiar changes in the bones*)[1891], by Thomas Cooley (1871–1945) and his associates. The Fanconi syndrome, familial congenital bone marrow hypoplasia with anaemia and other defects, was also described in 1927 – by Guido Fanconi (1892–1979)[1892].

At this same period there came three further significant advances in the knowledge of pernicious anaemia. Francis Weld Peabody (1881–1927) published on *The pathology of the bone marrow in pernicious anaemia*[1893] in 1927 and suggested that the disease was due to deficiencies in the making of the red blood cells, rather than in the presence of haemolysis; Peabody also suggested that the benefit of the raw liver diet was due to its helping the formation of erythrocytes. William Bosworth Castle then (in 1929) gave a now historic account of his *Observations on the etiologic relationship of achylia gastrica to pernicious anemia. I. The effect of the administration to patients with pernicious anemia of the contents of the normal human stomach recovered after the ingestion of beef muscle*[1894]. This was Castle's intrinsic factor, haemopoietin, present in the gastric juice and interacting with an extrinsic factor in meat and other foods to form the complete factor which both prevents and treats pernicious anaemia. The discovery led to the use of stomach preparations for the therapy of the condition. That the intrinsic factor resided in gastric tissue was shown by Cyrus Sturgis (1891–1966) and Raphael Isaacs in their paper of 1929 on the use of *Desiccated stomach in the treatment of pernicious anemia*[1895].

Maxwell Wintrobe's *Classification of the anemias on the basis of differences in the size and hemoglobin content of the red corpuscles*[1896] of 1930 forms a landmark in the scientific classification and understanding of the anaemias; it was already available when Lucy Wills (1888–1964) produced her account of the *Treatment of 'pernicious anaemia of pregnancy' and 'tropical anaemia', with special reference to yeast extract as a curative agent*[1897] – a paper which, in 1931, provided the first demonstration of the haemopoietic effect of folic acid.

The actual name of thalassaemia was given to the condition in the very fine account of its pathology in the *Mediterranean disease – thalassemia (erythroblastic anemia of Cooley); associated pigment abnormalities simulating hemochromatosis* (1936)[1898] by George Whipple and William Bradford. Almost immediately, in 1938, J. Caminopetros produced a study of the anthropology, aetiology and pathogenesis of thalassaemia and showed the disease to be genetically determined[1899].

Just before the mid-century, Tom Douglas Spies and his colleagues confirmed (1945) the haemopoietic capability of folic acid[1900] – and in 1946 Robert Crane Angier and his associates reported the determination of the structure, and the synthesis, of folic acid[1901]. The availability of this fine and useful drug was followed, in 1948, by the paper of Randolph West, *Activity of vitamin B_{12} in Addisonian pernicious anaemia*[1902], first showing the efficacy of the vitamin in this grave form of anaemia. Charles Ungley's report of *Vitamin B_{12} in pernicious anaemia: parenteral administration*[1903] appeared in 1949, completing the knowledge of the essential route of administration of the remedy. Folic acid remains widely used during pregnancy to prevent megaloblastic anaemia and it can also be given prophylactically in conditions, such as thalassaemia, in which there is chronic haemolysis; it must of course never be given in Addisonian pernicious anaemia or other vitamin B_{12} deficiency states in which it may precipitate the onset of subacute combined degeneration of the spinal cord. Thus, as most megaloblastic anaemias are due to deficiency of either vitamin B_{12} or folic acid, it is mandatory that the nature of the deficiency and its underlying cause be discovered in each individual case. Hydroxocobalamin has now replaced cyanocobalamin as the form of vitamin B_{12} for therapeutic use and this must surely be one of the most remarkable drugs of twentieth century medicine. The potency is such that once the usual five starting doses have been given, maintenance doses are of the order of 1 mg every 3 months. These produce a normal expectation of life from specific therapy in a previously lethal condition and do it with an admirable therapeutic margin of safety.

The knowledge of anaemias reached molecular level with the 1949 paper of Linus Carl Pauling who, with colleagues, published the results of their study of *Sickle cell anemia, a molecular disease*[1904], announcing the identification of the first structural variant haemoglobin to be recognized. Two of the great accounts of the struggle to understand the anaemias span the recent period but look back on the history of the achievement. Frederick Willius and Thomas Keys include much of the early material in their *Cardiac classics. A collection of classic work on the heart and circulation with comprehensive biographic accounts of the authors* (1941)[1905]. The 1961 edition, *Classics of cardiology*, brings the story, in its broad context, nearer the present. The splendid, recent account is *Blood, pure and eloquent. A story of discovery, of people, and of ideas*[1906], published in 1980 and edited by Maxwell Wintrobe.

Of the diseases of the reticuloendothelial system, Thomas Hodgkin (1798–1866), in his paper *On some morbid appearances of the absorbent glands and spleen*[1168] of 1832, described the lymphadenomatous condition which has come to bear his name. This first adequate description of Hodgkin's disease dates therefore from the period of outstanding clinical studies which came from Guy's Hospital at the time of Bright, Addison, and Hodgkin. The name of Hodgkin was first attached to the disease by Sir Samuel Wilks (1824–1911), also of Guy's[1907]. Theodor Langhans (1839–1915), in *Das maligne Lymphosarkom (Pseudoleukämie)*[1908] of 1872, recorded the presence of giant cells in the glands affected by Hodgkin's disease; these curious cells were again noted by William Greenfield (1846–1919) in 1878[1909] but their present designation as 'Dorothy Reed's giant cells' stems from that author's classical work *On the pathological changes in Hodgkin's disease, with especial reference to its relation to tuberculosis*[1910] published in *Johns Hopkins Hospital Reports* in 1902. The 'Pel–Ebstein fever', the remittent pyrexia characteristic of Hodgkin's disease, dates from the German publication of Pieter Pel (1852–1919) in 1885[1911] and Wilhelm Ebstein (1836–1912) 2 years later[1912]. The English *Clinical lecture on acute Hodgkin's disease*[1913] of 1892 by Julius Dreschfeld (1845–1907) and the German paper, *Ueber Lympho-Sarkomatosis*[1914] of 1893, by Hans Kundrat (1845–1893) differentiated Hodgkin's disease from lymphosarcoma and led to the European designation of the latter condition as 'Kundrat's disease'.

'Gaucher's disease', the lipid storage disease, characteristically familial, in which glucocerebroside accumulates in the histiocytes of the spleen, liver, and bone marrow, can produce an immense spleen with bone tumours leading to pathological fractures. It is probably inherited as an autosomal recessive and is due to a deficiency of the enzyme beta-glucocerebrosidase which splits glucocerebroside into glucose and ceramide. The infantile type often leads to rapid deterioration but the adult form may permit survival into old age. The condition was first described in a thesis of 1882[1915] by Philippe Gaucher (1854–1918).

Carl Sternberg's (1872–1935) classical account of lymphadenoma, differentiating it from aleukaemic leukaemia, is dated 1898[1916] but it was not until 1924 that Karl Aschoff (1866–1942) published his *Das reticulo-endotheliale system*[1917] – a work which led to the widespread adoption of the term 'reticuloendothelial system' which Aschoff had introduced 2 years before.

Of the means of therapy which relate to the growing knowledge of haematology, the technique of blood transfusion probably ranks as one of the greatest advances of the twentieth century. Although the surgeon had access to useful means of anaesthesia from the middle of the nineteenth century, and Leonard Landois (1837–1902) discovered the haemolysing effect of the serum of one species if it was transfused into another in 1874[1918], surgery had to wait for the period of the First World War for really significant advances in blood transfusion.

In 1914 (*Note sur une nouvelle méthode de transfusion*)[1919], Albert Hustin (1882–1967) showed the anticoagulant capability of sodium citrate and its potential for use in blood transfusion. The first to transfuse such citrated blood, in 1914–15, was Luis Agote (1868–1954)[1920]. At much the same time (1915), Richard Lewisohn (1875–1962), in New York, published on the use of citrate in transfusion[1921].

One of the first to use stored blood on battlefield casualties was Oswald Hope Robertson (1886–1966) who published his *Transfusion with preserved red blood cells*[1922] in Paris in 1917–1918. The modern technique of administering blood came in with the much later paper – of 1935 – on *Continuous drip blood transfusion*[1923], a publication in the *Lancet* by Hugh Marriottt and Alan Kekwick (1909–1974). Heparin was used in blood transfusion by the Scandinavian, Per Johannes Hedenius, whose *A new method of blood transfusion*[1924] appeared in 1936. Due to the shortage of material, Sergei Sergeievich Yudin (1891–1954) recorded the *Transfusion of cadaver blood*[1925] in 1936. This work was published in the *Journal of the American Medical Association* which, the following year printed the historic article, *The therapy of the Cook County Hospital. Blood preservation*[1926], by Bernard Fantus (1874–1940) describing the establishment of the first blood bank.

This concept had hardly preceded the outbreak of the Second World War – a conflict which stimulated further work on the practicalities of blood transfusion. In 1943, John Loutit and Patrick Mollison, in the *British Medical Journal*, published their account of the *Advantages of a disodium–citrate–glucose mixture as a blood preservative*[1927], and this work made it possible to store donated blood for periods approaching 3 weeks. The introduction of the plasma substitute, dextran, was due to Anders Grönwall and Björn Ingleman whose *Untersuchungen über Dextran und sein Verhalten bei parenteraler Zufuhr*[1928] appeared in 1944. This, by 6 years, preceded the *Prevention of haemolysis during freezing and thawing red blood-cells*[1929], a *Lancet* paper by Audrey Ursula Smith (1915–1981) showing that human blood diluted with glycerol in Ringer's lactate solution could be deep-frozen and thawed several weeks later without harm.

There is a fine article summarizing the *Histoy of blood transfusion*[1930], by Noble Maluf, in the *Journal of the History of Medicine* for 1954.

In addition to blood transfusion the last three-quarters of a century have seen the advent of the chemotherapy of haematological and reticuloendothelial disease. Phenylhydrazine hydrochloride in the management of polycythaemia vera was, in 1918, one of the early entrants in the field[1931]. It was followed by vitamin K in the treatment of haemorrhagic diathesis in cases of jaundice (1938)[1932], radiotherapy in Hodgkin's disease (1939)[1933], radioactive phosphorus in leukaemia (1939)[1934] and then the isolation of dicoumarol by Mark Stahmann and his colleagues (*Studies on the hemorrhagic sweet clover disease. V. Identification and synthesis of the hemorrhagic agent*)[1935] in 1941.

The modern era of the chemotherapy of malignant disease began immediately after the cessation of World War II. During the First World War medical attention first began to be focused on the vesicant effect on the skin, eyes and respiratory tract of sulphur mustard, first synthesized in 1854. It was soon realized that toxic effects of this kind were accompanied by profound leukopenia, bone marrow aplasia, and ulceration of the gastrointestinal tract. Clearly, the toxic effects were most intense on the tissues where cell replication was most rapid. This cytotoxic effect led, during World War II, to studies by Alfred Gilman, Louis S. Goodman and their assistants, on the action of nitrogen mustards on transplanted lymphosarcoma in mice. Goodman and Gilman, in their magnificent *The Pharmacological Basis of Therapeutics* (1975)[1936], comment that: 'In their early phases, all these investigations were conducted under secrecy restrictions imposed by the use of classified chemical-warfare agents. At the termination of World War II, however, the nitrogen mustards were declassified and a general review was presented...' This review was on *The biological actions and therapeutic applications of the β-chloroethylamines and sulfides*[1937] by Alfred Gilman and Frederick Philips and was dated 1946. The reports of the clinical studies appeared the same year and were followed by the still-unabated interest in the possibilities of developing compounds that would be lethal to the rapidly dividing cells of malignant tissue, and less so to the vulnerable tissues of the skin, bone marrow and gut wall.

There have been a number of such compounds, none of course by any means fully satisfactory, but allowing of effective therapy in some of the malignancies already discussed. These compounds can be represented by urethane[1938], used in the treatment of leukaemia in 1946; triethylene melamine[1939], used in Hodgkin's disease in 1950; 6-mercaptopurine[1940], synthesized in 1952; myleran, introduced for chronic myeloid leukaemia in 1953[1941]; chlorambucil, used in clinical studies of chronic lympatic leukaemia in 1955[1942]; the *Vinca* alkaloids, vinblastine used in Hodgkin's disease and vincristine in the acute leukaemias of childhood in 1963[1943]; and arabinosyl cytosine, found to be 'a useful agent in the treatment of acute leukemia in adults' in 1968[1944].

A second group of agents is represented by the oral anticoagulants. These include phenylindanedione[1945], first introduced by Jean Soulier and Jean Gueguen in 1947; and ethyl biscoumacetate, which was studied by Z. Reiniš and Mirko Kubík in 1948[1946].

Experimental studies of many different types have spanned the whole century. An early example is the transmission of fowl leukaemia by means of a filterable agent in a cell-free preparation. This production of transmissible neoplasia by means of a virus was achieved by Vilhelm Ellerman (1871–1924) and O. Bang as early as 1908[1947]. The studies of fairly recent years have included those on the blood platelets and the fibrinolytic system.

The blood platelets and the processes of blood clotting and fibrinolysis have one of their meeting places in the structure of the organized thrombus. The most simple terminology describes the 'white head', at the point of attachment of such a thrombus, as being largely composed of blood platelets. The 'red tail' is composed of a fibrin meshwork with the red cells, and other cells, entrapped in its interstices. The fibrin represents the end-point of the enzymatic cascade which produces coagulation – the last stage being the conversion of the soluble blood protein, fibrinogen, to insoluble fibrin by the enzyme thrombin.

Under favourable conditions such a thrombus is dissolved by the process of fibrinolysis: another soluble and freely available blood protein, plasminogen, is converted by enzymatic plasminogen activators (derived largely from the intima of the vein wall) to plasmin. This potent proteolytic enzyme, plasmin, then lyses the fibrin with the production of fibrin degradation products and the loss of integrity of the anatomical structure of the now-dissolving thrombus.

Sol Sherry and his colleagues made very significant preliminary observations on the blood plasminogen activator in 1959[1948]. A more direct demonstration of the presence of a specific kinase in normal blood was then achieved by Peter T. Flute in 1960[1948a]. The presence of fibrinolytic activity in the blood of normal subjects and the responsiveness of this activity to physical exertion was then shown, along with the fact that the normal fibrinolytic activity exhibits marked diurnal variation, in a long and careful series of studies beginning in 1957 and conducted by George R. Fearnley and his associates[1949].

It can be argued that the great difficulty with studies on subjects such as blood platelet behaviour and fibrinolysis is the demand to produce drugs before the physiology and pathology have been meaningfully explored. A drug then seeks for a disease. We still lack, even when laboratory tests for platelet effects and fibrinolytic and coagulation parameters are well worked out, the knowledge that would be provided by the use of these tests in large population prospective studies of normal and diseased persons. One of the observations that seems to have potential arises from the study on *Fibrinolytic activity and coronary artery disease*[1950], published by R. Chakrabarti and others of Fearnley's group in 1968. This study showed that survivors of proven myocardial infarction differ from sex and age-matched controls in having a significantly increased blood fibrinogen concentration. That those with proven arterial disease of this kind have such an abnormality of the protein so intimately concerned with coagulation and its related phenomena appears, if the observation is repeated, likely to be meaningful. It is also likely to offer therapeutic potential.

The interests of the haematologist and the oncologist overlap in respect of several of the diseases already mentioned. Organized laboratory work in the latter specialty can be said to have begun with the studies of Henri Morau whose *Inoculation en série d'une tumeur épithéliale de la souris blanche*[1951] appeared in 1891 and recorded the transfer of epitheliomata through successive generations of mice. Leo Loeb (1865–1959) reported *On transplantation of tumours*[1952] in 1901 and, by successfully transplanting a sarcomatous growth of the thyroid in rats, showed that the growth of the new tumour took place from its peripheral cells. Carl Oluf Jensen (1864–1934), in 1903, published the results of important experiments carrying a sarcoma through 40 generations of rats and showing that the tumour bred true in terms of histological structure[1953]. Then in an historic paper of 1910 and 1911, Francis Peyton Rous (1879–1970, a Nobel prizewinner of 1966) reported on *A transmissible avian neoplasm (sarcoma of the common fowl)*[1954]. This work showed that the Rous sarcoma could be transmitted to normal fowls by injection of cell-free preparations of the original growth. At the same time, in 1910, Alexis Carrel (1873–1944) and Montrose Burrows (1884–1947), using the Rous sarcoma, became the first to grow a malignant tissue *in vitro*[1955].

The same decade at the beginning of the present century saw also the beginnings of cancer therapy other than surgery. X-rays were first successfully used in the treatment of cancer by Tage Sjögren (1859–1939) who published his results in Stockholm in 1899[1956]. That agents which can arrest cancer can have the converse effect was recognized early, for in 1902 Ernst Frieben reported the carcinogenic effects of X-rays in man[1957]. These were the pioneer days of radiotherapy, Georg Perthes (1869–1927) reporting on the manner in which X-rays inhibit the growth of carcinomata in 1903[1958] and S. W. Goldberg and Efim London (1869–1939) announcing the first successful use of radium to treat cancer in the same year[1959].

The decade of the First World War saw attempts (1911) by Ernst Freund (1863–1946) and his colleagues[1960] to produce a serum reaction that would facilitate the diagnosis of cancer and the start of the work on the hormone dependence of some forms of new growth: in 1916, A. E. Lathrop and Leo Loeb (1869–1959) showed that removal of the ovaries in a strain of mice susceptible to spontaneous mammary cancer reduced the incidence and retarded the growth of these tumours[1961]. In 1912 this was followed by the demonstration of Henry Bayon (1876–1952) that epithelial proliferation and neoplastic change could be induced by the injection of gasworks tar[1962].

The complex issues involved in the induction of neoplasia soon became evident. Sir Ernest Kennaway (1881–1958), in *The formation of a cancer-producing substance from isoprene (2-methyl-butadiene)*[1963] of 1924 continued the work on carcinogenic tars and showed that some pure hydrocarbons can act as carcinogens. William Ewart Gye (1884–1952), in a paper on *The aetiology of malignant new growths* (1925)[1964], suggested that a virus, combined in its effects with those of an intrinsic chemical agent, was involved in the production of the Rous chicken sarcoma. Support for this theory was provided by a publication on *The microscopical examination of filterable viruses associated with malignant new growths* (1925)[1965] by Joseph Barnard (1870–1949). Studies on the metabolic characteristics of tumour tissues began, in respect of the utilization of glucose by such tissues by means of aerobic or anaerobic glycolysis, in the hands of Otto Warburg, who published on the subject in 1926[1966]. And then Maud Slye, in her work *Cancer and heredity*[1967] of 1928, showed that by selective breeding it was possible to produce highly resistant or highly susceptible mouse strains. Maud Slye's publications on this subject began in 1914 and strongly suggested that, in these animals, resistance to cancer is a Mendelian dominant and susceptibility a recessive characteristic, either of which could be bred into or out of successive generations.

All of these lines of investigation have proceeded and produced interesting results. The discovery of the carcinogenic properties of pure hydrocarbons was followed by the paper (1932) of Sir James Cook (1900–1975) and his colleagues showing the cancer-causing potential of dibenzanthracene compounds[1968]. The considerable number of natural and synthetic substances which can act as carcinogens has been extensively reviewed.

The work with hormones, now an established means of therapy in certain cases, has shown how complex are the issues involved. Georgiana Bonser (1898–1979), in a paper of 1937 on *The carcinogenic action of oestrone: induction of mammary carcinoma in female mice of a strain refractory to the spontaneous development of mammary tumours*[1969], showed how oestrone could favour malignancy; by contrast, Sir Alexander Haddow (1907–1976), with his co-workers, in 1944 showed that the clinical administration of synthetic oestrogens could cause regression of advanced malignant disease of the breast[1970].

Studies with the viruses concerned with tumour formation have led deep into the molecular biology of neoplasia. The Shope papilloma virus, described in the paper *A transmissible tumor-like condition of rabbits*[1971] published in 1932 by Richard Edwin Shope (1901–1966), provides an example of a benign tumour which is both transmissible and of viral origin. 'Bittner's milk factor' commemorates the paper *Some possible effects of nursing on the mammary gland tumor incidence in mice* (1936)[1972] by John Joseph Bittner (1904–1961) – the factor is concerned with the transmission of murine mammary cancer. The isolation of the papovavirus or polyomavirus was described in the 1957 publication by Sarah Elizabeth Stewart and her colleagues on *The induction of neoplasms with a substance released from mouse tumors by tissue culture*[1973]. This virus was shown to be capable of transforming cells in tissue culture by Marguerite Vogt who, working with Renato Dulbecco, wrote on the *Virus–cell interaction with a tumor-producing virus*[1974] in 1961. Almost 20 years ago Howard Martin Temin wrote on the *Nature of the provirus of Rous sarcoma*[1975] – the concept is that, following infection, a DNA provirus containing all of the genetic information of the RNA viral genome is synthesized.

Just before this, a previously almost unknown clinical condition was described by Denis Burkitt in his paper, *A sarcoma involving the jaws in African children* (1958–59)[1976]. The account was of 'Burkitt's tumour', or African lymphoma. Investigating this condition, Michael Anthony Epstein and Y. M. Barr (*Cultivation in vitro of human lymphoblasts from Burkitt's malignant lymphoma*[1977], in 1964, showed that a human herpes virus which could cause infectious mononucleosis was implicated in the causation of Burkitt's lymphoma. A little later, and again in the *Lancet* of 1964, Epstein and his colleagues reported on *Virus particles in cultured lymphoblasts from Burkitt's lymphoma*[1978]. Thomas Shope and his group then, in 1973, produced an animal model for the infection, publishing on *Malignant lymphoma in cotton-top marmosets after inoculation with Epstein–Barr virus*[1979].

As knowledge moves towards an increasing understanding of the molecular biology involved in these processes, David Baltimore, in 1970, wrote in *Nature* (London) on *RNA-dependent DNA polymerase in virions of RNA tumour viruses*[1980]; Howard Temin and Satoshi Mizutani published, again in *Nature* (London) in 1970, on *RNA-dependent DNA polymerase in virions of Rous sarcoma virus*[1981] and Renato Dulbecco (who shared the Nobel Prize with Baltimore and Temin for the discoveries on the interaction between tumour viruses and the cell genetic material) gave, in Stockholm, the 1975 Nobel Prize oration *From the molecular biology of oncogenic DNA viruses to cancer*[1982]. These publications are of the same vintage as the report on *Field trials with an attenuated cell associated vaccine for Marek's disease*[1983] by Peter Martin Biggs and his colleagues who, by showing that a vaccine could provide immunity against Marek's disease of chickens also demonstrated the aetiological relationship of this herpesvirus to cancer in this species.

The work in America on nitrogen mustard during World War II has already been mentioned[1937]. The clinical findings were reported by Louis Sanford Goodman and his associates in 1946[1984]. This was shortly after Cecilie Leuchtenberger and co-workers had shown (1944) that a concentrate of folic acid could inhibit tumour growth[1985]. Before long, aminopterin was introduced – the paper on *Temporary remissions in acute leukemia in children produced by folic acid antagonist 4-amethopteroylglutamic acid (aminopterin)*[1986] being published by Sidney Farber and his colleagues in 1948. Other drugs, uniformly toxic but of use in grave situations, have been cytosine arabinoside, a pyrimidine antagonist used in acute myeloblastic leukaemia (1951)[1986a]; chlorambucil, a nitrogen mustard used in several forms of cancer (1953)[1987]; cyclophosphamide, again for cancer chemotherapy (1958)[1988]; and the Vinca alkaloids (1963)[1943]. That the sensitivity of cancer cells to X-rays is much enhanced when they are irradiated in a highly-oxygenated medium was demonstrated in 1953[1988a] and the rather notable publication, *Combination chemotherapy in the treatment of advanced Hodgkin's disease*[1989], by Vincent DeVita and his colleagues appeared in 1970. These workers obtained improved results by using three cytotoxic agents at once in association with prednisone, a programme which they had been using for 5 or 6 years, and which, in its implications, has since attracted widespread attention.

Much of the practical laboratory medicine since the discovery of penicillin has been concerned, in the hands of the bacteriologist, with the study of resistance and sensitivity to antibiotics. Virology, as a subject, might be said to date from the demonstration by Friedrich Leoffler (1852-1915) and Paul Frosch (1860-1928), in 1898, that foot-and-mouth disease is due to a filter-passing virus[1990]. This was the first demonstration of a viral animal pathogen. Ultrafiltration methods were introduced by Heinrich Bechhold (1866-1937) in 1907[1991]; the use of graded collodion membranes for filterable virus studies and grading by size was brought in by William Elford (1900-1952) in 1931[1992], and Alice Woodruff with Ernest Goodpasture (1886-1960) introduced the use of the chorio-allantoic membrane of the chick embryo as a vital medium for the culture of viruses in 1931[1993].

Thus, these procedures were available when, in general microbiology, Rebecca Lancefield, in 1933, published on *A serological differentiation of human and other groups of hemolytic streptococci*[1994]. The important human pathogenic strains of these organisms fall into Group A of the Lancefield classification. The further classification of *Streptococcus pyogenes* by Frederick Griffith dates from 1934[1995].

The first isolation of a virus (tobacco-mosaic virus) in a crystalline form dates from 1935[1996], the isolation of cytomegalovirus from 1956[1997], and the detection of the Simian vacuolating virus SV_{40} from 1960[1998]. The discovery of the adenoviruses dates from the 1953 publication of the paper on the *Isolation of a cytopathogenic agent from human adenoids undergoing spontaneous degeneration in tissue culture*[1999] by Wallace Rowe and his associates.

The period around the mid-century marks the appearance, in 1949, of the very significant paper by Salvador Luria and Renato Dulbecco on *Genetic recombinations leading to production of active bacteriophage from ultraviolet inactivated bacteriophage particles*[2000]. Luria shared the 1969 Nobel Prize with Hershey and Delbrück for work on the genetics and the replication of bacteria. Work on the molecular manipulation of virus material has continued to advance, the first crystallization of an animal virus (purified MEF-1 poliomyelitis virus particles) being achieved in 1955[2001], and Heinz Ludwig Fraenkel-Conrat with Robley Williams reporting the quite remarkable *Reconstitution of active tobacco mosaic virus from its inactive protein and nucleic acid components in 1955*[2002].

Without following progress in these laboratory sciences which form part of modern medicine beyond the mid-century, it is perhaps worth observing that the rate of increasing knowledge has been such that whereas centuries of recorded experience lead up to the appearance in 1839 of Schwann's *Mikroskopische Untersuchungen* . . . , and its fundamental contribution to the doctrine of the cell structure of animal tissues, only 110 years separate that event from the genetic recombination of filter-passing bacteriophage reported by Luria and Dulbecco in 1949[2000].

Clinical medicine

The practice of bedside medicine in the early part of the present century was continuous with that of the preceding two or three decades, the turn of the century marking a quite arbitrary division and nothing changing, in any way that was fundamental, prior to the beginning of the era of chemotherapy and the onset of World War I.

Of the distinctive figures of the time, Sir Thomas Clifford Allbutt (1836–1925), Regius Professor of Physic at Cambridge, and Sir William Osler (1849–1919), form supreme examples.

Thomas Allbutt, in the Gulstonian Lectures of 1884, spoke on the subject of visceral neuroses[2003], providing a fairly early text on psychosomatic medicine. He described the histology of the cerebral arteries affected by syphilitic endarteritis in 1868[2004] and, in the following year, in a paper providing *Remarks on a case of locomotor ataxy with hydrarthrosis*[2005], gave an early description of the joint symptoms and signs in tabes dorsalis. Now that tertiary syphilis has become uncommon, Allbutt is probably more often remembered for his *Medical thermometry*[2006] of 1870, and for his contributions to the history of medicine, rather than for the rest of his clinical works. The 1870 paper introduced the modern clinical thermometer into everyday practice and provided Allbutt's most significant contribution to improving the methods of measurement in medicine.

Allbutt is now valued as a writer of great accomplishment on whole areas of medical history, the works including the Harveian Oration of 1900 (*Science and mediaeval thought*, 1901)[529], *The historical relations of medicine and surgery to the end of the sixteenth century* (1905)[2007] – a study which has been considered the best history of mediaeval surgery in English – and, as the FitzPatrick Lectures of 1909–10, the well known, *Greek medicine in Rome* (1921)[243]. Possibly, Allbutt's most important single stimulating concept in the latter work is his emphasis on the importance of Greek remaining the language of Magna Graecia until well into the Middle Ages. His later clinical work, and his original studies of the circulation, is contained in the two volume *Diseases of the arteries, including angina pectoris*[2008]. This contains his mechanical theory of the origin of cardiac pain in coronary artery disease and important insights into the psychosomatic manifestations of cardiac disease and what later came to be known as Da Costa's or the 'effort syndrome'.

Sir William Osler (Figure 138) is one of the most attractive of the figures of modern medical history. Originally of McGill University, to which he bequeathed his unsurpassed personal library of medicine, he later had a clinic at the Johns Hopkins where much important work was done, and in 1904 became Regius Professor of Medicine at Oxford. He was a contemporary of Allbutt and both

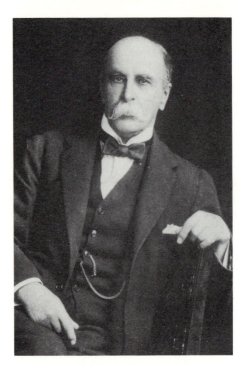

Figure 138   Sir William Osler (1849–1919). [*From: William Osler. Incunabula medica. Oxford, (1923).*]

were founders of the Section of the History of Medicine of the Royal Society of Medicine, London.

Osler's interest in clinical medicine was lifelong and his technical contributions to its literature of importance. They began with his account of the blood platelets in 1874[1836] and continued with his Gulstonian Lecture providing the first full description of subacute bacterial endocarditis in 1885[2009]. In 1877 he wrote the first complete account of pernicious anaemia[1879] and in 1892 published his splendid textbook on *The principles and practice of medicine*[2010]. This had its ninth edition in 1920 and was not only the best English work on medicine of its time but remains the choicest and most easily read portrait of the clinical practice of the Edwardian period. Osler's clinical papers continued with a study of multiple hereditary telangiectasis in 1901[2011] and an important account of polycythaemia vera of 1903[2012]. At the time this account was written Osler thought he was describing a new clinical entity; he later learnt of the earlier (1892) description of the condition by Louis Henri Vaquez (1860–1936)[2013]. Osler was editor of *Modern Medicine* (1910) and in 1908 became the founder and editor of the *Quarterly Journal of Medicine*. In the latter, in 1908–09, he published his account of *Chronic infectious endocarditis*[2014], thereby providing a classic description of subacute bacterial endocarditis and describing the tender subcutaneous nodules which form one of the features of the disease and are known as 'Osler's nodes'. He has also an important paper of 1919, the year of his death, recording his

INCUNABULA MEDICA

A Study of the Earliest
Printed Medical Books
1467—1480

BY

SIR WILLIAM OSLER, Bt., M.D., F.R.S.

REGIUS PROFESSOR OF MEDICINE, OXFORD

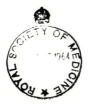

PRINTED FOR THE BIBLIOGRAPHICAL SOCIETY

AT THE OXFORD UNIVERSITY PRESS

1923

Figure 139 William Osler. Title page from: *Incunubula medica. Oxford*, (1923).

Observations on the severe anaemias of pregnancy and the postpartum state[1887].
    Osler had an outstanding knowledge of his subject, a reflective but humane manner, and an attractive style of writing which makes his works uniquely enjoyable. His book, *An Alabama student, and other biographical essays*[2015], published at Oxford in 1908, has become justifiably famous. In 1908 he published a typically polished study of *Thomas Linacre*[601] and, in 1921, followed this with

The evolution of modern medicine[19] – a work published at Yale but based on his Lectures on the Silliman Foundation of 1913. It is this work which is widely accounted the best book with which to begin the reading of the history of medicine.

At the height of his achievement Osler used his resources to gather together a medical library of great distinction and an accompanying knowledge of medical bibliography. He gave the presidential address to the Bibliographical Society in 1914 and, on this address based his *Incunabula medica. A study of the earliest printed medical books, 1467–1480*[2016]. In this work, of 1923, the introductory essay describes the influence of the early years of printing on the growth of medicine; Osler then lists 217 medical books printed before or during 1480.

Perhaps the greatest tribute to Osler's achievements was the production of an excellently annotated catalogue of his library. Upon this was based the *Bibliotheca Osleriana. A catalogue of books illustrating the history of medicine and science, collected, arranged, and annotated by Sir William Osler, Bt. and bequeathed to McGill University*[2017]. This work, published in Oxford in 1929 is of permanent value and its annotations provide a rich and intimate insight into Osler's knowledge and personality. Osler's other bequests included the only known copy of the 1476 edition of the *Almansor*[2018] of Rhazes (?850–?923). Osler purchased this unique piece in 1915 and made it his bequest to the British Museum. To the Royal Society of Medicine he left a distinguished collection of the letters of William Withering.

The portrait forming Figure 138 stands opposite the title page of his *Incunabula medica* . . . [2016] of 1923. The title page itself forms Figure 139.

The cardiovascular system

The atrioventricular bundle ('the bundle of His'), which conducts the contractile impulses between the auricles and ventricles, was independently discovered in 1893 by both Wilhelm His (1863–1934)[2019] and Albert Frank Kent (1863–1958)[2020]. Within a few years, Sir Arthur Keith (1866–1955) and Martin Flack (1882–1931) discovered the sinoatrial node[2021], the pacemaker of the normal heart, and Sunao Tawara described (1906) the atrioventricular node[2022]. Thus, by this date, the essential structures concerned with the transmission of the cardiac impulse had been described. A further understanding of the physiology of the heart was achieved by Ernest Henry Starling (1866–1927) whose 'all-or-none' law of the heart appeared in his *The Linacre lecture on the law of the heart*[2023] of 1918.

The standard methods of measuring the blood pressure date from the turn of the century. The first clinical use of the sphygmomanometer was recorded by Samuel Siegfried von Basch (1837–1905) in 1883[2024]. The standard clinical sphygmomanometer devised by Scipione Riva-Rocci (1863–1937) was brought into use in 1896[2025]. The following year Sir Leonard Hill (1866–1952) and Harold Barnard (1868–1908) published an account of their modification substituting a pressure gauge for the mercury manometer of the Riva-Rocci instrument[2026]. In 1905, Nikolai Sergeievich Korotkov (1874–1920) introduced the modern method of taking the blood pressure by applying the stethoscope to the brachial artery adjacent to biceps tendon[2027]; Korotkov also described the diagnostic sounds which carry his name and by which the blood pressure is measured. Thus, from 1905 the Riva-Rocci instrument and the knowledge of the Korotkov sounds became more and more widespread.

The understanding of the heart's action which can be obtained by comparing the arterial and venous pulse waves dates from the same period and is largely due to the fine work of Sir James Mackenzie (1853–1925). Mackenzie, in 1892, published the results of comparing simultaneous tracings of the jugular vein pulsation and the radial artery pulse[2028]. These tracings were made with a phlebograph, but from this Mackenzie developed a polygraph. With this instrument he made the observations which formed the basis for his classical monograph on *The study of the pulse* (1902)[2029].

Practical electrocardiography dates from the period shortly before World War I. Augustus Waller (1856–1922), in 1887, published *A demonstration in man of electromotive changes accompanying the heart's beat*[2030]. Using electrodes and electrical leads, Waller produced the first electrocardiogram recorded in man. In 1903–04, Willem Einthoven (1860–1927) published his paper on *The string galvanometer and the human electro-cardiogram*[2031] and this led to Einthoven's string galvanometer replacing the previously-used capillary electrometer. The great pioneer of the clinical application of the method was Sir Thomas Lewis (1881–1945) who wrote on *The mechanism of the heart beat* in 1911 and, in 1912, in three classic papers in the *British Medical Journal*, produced his work on *Electro-cardiography and its importance in the clinical examination of heart affections*[2032]. It is from these papers and this period, shortly before World War I, that practical clinical electrocardiography might be said to date. The book of 1911 appeared in its valuable second edition (*The mechanism and graphic registration of the heart beat*)[2033] in 1920; the third edition was of 1925.

The raised ST segment and inverted T wave forming Pardee's sign of recent myocardial infarction dates from a paper, *An electrocardiographic sign of coronary artery obstruction*[2034], published by Harold Ensign Pardee (1886–1972) in 1920. We have, therefore, something like 60 years experience of this famous ECG sign. Werner Theodor Forssmann (1904–1979) catheterized his own heart, published his findings in 1929[2035], and so began the modern practice of cardiac catheterization. He shared a Nobel Prize with Cournand and Richards in 1956. Aortography was also introduced in 1929[2036]. The electrocardiogram was improved by the use of chest leads in 1932[2037], the unipolar leads in 1934[2038], and the introduction of vectorcardiography in 1936[2039]. Angiocardiography dates from 1938 and a paper by George Robb and Israel Steinberg describing *A practical method of visualization of the chambers of the heart, the pulmonary circulation, and the great vessels in man*[2040]. Interest in the ballistocardiogram began with the work by Isaac Starr and his associates reporting *Studies on the estimation of cardiac output in man, and of abnormalities in cardiac function, from the heart's recoil and the blood's impacts; the ballistocardiogram*[2041] in 1939. The first use of cardiac catheterization as a means of practical clinical investigation was recorded in the report on *Catheterization of the right auricle in man* (1941)[2042] by André Cournand and Hilmert Ranges. And then, from this cluster of papers whose titles are even more than ordinarily informative, Sir John McMichael and Edward Sharpey-Schafer (1908–1963) wrote on the *Cardiac out-*

put in man by a direct Fick method[2043] in 1944 and John Samuel LaDue with Felix Wroblewski, in 1955, published their historic study, *The significance of the serum glutamic oxalacetic transaminase activity following acute myocardial infarction*[2044], which introduced this important diagnostic enzyme test into practical cardiology. The glutamic oxaloacetic transaminase has since become known as the aspartate aminotransferase; its serum levels begin to rise some 12 hours after infarction and reach a peak on the first or second day.

The development of these methods of measurement and of the increased understanding they gave, was preceded by a great deal of purely clinical descriptive cardiology. The first description of what later came to be known as 'Da Costa's syndrome' or the 'effort syndrome' of Sir Thomas Lewis was given in 1870 in a paper *On the etiology and prevalence of diseases of the heart among soldiers*[2045] by Arthur Bowen Myers (1838-1921). The actual paper of Jacob Mendes Da Costa (1833-1900) on this syndrome was entitled *On irritable heart; a clinical study of a form of functional cardiac disorder and its consequences*[2046]; it appeared in 1871 and showed that, from the beginning, the 'functional' or non-organic nature of the syndrome was recognized. The condition was to become of much prominence during the Great War.

Two of the cardiac murmers of diagnostic value date from the period when this syndrome was described. In 1871, Charles Hilton Fagge (1838-1883), in a paper *On the murmurs attendant on mitreal contraction*[2047], gave an excellent account of presystolic murmurs. In 1879, in Paris, Henri Roger (1809-1891) gave a good account of the congenital interventricular septal defect ('maladie de Roger')[2048] and described its characteristic murmur. The more complicated congenital defect of 'Fallot's tetralogy' was described by Etienne Louis Fallot (1850-1911) in 1888[2049]; it comprises pulmonary stenosis, ventricular septal defect, dextroposition of the aorta which overrides this defect, and right ventricular hypertrophy. Fallot described it as 'la maladie bleu (cyanose cardiaque) and this serves as a reminder that the tetralogy is the most common form of cyanotic congenital heart disease in children or adults.

Another of the classical murmurs was then described – this time by Graham Steell (1851-1942) whose paper of 1888-89, *The murmur of high-pressure in the pulmonary artery*[2050], provided the first description of this early diastolic murmur which occurs in the uncommon condition of pulmonary regurgitation and which is usually due to pulmonary hypertension. The 'Eisenmenger syndrome', with the congenital aortic abnormality overriding the patent interventricular septum and associated with right ventricular enlargement, was described in 1897[2051].

The first description of 'coronary thrombosis' diagnosed before death was given by Adam Hammer (1818-1878) in a German publication of 1878[2052]. This was followed by the initial account of myocardial infarction (*Ueber die pathologische Gerinnungs-Vorgänge*)[2053], given by Carl Weigert (1845-1904) in 1880. Osler, as has already been noted, gave the full description of subacute bacterial endocarditis in 1885[2009].

John MacWilliam (1857-1937) published on *Fibrillar contraction of the heart* in 1887[2054], thus discovering that fibrillation is due to a rapid sequence of uncoordinated contractions and clearly differentiating between auricular and ventricular fibrillation. In a paper on *Cardiac failure and sudden death*[2055] of 1889, MacWilliam gave the first recorded description of death resulting from ventricular fibrillation. The further arrhythmia of paroxysmal tachycardia was described by Léon Bouveret (1851-1929) in 1889[2056] and then 'Broadbent's sign', intercostal recession due to an adherent pericardium, was described in 1895[2057]. 'Ewart's sign' of pulmonary collapse at the left base in pericardial effusion was described by William Ewart (1848-1929) in 1896[2058] and in the same year Friedel Pick (1867-1926) gave an account of the cardiac type of pseudocirrhosis which has come to be called 'Pick's disease'[2059].

Thus, by the end of the nineteenth century, some forms of functional heart disease (psychoneurotic heart disease) had been described along with some of the classic murmurs of the valvular lesions, and the most obvious forms of arrhythmia. The commonest form of cyanotic congenital heart disease had been recognized, a good account of subacute bacterial endocarditis had been given, and the initial account of myocardial infarction had been written.

At the beginning of the twentieth century, Karl Albert Aschoff (1866-1942) published *Zur Myocarditisfrage*[2060] in 1904, so giving the classical account of rheumatic myocarditis and describing the characteristic lesion of the 'Aschoff nodule'. Auricular flutter was first described in the paper of 1905-06 by William Ritchie (1873-1945) on *Complete heart-block, with dissociation of the action of the auricles and ventricles*[2061]. Work up to the outbreak of the Great War then added considerably to the knowledge of the arrhythmias, bacterial endocarditis, and myocardial infarction.

Sir James Mackenzie, in papers on *New methods of studying affections of the heart* (1905)[2062] and in his *Diseases of the heart*[2063] of 1908 showed the action of digitalis in controlling the rate of auricular fibrillation and Arthur Cushny (1866-1926) published with Charles Edmunds (1873-1941) an essay of 1906 describing the first human study of auricular fibrillation, this having been observed in a case under their care in 1901[2064]. Sir Thomas Lewis, in 1909, wrote on *Auricular fibrillation; a common clinical condition*[2065] and William Jolly (1878-1939) with William Ritchie, in 1910, gave an account of *Auricular flutter and fibrillation*[2066]. In 1914, Karel Wenckebach (1864-1940) showed the value of quinine in treating some forms of fibrillation[2067] and 4 years later Walter Frey showed that quinidine was the most effective of the cinchona alkaloids in this effect[2068].

Of the cardiovascular infections, *Treponema pallidum* was first demonstrated in a diseased aorta (*Ueber Spirochaete pallida in der Aortenwand bei Hellerscher Aortitis*, 1906)[2069] by Karl Reuter. Osler's *Chronic infectious endocarditis* (1908-09)[2014], the 1909 classical paper on *Infective endocarditis, with an analysis of 150 cases*[2070] by Baron Thomas Jeeves Horder (1871-1955), and the 1910 publication on *The etiology of subacute infective endocarditis*[2071] by Emanuel Libman (1872-1946) and Herbert Celler (1878-1928) all antedate the First World War – as does the German paper by Hugo Schottmüller which, in 1910, showed that this author (who called the condition 'Endocarditis lenta') had become the first to isolate *Streptococcus viridans* from cases of subacute bacterial endocarditis[2072].

The first adequate description of bundle-branch block appears in *Zur Klinik des Elektrokardiogramms* (1910)[2073] by Hans Eppinger (1879-1946) and Oscar Stoerk (1870-1926) but the most significant development of the immediately pre-war period was the improved knowledge of coronary heart disease. The first complete account of coronary thrombosis with an ante-mortem diagnosis confirmed by autopsy was given in the paper *Zur Kenntniss der Thrombose der Koronararterien des Herzens*[2074] of 1910 by Vasilii Obraztsov (1849-1920) and Nikolai Strazhesko (1876-1952). The most distinguished full description in English is the study, *Clinical features of sudden obstruction of the coronary arteries*[2075], which appeared in the *Journal of the American Medical Association* in 1912 and was written by James Bryan Herrick (1861-1954).

Thus, the doctors of the World War I era knew of coronary thrombosis. They also met with cases of 'Da Costa's syndrome', called the 'effort syndrome' by Sir Thomas Lewis who, in 1917, wrote the official *Report upon soldiers returned as cases of 'disordered action of the heart' (D.A.H.) or 'valvular disease of the heart' (V.D.H.)*[2076]. Under one or other of these synonyms or euphemisms some soldiers with cardiac manifestations of what might now be considered to be psychoneurosis must have returned, hurt in their own way, from the war.

Between the wars, in the period starting with the first description of the heart in myxoedema (*Das Myxödemherz*)[2077] in 1918 by Hermann Zondek (1887-1979), the Keith-Wagener-Barker classification of the different types of essential hypertension appeared in 1929[2078], the Wolff-Parkinson-White syndrome was described in a paper on *Bundle-branch block with short P-R interval in healthy young people prone to paroxysmal tachycardia*[2079] of 1930, Sir Thomas Lewis wrote a classic account of vasovagal syncope and the carotid sinus mechanism in 1932[2080], and Henry Wagener and Norman Keith gave their diagnostically-important account of the grades of hypertensive retinopathy in a publication of 1939 on *Diffuse arteriolar disease with hypertension and the associated retinal lesions*[2081].

The mid-point of the century was marked by Ronald Christie's paper on *Penicillin in subacute bacterial endocarditis. Report to the Medical Research Council on 269 patients treated in 14 centres appointed by the Penicillin Clinical Trials Committee*[2082]. This report, of 1948, marked out one of the more spectacular pieces of progress in therapeutics of the era; it also represented one of the early great multicentre clinical trials which, organized by the MRC, became classics in their own right.

Myron Prinzmetal and his colleagues, in 1950, produced their notable paper on the *Mechanism of the auricular arrhythmias*[2083] and, in the same year, the great British cardiologist, Paul Hamilton Wood (1907-1962) offered a new and important classification in his study of *Congenital heart disease*[2084]. The external cardiac pacemaker, now so widely used, was brought in by Paul Maurice Zoll in his account, *Resuscitation of the heart in ventricular standstill by external electric stimulation*[2085], of 1952.

The experimental approaches to cardiology included the 'double-perfusion pump'[2086], an early (1928) attempt at producing a mechanical heart, by Sir Henry Dale (1875-1968) and Edgar Schuster (1899-1969), and the famous experiments of Harry Goldblatt whose first paper of the series was *Studies on experimental hypertension. 1. The production of persistent elevation of systolic blood pressure by means of renal ischemia*[2087]. This work with the Goldblatt clamp preceded, by 3 years, the 1937 report of Bernardo Houssay (1887-1971) and Juan Fasciolo showing that transplantation of a kidney from a hypertensive animal into a bilaterally nephrectomized animal would produce hypertension in the recipient animal[2088]. The same workers continued their studies and showed that the ischaemic kidneys of hypertensive dogs were a potent source of renin. Clifford Wilson and Frank Byrom produced their paper on *Renal changes in malignant hypertension; experimental evidence*[2089] in 1939 and this showed that, in the rat, experimental hypertension associated with renal arteriolar degeneration could be induced by unilateral constriction of a renal artery. This work led the way for the two great papers of 1940 – that on *The substance causing renal hypertension*[2090] by Eduardo Braun-Menendez, Juan Fasciolo and others, and the other reporting *A crystalline substance (angiotonin) resulting from the reaction between renin and renin-activator*[2091] by Irving Page and O. M. Helmer. Each of these papers announced the independent discovery of angiotensin, at first called angiotonin – a discovery leading to the introduction in recent years of the antihypertensive angiotensin-converting enzyme inhibitors.

The surgery of the heart goes back further than might perhaps be expected. Ludwig Rehn (1849–1930) is said to have been the first to achieve success in suturing a wound in the human heart (1896)[2092]. In Paris, Mathieu Jaboulay (1860–1913), in 1900, produced a paper on the *Chirurgie du grand sympathique et du corps thyroïde*[2093] recording his performance of sympathectomy. In 1905, Alexis Carrel (1873–1944) and Charles Guthrie (1880–1963) wrote on *The transplantation of veins and organs*[2094] after undertaking experimental cardiac transplantation in dogs. Alexis Carrel, in publications of 1902[2095] and 1907[2096] described his technique for the end-to-end anastomosis of divided arteries; in 1908[2097] and 1910[2098], seemingly years ahead of his time, this brilliant worker showed that it was possible to preserve segments of blood vessels in cold storage and some weeks later transplant them successfully.

French surgeons continued to make considerable progress with this subject, Eugène Doyen (1859–1916) discussing the *Chirurgie des malformations congénitales ou acquises du coeur*[2099] in 1913, Théodore Tuffier (1857–1929) providing an *Etude expérimentelle sur la chirurgie des valvules du coeur*[2100] in 1914, and Paul Hallopeau (1876–1924) recording *Un cas de cardiolyse*[2101] in 1921. These three publications gave accounts of Doyen's initial attempt at the surgery of congenital pulmonary stenosis, Tuffier's experiments to relieve chronic valvular disease, and Hallopeau's first pericardiectomy for constrictive pericarditis.

There is an historic paper, *Cardiotomy and valvulotomy for mitral stenosis. Experimental observations and clinical notes concerning an operated case with recovery*[2102], written by Elliott Cutler (1888–1947) and Samuel Levine in 1923 and describing, in Boston, the successful operative relief of mitral stenosis. Two years later, in 1925, the feat was repeated in England and Sir Henry Souttar (1875–1964) described a successful mitral valvotomy in a paper on *The surgical treatment of mitral stenosis*[2103] in the *British Medical Journal*.

The early attempts to provide surgical relief of cardiac ischaemia and severe angina pectoris included the implantation of part of the pectoral muscle into the pericardium[2104] and the attachment of a pedicled omental graft to the serous surface of the heart[2105]. The first of these methods of increasing blood flow and providing the means of a collateral circulation was devised by Claude Beck (1894–1971); the second technique was that of Laurence O'Shaughnessy (1900–1940).

By the time World War II began in 1939 work intended to permit open-heart surgery was well underway, and John Gibbon (1903–1973) in a report on *An oxygenator with a large surface–volume ratio* (1939)[2106], described the first successful use in an experimental animal of a heart–lung machine. The same year, Robert Gross and John Hubbard wrote on the *Surgical ligation of a patent ductus arteriosus: report of first successful case*[2107].

The year of the end of the war in Europe saw the appearance of three papers representing the attempts being made on both sides of the Atlantic to correct congenital heart disease. In America, Alfred Blalock (1899–1964) and Helen Taussig, one of the great pioneer teams of modern cardiac surgery, described the 'Blalock–Taussig' procedure; their paper was on *The surgical treatment of malformations of the heart in which there is pulmonary stenosis or pulmonary atresia*[2108]. Operative success with these operations was rewarded by improvement in the presenting cyanotic congenital heart disease. Clarence Crafoord and Karl Nylin wrote on *Congenital coarctation of the aorta and its surgical treatment*[2109] and Robert Gross on *Surgical correction for coarctation of the aorta*[2110]; these papers, both of 1945, introduced anastomotic procedures involving the aorta after resection of the coarctation.

In London, both Baron Russell Brock (1903–1980) and Sir Thomas Holmes Sellors wrote on the surgical treatment of pulmonary stenosis in 1948. Brock's account was of *Pulmonary valvulotomy for the relief of congenital pulmonary stenosis*[2111]; Holmes Sellors' was of *Surgery of pulmonary stenosis. A case in which the pulmonary valve was successfully divided*[2112]. In the same year (1948), in America, Edward Bland and Richard Sweet reported the first pulmonary-azygos vein operation in a paper describing *A venous shunt for marked mitral stenosis*[2113].

One of the historic works, one which marked the beginning of effective open heart surgery, was John Gibbon's *Application of a mechanical heart and lung apparatus to cardiac surgery*[2114], of 1954. This is almost exactly 30 years ago and followed from Gibbon's work, already noticed, of 1939. Successive publications, representing the progress since that time, include *Controlled cross circulation for direct-vision intracardiac surgery; correction of ventricular septal defects, atrio-ventricularis communis, and tetralogy of Fallot*[2115] by Clarence Lillehei in 1955; *Homologous aortic-valve-segment transplants as surgical treatment for aortic and mitral insufficiency*[2116] by Gordon Murray (1894–1976), describing the first successful aortic valve homograft in 1956; *Clinical use of an elastic Dacron prosthesis*[2117] by D. Emerick Szilagyi and his colleagues, reporting the use of an arterial prosthesis in 1958, and – as part of the animal surgical studies which have formed the basis for advances in clinical technique – the paper, *Studies on orthotopic homotransplantation of the canine heart*[2118], by Richard Lower and Norman E. Shumway in 1960. These authors reported several cardiac homotransplants performed in the dog.

The last two decades have seen the mitral valve replacement by the shielded ball valve prosthesis[2119] introduced in 1961 by Albert Starr and M. Lowell Edwards and homograft replacements of the aortic valve separately reported by Donald Ross in 1962[2120] and Sir Brian Barratt-Boyes in 1964[2121]. The first heart transplant in man was performed on December 3rd, 1967 by Christiaan Barnard whose paper *A human cardiac transplant: an interim report of a successful operation performed at Groote Schuur Hospital, Cape Town*[2122] appeared in the *South African Medical Journal* in the same year.

The first description of periarteritis nodosa was given by Adolf Kussmaul (1822–1902) and Rudolf Maier (1824–1888) as early as 1866[2123]. Of the other well-known diseases of the arteries, Felix von Winiwarter (1852–1931) gave an early account of what later came to be known as 'Buerger's disease' in 1879[2124]; Johann Mönckeberg (1877–1925) described 'Mönckeberg's medial sclerosis' in 1903[2125], and, in America, Leo Buerger (1879–1943) produced his classic paper on *Thrombo-angiitis obliterans; a study of the vascular lesions leading to presenile spontaneous gangrene*[2126] in 1908. This paper not only gave its present name to the disease but also provided the first full clinical and pathological account of it.

The use of nitrites for appropriate coronary artery indications started well before the end of the nineteenth century, Sir Thomas Lauder Brunton's report *On the use of nitrite of amyl in angina pectoris*[2127] introducing the use of amyl nitrite in 1867 and the paper on *Nitro-glycerine as a remedy for angina pectoris* by William Murrell (1853–1912) bringing trinitrin, glyceryl trinitrate, into practical therapeutics in 1879[2128].

Studies on experimental arteriosclerosis also began earlier than might perhaps have been expected. Alexander Ignatovski, in Russia, produced arteriosclerosis in rabbits fed a diet of milk and egg yolk and published the results in 1908 (there is a French translation of the same year)[2129]; Nikolai Anitschkov and S. S. Chalatov produced experimental arteriosclerosis with a cholesterol-rich diet in 1913[2130] and discussed the pathological processes involved. The history of the descriptions of cor pulmonale is interesting for the condition ('Ayerza's disease') was described[2131] in 1901 in lectures given by Abel Ayerza. He noted the cyanosis, dyspnoea, erythrocytosis and pulmonary artery changes characteristic of the condition but did not publish his findings. These were given in a thesis, *Cardiacos negros*[2132], produced in Buenos Aires in 1912 by Francisco Arrilaga and the disease was further discussed by Luis Ayerza in papers of 1925[2133].

The great study of angina pectoris was Sir James Mackenzie's fine book[2134] of 1923 which appeared a year before Martin Kirschner (1879–1942) published his paper on pulmonary embolectomy (*Ein durch die Trendelenburgsche Operation geheilter Fall von Embolie der Art. pulmonalis*)[2135] – thus adopting the heroic procedure suggested by Trendelenburg in 1908.

Of the treatments which remain in widespread use and antedate World War II, heparin is a notable example. Its clinical use as an anticoagulant was reported by Donald Murray and his colleagues in a paper, *Heparin and the thrombosis of veins following injury*[2136], of 1937.

Contrast radiographic methods of investigating the arterial tree in the living patient began with the first such angiogram in 1923[2137], the paper on *Intra-arterial injection of sodium iodid: preliminary report*[2138] by Barney Brooks in 1924 and, more recently, the 1962 study of *Cine-coronary arteriography*[2139] by Frank Sones and Earl K. Shirey. The latter work, on coronary arteriography, has been followed by important use of this technique.

In looking back at the rate of change in knowledge of the diseases of the cardiovascular system in the twentieth century, a number of drugs acting on the heart and vascular channels have already been mentioned. Those of the digitalis series remain among the more important. These glycosides have been studied throughout the century – an early example being the paper of 1904 by Max Cloetta (1868–1940), *Ueber Digalen (Digitoxinum solubile)*[2140], which introduced digalen. Digitoxin (Digitoxinum, *IP*) has already been mentioned as having the actions and uses of digitalis although, unlike digitalis, it is completely and readily absorbed when given by mouth. It is the most potent of the digitalis glycosides and the most cumulative in action. There is a Digalen-Neo in the Russian Pharmacopoeia; it is a purified aqueous extract of the leaves of *Digitalis ferruginea* of the Scrophulariaceae and is used in the USSR as it has similar actions and toxic effects to digitalis.

The work of the early part of the century on the cardiac glycosides continued with a notable study of 1916 by Walter Straub (1874–1944) who examined the effect of digitalis on the isolated frog heart[2141]. Between the World Wars, Arthur R. Cushny (1866–1926), when he was professor of pharmacology in the University of Edinburgh, wrote a full-length monograph on *The action and uses in medicine of digitalis and its allies*[2142]. Sydney Smith, in what many would think one of the most important papers to come from the laboratories of the Wellcome organization, followed Cushny's book of 1925 with a fundamental paper of 1930 on *Digoxin, a new digitalis glucoside*[2143]. This paper announced the isolation of digoxin from *Digitalis lanata*, Smith referring to work which had shown that the potency of the leaves of *Digitalis lanata* could be 3.5–4 times that of '*Digitalis purpurea*, the species used in medicine'. Digoxin has largely replaced all other digitalis preparations in Western medicine for it is readily and almost completely absorbed from the gastrointestinal tract and is rapidly distributed in the tissues; the drug is reported to have a half-life of 34–51 hours and it is excreted more rapidly and is less cumulative than digitalis.

Of the fairly early antihypertensive agents, reserpine is of special interest and remains widely used in North America. In the *Indian Journal of Medical Research*, October 1933, Ram Nath Chopra, J.C. Gupta and B. Mukherjee reported *The pharmacological action of an alkaloid obtained from Rauwolfia serpentia Benth. A preliminary note*[2144]. These authors reviewed the place of the drug in Indian folk-lore and, discussing 'its well-marked hypnotic and sedative properties' remarked 'No mention of these properties occurs in the old literature on Indian medicinal plants. The hypnotic and sedative action of the drug, however, appears to have been known to the poorer classes in Bihar and the practice of putting children to sleep by this drug is stated to be still present in certain parts of that province.' Having extracted a crystalline alkaloid from *Rauwolfia serpentina*, Chopra and his colleagues reached conclusions which included the following:

> The alkaloid is toxic to *Paramœcium caudatum* in concentrations of 1 in 20,000 and more. Its toxicity varies with different species of animals. The lethal doses for frogs, white mice, guinea-pigs and cats have been determined.
>
> The alkaloid has a stimulant effect on the plain muscle of the intestine and the uterus.
>
> The systemic blood-pressure falls due to dilatation of the blood vessels of the splanchnic area. The respiration is depressed, death occurring from failure of respiration due to the paralysing effect of the alkaloid on the respiratory centre.

The alkaloid has a pronounced effect on the central nervous system. In sublethal doses injected into the lymph sac of frogs narcosis quickly ensues. In mammals the alkaloid produces symptoms which are attributable to its depressing effect on various cerebral centres in the reverse order of their development. The short period of excitement seen in guinea-pigs and cats is probably due to the dissolution of the higher centres as is so often seen with morphine, chloroform and alcohol. There is also evidence to show that there is some depression of all nerve-cells in the body.

The alkaloid on account of its cerebral depressant properties should prove to be a valuable sedative drug. Its depressive effect on the respiratory centre should, however, be borne in mind. It lowers the blood-pressure and if administered in proper dosage should be of value as a remedy against hyperpiesis. Purgation is usually produced by the drug on account of its stimulant properties on the plain muscles of the gastro-intestinal tract. Its stimulant effect on the uterine movements, both virgin and pregnant, coupled with its pain-relieving properties should be useful during parturition. The drug is likely to be a valuable addition to the armamentarium of physicians and further work to place it on a definite therapeutic basis is in progress.

The possibilities of the alkaloid aroused industrial interest and, in 1952, from the laboratories of Ciba, Basel, J. M. Müller and co-workers reported that they had isolated the sedative principle of *Rauwolfia serpentia* Benth. in pure, crystalline form and studied its chemistry and pharmacology[2145].

Reserpine is now obtained from its natural sources or by synthesis. It has central depressant and sedative actions and an antihypertensive effect which is primarily peripheral in nature and accompanied by bradycardia. Its pharmacological effect is profound and results in depletion of noradrenaline stores in the peripheral sympathetic nerve terminals with depletion of the catecholamine and serotonin stores in the brain, heart and other organs. Its use in agitated pyschoses and in anxiety states has disappeared with the recognition that the doses needed can produce gross depression. It remains in use in treating mild hypertension, usually in combination with other suitable agents. Its most frequent side-effects include nasal congestion and gastrointestinal disturbances; it can produce suicidal depression, so that the lowest possible doses must be used. Some reports have proposed an association between the use of reserpine and breast neoplasia but the literature remains controversial; it is well reviewed by Martindale[2146].

Of the enyzmes which can possibly be used to effect fibrinolysis in the presence of intravascular thrombosis or coagulation, streptokinase has been most widely studied. This substance was recognized as a product of the growth of some haemolytic streptococci by William Tillett and Raymond Garner whose paper, *The fibrinolytic activity of hemolytic streptococci*[2147], was published in 1933. The work of these authors was elegant and, from the first, noted not only the identification of the action of a fibrinolytic principle but also its inactivation by natural immunological interactions and its inefficacy in the presence of a species-specific effect:

Broth cultures of hemolytic streptococci derived from patients are capable of rapidly liquefying normal human fibrin clot.

The active fibrinolytic principle is also contained in sterile, cell-free filtrates of broth cultures. The degree of activity of filtrates parallels the activity of whole broth cultures sufficiently closely to indicate that large amounts of the fibrinolytic substance are freely excreted into the surrounding medium and pass readily through Berkefeld V, Seitz, and Chamberland filters.

The plasma of many patients recovered from acute hemolytic streptococcus infections, when clotted in the presence of active cultures, is highly resistant to fibrinolysis. Furthermore, serum, derived from patients whose plasma clot is resistant, often confers on normal plasma clot an antifibrinolytic property.

In contrast to the susceptibility of normal human fibrin clot to liquefaction by active culture, normal rabbit fibrin clot is totally resistant to dissolution when tested under comparable conditions. The insusceptibility of rabbit fibrin clot is manifest provided the coagulum is composed of rabbit constituents. When human thrombin is used to clot rabbit plasma or fibrinogen in the present of active cultures, fibrinolysis is not prohibited. The rôle of thrombin in determining the resistance or susceptibility of rabbit fibrin to dissolution offers a suggestive approach to problems relating to the underlying mechanism.

Lauritz Christensen (*Streptococcal fibrinolysis. A proteolytic reaction due to a serum enzyme activated by streptococcal fibrinolysin*)[2148] in 1945 achieved the preparation and partial purification of the streptococcal fibrinolysin (streptokinase) which Tillett and Garner had detected. Christensen also put forward the vital concept of activation, suggesting 'that lysin factor exists in serum or plasma as a zymogen, and that it is activated by fibrinolysin, a kinase, in a manner similar to the activation of trypsinogen by enterokinase...'

One of the more fertile concepts of the pre-World War II period was the theory of competitive drug antagonism first formulated by Sir John Henry Gaddum (1900–1965). Gaddum, then at the Wellcome Physiological Research Laboratories, in a paper on *The action of adrenalin and ergotamine on the uterus of the rabbit* (1926)[2149], studied the action of varying concentrations of adrenalin and ergotamine on an isolated rabbit uterus preparation. This work showed that when, with the drugs examined, response to the drug was plotted against the logarithm of the drug concentration then an S-shaped curve was obtained. Gaddum comments that:

> The form of the curve is that which would be obtained on the assumption that the drugs are acting on a number of units whose susceptibility is distributed about a mean in accordance with a probability curve – it is the curve of the integral of the normal distribution.

Gaddum's later paper, of 1937, on *The quantitative effect of antagonistic drugs*[2150], investigated the laws by which the effects of drug antagonism could be expressed mathematically. He now showed that the S-shaped curve could be 'interpreted on the theory that the muscle contains a number of receptors with different thresholds, and that the logarithms of the thresholds of these receptors are normally distributed'. Competitive antagonism is now seen to be involved in the action of many drugs, including in some circumstances the sulphonamides, and Gaddum's work and contribution to receptor theory was of importance.

These pharmacological advances have been accompanied by studies elucidating complex chemical structures. One example is the work, recognized by the Nobel Prize in 1982, in which Sune Bergström and colleagues explored the chemical structure of the prostaglandins. The first of a series of papers was the study by Bergström and others on *The structure of prostaglandin E, F_1 and F_2*[2151] of 1962. At an earlier date, Bergström, working with U. S. von Euler and U. Hamberg, had reported the *Isolation of noradrenaline from the adrenal gland* (1949)[2152]. Noradrenaline was also independently isolated by B. F. Tullar (1950).

The most remarkable exponent of drug design using receptor theory and antagonism at receptor sites has been Sir James Whyte Black. In 1962, with J. S. Stephenson, Black reported the development of pronethalol, a specific adrenergic β-receptor antagonist relatively free from sympathomimetic activity on the cardiovascular system. Pronethalol, the lead candidate of the β-blocking anti-hypertensive, antianginal, antiarrhythmic drugs of today, was discarded due to clinical side-effects and the finding that it produced, in the mouse but not in the rat or dog, lymphosarcomas and reticulum-cell sarcomas. With pronethalol, these sarcomas were first seen in the thymus and began to appear, in the mice, after 10 weeks treatment.

A large number of compounds were then made and tested in order to develop a drug candidate with a wider therapeutic ratio and with no carcinogenic potential. Black and his colleagues, in a paper of 1964 on *A new adrenergic beta-receptor antagonist*[2153], introduced the resulting drug, propranolol. It was shown to be about ten times as active as pronethalol in blocking the inotropic action of isoprenaline in laboratory systems; it was also free of carcinogenic effect in a study of 66 weeks duration in mice. Propranolol became the compound which introduced the concept of the adrenergic β-blockers into practical clinical medicine. It thus has a major place in the history of twentieth century medicine. Known at the time by its laboratory designation, ICI 45,520, it was the product of the ingenious concept developed by Black at Alderley Park, Cheshire.

Propranolol has now been augmented by an extensive range of adrenergic β-blocking drugs, the more interesting of which are cardioselective in action; however, it remains in important and widespread use and there is now an extensive experience of its usefulness and safety. It features in the main list of the World Health Organization's Technical Report Series number 641.

This report, *The selection of essential drugs*[2154], was the second report of a WHO Expert Committee; it appeared in 1979 and provided a model list of essential drugs. It was expected that individual countries could use the list as a basis for identifying their own priorities in providing drug remedies. Clearly, the model list can also be used by the individual practitioner in identifying a personal pharmacopoeia.

The WHO selection provides a main list and a complementary list of alternatives. In some cases the drug listed is given as an example of a therapeutic category so that the least expensive available drug product in the category can be chosen. The main list for drugs affecting the blood and for cardiovascular drugs is the following:

Drugs affecting the blood
    Antianaemia drugs
        ferrous salt
        folic acid
        hydroxocobalamin

Anticoagulants and antagonists
  heparin
  phytomenadione
  protamine sulphate
  warfarin

Cardiovascular drugs
  Antianginal drugs
    glyceryl trinitrate
    isosorbide dinitrate
    propranolol
  Antiarrhythmic drugs
    lidocaine
    procainamide
    propranolol
  Antihypertensive drugs
    hydralazine
    hydrochlorothiazide
    propranolol
    sodium nitroprusside
  Cardiac glycosides
    digoxin
  Drugs used in shock or anaphylaxis
    dopamine
    epinephrine

This list can be compared with the contents of the *British Pharmacopoeia 1914*[2155]. This was the fifth BP and the preface noted that the General Council of Medical Education and Registration of the United Kingdom, in preparing the pharmacopoeia, had received 'through His Majesty's Privy Council, with the co-operation of the India Office and the Colonial Office, much help from the Dominions overseas...' It had thus been able to 'produce a British Pharmacopoeia suitable for the whole Empire'. The divisions of the British Empire which were to be dosed with the contents of the BP at the time of the outbreak of World War I were the following:

DIVISIONS OF THE BRITISH EMPIRE REFERRED TO IN
THE BRITISH PHARMACOPŒIA

India.—Ajmer-Merwara, The Andamans, Assam, Bengal, Bihar and Orissa, Bombay, Baluchistan, Burma, The Central Provinces and Berar, Coorg, Delhi, Madras, The North-West Frontier Province, the Punjab, United Provinces of Agra and Oudh.

African.—Basutoland, Bechuanaland Protectorate, Gambia, Gold Coast, Nigeria, Northern Rhodesia, Southern Rhodesia, Saint Helena, Sierra Leone, Swaziland, The Union of South Africa (provinces of Cape of Good Hope, Natal, Orange Free State, Transvaal).

Australasian.—New South Wales, Queensland, South Australia, Tasmania, Victoria, Western Australia, Northern Territory of Australia, Federal Capital Territory; forming the Commonwealth of Australia. New Zealand, Fiji Islands, Papua, Western Pacific.

544

Eastern.—Ceylon, Hong Kong, Labuan, Mauritius, Seychelles, Straits Settlements, Weihaiwei.

Mediterranean.—Cyprus, Gibraltar, Malta.

North American.—Alberta, British Columbia, Manitoba, New Brunswick, North-west Territories, Nova Scotia, Ontario, Prince Edward Island, Quebec, Saskatchewan, Yukon; forming the Dominion of Canada. Newfoundland.

West Indian.—Bahama Islands, Barbados, Bermuda Islands, British Guiana, British Honduras, Jamaica and Turks and Caicos Islands, Leeward Islands (Antigua, Dominica, Montserrat, Saint Christopher and Nevis, Virgin Islands), Trinidad and Tobago, Windward Islands (Grenada, Saint Lucia, Saint Vincent).

The Falkland Islands in the South Atlantic.

Looking through the long list of monographs of the BP 1914, the substances which might seem of use in difficult circumstances include: acetylsalicylic acid, phenol, salicylic acid, hydrous wool fat, adrenalin, purified ether, absolute alcohol, amyl nitrite, distilled water, toughened caustic, atropine sulphate, barbitone, calcium phosphate, chloral hydrate, chloroform, cocaine, codeine phosphate, flexible collodion, prepared chalk, diamorphine hydrochloride, digitalis leaves, ethyl chloride, liquid extract of male fern, ferrous sulphate, glucose, homatropine hydrobromide, hyoscine hydrobromide, hypodermic injection of ergot, hypodermic injection of morphine, iodine, ipecacuanha root, discs of homatropine, discs of physostigmine, lemon peel, solution of hydrogen peroxide, lithium carbonate, light magnesium carbonate, methyl salicylate, methylsulphonal, morphine hydrochloride, chaulmoogra oil, cod-liver oil, olive oil, opium, paraldehyde, pill of quinine sulphate, potassium bicarbonate, potassium iodide, refined sugar, santonin, hard soap, soft soap, senna pods, sodium bicarbonate, sodium carbonate, sodium chloride, sodium salicylate, lemon juice, trinitrin tablets, dry thyroid, strong tincture of iodine, salicylic acid ointment, tar ointment, sulphur ointment, zinc ointment and sherry.

This list is generous to the BP 1914. Today's doctor would surely be troubled to be limited to such a pharmacopoeia and, in terms of the drugs which affect the blood and cardiovascular system, the rate of progress has been such that the list of useful things from the BP 1914 and the WHO list of essential drugs of 1979 have only two items in common – these are ferrous sulphate and glyceryl trinitrate. In addition, the doctor of 1914 had digitalis in place of digoxin.

The respiratory system

Considering its difficulties the surgery of the lower respiratory tract infections seems to have begun rather earlier than might be expected. The first thoracotomy for empyema thoracis was undertaken by Ernst Küster (1839–1930) as early as 1889[2156]. The first thoracoplasty was undertaken by George Fowler (1848–1906) in 1893; the operation was performed in order to remove a large cicatricial fibrous mass resulting from an old empyema[2157]. Decortication of the lung as a treatment for chronic empyema was introduced by Edmond Delorme (1847–1929) in Paris in 1894[2158]. The first surgeon successfully to remove bronchiectatic lobes was Werner Körte (1853–1937) in 1909[2159].

Pneumonectomy and lobectomy when the lung was not necessarily fixed and adherent was developed in the decade beginning about 1930. Harold Brunn (1874-1950) wrote on the *Surgical principles underlying one-stage lobectomy*[2160] in 1929 and in Germany Rudolph Nissen described the successful excision of a bronchiectatic lung in 1931[2161]. The first pneumonectomy for malignancy was undertaken in America and reported by Evarts Graham (1883-1957) and Jacob Singer (1882-1954) in a paper, *Successful removal of entire lung for carcinoma of the bronchus*[2162], in 1933. In the same year, Howard Lilienthal (1861-1946) reported a *Pneumonectomy for sarcoma of the lung in a tuberculous patient*[2163].

Refinement of clinical descriptions took place in the first third of the century in parallel with those being written regarding cardiovascular disease. In 1903, Charles Emerson (1872-1938) wrote an account of *Pneumothorax; a historical, clinical, and experimental study*[2164] in *Johns Hopkins Hospital Reports*. William Pasteur (1856-1943) discovered and described atelectasis (*The Bradshaw Lecture on massive collapse of the lung*)[2165] in 1908. In a paper on *The nature of the 'oat-celled sarcoma' of the mediastinum* (1926)[2166], William Barnard (1892-1956) showed that this tumour was secondary to primary bronchial carcinoma. Of the allergic conditions, John Campbell, in 1932, described 'Farmer's lung' in a study of *Acute symptoms following work with hay*[2167]. In the next year, in the *Proceedings of the Mayo Clinic*, Charles Maytum gave an account of the hyper-ventilation syndrome (*Tetany caused by functional dyspnea with hyperventilation: report of a case*)[2168].

Of the now standard investigative techniques, direct bronchoscopy was introduced at the close of the nineteenth century by Gustav Killian (1860-1921) whose paper *Ueber directe Bronchoskopie*[2169] was dated 1898. Bronchography was begun in animals and then extended into clinical use: Charles Waters and a group of colleagues described *Roentgenography of the lung; roentgenographic studies in living animals after intratracheal injection of iodoform emulsion*[2170] in 1917 and this was followed, again using the intratracheal route for the contrast medium, by Jean Sicard (1872-1929) and Jacques Forestier in 1924[2171].

Work on the transmission of the common cold began before World War I and produced the report *Die Erreger von Husten und Schnupfen*[2172] of 1914 in which Walther Kruse (1864-1943) showed that colds could be transmitted to volunteers by intranasal instillation of cell-free filtrates of the nasal secretions of patients with colds. The detection of mycoplasma as a cause of human infection dates from somewhat later when, in 1937, Louis Dienes and Geoffrey Edsall reported on *Observations on L-organism of Klieneberger*[2173].

Prior to the availability of chemotherapy considerable efforts were made to find immunological methods of treatment. An example is the improved anti-pneumococcus serum described by Fred Neufeld (1861-1945) and Ludwig Haendel (1869-1939) in Germany in 1910[2174]. This work was contemporaneous with Ehrlich's development of the first agents of chemotherapy – agents which were to lessen interest in the antipneumococcal vaccines. Interest in the practical aspects of this subject continued until the use of antibiotics became widespread, Michael Heidelberger and Oswald Avery (1877-1955) studying the antigenic components of the pneumococcus and reporting on *The soluble specific substance of pneumococcus*[2175] in 1923 and 1924.

Other attempts at treatment included, for malignant lesions, the application of deep X-ray therapy. The positive findings include the report of Henri Coutard (1876–1950) who in 1921 described the cure of a carcinoma of the pharynx in a patient with secondary deposits in the lymphatic neck glands[2176].

Two of the medical treatments of the period soon after World War I remain in current use: David Israel Macht (1882–1961) and Giu-Ching Ting, in 1921, gave a pharmacological demonstration of the antispasmodic effect of theophylline on bronchial smooth muscle[2177]. The next year, in a clinical and experimental study, Samson Hirsch clearly demonstrated the value of this drug in the treatment of asthma[2178]. Then, in 1929, in *Guy's Hospital Reports,* Percy Camps (1877–1956) wrote *A note on the inhalation treatment of asthma*[2179] – this report recorded the first use of adrenaline by the respiratory route in the management of this condition.

Shortly before the Second World War, in 1936, Manoel de Abreu (1892–1962) introduced mass chest X-ray[2180]. Two years later, Gladys Evans and Wilfred Gaisford, in a *Lancet* paper on the *Treatment of pneumonia with 2-(p-amino-benzenesulphonamido) pyridine*[2181], introduced the historic compound M & B 693 (sulphapyridine) into the treatment of pneumonia. It is from this date, just before the second war, that the modern success in treating conditions such as lobar pneumonia can be said to have begun.

Since that time further clinical conditions and their causative agents have been described. Atypical pneumonia was described in America in 1938 by Hobart Reimann[2182], the 'Eaton agent' was isolated from cases of the condition and described, in 1944, by Monroe Eaton (*Studies on the etiology of primary atypical pneumonia. A Filterable agent transmissible to cotton rats, hamsters, and chick embryos)*[2183]; in 1962, Robert Chanock, showed that a mycoplasma was the cause of some cases of atypical pneumonia (*Growth on artificial medium of an agent associated with atypical pneumonia and its identification as a PPLO)*[2184]. Chanock has also shown the cause of the childhood infections due to the respiratory syncytial virus, describing this agent in a paper on *Recovery from infants with respiratory illness of a virus related to chimpanzee coryza agent (CCA)*[2185] of 1957.

Finally, the new form of pneumonia which has been the cause of widespread recent interest was given its first substantial account in the paper *Legionnaires' disease. Description of an epidemic of pneumonia*[2186] by David Fraser and eleven co-authors; in the following paper in the *New England Journal of Medicine,* Joseph McDade and his associates wrote on *Legionnaires' disease. Isolation of a bacterium and demonstration of its role in other respiratory diseases* (1977)[2187].

The surgery of the recent period has included the elegant dissection involved in the excision of individual bronchopulmonary segments. A notable paper on the subject is that of 1939 by Edward Delos Churchill (1895–1972) and Ronald Belsey (*Segmental pneumonectomy in bronchiectasis. The lingula segment of the left upper lobe)*[2188]. A convenient review of the subject at it presented up to 20 years ago is Richard Meade's *A history of thoracic surgery,* 1961[2189].

In terms of the Western World the greatest potential for lessening the mortality from respiratory disease must now lie in effective use of the findings which began when Franz Müller, as far back as 1939, found a statistically significant correlation between cigarette smoking and bronchial cancer[2190]. This finding has been confirmed in studies published in both Britain and America. Sir

Richard Doll and Sir Austin Bradford Hill reported the results of a comparison of 1465 cases of lung cancer and an equivalent number of matched controls in a paper on *Smoking and carcinoma of the lung. Preliminary report*[2191] published in the *British Medical Journal* in 1950; they confirmed their findings in later papers of 1952, 1956 and 1964. Ernest Wynder and Evarts Graham (1883–1957) established an association between prolonged, heavy cigarette smoking and bronchial carcinoma and published their findings, *Tobacco smoking as a possible etiologic factor in bronchogenic carcinoma*[2192], in the *Journal of the American Medical Association* in 1950.

Pulmonary tuberculosis is the disease which, as vividly as any other, shows the benefits of modern chemotherapy and the use of antibiotics. Until these new treatments transformed the clinical picture of the disease, its management depended largely on the sanatorium regime and the use of local methods of resting the lung in the hope that this would facilitate healing. The first to advocate the sanatorium treatment with rest and exposure to cold dry air was George Bodington (1799–1882) whose *Essay on the treatment and cure of pulmonary consumption*[2193] was published in London in 1840. Bodington's ideas met with an unsympathetic reception and it was not until 1859 that H. Brehmer established the first sanatorium at Görbersdorf.

The idea of inducing an artificial pneumothorax which would rest the lung by limiting its respiratory excursion was first discussed by Carlo Forlanini (1847–1918) in papers of 1882[2194]; he first adopted the technique in 1888 and there is an English translation of his contribution dated 1934–35. The emergency induction of an artificial pneumothorax by pleural incision was described in a paper of 1885, *A case of haemoptysis treated by the induction of pneumothorax so as to collapse the lung*[2195], by William Cayley (1836–1916).

As with other diseases of the chest, the early surgery remains somewhat remarkable. David Lowson (1850–1907), in a report on *A case of pneumonectomy*[2196] in 1893, described the treatment of a tuberculous patient. Théodore Tuffier (1857–1929), in Paris in 1897, described the excision of part of a lung in a book on the *Chirurgie du poumon en particulier dans les cavernes tuberculeuses et la gangrène pulmonaire*[2197]. Sir William Macewen (1848–1924), in an article *On some points in the surgery of the lung*[2198] in 1906, described the excision of a tuberculous left lung in 1895 of a patient who was still alive during World War II. And then, in 1908, Ludolph Brauer (1865–1951) gave an account of the first radical thoracoplasty[2199].

The typical feature of primary pulmonary tuberculosis, the 'Ghon focus' was first described, as early as 1876, by Joseph Parrot (1829–1883) who wrote on *Recherches sur les relations qui existent entre les lésions des poumons et celles des ganglions trachéo-bronchiques*[2200]. The features of the primary lesion of childhood, the peripheral discrete focus associated with infected hilar lymph glands, were again described by Anton Ghon (1866–1936). Ghon's book was called *Der primäre Lungenherd bei der Tuberkulose der Kinder*[2201]; it was published in 1912 but perhaps the English translation of 1916 led to Ghon's name becoming so firmly associated with the characteristic lesion.

Improvements in local therapy date from the period of World War I and the decade or two which followed. It was at this period that the sanatorium treatment was at its height, discipline being maintained despite a considerable mortality and the slow process of recovery being assisted by graded periods, measured by quite short periods of time, in which bed-rest was slowly replaced by sitting in a chair, walking, communal meals and a resumption of normal activity. The crushing or division of the phrenic nerve so that the paralysed hemi-diaphragm would restrict movement of the infected or cavitated lung was begun by Ernst Sauerbruch (1875–1951) in 1913[2202]. The operation whereby pleural adhesions were divided by a cautery so that an artificial pneumothorax could become effective was introduced by Hans Jacobaeus (1879–1937) in 1916[2203]. The artificial pneumo-peritoneum for the treatment of bilateral lung tuberculosis was introduced by Ludwig Vajda in 1933[2204] and, all three of these techniques having been developed by the German-speaking school, Andrew Banyai, in 1934, combined artificial pneumoperitoneum with phrenic nerve paralysis and published a paper on *Therapeutic pneumoperitoneum. A review of 100 cases*[2205] in the *American Review of Tuberculosis.*

The modern period of pulmonary resection for tuberculosis began with Samuel Freedlander's *Lobectomy in pulmonary tuberculosis. Report of a case*[2206] in 1935. In the same year, Carl Boye Semb described *Thoracoplasty with extrafascial apicolysis*[2207] – and this brought in the staged thoracoplasty in which the first stage provided for dissection of the 'Semb space' and limited rib resection, so splinting the difficult extreme lung apex by repositioning of the extrafascial chest wall structures. In a subsequent one or two stages, frequently under local anaesthesia, the thoraco-plasty was extended by further rib excision. It was this dissection of the Semb space which Sir Clement Price Thomas used to do so beautifully.

Of the textbooks of the era, the *Oxford University Press* volume of 1939, *Pulmonary tuberculosis. Pathology, diagnosis, management and prevention*[2208], by George Kayne (1901–1945), Walter Pagel and Laurence O'Shaughnessy, remains justifiably well-known. Its later edition, of 1935, was by Pagel, Simmonds, and Macdonald.

The two most dramatic aspects of the partial conquest of tuberculosis in the Western World have been the means of preventing the disease and its cure by chemotherapy. The decline in mortality due to tuberculosis proceeded, from 1900 to 1945, at about 3% per year in Britain. This was largely due to the better care of the public health and improvements in social conditions. Graphical expressions of this mortality show a marked break between 1945 and 1950 and, with the introduction of effective drug therapies, the annual reduction rose to approx-imately 15%. By 1960 the death rate was less than one-tenth that of 1940. As this change, due very largely to drug therapy, progressed, the specialty devoted to tuberculosis became reabsorbed within the profession and many of the chest hospitals and sanatoria became partly or completely converted to other purposes. Many of the clinical trials of the tuberculosis chemotherapies have an additional academic importance as exemplars of large-scale clinical research methodology.

One vastly important method of prevention has been the control of tuber-culosis in cattle and the avoidance of tuberculous milk carrying the bovine strain of the organism. A second means has been the isolation of infective human cases, detection by mass radiography, and such similar methods of hygiene. Of the immunological aspects, the diagnostic intradermal tuberculin test of Charles Mantoux (1877–1947) dates from this author's paper, *Intradermo-réaction de la tuberculine*[2209], of 1908.

The BCG (Bacille Calmette–Guérin) vaccine was first produced in 1906 and was subcultured for 13 years in order to produce a suitably attenuated strain. It was first used as a prophylactic agent against tuberculosis in children in 1921. Léon Charles Calmette (1863–1933), C. Guérin and B. Weill-Hallé published on the subject in their *Essai d'immunisation contre l'infection tuberculeuse*[2210] of 1924. Calmette and his colleagues provided a second important paper on their vaccine in 1927[2211].

The more modern adaptations of the diagnostic test for previous or present infection have included *The multiple-puncture tuberculin test*[2212] recorded by Frederick Roland Heaf (1894–1973) in 1951; the slightly later modification of the vaccine was announced in the paper of 1956 by Margaret Griffiths and Wilfrid Gaisford, who wrote on *Freeze-dried B.C.G. vaccination of newborn infants with a British vaccine*[2213].

The story of the chemotherapy of tuberculosis has to be ranked as one of the great embellishments of the twentieth century. In 1940, Selman Abraham Waksman (1888–1973), a Russian who had migrated to the United States and was working with H. B. Woodruff, discovered a new species of actinomyces; from it they isolated an antibiotic which they called actinomycin. This was found to have considerable antimicrobial activity but to be highly toxic.

In the same year William Hugh Feldman, H. C. Hinshaw and H. E. Moses, who had also been seeking drugs with antituberculous activity, published on *The effect of promin (sodium salt of P.P'-diamino-diphenyl-sulfone-N,N'-dextrose sulfonate) on experimental tuberculosis: a preliminary report* (1940)[2214]. Promin was sodium glucosulphone.

In 1944, Waksman, at Rutgers University, discovered another new species of fungus. This was later given the name *Streptomyces griseus* and from it Waksman isolated streptomycin, showing this to have a powerful antimicrobial action against a wide range of organisms and, more importantly, against the tubercule bacillus. Streptomycin was introduced by Albert Schatz, Elizabeth Bugie and Selman Waksman in a paper of early 1944, *Streptomycin, a substance exhibiting antibiotic activity against Gram-positive and Gram-negative bacteria*[2215], written from the New Jersey Agricultural Experiment Station, Rutgers University, Department of Soil Microbiology. Streptomycin was first tried out on a large scale in tuberculosis by another migrant to the United States, William Feldman, whose slightly earlier work on promin has already been noted. Feldman, originally of Glasgow, became professor of comparative pathology at the Mayo Foundation in the University of Minnesota. Horton Hinshaw and Feldman's paper on *Streptomycin in treatment of clinical tuberculosis: a preliminary report*[2216] appeared in the *Proceedings of the Mayo Clinic* in 1945. Feldman remained prominent in the work done to overcome the problems of resistance to streptomycin used in the treatment of tuberculosis. For his work on antibiotics and the streptomycin discovery, Waksman received a Nobel Prize in 1952.

It soon became obvious that the clinical improvement brought about by streptomycin was frequently transient: after some 6 or so weeks of treatment patients began to relapse and were found to produce strains of the tubercule bacillus resistant to the antibiotic. Then, in 1946, Jörgen Lehmann, a Swedish biochemist, showed that *para*-aminosalicylic acid (PAS) showed substantial activity against the tubercule bacillus both *in vitro* and in experimentally infected animals. Lehmann reported his findings in a paper, *Para-aminosalicyclic acid in the treatment of tuberculosis*[2217], in the *Lancet* of 1946 following an earlier communication to a Scandinavian journal. In the same year, Gerhard Domagk (1895–1964) and a group of co-workers introduced thiosemicarbazone[2218] in the treatment of tuberculosis and, in the *British Medical Journal*, Philip D'Arcy Hart produced an interesting review article on the *Chemotherapy of tuberculosis. Researches during the past 100 years*[2219]. Subsequent clinical trials by the Medical Research Council showed that streptomycin and PAS employed together provided a more effective means of treating the disease than either used alone and, moreover, combined use greatly delayed the emergence of resistant organisms. Once combination therapy with streptomycin and PAS was instituted there was a progressive decline in the mortality from reasonably acute and limited tuberculosis.

Further drugs continued to be discovered and, in 1949, Selman Waksman and Hubert Lechevalier reported the isolation of *Neomycin, a new antibiotic active against streptomycin-resistant bacteria, including tuberculosis organisms*[2220]. This agent was too toxic for any but topical use but in 1951 Alexander Finlay with 11 co-authors described *Viomycin, a new antibiotic active against mycobacteria*[2221]. Viomycin was discovered and developed independently by the industrial laboratories of Pfizer at Brooklyn, New York, and the Parke, Davis Company. It had a limited use as a reserve drug in tuberculosis.

In 1952 the third of the major antituberculous drugs was discovered. This was isoniazid, introduced by Edward Robitzek and his colleagues in a report, *Chemotherapy of human tuberculosis with hydrazine derivatives of isonicotinic acid (Preliminary report of representative cases)*[2222], in the *Quarterly Bulletin of the Sea View Hospital* for 1952. Major clinical trials, again organized by the Medical Research Council, soon showed the clinical activity of the drug. They also showed the need to use it in combination if resistance was to be delayed or prevented.

Ethionamide became known from the work of Noël Rist and his associates on *Experiments on the antituberculous activity of alpha-ethyl-thioisonicotinamide* (1959)[2223] and, in 1961, J. P. Thomas and his group announced yet another drug with useful activity in their paper, *A new synthetic compound with anti-tuberculous activity in mice: ethambutol (dextro-2,2'-(ethylenediimino)-di-l-butanol)*[2224].

Rifampicin is even more recent but has rapidly been acknowledged as one of the essential antituberculous drugs. Rifampicin and isoniazid are the most effective agents for the treatment of tuberculosis, although neither should ever be used alone due to the rapidity with which resistance develops. E. Atlas and M. Turck reported their *Laboratory and clinical evaluation of rifampicin*[2225] in 1968; C. M. Kunin and co-workers described their *Bacteriologic studies of rifampin, a new semisynthetic antibiotic*[2226] the following year. These studies showed that the drug inhibits the growth of most Gram-positive and many Gram-negative bacteria. The very considerable *in vitro* activity of the substance against the tubercule bacillus was shown by Verbist and Gyselen in 1968[2227] and by Lorian and Finland in 1969[2228]. The drug, as used clinically, is a semisynthetic derivative of rifamycin B, itself a member of the natural macrocyclic antibiotics produced by *Streptomyces mediterranei*.

This range of drugs permits the contemporary, and highly effective, therapy of tuberculosis. The current convention is for an initial phase, when at least three drugs are used to reduce the population of viable bacteria as rapidly as possible, and a continuation phase, using only two drugs, one of which, unless it is contraindicated, is always isoniazid. It is usually said that the treatment of choice in the initial phase, which is of at least 8 weeks duration, is the daily use of isoniazid and rifampicin augmented by ethambutol or streptomycin. Pyrazinamide can be added in order to achieve the most intense bactericidal effect possible during the initial phase. The second drug added to isoniazid during the continuation phase is usually rifampicin, ethambutol, or streptomycin. To those who knew tuberculosis before the advent of chemotherapy the most remarkable thing, apart from the response rate, is that when isoniazid and rifampicin are given daily throughout the treatment period, a 9-month course of therapy is adequate for the control of pulmonary tuberculosis, whatever its original extent; more intensive regimes can ensure that a 6-month course of treatment gives equally good results.

Parts of the pharmacopoeia

Even the most brief review of the landmarks in the progress of twentieth century cardiovascular and respiratory medicine shows how rapidly knowledge has advanced. In many of the infective diseases it has been exponential, providing a knowledge of the causative organisms and, in respect of many of the non-viral illnesses, reliable cures. In other areas, such as the arteriosclerotic degenerations of the great vessels and the pulmonary neoplasms of the non-smoker, knowledge of both causes and cures has advanced with much less assurance. A look back at the recent history in many other departments of medicine would provide the same general impression of spectacular·progress, but with great lacunae.

The bulk of the present day pharmacopoeia is, in historical terms, very recent indeed. Its main segments comprise the vitamins and the understanding of the diseases of deficiency; the substances natural to the body, especially its blood constituents and products, the steroids, and hormones; the hypnotics, sedatives and local and general anaesthetics; the chemotherapeutic agents, the antibiotics, and the diuretics, antidiabetic agents, and drugs for the treatment of mental disease that, in some instances, derived from the instruments of chemotherapy; the cardiovascular drugs; and, most ingeniously, the remedies that derived from the increased understanding of the autonomic nervous system, its pharmacology, and the receptor theory.

Of all of these great groups of drugs, the vitamins are amongst the most interesting. They are unique in being essential items of diet and both preventative and curative of a number of well defined and understood clinical conditions. Singer and Underwood, in the 1962 edition of their *A short history of medicine*[1520], give a particularly good account of this subject and Goodman and Gilman, in *The pharmacological basis of therapeutics* (1975)[1936], precede each of their monographs on the separate vitamins with a valuable account of its history.

As examples of the changes which have led to the other parts of the modern pharmacopoeia, some aspects of the chemotherapy and antibiotic practice of the present century and of the growth of knowledge of the autonomic nervous system and its receptors can be selected for discussion.

Until 1910 scientific medicine recognized as specific remedies (that is, drugs which could attack specifically the cause of the illness and not just influence its symptoms) only quinine, the alkaloid from cinchona which could eradicate certain malarial parasites; emetine, the alkaloid from ipecacuanha which could exterminate the protozoal organism causing amoebic dysentery; and mercury, which was more toxic to the spirochaete of syphilis than to the syphilitic.

The origins of the chemotherapeutic revolution lie in the experimental studies conducted by Paul Ehrlich (1854–1915; Figure 140) at the turn of the century. Ehrlich, of Strehlen, Silesia, became an assistant at Koch's Institute in Berlin and, in 1899, became director of the *Institut für experimentelle Therapie* at Frankfurt-on-Main. He experimented with dye-stuffs and tissue staining, discovered the mast cells and detected their granulations by basic aniline staining, divided the white blood corpuscles into their neutrophil, eosinophil and basophilic types, developed a fuchsin stain for tubercule bacilli, and in 1886 developed a method of intravital cellular staining. The enormous range of his studies is reflected in *The collected papers of Paul Ehrlich in four volumes including a complete bibliography . . .* [2229] This work, one of the more valuable recent sources, was compiled and edited by F. Himmelweit of the Wright–Fleming Institute at St. Mary's Hospital Medical School, London; it shows Ehrlich's interest in the possibilities of selective cellular stains, the selective affinity between chemical substances such as oxygen and the body tissues, and the outlines of the 'side-chain theory'. The latter was developed from August Kekulé's idea of the closed benzene ring (C_6H_6) in which the six carbon atoms are thought of as forming a stable hexagonal nucleus whilst, for each carbon atom, the fourth valency is assumed to be linked to an unstable side-chain based on the easily replacable hydrogen.

A subject of great controversy, this hypothesis led to fertile results in the hands of others, including Wassermann[2230], as well as Ehrlich. Ehrlich also reasoned that protozoan diseases needed to be treated by chemicals with a selective affinity for the parasite – a drug which could sterilize the pathogen without injuring the body tissues. In trying to treat trypanosomiasis in mice with such specific dyes, Ehrlich found that doses too small to kill the parasite would allow resistant variants to survive. In 1891, he administered methylene blue, a dye the biological actions of which he had studied for many years, to a malarial patient under the care of Paul Guttmann (1834–1893). Ehrlich thought that benefit resulted – and this was the first clinical demonstration of 'chemotherapy' in the sense in which Ehrlich developed the term.

At this point Ehrlich's interest in the aniline dyes was diverted to the organic compounds of arsenic by the discovery of the Liverpool School for Tropical Medicine that atoxyl, a synthetic organic arsenical, was more active against experimental infections due to trypanosomes than inorganic arsenic. Ehrlich confirmed this and set about modifying atoxyl in order to produce a compound that would kill all of the infecting trypanosomes so rapidly that none would survive to develop resistance.

By 1907 Ehrlich had synthesized and tested over 600 arsenical compounds. Number 418 in the series proved to be highly effective against experimental trypanosomiasis in laboratory animals. Number 606 was tested against the *Treponema pallidum* (already described as the causative organism of syphilis)[2231], [2232] and reported to be inactive but in 1909 Sahachiro Hata (1873–1938), a

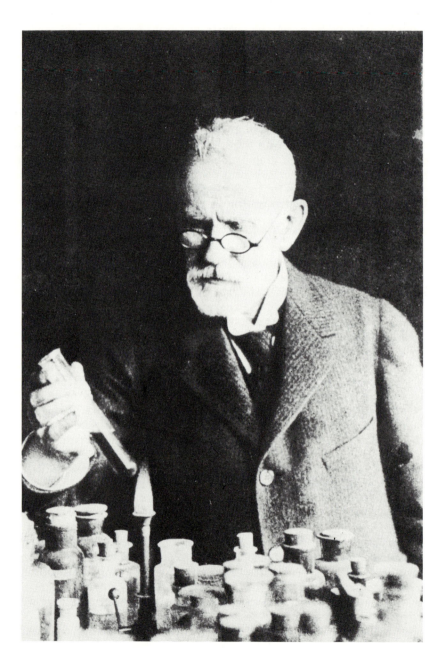

Figure 140   Paul Ehrlich (1854–1915).

Japanese bacteriologist who had developed a method of transmitting syphilis to rabbits, began to work as an assistant to Ehrlich. Hata, retesting the whole of Ehrlich's synthetic series, showed that, *in vivo*, compound number 606 was highly active[2233]. It was named 'Salvarsan' and in 1911 was first used in the treatment of human syphilis. In the same year Hideyo Noguchi (1876–1928) first obtained pure cultures of *Treponema pallidum*[2234].

The fortunate availability of a valid laboratory screen for substances active *in vivo* against the spirochaete of syphilis seems to have been important in the discovery of Salvarsan (arsphenamine) which revolutionized the treatment of syphilis. However, the compound was only sparingly soluble and the dose required necessitated a large volume of solvent. Ehrlich overcame this disadvantage with the introduction of his compound 914, Neosalvarsan, now called neoarsphenamine[2235].

Salvarsan, compound 606, arsphenamine is 3,3'-diamino-4,4'-dihydroxy-arsenobenzene dihydrochloride dihydrate. It had to be stored below 15 °C in sealed containers from which the air had been exhausted or replaced by inert gas; it also needed to be protected from the light. It was given intravenously and was replaced by the somewhat less toxic neoarsphenamine and the arsenoxides – until all were displaced by the antibiotics.

Neosalvarsan, compound 914, neoarsphenamine consists mainly of sodium 3-amino-4,4'-dihydroxy-3'-sulphinomethylamino-arsenobenzene and contains 18–21% of arsenic. Its more severe side-effects included exfoliative dermatitis, severe nephritis, acute yellow atrophy, acute purpura, aplastic anaemia, agranulocytosis, and, on prolonged administration, major central nervous system disturbances. In the treatment of syphilis it has now been completely replaced by penicillin[2236].

In other hands the continued search for drugs with which to treat trypanosomiasis led to the introduction in 1919 of tryparsamide by Walter Jacobs (1883–1967) and a group of colleagues from the laboratories of The Rockefeller Institute for Medical Research in New York[2237]. In 1926, in a paper *On the chemotherapy of neurosyphilis and trypanosomiasis*[2238], Arthur Loevenhart (1878–1929) and W. K. Stratman-Thomas 'discussed the relation of chemical constitution of a series of twelve drugs to their activity in neurosyphilis and trypanosomiasis, with special reference, however, to tryparsamide'. This paper is of interest in providing a fairly early discussion of structure–activity relationships.

Although the search for chemotherapeutic agents continued, almost a generation elapsed before the modern era of sustained progress began. Salvarsan had been first used in human syphilis in 1911 – just prior to World War I. For the next 25 years the known chemotherapeutic drugs were active only against protozoal parasites and the organism of syphilis. Then, in 1935, shortly before World War II, Gerhard Domagk (1895–1964), who had reverted to a study of the biological effects of dyes, published his results with prontosil red, one of the newer synthetic dye-stuffs, showing that it would protect mice experimentally infected with streptococci. This paper, *Ein Beitrag zur Chemotherapie der bakteriellen Infektionen*[2239] of 1935, is one of the historically important papers in medicine; it introduced Prontosil, the first drug containing a sulphanilamide, into the literature and began the era of chemotherapeutic drugs active in the living organism against bacteria.

The two phases of the beginnings of chemotherapy were marked by the award of the Nobel Prize to Ehrlich in 1908 and to Domagk in 1939.

J. and Mme J. Tréfouël, N. Nitti and D. Bovet, in a work reporting the *Activité du p-aminophénylsulfamide sur les infections streptococciques expéri-mentales de la souris et du lapin*[2240], of 1935, confirmed Domagk's experimental work but showed that the effectiveness of prontosil red was due to its conversion in the body to sulphanilamide, a member of the chemical group known as the sulphonamides. It was shown that the drugs of this group, although possessed of only slight antimicrobial activity *in vitro*, produced remarkable protection against experimental infection with several micro-organisms *in vivo*. The concept that a dye, as such, was necessary was exploded and large numbers of new sulphonamides, in simple and modified forms, were soon made and exploited.

The experimental proof of the efficacy of sulphapyridine, more widely known in its early days as M & B 693, was provided by Sir Lionel Whitby (1895–1956) in a *Lancet* paper of 1938 on the *Chemotherapy of pneumococcal and other infections with 2-(p-amino-benzenesulphonamido) pyridine*[2241]. Whitby was then assistant pathologist at the Bland–Sutton Institute at Middlesex Hospital. Clinical proof of the value of the drug in pneumonia came with the publication of Gladys Evans and Wilfred Gaisford of the Dudley Road Hospital, Birmingham; these authors summarized their findings of 1938 by saying that 'The results of treatment of 100 cases of lobar pneumonia with M & B 693 are given. The case-mortality rate was 8% as compared with 27% in a control series observed at the same time'[2242]. Apart from the demonstration of the usefulness of the drug, the doctor of today might be surprised to note that 200 cases of lobar pneumonia were admitted to the Dudley Road Hospital in the period from March to the middle of June 1938; by today's standards the loss of roughly one in four of the patients in the comparison series is astounding and a reminder of the frequent comment of the physicians of a generation ago that there was always someone on the ward dying of lobar pneumonia.

With the war in Europe in progress, the first major trial of sulphathiazole was published from the Kantonsspital St. Gallen in Switzerland in 1940. The paper, *Chemotherapie akuter Infektionskrankheiten durch Ciba 3714 (Sulfanilamido-thiazol)*[2243] by Otto Gsell, showed the broadening activity with this group of drugs of the pharmaceutical industry. The introduction of sulphadiazine took place the following year with a paper by Maxwell Finland, Elias Strauss and Osler Peterson reporting, in 1941, the results of treating 446 adult patients treated with the drug in the Boston City Hospital[2244]. One of the major early trials of sulphadimidine, the drug having been supplied by ICI, was the paper of 1942 by Donald Macartney and his colleagues of the Crumpsall Hospital, Manchester: in their report, *Sulphamethazine, clinical trial of a new sulphonamide*[2245], these workers noted the efficacy of the drug in 73 cases of lobar pneumonia and a few cases of meningococcal meningitis and gonorrhoea; they also commented that renal damage with the compound was unlikely due to its high solubility.

We are now within a very short period of the 50th anniversary of Domagk's historic paper of February 15th, 1935 introducing prontosil red[2239] and ushering in the modern chemotherapeutic era. Looking back over those 50 years it is apparent that the discovery of the sulphonamides was, from some points of view, the most notable therapeutic advance of the period. The availability of this group of drugs had an immediate effect upon the treatment of susceptible infectious diseases; it transformed the mortality from lobar pneumonia and provided the first drugs which were effective against puerperal fever, cerebrospinal meningitis and septicaemia. The sulphonamides also led to the development of some other classes of drugs, including the early orally-active diuretics and oral hypoglycaemic agents. Finally, they had a major impact on the growth of the pharmaceutical industry: they began the era of sophisticated, large-scale, precision manufacturing techniques to exact product specifications and led to the growth of high-investment manufacturing plant. They also swept away the earlier use of serums and vaccines for the treatment of pneumonia.

Domagk was a research director at the I. G. Farbenindustrie A. G. Werk Elberfeld where in 1932 a German patent had been issued to Klarer and Mietzsch covering Prontosil and several other azo dyes containing a sulphonamide group. The great contribution of the Tréfouëls, Nitti, and Bovet (1935) at the Pasteur Institute in Paris, was to show that in the tissues the azo linkage was split so that Prontosil yielded *para*-aminobenzenesulphonamide, the chemotherapeutic moiety of the molecule[2240]. Many more than 5000 congeneric substances were made and examined in the decade that followed the discovery of sulphanilamide and, although only a handful of them achieved clinical importance, their consequences in the development of other groups of drugs became considerable.

M. Janbon and co-workers, in 1942, whilst conducting studies on the treatment of typhoid fever, found that a sulphonamide induced hypoglycaemia; they published their results in a paper on *Accidents hypoglycémiques graves par un sulfamidothiadiazol (le VK57 ou 2254RP)*[2246]. Janbon's colleague, A. Loubatières, then made the fundamentally important discovery that the compound exerted no such effect in the animal which had undergone pancreatectomy[2247]; Loubatières therefore suggested that the hypoglycaemic effect was due to stimulation of the pancreas with the secretion of insulin[2248]. These findings led to the demonstration that the antibacterial agent, carbutamide, was useful in the treatment of diabetes mellitus[2249] and, soon after this, to the introduction of tolbutamide – a substance which is not an antimicrobial but was the practical lead member of the orally-active, antidiabetic agents known as the sulphonylureas[2250].

A second ramification of Domagk's discovery was that when sulphanilamide was introduced as a chemotherapeutic agent, metabolic acidosis was soon recognized as a side-effect. The drug was found to inhibit carbonic anhydrase, the enzymatic effects of which had already been described, *in vitro*; it was also found to inhibit the normal acidification of the urine *in vivo*. The later studies showed the part played by carbonic anhydrase in renal transport – and, in the event, the benzothiadiazides were first synthesized as an outgrowth of the studies on carbonic anhydrase inhibitors.

Thus, studies of the sulphonamides led not only to the orally-active, sulphonylurea antidiabetic agents but also to the chlorothiazide-type diuretic agents which now form the mainstay of antihypertensive therapy.

The search for other antimicrobial substances continued and, in 1944, Matthew Dodd and William Stillman, in a paper on *The in vitro bacteriostatic action of some simple furan derivatives*[2251], introduced nitrofuran, the preferred member of the 42 furan compounds which they had examined. A somewhat more interesting compound is trimethoprim, 2,4-diamino-5-(3,4,5-trimethoxybenzyl) pyrimidine, a highly active broad-spectrum antibacterial agent structurally related to the antimalarial compound, pyrimethamine. The substance has an anti-bacterial spectrum somewhat like that of the sulphonamides, but is markedly more potent. Since 1969, trimethoprim has been extensively used in combination with sulphamethoxazole, as co-trimoxazole. The rationale for the combination was the synergy and bactericidal activity shown by the two drugs when tested against human pathogens *in vitro*. This synergy under laboratory conditions was shown by Bushby and Hitchings (*Trimethoprim, a sulphonamide potentiator*)[2252] in 1968; the later work of Bushby (1973) and a number of other workers led to the interesting concept that the enhanced effects of trimethoprim when combined with a sulphonamide are due to sequential blockade of bacterial folic acid synthesis[2253]. The synergy was never satisfactorily shown *in vivo* or in clinical studies and, following extensive clinical trials of trimethoprim used alone (Kasanen and colleagues, 1979)[2254], the substance was introduced as a single-treatment agent in the United Kingdom (Mann and Jones, *Trimethoprim in the treatment of urinary tract infections*, 1980)[2255].

In terms of their direct effect on clinical practice – even though the discovery of the sulphonamides had widespread repercussions – the development of the antibiotics has, without doubt, provided the greatest contribution to twentieth century therapeutics. The term 'antibiosis' was introduced at the end of nineteenth century to indicate antagonism between one organism and another. The early observations date from that time. John Tyndall (1820–1893) not only invented a somewhat curious method of disinfection but also wrote (1876): 'I wished to free my mind . . . from the uncertainty and confusion which now beset the doctrine of "spontaneous generation". Pasteur has pronounced it "a chimera", and expressed the undoubting conviction that this being so it is possible to remove parasitic diseases from the earth.'[2256] Tyndall's own observations on putrefaction and infection showed that certain members of the *Penicillium* could inhibit bacteria but *Pseudomonas pyocyanea* were resistant to this effect. Pasteur and Jules Joubert in 1877 noted the antagonism between *Bacillus anthracis* and other bacteria being grown in cultures[1500]; they may there-fore have come close to realizing that one organism could be set against another in a way that would deliberately inhibit growth. Rudolf Emmerich (1852–1914) and Oscar Löw, in a paper of 1899, went further and recorded that they had prepared a water-soluble bacteriolytic enzyme from cultures of *Pseudomonas aeruginosa*[2257].

In 1921, Sir Alexander Fleming (1881–1955), of St. Mary's Hospital, cultured nasal mucus from a person suffering from an acute cold and detected what he described as 'an extraordinary bacteriolytic phenomenon' in the cultures. He called the substance responsible for this effect 'lysozyme' and, when President of the Section of Pathology of the Royal Society of Medicine in 1932, he summarized his findings by saying[2258]:

(1) That lysozyme is a widely distributed antibacterial ferment which is probably inherent in all animal cells and constitutes a primary method of destroying bacteria.

(2) That lysozyme, while acting most strikingly on non-pathogenic bacteria, yet can, when allowed to act in the full strength in which it occurs in some parts of the body, attack pathogenic organisms.

(3) That it is very easy to make bacteria relatively resistant to lysozyme, so that any pathogenic microbe isolated from the body where it has been growing in the presence of a non-lethal concentration of lysozyme, must have acquired increased resistance to the ferment.

(4) That there are some differences in the lysozyme of different tissues and in different animals whereby bacteria are susceptible to different lysozymes in varying degrees.

Lysozyme still appears in our dictionaries as 'a bacteriolytic enzyme present in some plants, animal secretions (e.g. tears), egg-white, etc.' – but it is nothing like as well known as Fleming's discovery of 1928, 7 years before Domagk announced his discovery of the chemotherapeutic value of Prontosil.

In his paper of 1929, *On the antibacterial action of cultures of a Penicillium, with special reference to their use in the isolation of B. influenzae*[2259], Fleming described the circumstances of his great discovery in the following paragraphs:

> While working with staphylococcus variants a number of culture-plates were set aside on the laboratory bench and examined from time to time. In the examinations these plates were necessarily exposed to the air and they became contaminated with various micro-organisms. It was noticed that around a large colony of a contaminating mould the staphylococcus colonies became transparent and were obviously undergoing lysis (see Fig. 1).
>
> Subcultures of this mould were made and experiments conducted with a view to ascertaining something of the properties of the bacteriolytic substance which had evidently been formed in the mould culture and which had diffused into the surrounding medium. It was found that broth in which the mould had been grown at room temperature for one or two weeks had acquired marked inhibitory, bactericidal and bacteriolytic properties to many of the more common pathogenic bacteria.

Fleming's 'Fig. 1' is, in this text, reproduced as Figure 141; he ends his historic paper with the following summary:

1. A certain type of penicillium produces in culture a powerful antibacterial substance. The antibacterial power of the culture reaches its maximum in about 7 days at 20 °C and after 10 days diminishes until it has almost disappeared in 4 weeks.
2. The best medium found for the production of the antibacterial substance has been ordinary nutrient broth.
3. The active agent is readily filterable and the name ''penicillin'' has been given to filtrates of broth cultures of the mould.
4. Penicillin loses most of its power after 10 to 14 days at room temperature but can be preserved longer by neutralization.
5. The active agent is not destroyed by boiling for a few minutes but in alkaline solution boiling for 1 hour markedly reduces the power. Autoclaving for 20 minutes at 115 °C practically destroys it. It is soluble in alcohol but insoluble in ether or chloroform.
6. The action is very marked on the pyogenic cocci and the diphtheria group of bacilli. Many bacteria are quite insensitive, *e.g.* the coli-typhoid group, the influenza-bacillus group, and the enterococcus.

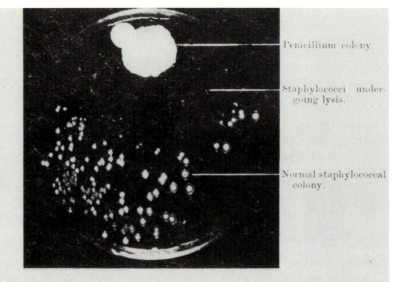

Penicillium colony.

Staphylococci undergoing lysis.

Normal staphylococcal colony.

Fig. 1.—Photograph of a culture-plate showing the dissolution of staphylococcal colonies in the neighbourhood of a penicillium colony.

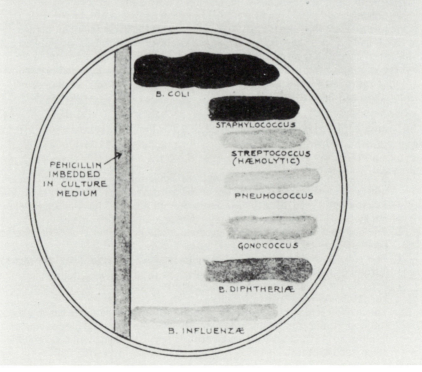

Figure 141 Alexander Fleming. Figure 1 from: *On the antibacterial action of cultures of a Penicillium* ... (1929).

7. Penicillin is non-toxic to animals in enormous doses and is non-irritant. It does not interfere with leucocytic function to a greater degree than does ordinary broth.
8. It is suggested that it may be an efficient antiseptic for application to, or injection into, areas infected with penicillin-sensitive microbes.
9. The use of penicillin on culture plates renders obvious many bacterial inhibitions which are not very evident in ordinary cultures.
10. Its value as an aid to the isolation of *B. influenzæ* has been demonstrated.

Apart from his knowledge of the literature, Fleming had, due to his work on lysozymes, been familiar for some 6 or 7 years with bacteriolytic substances of natural origin. It is, therefore, perhaps not so serendipitidous as is sometimes made out that he should notice this lytic event on a bacterial plate contaminated by a mould.

However, his conclusion number 8 is striking. Although he recognizes that 'Penicillin is non-toxic to animals in enormous doses and is non-irritant', Fleming suggests that 'it may be an efficient antiseptic for application to, or injection into, areas infected with penicillin-sensitive microbes.' Thus, there was no initial emphasis on the systemic use of this non-toxic antibiotic.

Reasonably effective topical antiseptics were already available, and penicillin remained a laboratory curiosity and bench reagent for over a decade. In 1939, René Dubos (1901–1982), from the Hospital of the Rockefeller Institute for Medical Research in New York City, reported the isolation of gramicidin[2260]. In the same year, Albert Oxford, Harold Raistrick and Paul Simonart, from the London School of Hygiene and Tropical Medicine, reported the isolation of griseofulvin[2261]. Thus, with other antibiotics already known, serious interest in penicillin was rekindled by the outbreak of World War II and the tensions of the period that preceded it.

In Oxford, Sir Ernst Chain (1906–1979) and Lord Florey decided to undertake a systematic study of the antibacterial substances produced by moulds and bacteria. Their investigation was begun by examining the antibacterial properties of the mould described by Fleming in 1929. They obtained what they described as 'a considerable yield of penicillin' in the form of a brown powder soluble in water. Chain, Florey and their co-workers from the Sir William Dunn School of Pathology, Oxford provided proof of the therapeutic action of penicillin *in vivo* in a *Lancet* paper, *Penicillin as a chemotherapeutic agent*[2262], of August, 1940. The limitation of penicillin, that some organisms were resistant to it because they produced a penicillinase which destroyed the antibiotic, was reported in December, 1940 in a paper, *An enzyme from bacteria able to destroy penicillin*[2263], published by Sir Edward Abraham and Sir Ernst Chain.

The classic paper is that providing *Further observations on penicillin*[2264] by Abraham, Chain, Florey and their colleagues from the Sir William Dunn School of Pathology and the Radcliffe Infirmary at Oxford. This paper of August, 1941 described the cultural and other conditions needed for the small-scale mass production of penicillin from *Penicillium notatum*; it also described the results in the first ten clinical cases.

Under wartime conditions scale-up to large volume production was undertaken by pharmaceutical operations in the United States and, once adequate quantities were produced and made clinically available, the transformation to be wrought by penicillin upon susceptible infections began. More information on penicillamine was produced from the group at Oxford in 1943[2265] and, marking one of the greatest events of medicine, Fleming, Chain and Florey shared the Nobel Prize in 1945.

The crucial advance in the large-scale production of penicillin was the deep-fermentation process developed at the Northern Regional Research Laboratories of the American Department of Agriculture in Peoria, Illinois. The early, improvised methods of manufacture developed at Oxford had yielded so little material that in Case 1 of the classic 1941 report[2264], a policeman suffering from a severe mixed staphylococcal and streptococcal infection, some of the penicillin used had been recovered from the urine of other patients given the drug. With the deep-fermentation method production increased so that something like 150 tons of penicillin were being produced by 1950.

In the early years, all of the penicillin came from subcultures of Fleming's original strain of *Penicillium notatum*. During World War II great efforts were made to find more productive strains. These resulted in the isolation of *Penicillium chrysogenum*, originally obtained from the stem of a mouldy cantaloupe melon. The exposure of this organism to X-rays produced the mutant strain, X-1612, with its capability for a characteristically high penicillin yield.

The standard system for describing the potency of penicillin was derived at the International Conference on the Standardization of Penicillin held in London in 1944. This established the international unit of penicillin and, from a sample of the crystalline sodium salt of penicillin G, laid down the international penicillin master standard. The unit was defined as the specific penicillin activity of $0.6\,\mu g$ of the master standard. Today, the dosage and antimicrobial potency of the semi-synthetic penicillins are almost always expressed in terms of weight.

The basic structure of the penicillins is that of a thiazolidine ring (shown as A in Figure 142), joined to a β-lactam ring (B), to which is attached a side-chain (R). The penicillin nucleus is the source of the useful antibiotic effect. The side-chain and its substitutions determine the differences in antimicrobial spectrum and pharmacological characteristics which differentiate the various penicillins. The parent form of penicillin, penicillin G, is benzylpenicillin. It was the discovery that 6-aminopenicillanic acid could be obtained from cultures of *Penicillium chrysogenum* that were depleted of side-chain precursors which, by allowing side-chain substitutions, led to the splendid development of the semisynthetic penicillins which have now received such widespread use. 6-aminopenicillanic acid is now produced in massive quantities by cleavage (as shown in Figure 142) with an amidase from *Penicillium chrysogenum*. The mechanism, involving splitting of the peptide linkage by which the side-chain of penicillin is joined to 6-aminopenicillanic acid, is explained by J. M. T. Hamilton-Miller in a paper of 1966 on *Penicillinacylase*[2266]. The penicillinase-resistant semisynthetic penicillins now in extensive clinical use are made by side-chain substitutions which alter the susceptibility of the final compounds to cleavage of the β-lactam ring.

The antibiotics discovered after penicillin have come from many sources. Balbina A. Johnson and colleagues from the College of Physicians and Surgeons of Columbia University reported the discovery of *Bacitracin: a new antibiotic produced by a member of the B. subtilis group*[2267] in a paper of 1945; the strain of

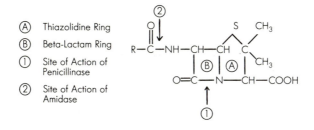

Ⓐ Thiazolidine Ring
Ⓑ Beta-Lactam Ring
① Site of Action of Penicillinase
② Site of Action of Amidase

Figure 142   The basic structure of the penicillins.

the organism from which the antibiotic was produced was isolated from tissue debrided from a compound fracture of the tibia; it was named Tracy I after the patient concerned. In 1947, from the Wellcome Physiological Research Laboratories at Beckenham, Kent, G. C. Ainsworth, Annie Brown and George Brownlee reported '*Aerosporin', an antibiotic produced by Bacillus aerosporus Greer*[2268]. This antibiotic-producing organism was isolated from the soil of a market garden in Surrey during February 1946 and afterwards from a Yorkshire soil and from the air; it got its name from the latter happenstance.

Aerosporin, later known as polymyxin A, and polymyxin D[2269] (as it is now known) were independently discovered in 1947. Both are examples of novel antibiotics resulting from the search for such substances conducted by the pharmaceutical industry. Chloramphenicol came from a similar source. It was isolated in the Osborn Botanical Laboratory of Yale University by Paul R. Burkholder from a soil sample obtained from a mulched field near Caracas, Venezuela; it was reported in a paper *Chloromycetin, a new antibiotic from a soil Actinomycete* (1947)[2270] by John Ehrlich and his colleagues from Parke, Davis and Company, Detroit, who wrote in joint authorship with Paul Burkholder. The organism from which these workers had produced chloramphenicol became known as *Streptomyces venezuelae*. Chloramphenicol, in experimental rickettsial and other infections[2271], was introduced by Joseph Smadel and Elizabeth Jackson in 1947.

Attempts to prolong the duration of action of penicillin and sustain its blood levels included the intramuscular injection of penicillin calcium in beeswax and peanut oil. Preparations of this type were, in 1947, displaced by procaine penicillin. Pharmacological studies of this substance, prepared by Eli Lilly and Company which had combined one molecule of procaine base with one molecule of penicillin, were reported in a paper on *Procaine penicillin G (Duracillin): a new salt of penicillin which prolongs the action of penicillin*[2272]; this communication was made by Wallace E. Herrell in the *Proceedings of the Staff Meetings of the Mayo Clinic* – it began the widespread use of an important form of penicillin.

The discoveries continued. Chlortetracycline, and its discovery and clinical application, was announced in a symposium, *Aureomycin – a new antibiotic*[2273], published on November 30th, 1948 by means of a grant from the Lederle

Laboratories Division, American Cyanamid Company. It was known that a few antibiotics, including streptomycin, could prevent bacteriophage action and methods of both testing and isolating for such a capability were described in a paper, *An antiphage agent isolated from Aspergillus sp.*[2274], published by Frederick Hanson and Thomas Eble of the Upjohn Company, Kalamazoo, Michigan in 1949. The isolation of a new actinomycete, *Streptomyces rimosus*, from a soil sample and the preparation of a crystalline antibiotic, oxytetracycline, from broth cultures of this organism were reported in 1950 in a paper on *Terramycin, a new antibiotic*[2275] by Alexander Finlay, Gladys Hobby and their associates of Chas. Pfizer and Company of Brooklyn, New York. In 1951 two antibiotics appeared from non-industrial laboratories. The first of these was nystatin, the isolation of which was reported by Elizabeth Hazen and Rachel Fuller Brown of the Division of Laboratories and Research, New York State Department of Health, Albany; in their paper on *Fungicidin, an antibiotic produced by a soil actinomycete*[2276], these two workers noted that Fungicidin (nystatin) was both fungicidal and fungistatic although it lacked antibacterial activity. The second of these two antibiotics of 1951 was reported by H. S. Burton and Sir Edward Abraham; from the Sir William Dunn School of Pathology at Oxford these two authors wrote on the *Isolation of antibiotics from a species of Cephalosporium. Cephalosoprins P₁, P₂, P₃, P₄ and P₅*[2277]. In this work Abraham and his colleagues described the isolation and some of the properties of a whole group of antibiotics obtained from the active culture filtrates of a species of *Cephalosporium* originally isolated from the sea near Sardinia by G. Brotzu.

From a soil sample collected in the Philippine Archipelago an actinomycete of the genus *Streptomyces* was isolated and identified as *Streptomyces erythreus* by James McGuire and a number of co-workers of the Lilly Research Laboratories, Indianapolis, Indiana; from this organism the isolation and development of erythromycin was reported in a publication of 1952 on *'Ilotycin', a new antibiotic*[2278]. Continued work on the *Cephalosporium* isolated by Brotzu from a sewage outfall off Sardinia led to the 1954 note of the *Purification and some properties of cephalosporin N, a new penicillin*[2279] by Abraham and the Oxford group which, the following year (Newton and Abraham, 1955), reported the isolation of *Cephalosporin C, a new antibiotic containing sulphur and D-α-aminoadipic acid*[2280].

The great spate of discoveries slowed at the beginning of the decade starting with 1960. From the Squibb Institute for Medical Research at New Brunswick, New Jersey, two new antibiotics were described in the paper *Amphotericins A and B, antifungal antibiotics produced by a streptomycete*[2281] by W. Gold and associates (1955–56). The very productive group led by Hamao Umezawa at the National Institute of Health, Tokyo, in 1957, reported the *Production and isolation of a new antibiotic, kanamycin*[2282] and then, in 1963, from the laboratories of the Schering Corporation at Bloomfield, New Jersey, Marvin Weinstein and his colleagues described the isolation of *Gentamicin, a new antibiotic complex from Micromonospora*[2283].

The two decades that began with the year 1940 saw, even in terms of the limited number of examples considered above, the discovery and development of a range of antibiotics which, with their different antimicrobial spectra, transformed the clinical picture of bacterial infectious diseases. A comparison of mortality by cause, age and sex in England and Wales [2284] (Figure 143) shows that in 1931 the pattern was not very different between males and females – in both 10- and 20-year-old subjects, whether boys or girls, infective diseases accounted for very roughly 40% of total deaths. In 1973, a figure of between 2 and 4% would provide a better approximation of the percentage of deaths due to infective diseases in these young age groups; accidents have now come to provide half or more of the total deaths in young adults.

Neoplasia is now responsible for something like half the deaths in 50–54-year-old women, with cardiovascular causes killing something like an equal proportion of men of the same age. In both sexes, cardiovascular diseases are now the most common cause of death in people over 70, neoplasia and respiratory diseases sharing, roughly equally, the remaining percentage of total deaths.

Even if improvements in nutrition and social circumstances and the great unmeasurable alterations in the pathogenesis of individual diseases have combined to contribute to this improvement, the use of the antibiotics must be judged to have brought benefits on a vast scale. It must seem that this group of drugs, which gained most of its strength in the decades that fell either side of the mid-century, represents the most singular therapeutic achievement of medical science. Whether it is better to have been able to discover Jenner's smallpox vaccine and use it as a prophylactic to eradicate smallpox; or discover anaesthetics, and so permit the developments of modern surgery; or discover and develop antibiotics, and thereby be able to treat most bacterial infectious diseases, is a point of speculative debate. Jenner's vaccine in the eighteenth century, the inhalational anaesthetics in the nineteenth century, and the antibiotics in the twentieth century, represent the pinnacles of the application of medical science. Even if the hygiene taught at the Broad Street pump and by the social reformers is of greater ultimate importance, the antibiotics remind us that 'The Lord hath created medicines out of the earth; and he that is wise will not abhor them.' [2285]

Many of the important drugs of modern therapeutics influence physiological functions or provide symptomatic relief of disease, unlike the curative and sometimes life-saving antibiotics. Many of these drugs affect the autonomic nervous system and the receptor sites – modern knowledge of which is largely rooted in the work, begun in the last years of the nineteenth century, which culminated in Walter Gaskell's *The involuntary nervous system* (1916) [1387] and the twentieth century classic, John Langley's *The autonomic nervous system* (1921) [1391]. The work of these two Cambridge physiologists has been previously mentioned, for Langley, in 1905, introduced the vital concept of the receptor site with which a drug has to interact in order to exert its biological effect. This concept is so important that it is worth recalling part [2286] of the 'general results and conclusions' from Langley's paper of 1905–6 *On the reaction of cells and of nerve-endings to certain poisons, chiefly as regards the reaction of striated muscle to nicotine and to curari* [1390]:

> Nicotine causes in certain muscles of the fowl prolonged contraction. The muscular contraction is also obtained after section of the nerves to the muscle and after paralysis of the nerves by nicotine or by curari.
>
> The nicotine contraction is diminished by injection of a sufficient dose of

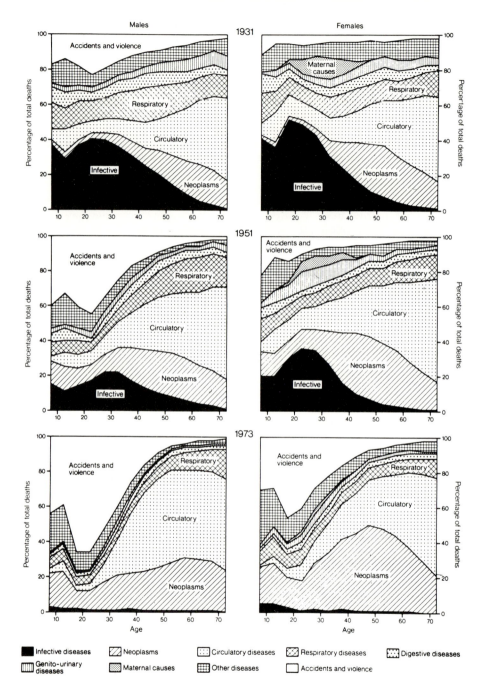

Figure 143 Mortality by cause, age and sex, 1931, 1951 and 1973. [*From: Office of Population Censuses and Surveys. Trends in mortality 1951–1975. HMSO (1978).*]

curari. The two poisons are mutually antagonistic as regards stimulating effect on the muscles; but the action of nicotine is more powerful than that of curari.

At the height of the nicotine contraction a galvanic current causes partial inhibition.

Degeneration of the nerves supplying the muscles leaves essentially unaltered the effects described above; but there is evidence of an increased responsiveness to nicotine. The action of curari is less marked, but that may be due to an increased sensitiveness to nicotine.

Since there is evidence that the axon-endings in skeletal muscle degenerate after section of the nerves supplying the muscle, I conclude that nicotine and curari do not act on the axon-endings but on the muscle itself. Further, since both nicotine and curari prevent nervous impulses from affecting the contractile substance, but do not prevent the muscle from contracting on direct stimulation, I conclude that the poisons do not act directly on the contractile substance, but on other substances in the muscle which may be called receptive substances.

The evidence with regard to striated muscle seems to me to be on a sufficiently firm basis to allow the deductions drawn from it to be applied to other cells, with regard to which there is more or less evidence of a similar kind.

Thus there is evidence that the majority of substances which are ordinarily supposed to act upon nerve-endings (as nicotine, curari, atropine, pilocarpine, strychnine) act upon the receptive substances of the cells.

And as adrenalin, an internal secretion, acts upon receptive substance, it is probable that secretin, thyroidin, and the internal secretion formed by the generative organs, also act on receptive substances, although in these cases the cells may be unconnected with nerve fibres.

So we may suppose that in all cells two constituents at least are to be distinguished, a chief substance, which is concerned with the chief function of the cell as contraction and secretion, and receptive substances which are acted upon by chemical bodies and in certain cases by nervous stimuli. The receptive substance affects or is capable of affecting the metabolism of the chief substance.

A study of the action of different poisons shows – on the theory just given – that the receptive substance of cells, even of the same class, varies considerably. This I consider is mainly due to an inherent tendency to variation in the chemical nature of the cells, so that even in the same class of cell the receptive substances formed are commonly not identical.

In unstriated muscle and glands the innervation varies widely in degree, and in some cases no nervous action can be shown; this difference may, I think, reasonably be attributed primarily to a different responsiveness to nervous stimuli of the receptive substances, and it seems to me possible that in some cases nerve-endings are present which are unable to influence the cell. No doubt such ineffective nerves would tend to disappear by natural selection. No doubt also, when a nerve is effective, the frequency with which it is put in action would tend to increase the receptive substance by use (just as the cell as a whole is increased by use) and so to check the tendency in the cell to further chemical change.

The different degree of tone of the tissues is probably also in part due to the responsiveness of the receptive substance.

Many chemical bodies show a more or less marked preference for the receptive substance connected with certain classes of nerves. And this is the case also, when a tissue (unstriated muscle and gland cell) is innervated from two different systems of nerves. This preference I connect with a similarity in the receptive substance due to each system of nerves becoming functionally connected with cells at approximately the same time in phylogenetic development. The conditions leading to the formation of receptive substance would be in general similar, and the receptive substance of many of the cells would have common characters. These tend to become fixed by use.

In 1901 Langley had pointed out that stimulation of nerves belonging to the sympathetic division of the autonomic nervous system produced results which closely resembled the actions of adrenaline. At this time two other drugs were in frequent experimental use in the laboratories of physiology, like that at Cambridge. One was muscarine, the active principle of the fungus, *Amanita muscaria*; the other was nicotine, the main alkaloid of tobacco. The active alkaloid muscarine was thought to be related to choline and was shown experimentally to produce effects very like those resulting from stimulation of the parasympathetic nerves. Although it is now recognized that muscarine does not occur in the animal body it is acknowledged that muscarine is one of the cholinergic alkaloids which (like pilocarpine) acts selectively on end-organs that respond to acetylcholine. Thus it was known that adrenaline produced an effect like that of stimulating the sympathetic system, and muscarine an effect like that of stimulating the parasympathetic system. Nicotine was shown to stimulate either sympathetic or parasympathetic ganglia.

In 1904, Thomas Elliott (1877–1961), who had Henry Dale as a fellow-student at Cambridge, in a short preliminary paper *On the action of adrenaline*[2287], suggested that sympathetic fibres might act indirectly on the cells of plain muscle and the glands innervated by them by liberating adrenaline. This was the first intimation, based on experimental work, of the chemical transmission of a nerve impulse. Elliott very shortly showed that the adrenal medulla is a homologue of the sympathetic ganglia. At this stage, George Barger (1878–1939), with F. H. Carr and Henry Dale, isolated ergotoxine reporting this in a paper *An active alkaloid from ergot*[2288] of 1906 and noting that all active preparations of ergot not only had the well-known effects such as contraction of the uterus but showed also 'a secondary selective paralysis of certain myoneural junctions of the true sympathetic system, whereby the normal motor effects of sympathetic nerves and of the suprarenal active principle are abolished or replaced by inhibition.'

It was also suggested, by Walter Dixon (1871–1931) of Cambridge, that the parasympathetic nerves must also release a chemical transmitter. Publishing in the *American Journal of Physiology* in 1905–6, William Howell (1860–1945), in a paper on the *Vagus inhibition of the heart in its relation to the inorganic salts of the blood*[2289], suggested that nerve impulses exert an indirect effect by increasing the amount of diffusible potassium in the heart tissue. This work provides one of the early examples of interest in the electrolyte migrations which have become relevant to drug action. It was contemporary with the demonstration of the hypotensive effect of acetylcholine by Reid Hunt (1870–1948) and René de M. Taveau (*On the physiological action of certain cholin derivatives and new methods for detecting cholin,* 1906)[2290] and was only slightly earlier than the report of Walter Dixon and Philip Hamill (1883–1959) on *The mode of action of specific substances with special reference to secretin* (1908–9)[2291] in which emphasis was given to the similarity of effect between drugs, such as muscarine, acting on the heart and the stimulation of nerves affecting the heart.

The synthesis of histamine in 1907, by Adolf Windaus (1876–1959) and Karl Vogt[2292], was also of this period. Histamine became of great importance in another context but was of great current interest at the time when early knowledge was accumulating on the chemical transmission of the nerve impulse in the autonomic nervous system and its divisions. George Barger (1878–1939) and Sir Henry Dale wrote on the *Chemical structure and sympathomimetic action of amines*[2293] in 1910 and announced the discovery of histamine in an extract of ergot. Dale, with Sir Patrick Laidlaw (1881–1940), noted the effects of histamine in a paper on *The physiological action of β-iminoazolylethylamine* (1910)[2294] and Barger and Dale (1911) reported their isolation of histamine from animal tissues in an important publication on *β-iminozolyethylamine a depressor constituent of intestinal mucosa*[2295]. Both George Barger and Henry Dale were, at the time of these studies, working at the Wellcome Physiological Research Laboratories.

While these studies in England were in progress, Reid Hunt and René de M. Taveau, of the Public Health and Marine Hospital Service in Washington DC, studied the relationship between the toxicity and chemical constitution of a number of derivatives of choline and a series of analogous compounds. Their paper, of 1909, provides another interesting early example of the study of structure–activity relationships for they made a comparison of the effect of a series of substitutions and the average fatal dose in experimental animals[2296].

Knowledge of *The plant alkaloids*[2297] just before World War I was well summarized in a book of that title, dated 1913, and written by Thomas Henry (1873–1958), Director of the Wellcome Chemical Research Laboratories when the second edition of this work appeared in 1924. Sir Henry Dale continued the particular lines of research he had developed on plant substances and, in 1914, found in an ergot extract certain activities which were not explained by any known constituent of the ergot fungus. These activities resembled those of muscarine and Dale then published on *The action of certain esters and ethers of choline, and their relation to muscarine* (1914)[2298]. When the active principle responsible for these unexplained actions was isolated by Dale's colleague, Arthur James Ewins (1882–1957), it proved to be acetylcholine. The findings were noted in a paper on *Acetylcholine, a new active principle of ergot*[2299] written by Ewins in 1914 but they caused little interest. The acetyl ester of choline was not a new substance, having been first synthesized in 1867 or 1894, and it was known to occur widely in the animal and vegetable kingdoms. It has a depressor action which slows the heart, increases the intestinal movements, and augments the secretions of the lacrymal and salivary glands. It was known to be chemically related to muscarine and to have actions which are similar.

Dale, during the course of this work, had noted that the depressor effect of acetylcholine in slowing the heart was very transient; he suggested that this was due to rapid hydrolysis of the acetylcholine with the production of choline and acetic acid. Dale also showed that these evanescent biological effects of acetylcholine closely resembled the consequences of stimulating the postganglionic fibres of the parasympathetic nerves. Dale and his colleagues had been fortunate to find acetylcholine in their ergot extract for it is uncommon in this situation. Their papers of 1914 were followed by that on *Vasodilator reactions*[2300] in which, in 1918, Reid Hunt demonstrated that the tissues are more responsive to acetylcholine after exposure to eserine (physostigmine).

The isolation of ergotamine was achieved by Karl Spiro (1867–1932) and Arthur Stoll (1887–1971) in 1921[2301] – the year which saw the next major advance in the understanding of the chemical transmission of the nerve impulse. In 1921, Otto Loewi, then professor of pharmacology at Graz, conducted some of the definitive experiments of the science. He isolated the hearts of two frogs, stimulated the vagus (parasympathetic) nerve to the first heart after introducing Ringer's solution into its cavities, noted the expected slowing of the first heart due to vagal stimulation, and then transferred the Ringer's solution to the second un-stimulated heart. When this was found to undergo inhibition it was clear that a chemical mediator of response had been transferred with the Ringer's solution. Loewi recorded his work in papers (*Ueber humorale Uebertragbarkeit der Herz-nervenwirkung*)[2302] of 1921, 1922 and 1924 and showed that each stimulation of the vagus produced the chemical transmitter within the cavity of the heart. In additions of 1924 and 1926[2303] to the same paper, Loewi, with E. Navratil showed that the transmitter, the 'vagal substance', was rapidly destroyed by an esterase in the heart muscle. He also showed that eserine (physostigmine) inhibted the action of the esterase.

Sir Henry Hallett Dale (1875–1968) and Otto Loewi (1873–1961), for their work on the chemical mediation of the nervous impulse, shared the Nobel Prize for physiology in 1936.

If we glance aside to recall other developments in the materia medica and therapeutics of the early and mid years of the decade starting in 1920, special note would be made of the paper by Sir Frederick Grant Banting (1891–1941) and Charles Herbert Best (1899–1978) on *The internal secretion of the pancreas* (1922)[2304]. This paper's conclusions included the statements that 'Intravenous injections of extract from dog's pancreas, removed from 7 to 10 weeks after ligation of the ducts, invariably exercises a reducing influence upon the per-centage sugar of the blood and the amount of sugar excreted in the urine'; 'pancreatic juice destroys the active principle of the extract.' Banting, instru-mental in the discovery of insulin for the treatment of diabetes, shared in a Nobel Prize of 1923. Knowledge of the pharmacological action of optical isomers had reached the point that Arthur Robertson Cushny (1866–1926) was able to contribute his *Biological relations of optically isomeric substances*[2305] in 1926. Of the everyday and important drugs of medicine, the information on the *Actions and uses of the salicylates and cinchophen in medicine*[2306], a paper by Paul John Hanzlik (1885–1951), was of almost book size when it was published in 1926. And, from the Wellcome Physiological Research Laboratories, J. W. Trevan (1887–1955) produced, in 1927, a paper on *The error determination of toxicity*[2307] which represents the beginning of the modern, mathematically-based, methods of estimating drug toxicity. This notable paper showed the Gaussian distribution of variation in the graded response of living organisms to the same dose of a drug.

In the year of Trevan's paper, Charles Herbert Best, with Dale, Dudley and Thorpe, wrote, now from the National Institute for Medical Research at Hampstead, on *The nature of the vasodilator constituents of certain tissue extracts*[2308], they reported that 'Histamine and choline have been isolated from alcoholic extracts of fresh liver and lung, in quantities sufficient to account for the immediate vasodilator activities of those extracts. Histamine is responsible for the greater part of this activity, and is present in remarkably large amount in the extract from lung.' Dale and Dudley showed the ubiquitous distribution of these biogenic substances in a paper on the *Presence of histamine and acetylcholine in the spleen of ox and horse* (1929)[2309] and Alfred Clark (1885–1941), professor of materia medica in the University of Edinburgh, drew together many of the biologial and mathematical strands of these enquiries in a study on *The Mode of action of drugs on cells* (1933)[2310]. Despite these advances, it was not until 1934 that Wilhelm Feldberg and Sir John Henry Gaddum (1900–1965) produced the final evidence that acetylcholine is the chemical transmitter involved in the transfer of the nerve impulse from neuron to neuron in the sympathetic nerve ganglia[2311].

Of the transmitters now considered to be involved in the functioning of central pathways, 'enteramine', later found to be identical with 5-hydroxytryptamine, was reported by Maffo Vialli and Vittorio Erspamer of the University of Pavia in 1933[2312]; in 1948 the substance was isolated and named 'serotonin'. Of the peripheral sites of action of the biogenic amines, Sir George Lindor Brown (1903–1971), with Dale and Feldberg, described the *Reactions of the normal mammalian muscle to acetylcholine and to eserine*[2313] in 1936 and then, as attention turned to the therapeutic exploitation of the new knowledge as it related to histamine, Daniel Bovet and Mlle Anne-Marie Staub, in a paper of 1937 on the *Action protectrice des éthers phénoliques au cours de l'intoxication histaminique*[2314] gave an account of the structure and action of the first antihistamine.

Dale had by this time proposed that the anatomical origin of the postganglionic fibres of the autonomic nervous system should be disregarded, the fibres being classified as 'adrenergic' or 'cholinergic' according to the nature of the transmitter released on stimulation. Thus, postganglionic parasympathetic fibres came to be regarded as being predominantly, if not completely, cholinergic. The postganglionic sympathetic fibres were regarded as predominantly, though not entirely, adrenergic. Most of the preganglionic fibres of the autonomic nervous system, in both its parasympathetic and sympathetic divisions, were considered to be cholinergic.

About the time of the beginning of World War II, James Gunn (1822–1958), then professor of therapeutics at Oxford, wrote on the pharmacological actions and therapeutic uses of some compounds related to adrenaline[2315]. The compounds he considered included β-phenylethylamine, tyramine, adrenaline, benzedrine and ephedrine and he concluded that one action which is retained by compounds based on phenylethylamine, even if the molecular structure is considerably modified, is an action on smooth muscle – hence, due to the action on vascular smooth muscle, the pressor, hypertensive side-effects of this group of substances.

By 1946, Ulf von Euler, who shared the Nobel Prize in 1970 with Katz and Axelrod, had shown that noradrenaline is the predominant transmitter of the postganglionic sympathetic nerve fibres[2316]. The methonium compounds came to notice with the report of Sir William Paton and Eleanor Zaimis on the *Curare-like action of polymethylene bis-quarternary ammonium salts* (1948)[2317] and one year later, the discovery of bradykinin was announced in a paper by Mauricio Rocha E Silva and colleagues[2318].

The recent history of both the chemical transmitters of the nerve impulse in the autonomic system, and of the pathways involved in the biological actions of histamine, has been productive of important therapeutic implications.

Since the early years of the study of the subject it was known that the peripheral, vasoconstrictive effects of adrenaline could be prevented, whereas the peripheral vasodilatatory and cardiac stimulant actions of adrenaline could not be prevented by the antagonists (ergot alkaloids, phenoxybenzamine) then available. In 1948, R. P. Ahlquist (*A study of adrenotropic receptors*)[2319] introduced a hypothesis which accounted for this by postulating the existence of two different types, α and β, of adrenoreceptors.

For something like 10 years after the proposal of Ahlquist's hypothesis, only antagonists of α-receptor effects were known; these α-adrenoceptor blocking drugs now include phentolamine, phenoxybenzamine and thymoxamine. Then, in 1958, dichloroisoprenaline was discovered – this proved to be the first substance able to selectively and competitively prevent β-receptor effects; although unsuitable for clinical use it was the first of the now numerous β-adrenoceptor blockers. In 1962, pronethalol was added to the list of these drugs but had to be abandoned due to its proven carcinogenicity in mice. Its replacement by propranolol has already been mentioned[2153].

In 1969, Sir Bernard Katz produced his important study, *The release of neural transmitter substances*[2320]. This book was printed by the University Press, Liverpool, the year before Katz shared the Nobel Prize with U. S. von Euler and J. Axelrod for his research into the processes of chemical neurotransmission.

It has been shown by A. M. Lands and his co-workers (1967)[2321] that differences in the sensitivity of the β-receptors to both stimulant and blocking drugs of varied chemical composition are such as to differentiate two distinct types of β-receptor: these are β_1 in the heart and small intestine and β_2 in the bronchi, vascular beds, and uterus. Thus, as shown by B. Levy and B. E. Wilkenfield (1969)[2322], there are β-blocking drugs which are selective enough to block either β_1 or β_2 receptors without much affecting the other type of β-receptor. In the same way, as shown by Y. F. J. Choo-Kang and associates (1970)[2323], salbutamol – now extensively used to treat bronchial asthma – selectively activates β_2 receptors and relaxes bronchial smooth muscle without producing unwanted cardiac stimulation.

The principal agonists, or activators of the sympathetic system are adrenaline, noradrenaline and isoprenaline. Their effects vary according to their selectivity for the α- or β-receptors. Adrenaline has both α and β effects; the β stimulation relaxing the bronchi is useful in asthma, the mixed effects make it useful in anaphylactic shock. Noradrenaline has predominantly α effects which, acting on the arterioles, produce vasoconstriction giving it a historical place in the treatment of shock. Isoprenaline has predominantly β effects which, exerted on the bronchi, made it useful in asthma, although it has a powerful effect on the heart; the latter effect, a β action on the conducting tissue, led to its use in heart block.

It is apparent that the last 20 years have seen a remarkable advance in the availability of drugs with selective and useful actions on the different types of receptors disclosed by the studies of the chemical messengers of nerve impulse transmission; the same period has seen a much increased understanding of the mode of action of drugs, such as adrenaline, which have been available for several decades. The result has been improvement in the treatment of diseases, such as asthma and hypertension, in which the opportunities to use selective and appropriate agonists or antagonists of nerve impulse transmission at its receptor sites can be exploited.

We can conclude by referring to the developments of a decade ago which resulted in the introduction of cimetidine. The knowledge of histamine developed alongside that of the nerve impulse transmission but it was not until 1947 that the first group of drugs which competitively blocked histamine receptors was introduced. These comprised the conventional antihistamines which inhibit the increased capillary permeability, flare and discomfort of the local response to histamine. They also have some action on the effects of histamine on vascular smooth muscle, thereby limiting the hypotensive response to histamine – but they have no effect of histamine-induced gastric acid output. This fact was made use of in testing for the ability to produce gastric acid by the histamine fractional test-meal technique: histamine was injected after giving a full dose of an antihistamine which was expected to block the unwanted effects of histamine on organs other than the stomach.

It seemed that there must be more than one kind of histamine receptor and in 1964 studies were begun to find substances which would block the effects of histamine spared by the conventional antihistamines. These were conducted by James Whyte Black and, in 1972, were reported by Black and his associates from the Research Institute of Smith Kline and French Laboratories in Welwyn Garden City. Black's previous work at Alderley Park, Cheshire had led to the introduction of propranolol[2153], thus establishing the place of the β-blocking agents in therapeutics.

Black, in his report of 1972 on the *Definition and antagonism of histamine H$_2$-receptors*[2324], noted that the pharmacological receptors involved in the histamine responses which could be blocked by a conventional antihistamine, such as mepyramine, might be termed H$_1$-receptors. He continued: 'Histamine also stimulates the secretion of acid by the stomach, increases the heart rate and inhibits contractions in the rat uterus; these actions cannot be antagonized by mepyramine and related drugs. This article is concerned with the classification and specific blockade of the receptors involved in mepyramine-insensitive, non-H$_1$, histamine responses. Work was started in 1964, based on a simple analogy with catecholamine β-receptors and their antagonists and on the structure of histamine. Since then about 700 compounds have synthesized and tested.'

The work led to the identification of the histamine receptors as being of two kinds: the H$_1$-receptors where the responses to histamine were blocked by conventional antihistamines, and the H$_2$-receptors which were not blocked by the conventional drugs such as mepyramine. It resulted also in the introduction of cimetidine, the first of the clinically-useful H$_2$-blocking agents, and thereby established in clinical practice the first specific drug that could, with a high rate of short-term efficacy, induce peptic ulcer healing.

References

1704. Mendel, Gregor Johann. Versuche über Pflanzen-Hybriden. *Verh. Naturf. Vereines Brünn* (1865), 1866, **4**, 3–47

1705. Bateson, William. Mendel's principles of heredity. Cambridge, *Univ. Press,* 1909

1706. Vries, Hugo Marie de. Die Mutationstheorie. 2 vols. Leipzig, *Veit & Co.,* 1901–3

1707. Galton, Sir Francis. Natural inheritance. London, *Macmillan & Co.,* 1889

1708. Bateson, William. Materials for the study of variation treated with especial regard to discontinuity in the origin of species. London, *Macmillan & Co.,* 1894

1709. Johannsen, Wilhelm Ludwig. Ueber Erblichkeit in Populationen und in reinen Linien. Jena, *G. Fischer,* 1903

1710. Sutton, Walter Stanborough. The chromosomes in heredity. *Biol. Bull.,* 1903, **4**, 231–51

1711. Morgan, Thomas Hunt. Sex-linked inheritance in *Drosophilia. Science,* 1910, **32**, 120–22

1712. Sturtevant, Alfred Henry. The linear arrangement of six sex-linked factors in *Drosophila,* as shown by their mode of association. *J. Exp. Zool.,* 1913, **14**, 43–59

1713. Morgan, Thomas Hunt *et al.* The mechanism of Mendelian heredity. New York, *H. Holt,* 1915

1714. Muller, Hermann Joseph. Artificial transmutation of the gene. *Science,* 1927, **66**, 84–7

1715. Timoféeff-Ressovsky, Nikolai Vladimirovich. *et al.* Ueber die Natur der Genmutation und der Genstruktur. *Nachr. Ges. Wiss. Göttingen, Math.-Fis. Kl.,* Fachgr. 6, 1935, **1**, 189–245

1716. Avery, Oswald Theodore *et al.* Studies on the chemical nature of the substance inducing transformation of pneumococcal types. Induction of transformation by a desoxyribonucleic acid fraction from pneumococcus type III. *J. Exp. Med.,* 1944, **79**, 137–58

1717. Lederberg, Joshua and Tatum, Edward Lawrie. Gene recombination in *Escherichia coli. Nature (Lond.),* 1946, **158**, 558

1718. Barr, Murray Llewellyn and Bertram, Ewart George. A morphological distinction between neurones of the male and female, and the behaviour of the nucleolar satellite during accelerated nucleo-protein synthesis. *Nature (Lond.),* 1949, **163**, 676–7

1719. Hershey, Alfred Day and Chase, Martha Cowles. Independent functions of viral protein and nucleic acid in growth of bacteriophage. *J. Gen. Physiol.,* 1952, **36**, 39–56

1720. Tjio, Joe Hin and Levan, Albert. The chromosome number of man. *Hereditas (Lund),* 1956, **42**, 1–6

1721. Baker, John Randal. The cell-theory: a restatement, history, and critique. *Q. J. Micr. Sci.,* 1948, **89**, 103–25; 1949, **90**, 87–108; 1952, **93**, 157–90

1722. Nuttall, George Henry Falkiner. Experimente über die bacterienfeindlichen Einflüsse des thierischen Körpers. *Z. Hyg. InfektKr.,* 1888, **4**, 353–94

1723. Buchner, Hans. Ueber die bakterientödtende Wirkung des zellenfreien Blutserums. *Zbl. Bakt.,* 1889, **5**, 817–23; **6**, 1–11

1724. Sternberg, George Miller. Practical results of bacteriological researches. *Trans. Ass. Am. Phycns.,* 1892, **7**, 68–86

1725. Bordet, Jules Jean Baptiste Vincent. Contribution à l'étude du sérum chez les animaux vaccinés. *Ann. Soc. R. Sci. Méd. Nat. Brux.,* 1895, **4**, 455–530

1726. Bordet, Jules Jean Baptiste Vincent. Sur l'agglutination et la dissolution des globules rouges par le sérum d'animaux injectés de sang défibriné. *Ann. Inst. Pasteur,* 1898, **12**, 688–95; 1899, **13**, 225–50

1727. Widal, Georges Fernand Isidor and Sicard, Arthur. Recherches de la réaction agglutinante dans le sang et le sérum desséchés des typhiques et dans la sérosité des vésicatoires. *Bull. Mém. Soc. Méd. Hôp. Paris,* 1896, 3 sér., **13**, 681–82

1728. Bordet, Jules Jean B.P. and Gengou, Octave. Sur l'existence de substances sensibilisatrices dans la plupart des sérums antimicrobiens. *Ann. Inst. Pasteur,* 1901, **15**, 289–302

1729. Metchnikoff, Elie. L'immunité dans les maladies infectieuses. Paris, *Masson,* 1901

1730. Breinl, Friedrich and Haurowitz, Felix. Chemische Untersuchung des Präzipitates aus Hämoglobin und Anti-Hämoglobin-Serum und Bemerkungen über die Natur der Antikörper. *Hoppe-Seyl. Z. Physiol. Chem.,* 1930, **192**, 45–57

1731. Landsteiner, Karl. Die Spezifizität der serologischen Reaktionen. Berlin, *Springer,* 1933

1732. Tiselius, Arne Wilhelm Kaurin and Kabat, Elvin Abraham. An electrophoretic study of immune sera and purified antibody preparations. *J. Exp. Med.,* 1939, **69,** 119–31

1733. Freund, Jules Thomas and McDermott, Katherine. Sensitization to horse serum by means of adjuvants. *Proc. Soc. Exp. Biol. (N.Y.),* 1942, **49,** 548–53

1734. Landsteiner, Karl and Chase, Merrill Wallace. Experiments on transfer of cutaneous sensitivty to simple compounds. *Proc. Soc. Exp. Biol. (N.Y.),* 1942, **49,** 688–90

1735. Coons, Albert Hewett and Kaplan, Melvin H. Localization of antigen in tissue cells. II. Improvements in a method for the detection of antigen by means of fluorescent antibody. *J. Exp. Med.,* 1950, **91,** 1–13

1736. Grabar, Pierre and Williams, C. A. Méthode permettant l'étude conjugée des propriétés électrophorétiques et immunochimiqes d'un mélange de protéines. Application au sérum sanguin. *Biochim. Biophys. Acta,* 1953, **10,** 193–4

1737. Mayer, Manfred Martin and Levine, Lawrence. Kinetic studies on immune hemolysis. II–IV. *J. Immunol.,* 1954, **72,** 511–30

1737a Yalow, Rosalyn Sussman and Berson, Solomon. Immunoassay of endogenous plasma insulin in man. *J. Clin. Invest.,* 1960, **39,** 1157–75

1738. Twort, Frederick William. An investigation on the nature of ultra-microscopic viruses. *Lancet,* 1915, **2,** 1241–43

1739. d'Herelle, Félix Hubert. Sur une microbe invisible antagoniste des bacilles dysentérique. *C. R. Acad. Sci. (Paris),* 1917, **165,** 373–75

1740. Gierer, Alfred and Schramm, Gerhard. Infectivity of ribonucleic acid from tobacco mosaic virus. *Nature (Lond.),* 1956, **177,** 702–03

1741. Roitt, Ivan Maurice *et al.* Autoantibodies in Hasimoto's disease (lymphadenoid goitre). *Lancet,* 1956, **2,** 820–21

1742. Isascs, Alick and Lindenmann, Jean. Virus interference. I. The interferon. *Proc. R. Soc. B,* 1957, **147,** 258–67

1743. Uhlenhuth, Paul Theodor. Zur Lehre von der Unterscheidung verschiedener Eiweissarten mit Hilfe spezifischer Sera. In *Festschrift zur sechzigsten Geburstage von Robert Koch.* Jena, *G. Fischer,* 1903, pp. 49–74

1744. Little, Clarence Cook and Tyzzer, Ernest Edward. Further experimental studies on the inheritance of susceptibility to a transplantable tumour, carcinoma (J.W.A.) of the Japanese waltzing mouse. *J. Med. Res.,* 1916, **33,** 393–427

1745. Little, Clarence Cook. The genetics of tissue transplantation in mammals. *J. Cancer Res.,* 1924, **8,** 75–95

1746. Gorer, Peter Alfred. The genetic and antigenic basis of tumour transplantation. *J. Pathol. Bact.,* 1937, **44,** 691–7; 1938, **47,** 231–52

1747. Gibson, Thomas and Medawar, Sir Peter Brian. The fate of skin homografts in man. *J. Anat. (Lond.),* 1943, **77,** 299–310

1748. Burnet, Sir Frank Macfarlane and Fenner, Frank John. The production of antibodies. 2nd edn. Melbourne, *Macmillan,* 1949

1749. Billingham, Rupert Everett *et al.* 'Activity acquired tolerance' of foreign cells. *Nature (Lond.),* 1953, **172,** 603–06

1750. Billingham, Rupert Everett *et al.* Quantitative studies on tissue transplantation immunity. I. The survival times of skin homografts exchanged between members of different inbred strains of mice. II. The origin, strength and duration of actively and adoptively acquired immunity. *Proc. R. Soc. B,* 1954, **143,** 43–80

1751. Burnet, Sir Frank Macfarlane. The clonal selection theory of acquired immunity. Nashville, *Vanderbilt University Press,* 1959

1752. Medawar, Sir Peter Brian. The homograft reaction. *Proc. R. Soc. B.,* 1958, **149,** 145–66

1753. Payne, Rose Marise. Leukocyte agglutinins in human sera. Correlations between blood transfusions and their development. *Arch. Intern. Med.,* 1957, **99,** 587–606

1754. Rood, J. J. van *et al.* Leucocyte antibodies in sera from pregnant women. *Nature (Lond.),* 1958, **181,** 1735–6

1755. Dausset, Jean. Iso-leuco-anticorps. *Acta Haemat. (Basel),* 1958, **20,** 156–66

1756. Snell, George Davis. Histocompatibility genes of the mouse. *J. Nat. Cancer Inst.,* 1958, **20,** 787–824; **21,** 843–75

1757. Benacerraf, Baruj and McDevitt, Hugh O'Neill. Histocompatibility-linked immune response genes. *Science,* 1972, **175,** 273–79

1758. Miller, Jacques Francis Albert Pierre. Immunological function of the thymus. *Lancet,* 1961, **2,** 748–49

1759. Gowans, James Learmonth *et al.* Initiation of immune responses by small lymphocytes. *Nature (Lond.),* 1962, **196,** 651–5

1760. Edelman, Gerald Maurice *et al.* The covalent structure of an entire γG immunoglobulin molecule. *Proc. Nat. Acad. Sci. (Wash.),* 1969, **63,** 78–85

1761. Portier, Paul and Richet, Charles Robert. De l'action anaphylactique de certains venins. *C. R. Soc. Biol. (Paris),* 1902, **54,** 170–72

1762. Arthus, Nicolas Maurice. Injections répétées de sérum de cheval chez le lapin. *C. R. Soc. Biol. (Paris),* 1903, **55,** 817–20

1763. Auer, John and Lewis, Paul A. The physiology of the immediate reaction of anaphylaxis in the guinea-pig. *J. Exp. Med.,* 1910, **12,** 151–75

1764. Hamburger, Franz and Moro, Ernst. Ueber die biologisch nachweisbaren Veränderungen des menschlichen Blutes nach den Seruminjektion. *Wien. Klin. Wschr.,* 1903, **16,** 445–7

1765. Pirquet von Cesenatico, Clemens Peter and Schick, Bela. Die Serumkrankheit. Wien, *F. Deuticke,* 1905

1766. Pirquet von Cesenatico, Clemens Peter. Klinische Studien über Vakzination und vakzinale Allergie. Leipzig, Wien, *F. Deuticke,* 1907

1767. Lewis, Sir Thomas and Grant, Ronald Thomson. Vascular reactions of the skin to injury. II. The liberation of a histamine-like substance in injured skin; the underlying cause of factitious urticaria and of wheals produced by burning; and observations upon the nervous control of certain skin reactions. *Heart,* 1924, **11,** 209–65

1768. Lewis, Sir Thomas. The blood-vessels of the human skin and their responses. London, *Shaw,* 1927

1769. Dragstedt, Carl Albert and Gebauer-Fuelnegg, Erich. Studies in anaphylaxis. *Am. J. Physiol.,* 1932, **102,** 512–26

1770. Storm van Leeuwen, Willem. Allergic diseases; diagnosis and treatment of bronchial asthma, hay-fever, and other allergic diseases. Philadelphia, *J. B. Lippincott,* 1925

1771. Heimstädt, Oskar. Das Fluoreszenzmikroskop. *Z. Wiss. Mikr.,* 1911, **28,** 330–37

1772. Knoll, Max and Ruska, Ernst. Beitrag zur geometrischen Elektronenoptik. *Ann. Physik,* 1932, **12,** 607–61

1773. Zernike, Frits. Das Phasenkontrastverfahren b.d. mikroskopischen Beobachtung. *Phys. Z.,* 1935, **36,** 848–51

1774. Ehrenberg, Werner and Spear, W. E. An electrostatic focussing system and its application to a fine focus X-ray tube. *Proc. Phys. Soc. (Lond.), B,* 1951, **64,** 67–75

1775. Spemann, Hans and Mangold, Hilde. Über Induktion von Embryonalanlagen durch Implantation artfremder Organisatoren. *Wilhelm Roux Arch. EntwMech. Org.,* 1924, **100,** 599–638

1776. Holtfreter, Johannes. Gewebeaffinität, ein Mittel der embryonalen Formbildung. *Arch. Exp. Zellforsch.,* 1939, **23,** 169–209

1777. Ehrlich, Paul. Collected papers of Paul Ehrlich. Compiled and edited by F. Himmelweit. 3 vols. London, *Pergamon Press,* 1956–60

1778. Ehrlich, Paul. Beiträge zur Kenntniss der granulirten Bindegewebszellen und der eosinophilen Leukocythen. *Arch. Anat. Physiol., Physiol. Abt.,* 1879, 166–69

1779. Ehrlich, Paul. Ueber die Methylenblaureaction der lebenden Nervensubstanz. *Dtsch. Med. Wschr.,* 1886, **12,** 49–52

1780. Harrison, Ross Granville. The outgrowth of the nerve fibre as a mode of protoplasmic movement. *J. Exp. Zool.,* 1910, **9,** 787–846

1781. Carrel, Alexis. Rejuvenation of cultures of tissues. *J. Am. Med. Assoc.,* 1911, **57,** 1611

1782. Ramón Y Cajal, Santiago. Degeneration and regeneration of the nervous system. 2 vols. London, *Humphrey Milford,* 1928

1783. Fell, Dame Honor Bridget and Robison, Robert. The growth, development and phosphatase activity of embryonic avian femora in limb-buds cultivated *in vitro. Biochem. J.,* 1929, **23,** 767–84

1784. Sanford, Katherine Koontz *et al.* The growth in vitro of single isolated tissue cells. *J. Nat. Cancer Inst.,* 1948, **9,** 229–46

1785. Aterman, Kurt. Some local factors in the restoration of the rat's liver after partial hepatectomy. 1. Glycogen; the Golgi apparatus; sinusoidal cells; the basement membranes of the sinusoids. *Arch. Pathol. (Chicago),* 1952, **53,** 197–208

1786. Brian, Thomas. The Pisse-prophet or certaine pissepot lectures. London, *E. P. for R. Thrale,* 1637

1787. Bush, Ronnie Beth. Urine is an harlot, or a lier. *J. Am. Med. Assoc.,* 1969, **208,** 131–134

1788. Rouelle, Hilaire Marie. Observations sur l'urine humaine. *J. Méd. Chir. Pharm.,* 1773, **40,** 451–68

1789. Scheele, Carl Wilhelm. Undersökning om blåsestenen. *Kongl. Vetenskaps-Acad. Handl.,* 1776, **37,** 327–32

1790. Wollaston, William Hyde. On cystic oxide, a new species of urinary calculus. *Phil. Trans.,* 1810, **100,** 223–30

1791. Chevreul, Michel Eugène. Recherches chimiques sur plusieurs corps gras, et particulièrement sur leurs combinations avec les calculs. Cinquième mémoire. Des corps qu'on a appelés adipocire, c'est-à-dire, de la substance cristallisée des calculs biliaires humains, du spermacéti et de la substance grasse des cadavres. *Ann. Chim. (Paris),* 1815, **95,** 5–50

1792. Braconnot, Henri. Mémoire sur la conversion des matières animales en nouvelles substances par le moyen de l'acide sulfurique. *Ann. Chim. Phys.,* 1820, Sér. 2, **13,** 113–25

1793. Chevreul, Michel Eugène. Recherches chimiques sur les corps gras d'origine animale. Paris, *F. G. Levrault,* 1823

1794. Chevreul, Michel Eugène. Neues eigenthümliches stickstoffhaltiges Princip, in Muskelfleisch gefunden. *J. Chem. Physik,* 1832, **65,** 455–56

1795. Pettenkofer, Max Josef von. Notiz über eine neue Reaction auf Galle und Zucker. *Ann. Chem. Pharm.,* 1844, **52,** 90–96

1796. Fehling, Hermann Christian von. Quantitative Bestimmung des Zuckers im Harn. *Arch. Physiol. Heilk.,* 1848, **7,** 64–73

1797. Marcet, William. On the immediate principles of human excrements in the healthy state. *Phil. Trans.,* 1857, **147,** 403–13

1798. Jaffé, Max. Beitrag zur Kenntniss der Gallen- und Harnpigmente. *J. Prakt. Chem.,* 1868, **104,** 401–06

1799. Kühne, Willy. Erfahrungen und Bemerkungen über Enzyme und Fermente. *Untersuch. Physiol. Inst. Univ. Heidelberg.,* 1878, **1,** 291–324

1800. Kjeldahl, Johann. En ny Methode til kvaelstofbestemmelse i organiske Stoffer. *Medd. Carlsberg Lab. (Kbh.),* 1883, **2,** 1–27

1801. Hay, Matthew. Test for the bile acids. In Landois and Stirling: *Text-book of Human Physiology,* 2nd edn., London, 1886, **1,** 381

1802. Jaffé, Max. Ueber den Niederschlag, welchen Pikrinsäure in normalen Harn erzeugt und über eine neue Reaction des Kreatinins. *Hoppe-Seyl. Z. Physiol. Chem.,* 1886, **10,** 391–400

1803. Hopkins, Sir Frederick Gowland. On the estimation of uric acid in the urine. *J. Pathol. Bact.,* 1892–93, **1,** 451–59

1804. Buchner, Eduard. Alkoholische Gärung ohne Hefezellen. *Ber. Dtsch. Chem. Ges.,* 1897, **30,** 117–24, 1110–13, 2668–78

1805. Dutrochet, Réné Joachim Henri. Nouvelles observations sur l'endosmose et l'exosmose. *Ann. Chim. Phys.,* 1827, **35,** 393–400; 1828, **37,** 191–201; 1832, **49,** 411–37; **51,** 159–66; 1835, **60,** 337–68

1806. Miescher, Johann Friedrich. Ueber die chemische Zusammensetzung der Eiterzellen. In F. Hoppe-Seyler: *Medicinisch-chemische Untersuchungen,* Berlin, 1871, Heft 4, 441–60

1807. Kossel, Albrecht. Zur Chemie des Zellkerns. *Hoppe-Seyl. Z. Physiol. Chem.,* 1882–83, **7,** 7–22; 1886, **10,** 248–64; 1896–97, **22,** 176–87

1808. Arrhenius, Svante August. Ueber die Dissociation der in Wasser gelösten Stoffe. *Z. Physikal. Chem.,* 1887, **1,** 631–48

1809. Kossel, Albrecht. Ueber die Eiweisstoffe. *Dtsch. Med. Wschr.,* 1898, **24,** 581–82

1810. Levene, Phoebus Aaron Theodore. Darstellung und Analyse einiger Nucleinsäuren. *Hoppe-Seyl. Z. Physiol. Chem.,* 1903, **39,** 4–8, 133–35, 479–83

1811. Fischer, Emil. Untersuchungen über Aminosäuren, Polypeptide und Proteine. Berlin, *J. Springer,* 1906

1812. Willock, Edith Gertrude and Hopkins, Sir Frederick Gowland. The importance of individual amino-acids in metabolism. *J. Physiol. (Lond.),* 1906, **35,** 88–102

1813. Fletcher, Sir Walter Morley and Hopkins, Sir Frederick Gowland. Lactic acid in amphibian muscle. *J. Physiol. (Lond.), 1907, 35,* 247–309

1814. Hasselbalch, Karl Albert and Lundsgaard, Christen. Elektrometrische Reaktionsbestimmung des Blutes bei Körpertemperatur. *Biochem. Z.* 1912, **38**, 77–91

1815. Fiske, Cyrus Hartwell and Subbarow, Yellapragada. Phosphorus compounds of muscle and liver. *Science,* 1929, **70**, 381–382

1816. Keilin, David. Cytochrome and respiratory enzymes. *Proc. R. Soc. B,* 1929, **104**, 206–52

1817. Meldrum, Norman Urquhart and Roughton, Fancis John Worsley. Carbonic anhydrase. Its preparation and properties. *J. Physiol. (Lond.),* 1933, **80**, 113–42

1818. Krebs, Sir Hans Adolf and Johnson, William Arthur. Citric acid in intermediate metabolism in animal tissues. *Enzymologia,* 1937, **4**, 148–56

1819. Chargaff, Erwin. Chemical specificity of nucleic acids and the mechanism of their enzymatic degradation. *Experientia (Basel),* 1950, **6**, 201–9

1820. Watson, James Dewey and Crick, Francis Harry Compton. Molecular structure of nucleic acids. A structure for deoxyribose nucleic acid. *Nature (Lond.),* 1953, **171**, 737–38

1821. Wilkins, Maurice Hugh Frederick *et al.* Helical structure of crystalline deoxypentose nucleic acid. *Nature (Lond.),* 1953, **172**, 759–62

1822. Watson, James Dewey and Crick, Francis Harry. Genetical implications of the structure of deoxyribonucleic acid. *Nature (Lond.),* 1953, **171**, 964–67

1823. Grunberg-Manago, Marianne and Ochoa de Albornoz, Severo. Enzymatic synthesis and breakdown of polynucleotides; polynucleotide phosphorylase. *J. Am. Chem. Soc.,* 1955, **77**, 3165–66

1824. Kornberg, Arthur *et al.* Enzymic synthesis of deoxyribonucleic acid. *Biochim. Biophys. Acta,* 1956, **21**, 197–98

1825. Theorell, Axel Hugo Teodor. The nature and mode of action of oxidation enzymes. Nobel Lecture, December 12, 1955. In *Festschrift Arthur Stoll,* Basel, Birkhäuser, 1957, pp. 35–47

1826. Gilham, Peter Thomas and Khorana, Har Gobind. Studies on polynucleotides. I. A new and general method for the chemical synthesis of the C_5'-C_3' internucleotide linkage. Synthesis of deoxyribo-denucleotides. *J. Am. Chem. Soc.,* 1958, **80**, 6212–22

1827. Brenner, Sydney *et al.* An unstable intermediate carrying information from genes to ribosomes for protein synthesis. *Nature (Lond.),* 1961, **190**, 576–80

1828. Matthaei, J. Heinrich and Nirenberg, Marshall Warren. Characteristics and stabilization of DNAase-sensitive protein synthesis in *E. coli* extracts. *Proc. Nat. Acad. Sci. (Wash.),* 1961, **47**, 1580–88

1829. Holley, Robert William *et al.* Structure of a ribonucleic acid. *Science,* 1965, **147**, 1462–65

1830. Robson, George Alan, Butcher, Reginald William and Sutherland, Earl Wilber. Cyclic AMP. *Ann. Rev. Biochem.,* 1968, **37**, 149–74

1831. Tabin, Clifford J. *et al.* Mechanism of activation of a human oncogene. *Nature (Lond.),* 1982, **300**, 143–149

1832. Reddy, E. Premkumar *et al.* A point mutation is responsible for the acquisition of transforming properties by the T24 human bladder carcinoma oncogene. *Nature (Lond.),* 1982, **300**, 149–152

1833. Euler, Ulf Svante Hansson von. Zur Kenntnis der pharmakologischen Wirkungen von Nativsekreten und Extrakten männlicher accessorischer Geschlechtdrüsen. *Arch. Exp. Pathol., Pharmak.,* 1934, **175**, 78–84

1834. Hamberg, Mats *et al.* Thromboxanes: a new group of biologically active compounds derived from prostaglandin endoperoxides. *Proc. Nat. Acad. Sci. (Wash.),* 1975, **72**, 2994–98

1835. Vane, John R. Prostacyclin. *J. R. Soc. Med.,* 1983, **76**, 245–249

1836. Osler, Sir William, Bart. An account of certain organisms ocurring in the liquor sanguinis. *Proc. R. Soc. (Lond.),* (1873), 1874, **22**, 391–98

1837. Bizzozero, Giulio. Su di un nuovo elemento morfologico del sangue dei mammiferi e della sua importanza nella trombosi e nella coagulazione. *Osservatore,* 1882, **17**, 785–87; **18**, 97–99

1838. Wright, James Homer. The origin and nature of the blood plates. *Boston Med. Surg. J.,* 1906, **154**, 643–45

1839. Hammarsten, Olof. Undersökningar af de s.k. fibringeneratorerna fibrinet samt fibrinogenets koagulation. *Upsala LäkFören. Förh.,* 1875–76, **11**, 538–79

1840. Arthus, Nicolas Maurice and Pagès, Calixte. Nouvelle théorie chimique de la coagulation du sang. *Arch. Physiol. Norm. Pathol.*, 1890. 5 ser. 2, 732–46

1841. Howell, William Henry. The preparation and properties of thrombin, together with observations on antithrombin and prothrombin. *Am. J. Physiol.*, 1910, **26**, 453–73

1842. Howell, William Henry. The role of antithrombin and thromboplastin (thromboplastic substance) in the coagulation of blood. *Am. J. Physiol.*, 1911-12, **29**, 187–209

1843. McLean, Jay. The thromboplastic action of cephalin. *Am. J. Physiol.*, 1916, **41**, 250–57

1844. Howell, William Henry and Holt, Luther Emmett. Two new factors in blood coagulation – heparin and pro-antithrombin. *Am. J. Physiol.*, 1918-19, **47**, 328–41

1845. Ehrlich, Paul. Methodologische Beiträge zur Physiologie und Pathologie der verschiedenen Formen der Leukocyten. *Z. Klin. Med.*, 1879-80, **1**, 553–560

1846. Haldane, John Scott. The colorimetric determination of haemoglobin. *J. Physiol. (Lond.)*, 1901, **26**, 497–504

1847. Vaughan, Victor Clarence. On the appearance and significance of certain granules in the erythrocytes of man. *J. Med. Res.*, 1903, **10**, 342–66

1848. Price-Jones, Cecil. The variation in the sizes of red blood cells. *Br. Med. J.*, 1910, **2**, 1418–19

1849. Keith, Norman Macdonnell *et al.* A method for the determination of plasma and blood volume. *Arch. Intern. Med.*, 1915, **16**, 547–76

1850. Landsteiner, Karl. Zur Kenntniss der antifermentativen, lytischen und agglutinierenden Wirkungen des Blutserums und der Lymphe. *Zbl. Bakt.*, 1900, **27**, 357–62

1851. Janský, Jan. Haematologické studie u psychotiku. *Sborn. Klinický*, 1906-07, **8**, 85–139

1852. Moss, William Lorenzo. Studies on isoagglutinins and isohemolysins. *Johns Hopk. Hosp. Bull.*, 1910, **21**, 63–70

1853. Morton, Leslie T. A medical bibliography (Garrison and Morton). 4th edn. Aldershot, *Gower*, 1983, p. 117

1854. Landsteiner, Karl and Levine, Philip. A new agglutinable factor differentiating individual human bloods. *Proc. Soc. Exp. Biol. (N.Y.)*, 1927, **24**, 600–02

1855. Levine, Philip and Stetson, Rufus E. An unusual case of intra-group agglutination. *J. Am. Med. Assoc.*, 1939, **113**, 126–27

1856. Moureau, Paul. Recherches sur un nouvel hémo-agglutinogène du sang humain. *Acta Biol. Belg.*, 1941, **1**, 123–28

1857. Landsteiner, Karl and Wiener, Alexander Solomon. An agglutinable factor in human blood recognized by immune sera for Rhesus blood. *Proc. Soc. Exp. Biol. (N.Y.)*, 1940, **43**, 223

1858. Cohn, Edwin Joseph *et al.* Chemical, clinical and immunological studies on the products of human plasma fractionation. *J. Clin. Invest.*, 1944, **23**, 417–606

1859. Friedreich, Nikolaus. Ein neuer Fall von Leukämie. *Virchows Arch. Pathol. Anat.*, 1857, **12**, 37–58

1860. Henoch, Eduard Heinrich. Über den Zusammenhang von Purpura und Intestinalstörungen. *Berl. Klin. Wschr.*, 1868, **5**, 517–19

1861. Ehrlich, Paul. Farbenanalytische Untersuchungen zur Histologie und Klinik. Berlin, *A. Hirschwald*, 1891

1862. Brown, Philip King and Ophüls, William. A fatal case of acute primary infectious pharyngitis. *Trans. Med. Soc. Calif.*, 1901, 93–101

1863. Türk, Wilhelm. Septische Erkrankungen bei Verkümmerung des Granulozytensystems. *Wien. Klin. Wschr.*, 1907, **20**, 157–62

1864. Schultz, Werner. Gangräneszierende Prozesse und Defekt des Granulocytensystems. *Dtsch. Med. Wschr*, 1922, **48**, 1495–96

1865. Bulloch, William and Fildes, Sir Paul. Haemophilia. London, *Dulau & Co.*, 1911

1866. Willebrand, Erik Adolf von. Hereditär pseudohemofili. *Fin. Läk.-Sallsk. Handl.*, 1926, **68**, 87–112

1867. Patek, Arthur Jackson and Taylor, Francis Henry Laskey. Hemophilia. II. Some properties of a substance obtained from normal human plasma effective in accelerating the coagulation of hemophilic blood. *J. Clin. Invest.*, 1937, **16**, 113–24

1868. Biggs, Rosemary Peyton *et al.* Christmas disease, a condition previously mistaken for haemophilia. *Br. Med. J.*, 1952, **2**, 1378–82

1869. Reschad, Hassan and Schilling-Torgau, V. Ueber eine neue Leukämie durch echte Uebergangsformen (Splenozytenleukämie) und ihre Bedeutung für die Selbständigkeit dieser Zellen. *Münch. Med. Wschr.,* 1913, **60**, 1981–84

1870. Levine, Philip *et al.* The rôle of iso-immunization in the pathogenesis of erythroblastosis fetalis. *Am. J. Obstet. Gynec.,* 1941, **42**, 925–37

1871. Hart, Alfred Purvis. Familial icterus gravis of the new-born and its treatment. *Can. Med. Assoc. J.,* 1925, **15**, 1008 112

1872. Diamond, Louis Klein. Replacement transfusion as a treatment for erythroblastosis fetalis. *Pediatrics,* 1948, **2**, 520–24

1873. Liley, Albert William. Intrauterine transfusion of foetus in haemolytic disease. *Br. Med. J.,* 1963, **2**, 1107–9

1874. Freda, Vincent J. *et al.* Successful prevention of experimental Rh sensitization in man with an anti-Rh gamma$_2$-globulin antibody preparation. *Transfusion,* 1964, **4**, 26–32

1875. Westergren, Alf Vilhelm. Studies of the suspension stability of the blood in pulmonary tuberculosis. *Acta Med. Scand.,* 1921, **54**, 247–82

1876. Wintrobe, Maxwell Myer and Landsberg, J. Walter. A standardized technique for the blood sedimentation test. *Am. J. Med. Sci.,* 1935, **189**, 102–15

1877. Quick, Armand James. The prothrombin in hemophilia and in obstructive jaundice. *J. Biol. Chem.,* 1935, **109**, lxxiii–lxxix

1878. Coombs, Robin Royston Amos *et al.* Detection of weak and "incomplete" Rh agglutinins: a new test. *Lancet,* 1945, **2**, 15–16

1879. Gardner, William and Osler, Sir William, Bart. A case of progressive pernicious anaemia, (idiopathic of Addison). *Can. Med. Surg. J.,* 1877, **5**, 383–404

1880. Ehrlich, Paul. Über einige Beobachtungen am anämischen Blut. *Berl. Klin. Wschr.,* 1881, **18**, 43

1881. Banti, Guido. Dell' anemia splenica. Firenze, *succ. Le Monnier,* 1882

1882. Leichtenstern, Otto. Ueber progressive perniciöse Anämie bei Tabeskranken. *Dtsch. Med. Wschr.,* 1884, **10**, 849

1883. Ehrlich, Paul. Ueber einen Fall von Anämie mit Bemerkungen über regenerative Veränderungen des Knochenmarks. *Charité-Ann.,* 1888, **13**, 300–09

1884. Bunge, Gustav von. Ueber die Eisentherapie. *Verh. Congr. Inn. Med.,* 1895, **13**, 133–47

1885. Herrick, James Bryan. Peculiar elongated and sickle-shaped red blood corpuscles in a case of severe anemia. *Arch. Intern. Med.,* 1910, **6**, 517–21; *Trans. Assoc. Am. Phys.,* 1910, **25**, 553–61

1886. Faber, Knud Helge. Anämische Zustände bei der chronischen Achylia gastrica. *Berl. Klin. Wschr.,* 1913, **50**, 958–62

1887. Osler, Sir William, Bart. Observations on the severe anaemias of pregnancy and the post-partum state. *Br. Med. J.,* 1919, **1**, 1–3

1888. Mason, Verne Rheem. Sickle cell anemia. *J. Am. Med. Assoc.,* 1922, **79**, 1318–20

1889. Robscheit-Robbins, Frieda Saur and Whipple, George Hoyt. Blood regeneration in severe anaemia. II. Favourable influence of liver, heart and skeletal muscle in diet. *Am. J. Physiol.,* 1925, **72**, 408–18

1890. Minot, George Richards and Murphy, William Parry. Treatment of pernicious anemia by a special diet. *J. Am. Med. Assoc.,* 1926, **87**, 470–76

1891. Cooley, Thomas Benton *et al.* Anemia in children, with splenomegaly and peculiar changes in the bones. *Am. J. Dis. Child.,* 1927, **34**, 347–63

1892. Fanconi, Guido. Familiäre infantile perniziosaartige Anämie (perniziöses Blutbild und Konstitution). *Jb. Kinderheilk.,* 1927, **117**, 257–80

1893. Peabody, Francis Weld. The pathology of the bone marrow in pernicious anaemia. *Am. J. Pathol.,* 1927, **3**, 179–202

1894. Castle, William Bosworth. Observations on the etiologic relationship of achylia gastrica to pernicious anemia. I. The effect of the administration to patients with pernicious anemia of the contents of the normal human stomach recovered after the ingestion of beef muscle. *Am. J. Med. Sci.,* 1929, **178**, 748–64

1895. Sturgis, Cyrus Cressey and Issacs, Raphael. Desiccated stomach in the treatment of pernicious anemia. *J. Am. Med. Assoc.,* 1929, **93**, 747–49

1896. Wintrobe, Maxwell Myer. Classification of the anemias on the basis of differences in the size and hemoglobin content of the red corpuscles. *Proc. Soc. Exp. Biol. (N.Y.),* 1930, **27,** 1071–73

1897. Wills, Lucy. Treatment of "pernicious anaemia of pregnancy" and "tropical anaemia", with special reference to yeast extract as a curative agent. *Br. Med. J.,* 1931, **1,** 1059–64

1898. Whipple, George Hoyt and Bradford, William L. Mediterranean disease – thalassemia (erythroblastic anemia of Cooley); associated pigment abnormalities simulating hemochromatosis. *J. Pediatr.,* 1936, **9,** 279–311

1899. Caminopetros, J. Recherches sur l'anémie érythroblastique infantile des peuples de la Méditerranée orientale. Étude anthropologique, étiologique et pathogenique. La transmission héréditaire de la maladie. *Ann. Méd.,* 1938, **43,** 104–25

1900. Spies, Tom Douglas *et al.* Observations of the anti-anemic properties of synthetic folic acid. *Sth. Med. J. (Nashville),* 1945, **38,** 707–09

1901. Angier, Robert Crane *et al.* Structure and synthesis of liver *L. casei* factor. *Science,* 1946, **103,** 667–69

1902. West, Randolph. Activity of vitamin B_{12} in Addisonian pernicious anemia. *Science,* 1948, **107,** 398

1903. Ungley, Charles Cady. Vitamin B_{12} in pernicious anaemia: parenteral administration. *Br. Med. J.,* 1949, **2,** 1370–77

1904. Pauling, Linus Carl *et al.* Sickle cell anemia, a molecular disease. *Science,* 1949, **110,** 543–48

1905. Willius, Frederick Arthur and Keys, Thomas Edward. Cardiac classics. A collection of classic works on the heart and circulation with comprehensive biographic accounts of the authors. St. Louis, *C. V. Mosby Co.,* 1941

1906. Wintrobe, Maxwell Myer. Blood, pure and eloquent. A story of discovery, of people, and of ideas. New York, *McGraw-Hill,* 1980

1907. Wilks, Sir Samuel, Bart. Cases of a peculiar enlargement of the lymphatic glands frequently associated with disease of the spleen. *Guy's Hosp. Rep.,* 1856, 3 ser. **2,** 114–32; 1865, 3 ser. **11,** 56–67

1908. Langhans, Theodor. Das maligne Lymphosarkom (Pseudoleukämie). *Virchows Arch. Pathol. Anat.,* 1872, **54,** 509–37

1909. Greenfield, William Smith. Specimens illustrative of the pathology of lymphadenoma and leucocythemia. *Trans. Pathol. Soc. Lond.,* 1878, **29,** 272–304

1910. Reed, Dorothy. On the pathological changes in Hodgkin's disease, with especial reference to its relation to tuberculosis. *Johns Hopk. Hosp. Rep.,* 1902, **10,** 133–96

1911. Pel, Pieter Klazes. Zur Symptomatologie der sog. Pseudo-Leukämie. *Berl. Klin. Wschr.,* 1885, **22,** 3–7

1912. Ebstein, Wilhelm. Das chronische Rückfallsfieber, eine neue Infektionskrankheit. *Berl. Klin. Wschr.,* 1887, **24,** 565–68

1913. Dreschfeld, Julius. Clinical lecture on acute Hodgkin's disease. *Br. Med. J.,* 1892, **1,** 893–96

1914. Kundrat, Hans. Ueber Lympho-Sarkomatosis. *Wien. Klin. Wschr.,* 1893, **6,** 211–13, 234–39

1915. Gaucher, Philippe Charles Ernest. De l'épithélioma primitif de la rate, hypertrophie idiopathique de la rate sans leucémie. Paris, *Thèse,* 1882

1916. Sternberg, Carl. Ueber eine eigenartige, unter dem Bilde der Pseudoleukämie verlaufende Tuberkulose des lymphatischen Apparates. *Z. Heilk.,* 1898, **19,** 21–90

1917. Aschoff, Karl Albert Ludwig. Das reticulo-endotheliale System. *Ergebn. Inn. Med.,* 1924, **26,** 1–118

1918. Landois, Leonard. Auflösung der rothen Blutzellen. *Zbl. Med. Wiss.,* 1874, **12,** 419–22

1919. Hustin, Albert. Note sur une nouvelle méthode de transfusion. *Bull. Soc. R. Sci. Méd. Brux.,* 1914, **72,** 104–11

1920. Agote, Luis. Nuevo procedimiento para la transfusion de la sangre. *An. Inst. Mod. Clin. Méd. (B. Aires),* 1914–15, **1,** 24–31

1921. Lewisohn, Richard. A new and greatly simplified method of blood transfusion. A preliminary report. *Med. Rec. (N.Y.),* 1915, **87,** 141–42

1922. Robertson, Oswald Hope. Transfusion with preserved red blood cells. *Med. Bull. (Paris),* 1917–1918, **1,** 436–40

1923. Marriott, Hugh Leslie and Kekwick, Alan. Continuous drip blood transfusion. *Lancet,* 1935, **1**, 977–81

1924. Hedenius, Per Johannes. A new method of blood transfusion. *Acta Med. Scand.,* 1936, **89**, 263–267

1925. Yudin, Sergei Sergeievich. Transfusion of cadaver blood. *J. Am. Med. Assoc.,* 1936, **106**, 997–99

1926. Fantus, Bernard. The therapy of the Cook County Hospital. Blood preservation. *J. Am. Med. Assoc.,* 1937, **109**, 128–31

1927. Loutit, John Freeman and Mollison, Patrick Loudon. Advantages of a disodium-citrate-glucose mixture as a blood preservative. *Br. Med. J.,* 1943, **2**, 744–5

1928. Grönwall, Anders Johan Troed and Ingleman, Björn. Untersuchungen über Dextran und sein Verhalten bei parenteraler Zufuhr. *Acta Physiol. Scand.,* 1944, **7**, 97–107

1929. Smith, Audrey Ursula. Prevention of haemolysis during freezing and thawing red blood-cells. *Lancet,* 1950, **2**, 910–11

1930. Maluf, Noble Suydam R. History of blood transfusion. *J. Hist. Med.,* 1954, **9**, 59–107

1931. Eppinger, Hans and Kloss, Karl. Zur Therapie der Polyzythämie. *Therap. Mh.,* 1918, **32**, 322–26

1932. Butt, Hugh Roland and Snell, Albert Markley. The use of vitamin K and bile in treatment of the hemorrhagic diathesis in cases of jaundice. *Proc. Mayo Clin.,* 1938, **13**, 74–80

1933. Gilbert, René. Radiotherapy in Hodgkin's disease (malignant granulomatosis). Anatomic and clinical foundations; governing principles; results. *Am. J. Roentgenol.* 1939, **41**, 198–241

1934. Lawrence, John Hundale *et al.* Studies on leukemia with the aid of radioactive phosphorus. *N. Int. Clin.,* 1939, n.s., **2**, vol. 3, 33–58

1935. Stahmann, Mark Arnold *et al.* Studies on the hemoorrhagic sweet clover disease. V. Identification and synthesis of the hemorrhagic agent. *J. Biol. Chem.,* 1941, **138**, 513–27

1936. The pharmacological basis of therapeutics. Eds. Goodman, louis S. and Gilman, Alfred. 5th edn. New York, *Macmillan,* 1975, p. 1254

1937. Gilman, Alfred and Philips, Frederick Stanley. The biological actions and therapeutic applications of the β-chloroethyl amines and sulfides. *Science,* 1946, **103**, 409–15

1938. Paterson, Edith *et al.* Leukaemia treated with urethane compared with deep X-ray therapy. *Lancet,* 1946, **1**, 677

1939. Rhoads, Cornelius Packard *et al.* Triethylene melamine in the treatment of Hodgkin's disease and allied neoplasms. *Trans. Assoc. Am. Phycns,* 1950, **63**, 136–46

1940. Elion, Gertrude B. *et al.* Condensed pyrimidine system. IX. The synthesis of 6-substituted pyrimidines. *J. Am. Chem. Soc.,* 1952, **74**, 411–14

1941. Haddow, Sir Alexander and Timmis, Geoffrey Millward. Myleran in chronic myeloid leukaemia: chemical constitution and biological action. *Lancet,* 1953, **1**, 207–8

1942. Galton, David Abraham Goiten *et al.* Clinical trials of p-(DI-2-chlorethylamino)-phenyl-butyric acid (CB 1348) in malignant lymphoma. *Br. Med. J.,* 1955, **2**, 1172–76

1943. Johnson, Irving Stanley *et al.* The Vinca alkaloids: a new class of oncolytic agents. *Cancer Res.,* 1963, **23**, 1390–1427

1944. Ellison, Rose Ruth *et al.* Arabinosyl cytosine. A useful agent in the treatment of acute leukemia in adults. *Blood,* 1968, **32**, 507–23

1945. Soulier, Jean Pierre and Gueguen, Jean. Action hypoprothrombinémiante (anti-K) de la phényl-indanedione étudiée expérimentalement chez le lapin. Son application chez l'homme. *C. R. Soc. Biol. (Paris),* 1947, **141**, 1007–11

1946. Reinis, Z. and Kubík, Mirko. Klinische Erfahrungen mit einem neuen Präparat der Cumarinreihe. *Schweiz. Med. Wschr.,* 1948, **78**, 785–90

1947. Ellermann, Vilhelm and Bang, O. Experimentelle Leukämie bei Hühnern. *Zbl. Bakt.,* 1908, Abt. I, Orig., **46**, 595–609

1948. Sherry, Sol *et al.* Studies on enhanced fibrinolytic activity in man. *J. Clin. Invest.,* 1959, **38**, 810–822

1948a Flute, Peter T. The fibrinolytic system of human plasma. Thesis, MD, University of London, 1960

1949. Fearnley, George R. Evidence of a diurnal fibrinolytic rhythm; with a simple method of measuring natural fibrinolysis. *Clin. Sci.,* 1957, **16**, 645–650

1950. Chakrabarti, R., Hocking, E.D., Fearnley, G.R., Mann, R.D., Attwell, T.N. and Jackson, D. Fibrinolytic activity and coronary artery disease. *Lancet,* 1968, **1**, 1987–1990

1951. Morau, Henri. Inoculation en série d'une tumeur épithéliale de la souris blanche. *C.R. Soc. Biol.,* 1891, **43**, 289–90

1952. Loeb, Leo. On transplantation of tumors. *J. Med. Res.,* 1901, **6**, 28–38

1953. Jensen, Carl Oluf. Experimentelle Untersuchungen über Krebs bei Mäusen. *Zbl. Bakt.,* 1903, Abt. I, Orig., **34**, 28–34, 122–43

1954. Rous, Francis Peyton. A transmissible avian neoplasm (sarcoma of the common fowl). *J. Exp. Med.,* 1910, **12**, 696–705; 1911, **13**, 397–411

1955. Carrel, Alexis and Burrows, Montrose Thomas. Cultures de sarcoma en dehors de l'organisme. *C.R. Soc. Biol. (Paris),* 1910, **69**, 332–34

1956. Sjögren, Tage Anton Ultimus. Fall af epiteliom behandladt med Roentgenstråler. *Förh. Svenska Läkare-Sallskapets Sammankomster,* Stockholm, 1899, p. 208

1957. Frieben, Ernst August Franz Albert. Cancroid des rechten Handrückens. *Dtsch. Med. Wschr.,* 1902, **28**, Vereins-Beilage, 335

1958. Perthes, Georg Clemens. Ueber den Einfluss der Röntgenstrahlen auf epitheliale Gewebe, insbesondere auf das Carcinom. *Arch. Klin. Chir.,* 1903, **71**, 955–1000

1959. Goldeberg, S.W. and London, Efim Semenovic. Zur Frage der Beziehungen zwischen Becquerelstrahlen und Hautaffectionen. *Derm. Z.,* 1903, **10**, 457–62

1960. Freund, Ernst and Kaminer, Gisa. Zur Diagnose des Karzinoms. *Wien. Klin. Wschr.,* 1911, **24**, 1759–64

1961. Lathrop, A.E.C. and Loeb, Leo. Further investigations on the origin of tumors in mice. III. On the part played by internal secretion in the spontaneous development of tumors. *J. Cancer Res.,* 1916, **1**, 1–19

1962. Bayon, Henry Peter George. Epithelial proliferation induced by the injection of gasworks tar. *Lancet,* 1912, **2**, 1579

1963. Kennaway, Sir Ernest Laurence. The formation of a cancer-producing substance from isoprene (2-methyl-butadiene). *J. Pathol., Bact.,* 1924, **27**, 233–38

1964. Gye, William Ewart. The aetiology of malignant new growths. *Lancet,* 1925, **2**, 109–17

1965. Barnard, Joseph Edwin. The microscopical examination of filterable viruses associated with malignant new growths. *Lancet,* 1925, **2**, 117–23

1966. Warburg, Otto Heinrich. Ueber den Stoffwechsel der Tumoren. Berlin, *J. Springer,* 1926

1967. Slye, Maud. Cancer and heredity. *Ann. Intern. Med.,* 1928, **1**, 951–76

1968. Cook, Sir James Wilfred *et al.* The production of cancer by pure hydrocarbons. *Proc. R. Soc. B,* 1932, **111**, 455–96

1969. Bonser, Georgiana May *et al.* The carcinogenic action of oestrone: induction of mammary carcinoma in female mice of a strain refractory to the spontaneous development of mammary tumours. *J. Pathol. Bact.,* 1937, **45**, 709–14

1970. Haddow, Sir Alexander *et al.* Influence of synthetic oestrogens upon advanced malignant disease. *Br. Med. J.,* 1944, **2**, 393–98

1971. Shope, Richard Edwin. A transmissible tumor-like condition in rabbits. *J. Exp. Med.,* 1932, **56**, 793–802

1972. Bittner, John Joseph. Some possible effects of nursing on the mammary gland tumor incidence in mice. *Science,* 1936, **84**, 162

1973. Stewart, Sarah Elizabeth *et al.* The induction of neoplasms with a substance released from mouse tumors by tissue culture. *Virology,* 1957, **3**, 380–400

1974. Vogt, Marguerite and Dulbecco, Renato. Virus-cell interaction with a tumor-producing virus. *Proc. Nat. Acad. Sci. (Wash.),* 1961, **46**, 365–70

1975. Temin, Howard Martin. Nature of the provirus of Rous sarcoma. *National Cancer Institute Monograph 17.* Bethesda, Md., *National Cancer Institue,* 1964, pp. 557–70

1976. Burkitt, Denis. A sarcoma involving the jaws in African children. *Br. J. Surg.,* 1958–59, **46**, 218–23

1977. Epstein, Michael Anthony and Barr, Y.M. Cultivation in vitro of human lymphoblasts from Burkitt's malignant lymphoma. *Lancet,* 1964, **1**, 252–3

1978. Epstein, Michael Anthony *et al.* Virus particles in cultured lymphoblasts from Burkitt's lymphoma. *Lancet,* 1964, **1**, 702–3

1979. Shope, Thomas *et al.* Malignant lymphoma in cotton-top marmosets after inoculation with Epstein-Barr virus. *Proc. Nat. Acad. Sci. (Wash.),* 1973, **70**, 2487–91

1980. Baltimore, David. RNA-dependent DNA polymerase in virions of RNA tumour viruses. *Nature (Lond.)*, 1970, **226**, 1209–11

1981. Temin, Howard Martin and Mizutani, Satoshi. RNA-depenent DNA polymerase in virions of Rous sarcoma virus. *Nature (Lond.)*, 1970, **226**, 1211–13

1982. Dulbecco, Renato. From the molecular biology of oncogenic DNA viruses to cancer. *Les Prix Nobel en 1975*, Stockholm, pp. 172–80

1983. Biggs, Peter Martin *et al.* Field trials with an attenuated cell associated vaccine for Marek's disease. *Vet. Rec.*, 1970, **87**, 704–9

1984. Goodman, Louis Sanford *et al.* Nitrogen mustard therapy. Use of methyl-bis (beta-chloroethyl(amine) hydrochloride and tris (beta-chloroethyl)amine hydrochloride for Hodgkin's disease, lymphosarcoma, leukemia and certain allied and miscellaneous disorders. *J. Am. Med. Assoc.*, 1946, **132**, 126–32

1985. Leuchtenberger, Cecilie *et al.* "Folic acid" a tumour growth inhibitor. *Proc. Soc. Exp. Biol. (N.Y.)*, 1944, **55**, 204–05

1986. Farber, Sidney *et al.* Temporary remissions in acute leukemia in children produced by folic acid antagonist 4-amethopteroylglutamic acid (aminopterin). *New Engl. J. Med.*, 1948, **238**, 787–93

1986a Bergmann, Werner and Feeney, Robert J. Contributions to the study of marine products. XXXII. The nucleosides of sponges. I. *J. Org. Chem.*, 1951, **16**, 981–7

1987. Everett, James Lionel *et al.* Aryl-2-halogenoalkylamines. Part XII. Some carboxylic derivatives of *NN*-Di-2-chloroethylaniline. *J. Chem. Soc.*, 1953, 2386–92

1988. Arnold, Herbert *et al.* Neuartige Krebs-Chemotherapeutica aus der Gruppe der zyklischen N-Lost-Phosphamidester. *Naturwissenschaften*, 1958, **45**, 64–66

1988a Gray, Louis Harold *et al.* The concentration of oxygen dissolved in tissues at the time of irradiation as a factor in radiotherapy. *Br. J. Radiol.*, 1953, **26**, 638–48

1989. DeVita, Vincent T. *et al.* Combination chemotherapy in the treatment of advanced Hodgkin's disease. *Ann. Intern. Med.*, 1970, **73**, 881–95

1990. Loeffler, Friedrich August Johann and Frosch, Paul. Bericht der Kommission zur Erforschung der Maul- und Klauenseuche bei dem Institut für Infektionskrankheiten. *Zbl. Bakt.*, 1898, I. Abt., **23**, 371–91

1991. Bechhold, Heinrich. Kolloidstudien mit der Filtrationsmethode. *Z. Phys. Chem.*, 1907, **60**, 257–318

1992. Elford, William Joseph. A new series of graded collodion membranes suitable for general bacteriological use, especially in filterable virus studies. *J. Pathol. Bact.*, 1931, **34**, 505–21

1993. Woodruff, Alice Miles and Goodpasture, Ernest William. The susceptibility of the chorioallantoic membrane of chick embryos to infection with the fowl-pox virus. *Am. J. Pathol.*, 1931, **7**, 209–22

1994. Lancefield, Rebecca Craighill. A serological differentiation of human and other groups of hemolytic streptococci. *J. Exp. Med.*, 1933, **57**, 571–95

1995. Griffith, Frederick. The serological classification of *Streptococcus pyogenes*. *J. Hyg. (Camb.)*, 1934, **34**, 542–84

1996. Stanley, Wendell Meredith. Isolation of a cyrstalline protein possessing the properties of tobacco-mosaic virus. *Science*, 1935, **81**, 644–45

1997. Smith, Margaret G. Propagation in tissue culture of a cytopathogenic virus from human salivary gland virus (SGV) disease. *Proc. Soc. Exp. Biol. Med.*, 1956, **92**, 424–30

1998. Sweet, Benjamin Hersh and Hilleman, Maurice Ralph. The vacuolating virus SV_{40}. *Proc. Soc. Exp. Biol. (N.Y.)*, 1960, **105**, 420–27

1999. Rowe, Wallace Prescott *et al.* Isolation of a cytopathogenic agent from human adenoids undergoing spontaneous degeneration in tissue culture. *Proc. Soc. Exp. Biol. (N.Y.)*, 1953, **84**, 570–73

2000. Luria, Salvador Edward and Dulbecco, Renato. Genetic recombinations leading to production of active bacteriophage from ultraviolet inactivated bacteriophage particles. *Genetics*, 1949, **34**, 93–125

2001. Schaffer, Frederick Leland and Schwerdt, Carlton Everett. Crystallization of purified MEF-1 poliomyelitis virus particles. *Proc. Nat. Acad. Sci. (Wash)*, 1955, **41**, 1020–23

2002. Fraenkel-Conrat, Heinz Ludwig and Williams, Robley Cook. Reconstitution of active tobacco mosaic virus from its inactive protein and nucleic acid components. *Proc. Nat. Acad. Sci. (Wash)*, 1955, **41**, 690–98

2003. Allbutt, Sir Thomas Clifford. On visceral neuroses. London, *J. & A. Churchill,* 1884

2004. Allbutt, Sir Thomas Clifford. Case of cerebral disease in a syphilitic patient. *St. George's Hosp. Rep.,* 1868, **3**, 55–65

2005. Allbutt, Sir Thomas Clifford. Remarks on a case of locomotor ataxy with hydrarthrosis. *St. George's Hosp. Rep.,* 1869, **4**, 259–60

2006. Allbutt, Sir Thomas Clifford. Medical thermometry. *Br. For. Med.-Chir. Rev.,* 1870, **45**, 429–41

2007. Allbutt, Sir Thomas Clifford. The historical relations of medicine and surgery to the end of the sixteenth century. London, *Macmillan & Co.,* 1905

2008. Allbutt, Sir Thomas Clifford. Diseases of the arteries, including angina pectoris. 2 vols. London, *Macmillan & Co.,* 1915

2009. Osler, Sir William, Bart. The Gulstonian Lectures, on malignant endocarditis. *Br. Med. J.,* 1885, **1**, 467–70, 522–26, 577–79

2010. Osler, Sir William, Bart. The principles and practice of medicine. New York, *D. Appleton,* 1892

2011. Osler, Sir William, Bart. On a family form of recurring epistaxis, asociated with multiple telangiectases of the skin and mucous membranes. *Johns Hopk. Hosp. Bull.,* 1901, **12**, 333–37

2012. Osler, Sir William, Bart. Chronic cyanosis, with polycythaemia and enlarged spleen: a new clinical entity. *Am. J. Med. Sci.,* 1903, **126**, 187–201

2013. Vaquez, Louis Henri. Sur une forme spéciale de cyanose s'accompagnant d'hyperglobulie excessive et persistante. *C. R. Soc. Biol. (Paris),* 1892, **44**, 384–88

2014. Osler, Sir William, Bart. Chronic infectious endocarditis. *Q. J. Med.,* 1908–09, **2**, 219–30

2015. Osler, Sir William, Bart. An Alabama student, and other biographical essays. London. *Oxford Univ. Press,* 1908

2016. Osler, Sir William, Bart. Incunabula medica. A study of the earliest printed medical books, 1467–1480. Oxford, *Univ. Press,* 1923

2017. Osler, Sir William, Bart. Bibliotheca Osleriana. A catalogue of books illustrating the history of medicine and science, collected, arranged, and annotated by Sir William Osler, Bt. and bequeathed to McGill University. Oxford, *Clarendon Press,* 1929

2018. Rhazes (Abū Bakr Muhammad ibn Zakarīya al-Rāzī). Liber nonus ad Almansorem, cum commentario Sillani di Nigris. (Padua, *B. Valdezochius),* 1476

2019. His, Wilhelm, Jnr. Die Thätigkeit des embryonalen Herzens und deren Bedeutung für die Lehre von der Herzbewegung beim Erwachsenen. *Arb. Med. Klin. Leipzig,* 1893, 14–50

2020. Kent, Albert Frank Stanley. Researches on the structure and function of the mammalian heart. *J. Physiol. (Lond.),* 1893, **14**, 233–54

2021. Keith, Sir Arthur and Flack, Martin William. The form and nature of the muscular connections between the primary divisions of the vertebrate heart. *J. Anat. Physiol. (Lond.),* 1906–07, **41**, 172–89

2022. Tawara, Sunao. Das Reizleitungssystem des Säugethierherzens. Jena, *G. Fischer,* 1906

2023. Starling, Ernest Henry. The Linacre lecture on the law of the heart. London, *Longmans, Green & Co.,* 1918

2024. Basch, Samuel Siegfried von. Ein Metall-Sphygmomanometer. *Wien. Med. Wschr.,* 1883, **33**, 673–675

2025. Riva-Rocci, Scipione. Un nuovo sfigmomanometro. *Gaz. Med. Torino,* 1896, **47**, 981–96, 1001–17

2026. Hill, Sir Leonard Erskine and Barnard, Harold Leslie. A simple and accurate form of sphygmomanometer or arterial pressure gauge contrived for clinical use. *Br. Med. J.,* 1897, **2**, 904

2027. Korotkov, Nikolai Sergeievich. (On methods of studying blood pressure.) *Izvest. imp. voyenno-med. Akad. St. Petersburg,* 1905, **11**, 365

2028. Mackenzie, Sir James. Pulsation in the veins, with the description of a method for graphically recording them. *J. Pathol. Bact.,* 1892, **1**, 53–89

2029. Mackenzie, Sir James. The study of the pulse. Edinburgh, *Y. J. Pentland,* 1902

2030. Waller, Augustus Désiré. A demonstration in man of electromotive changes accompanying the heart's beat. *J. Physiol. (Lond.),* 1887, **8**, 299–34

2031. Einthoven, Willem. The string galvanometer and the human electro-cardiogram. *K. Akad Wet. Amst., Proc. Sect. Sci.,* 1903–04, **6**, 107–15

2032. Lewis, Sir Thomas. Electro-cardiography and its importance in the clinical examination of heart affections. *Br. Med. J.,* 1912, **1**, 1421–23, 1479–82; **2**, 65–67

2033. Lewis, Sir Thomas. The mechanism and graphic registration of the heart beat. London, *Shaw & Sons,* 1920

2034. Pardee, Harold Ensign Bennett. An electrocardiographic sign of coronary artery obstruction. *Arch. Intern. Med.,* 1920, **26**, 244–57

2035. Forssmann, Werner Theodor Otto. Die Sondierung des rechten Herzens. *Klin. Wschr.,* 1929, **8**, 2085–87, 2287

2036. Santos, Reynaldo dos *et al.* L'artériographie des membres de l'aorte et de ses branches abdominales. *Med. Contemp. (Lisboa),* 1929, **47**, 93–96

2037. Wolferth, Charles Christian and Wood, Francis Clark. The electrocardiographic diagnosis of coronary occlusion by the use of chest leads. *Am. J. Med. Sci.,* 1932, **183**, 30–35

2038. Wilson, Frank Norman *et al.* Electrocardiograms that represent the potential variations of a single electrode. *Am. Heart J.,* 1934, **9**, 447–58

2039. Schellong, Fritz. Elektrographische Diagnostik der Herzmuskelerkrankungen. *Verh. Dtsch. Ges. Inn. Med.,* 1936, **48**, 288–310

2040. Robb, George Porter and Steinberg, Israel. A practical method of visualization of the chambers of the heart, the pulmonary circulation, and the great vessels in man. *J. Clin. Invest.,* 1938, **17**, 507

2041. Starr, Isaac *et al.* Studies on the estimation of cardiac output in man, and of abnormalities in cardiac function, from the heart's recoil and the blood's impacts; the ballistocardiogram. *Am. J. Physiol.,* 1939, **127**, 1–28

2042. Cournand, André Frédéric and Ranges, Hilmert Albert. Catheterization of the right auricle in man. *Proc. Soc. Exp. Biol. (N.Y.),* 1941, **46**, 462–66

2043. McMichael, Sir John and Sharpey-Schafer, Edward Peter. Cardiac output in man by a direct Fick method. *Br. Heart J.,* 1944, **6**, 33–40

2044. LaDue, John Samuel and Wroblewski, Felix. The significance of the serum glutamic oxalacetic transaminase activity following acute myocardial infarction. *Circulation,* 1955, **11**, 871–77

2045. Myers, Arthur Bowen Richards. On the etiology and prevalence of diseases of the heart among soldiers. London, *J. Churchill,* 1870

2046. Da Costa, Jacob Mendes. On irritable heart; a clinical study of a form of functional cardiac disorder and its consequences. *Am. J. Med. Sci.,* 1871, n.s. **61**, 17–52

2047. Fagge, Charles Hilton. On the murmurs attendant on mitral contraction. *Guy's Hosp. Rep.,* 1871, 3 ser., **16**, 247–342

2048. Roger, Henri. Recherches cliniques sur la communication congénitale des deux coeurs par inocclusion du septum interventriculare. *Bull. Acad. Méd. (Paris),* 1879, 2 sér., **8**, 1074–94, 1189–91

2049. Fallot, Etienne Louis Arthur. Contribution à l'anatomie pathologique de la maladie bleu (cyanose cardiaque). *Marseille Méd.,* 1888, **25**, 77–93, 138–58, 207–23, 270–86, 341–54, 403–20

2050. Steell, Graham. The murmur of high-pressure in the pulmonary artery. *Med. Chron. (Manch.),* 1888–89, **9**, 182–88

2051. Eisenmenger, Victor. Die angeborenen Defecte der Kammerscheidewand des Herzens. *Z. Klin. Med.,* 1897, **32**, Suppl.-Heft, 1–28

2052. Hammer, Adam. Ein Fall von thrombotischem Verschlusse einer der Kranzarterien des Herzens. *Wien. Med. Wschr.,* 1878, **28**, 97–102

2053. Weigert, Carl. Ueber die pathologische Gerinnungs-Vorgänge. *Virchows Arch. Pathol., Anat.,* 1880, **79**, 87–123

2054. MacWilliam, John Alexander. Fibrillar contraction of the heart. *J. Physiol. (Lond.),* 1887, **8**, 296–310

2055. MacWilliam, John Alexander. Cardiac failure and sudden death. *Br. Med. J.,* 1889, **1**, 6–8

2056. Bouveret, Léon. Da la tachycardie essentielle paroxystique. *Rev. Médecine,* 1889, **9**, 753–93, 837–55

2057. Broadbent, Walter. An unpublished physical sign. *Lancet,* 1895, **2**, 200–01

2058. Ewart, William. Practical aids in the diagnosis of pericardial effusion, in connection with the question as to surgical treatment. *Br. Med. J.,* 1896, **1**, 717–21

2059. Pick, Friedel. Ueber chronische unter dem Bilde der Leberzirrhose verlaufende Perikarditis (perikarditische Pseudoleberzirrhose) nebst Bemerkungen über die Zuckergussleber. *Z. Klin. Med.,* 1896, **29**, 385–410

2060. Aschoff, Karl Albert Ludwig. Zur Myocarditisfrage. *Verh. Dtsch. Pathol. Ges.,* 1904, **8**, 46–53

2061. Ritchie, William Thomas. Complete heart-block, with dissociation of the action of the auricles and ventricles. *Proc. R. Soc. Edinb.,* 1905–06, **25**, 1085–91

2062. Mackenzie, Sir James. New methods of studying affections of the heart. *Br. Med. J.,* 1905, **1**, 519–21, 587–89, 702–05, 759–62, 812–15

2063. Mackenzie, Sir James. Diseases of the heart. London, *H. Frowde,* 1908

2064. Cushny, Arthur Robertson and Edmunds, Charles Wallis. Paroxysmal irregularity of the heart and auricular fibrillation. In *Studies in pathology written . . . to celebrate the quatercentenary of Aberdeen University.* Edited by W. Bullock, Aberdeen, 1906, pp. 95–110

2065. Lewis, Sir Thomas. Auricular fibrillation; a common clinical condition. *Br. Med. J.,* 1909, **2**, 1528

2066. Jolly, William Adam and Ritchie, William Thomas. Auricular flutter and fibrillation. *Heart,* 1910, **2**, 177–221

2067. Wenckebach, Karel Frederik. Die unregelmässige Herztätigkeit und ihre klinische Bedeutung. Leipzig, Berlin, *W. Engelmann,* 1914

2068. Frey, Walter. Ueber Vorhofflimmern beim Menschen und seine Beseitigung durch Chinidin. *Berl. Klin. Wschr.,* 1918, **55**, 450–52

2069. Reuter, Karl. Ueber Spirochaete pallida in der Aortenwand bei Hellerscher Aortitis. *Münch. Med. Wschr.,* 1906, **53**, 778

2070. Horder, Thomas Jeeves, 1st Baron Horder. Infective endocarditis, with an analysis of 150 cases. *Q. J. Med.,* 1909, **2**, 289–324

2071. Libman, Emanuel and Celler, Herbert Louis. The etiology of subacute infective endocarditis. *Am. J. Med. Sci.,* 1910, **140**, 516–27

2072. Schottmüller, Hugo. Endocarditis lenta. Zugleich ein Beitrag zur Artunterscheidung der pathogenen Streptokokken. *Münch. Med. Wschr.,* 1910, **57**, 617–20, 697–99

2073. Eppinger, Hans and Stoerk, Oscar. Zur Klinik des Elektrokardiogramms. *Z. Klin. Med.,* 1910, **71**, 157–164

2074. Obraztsov, Vasillii Parmenovich and Strazhesko, Nikolai Dmitrievich. Zur Kenntniss der Thrombose der Koronararterien des Herzens. *Z. Klin. Med.,* 1910, **71**, 116–32

2075. Herrick, James Bryan. Clinical features of sudden obstruction of the coronary arteries. *J. Am. Med. Assoc.,* 1912, **59**, 2015–20

2076. Lewis, Sir Thomas. Report upon soldiers returned as cases of "disordered action of the heart" (D.A.H.) or "valvular disease of the heart" (V.D.H.). London, *HMSO,* 1917

2077. Zondek, Hermann. Das Myxödemherz. *Münch. Med. Wschr.,* 1918, **65**, 1180–82

2078. Keith, Norman Macdonnell *et al.* Some different types of essential hypertension: their course and prognosis. *Am. J. Med. Sci.,* 1929, **197**, 332–43

2079. Wolff, Louis, Parkinson, Sir John and White, Paul Dudley. Bundle-branch block with short P–R interval in healthy young people prone to paroxysmal tachycardia. *Am. Heart J.,* 1930, **5**, 685–704

2080. Lewis, Sir Thomas. A lecture on vaso-vagal syncope and the carotid sinus mechanism. *Br. Med. J.,* 1932, **1**, 873–76

2081. Wagener, Henry Patrick and Keith, Norman Macdonnell. Diffuse arteriolar disease with hypertension and the associated retinal lesions. *Medicine,* 1939, **18**, 317–430

2082. Christie, Ronald Victor. Penicillin in subacute bacterial endocarditis. Report to the Medical Research Council on 269 patients treated in 14 centres appointed by the Penicillin Clinical Trials Committee. *Br. Med. J.,* 1948, **1**, 1–4

2083. Prinzmetal, Myron *et al.* Mechanism of the auricular arrhythmias. *Circulation,* 1950, **1**, 241–45

2084. Wood, Paul Hamilton. Congenital heart disease. *Br. Med. J.,* 1950, **2**, 639–45, 693–98

2085. Zoll, Paul Maurice. Resuscitation of the heart in ventricular standstill by external electric stimulation. *New Engl. J. Med.,* 1952, **247**, 768–71

2086. Dale, Sir Henry Hallett and Schuster, Edgar Hermann Joseph. A double perfusion-pump. *J. Physiol. (Lond.),* 1928, **64**, 356–64

2087. Goldblatt, Harry *et al.* Studies on experimental hypertension. 1. The production of persistent elevation of systolic blood pressure by means of renal ischemia. *J. Exp. Med.,* 1934, **59**, 347–79

2088. Houssay, Bernardo Alberto and Fasciolo, Juan Carlos. Secreción hipertensora del rinón isquemiado. *Rev. Soc. Argent. Biol.,* 1937, **13**, 284–94

2089. Wilson, Clifford and Byrom, Frank Burnet. Renal changes in malignant hypertension; experimental evidence. *Lancet,* 1939, **1**, 136–39

2090. Braun-Menendez, Eduardo *et al.* The substance causing renal hypertension. *J. Physiol. (Lond.),* 1940, **98**, 283–98

2091. Page, Irving Heinly and Helmer, O. M. A crystalline substance (angiotonin) resulting from the reaction between renin and renin-activator. *J. Exp. Med.,* 1940, **71**, 29–42

2092. Rehn, Ludwig. Fall von penetrirender Stichverletzung des rechten Ventrikel's. Herznaht. *Zbl. Chir.,* 1896, **23**, 1048–49

2093. Jaboulay, Mathieu. Chirurgie du grand sympathique et du corps thyroïde. Paris, *O. Doin,* 1900

2094. Carrel, Alexis and Guthrie, Charles Claude. The transplantation of veins and organs. *Am. Med.,* 1905, **10**, 1101–2

2095. Carrel, Alexis. La technique opératoire des anastomoses vasculaires et la transplantation des viscères. *Lyon Méd.,* 1902, **98**, 859–64

2096. Carrel, Alexis. The surgery of blood vessels, etc. *Johns Hopk. Hosp. Bull.,* 1907, **18**, 18–28

2097. Carrel, Alexis. Results of the transplantation of blood vessels, organs and limbs. *J. Am. Med. Assoc.,* 1908, **51**, 1662–67

2098. Carrel, Alexis. Latent life of arteries. *J. Exp. Med.,* 1910, **12**, 460–86

2099. Doyen, Eugène Louis. Chirurgie des malformations congénitales ou acquises du coeur. *Congr. Franç. Chir., Proc.-Verb.,* 1913, **26**, 1062–65; *Presse Méd.,* 1913, **21**, 860

2100. Tuffier, Théodore. Etude expérimentelle sur la chirurgie des valvules du coeur. *Bull. Acad. Méd. (Paris),* 1914, 3 sér., **71**, 293–95

2101. Hallopeau, Paul. Un cas de cardiolyse. *Bull. Mém. Soc. Chir. Paris,* 1921, **47**, 1120–21

2102. Cutler, Elliott Carr and Levine, Samuel Albert. Cardiotomy and valvulotomy for mitral stenosis. Experimental observations and clinical notes concerning an operated case with recovery. *Boston Med. Surg. J.,* 1923, **188**, 1023–27

2103. Souttar, Sir Henry Sessions. The surgical treatment of mitral stenosis. *Br. Med. J.,* 1925, **2**, 603–06

2104. Beck, Claude Schaeffer. The development of a new blood supply to the heart by operation. *Ann. Surg.,* 1935, **102**, 801–13

2105. O'Shaughnessy, Laurence. An experimental method of providing a collateral circulation to the heart. *Br. J. Surg.,* 1936, **23**, 665–70

2106. Gibbon, John Heysham. An oxygenator with a large surface-volume ratio. *J. Lab. Clin. Med.,* 1939, **24**, 1192–98

2107. Gross, Robert Edward and Hubbard, John Perry. Surgical ligation of a patent ductus arteriosus: report of first successful case. *J. Am. Med. Assoc.,* 1939, **112**, 729–31

2108. Blalock, Alfred and Taussig, Helen Brooke. The surgical treatment of malformations of the heart in which there is pulmonary stenosis or pulmonary atresia. *J. Am. Med. Assoc.,* 1945, **128**, 189–202

2109. Crafoord, Clarence and Nylin, Karl Gustav Vilhelm. Congenital coarctation of the aorta and its surgical treatment. *J. Thorac. Surg.,* 1945, **14**, 347–61

2110. Gross, Robert Edward. Surgical correction for coarctation of the aorta. *Surgery,* 1945, **18**, 673–8

2111. Brock, Russell Claude, Baron Brock of Wimbledon. Pulmonary valvulotomy for the relief of congenital pulmonary stenosis. Report of three cases. *Br. Med. J.,* 1948, **1**, 1121–26

2112. Sellors, Sir Thomas Holmes. Surgery of pulmonary stenosis. A case in which the pulmonary valve was successfully divided. *Lancet,* 1948, **1**, 988–9

2113. Bland, Edward Franklin and Sweet, Richard Harwood. A venous shunt for marked mitral stenosis. *Am. Practit.,* 1948, **2**, 756–61

2114. Gibbon, John Heysham. Application of a mechanical heart and lung apparatus to cardiac surgery. *Minn. Med.,* 1954, **37**, 171–80, 185

2115. Lillehei, Clarence Walton. Controlled cross circulation for direct-vision intracardiac surgery; correction of ventricular septal defects, atrioventricularis communis, and tetralogy of Fallot. *Postgrad. Med.,* 1955, **17,** 388–96

2116. Murray, Gordon Donald Walter. Homologous aortic-valve-segment transplants as surgical treatment for aortic and mitral insufficiency. *Angiology,* 1956, **7,** 466–71

2117. Szilagyi, D. Emerick *et al.* Clinical use of an elastic Dacron prosthesis. *Arch. Surg.,* 1958, **77,** 538–51

2118. Lower, Richard Rowland and Shumway, Norman E. Studies on orthotopic homotransplantation of the canine heart. *Surg. Forum,* 1960, **11,** 18–19

2119. Starr, Albert and Edwards, M. Lowell. Mitral replacement: the shielded ball valve prosthesis. *J. Thorac. Cardiovasc. Surg.,* 1961, **42,** 673–82

2120. Ross, Donald Nixon. Homograft replacement of the aortic valve. *Lancet,* 1962, **2,** 487 (only)

2121. Barratt-Boyes, Sir Brian Gerald. Homograft aortic valve replacement in aortic incompetence and stenosis. *Thorax,* 1964, **19,** 131–50

2122. Barnard, Christiaan Neethling. A human cardiac transplant: an interim report of a successful operation performed at Groote Schuur Hospital, Cape Town. *S. Afr. Med. J.,* 1967, **41,** 1271–4

2123. Kussmaul, Adolf and Maier, Rudolf. Ueber eine bisher noch nicht beschriebene eigenthümliche Arterienerkrankung (Periarteritis nodosa), die mit Morbus Brightii und rapid fortschreitender allgemeiner Muskellähmung einhergeht. *Dtsch. Arch. Klin. Med.,* 1866, **1,** 484–518

2124. Winiwarter, Felix von. Ueber eine eigenthümliche Form von Endarteriitis und Endophlebitis mit Gangrän des Fusses. *Arch. Klin. Chir.,* 1879, **23,** 202–26

2125. Mönckeberg, Johann Georg. Ueber die reine Mediaverkalkung der Extremitätenarterien und ihr Verhalten zur Arteriosklerose. *Virchows Arch. Pathol. Anat.,* 1903, **171,** 141–67

2126. Buerger, Leo. Thrombo-angiitis obliterans; a study of the vascular lesions leading to presenile spontaneous gangrene. *Am. J. Med. Sci.,* 1908, **136,** 567–580

2127. Brunton, Sir Thomas Lauder. On the use of nitrite of amyl in angina pectoris. *Lancet,* 1867, **2,** 97–98

2128. Murrell, William. Nitro-glycerine as a remedy for angina pectoris. *Lancet,* 1879, **1,** 80–81, 113–15, 151–52, 225–27

2129. Ignatovski, Alexander. (Influence of animal food on the organism of rabbits.) *Izvest. imp. vo.-med. Akad. St. Petersburg,* 1908, **16,** 154–76. French translation in *Arch. Méd. Exp. Anat. Pathol.,* 1908, **20,** 1–20

2130. Anitschkov, Nikolai and Chalatov, S. S. Ueber experimentelle Cholesterinsteatose und ihre Bedeutung für die Entstehung einiger pathologischer Prozesse. *Zbl. Allg. Pathol. Pathol. Anat.,* 1913, **24,** 1–9

2131. Morton, Leslie T. (1983). As ref. 1853 but p. 390

2132. Arrilaga, Francisco C. Cardiacos negros. Buenos Aires, *Thesis No.* 2536, 1912

2133. Ayerza, Luis. Consideraciones sobre la denominación de "Enfermedad de Ayerza." *Semana Méd.,* 1925, **32,** pt. 2. 386–88

2134. Mackenzie, Sir James. Angina pectoris. London, *H. Frowde,* 1923

2135. Kirschner, Martin. Ein durch die Trendelenburgsche Operation geheilter Fall von Embolie der Art. pulmonalis. *Arch. Klin. Chir.,* 1924, **133,** 312–59

2136. Murray, Donald Walter Gordon *et al.* Heparin and the thrombosis of veins following injury. *Surgery,* 1937, **2,** 163–87

2137. Berberich, Josef and Hirsch, S. Die röntgenographische Darstellung der Arterien und Venen am lebenden Menschen. *Klin. Wschr.,* 1923, **2,** 2226–28

2138. Brooks, Barney. Intra-arterial injection of sodium iodid: preliminary report. *J. Am. Med. Assoc.,* 1924, **82,** 1016–19

2139. Sones, Frank Mason and Shirey, Earl K. Cine-coronary arteriography. *Mod. Conc. Cardiovasc. Dis.,* 1962, **31,** 735–38

2140. Cloetta, Max. Ueber Digalen (Digitoxinum solubile). *Münch. Med. Wschr.,* 1904, **51,** 1466–68

2141. Straub, Walter. Digitaliswirkung am isolierten Vorhof des Frosches. *Arch. Exp. Pathol. Pharmak.,* 1916, **79,** 19–29

2142. Cushny, Arthur Robertson. The action and uses in medicine of digitalis and its allies. London, *Longmans, Green & Co.,* 1925

2143. Smith, Sydney. Digoxin, a new digitalis glucoside. *J. Chem. Soc.,* 1930, 508-10

2144. Chopra, Ram Nath *et al.* The pharmacological action of an alkaloid obtained from *Rauwolfia serpentina* Benth. A preliminary note. *Indian J. Med. Res.,* 1933, **21,** 261-71

2145. Müller, J.M. *et al.* Reserpin, der sedative Wirkstoff aus *Rauwolfia serpentina* Benth. *Experientia (Basel),* 1952, **8,** 338

2146. Martindale (1977). As ref. 1 but p. 675

2147. Tillett, William Smith and Garner, Raymond Loraine. The fibrinolytic activity of hemolytic streptococci. *J. Exp. Med.,* 1933, **58,** 485-502

2148. Christensen, Lauritz Royal. Streptococcal fibrinolysis. A proteolytic reaction due to a serum enzyme activated by streptococcal fibrinolysin. *J. Gen. Physiol.,* 1945, **28,** 363-83

2149. Gaddum, Sir John Henry. The action of adrenalin and ergotamine on the uterus of the rabbit. *J. Physiol. (Lond.),* 1926, **61,** 141-50

2150. Gaddum, Sir John Henry. The quantitative effect of antagonistic drugs. *J. Physiol. (Lond.),* 1937, **89,** 7P-9P

2151. Bergström, Sune *et al.* The structure of prostaglandin E, F_1 and F_2. *Acta Chem. Scand.,* 1962, **16,** 501-2

2152. Bergström, Sune *et al.* Isolation of *nor*-adrenaline from the adrenal gland. *Acta Chem. Scand.,* 1949, **3,** 305-6

2153. Black, James Whyte *et al.* A new adrenergic beta-receptor antagonist. *Lancet,* 1964, **1,** 1080-81

2154. World Health Organization. Technical Report Series 641. The selection of essential drugs. Geneva, *World Health Organization,* 1979

2155. The British Pharmacopoeia 1914 published under the direction of the General Council of Medical Education and Registration of the United Kingdom. London, *General Medical Council,* 1914

2156. Küster, Ernst Georg Ferdinand von. Ueber die Grundsätze der Behandlung von Eiterungen in starrwandigen Höhlen, mit besonderer Berücksichtigung des Empyems der Pleura. *Dtsch. Med. Wschr.,* 1889, **15,** 185-87

2157. Fowler, George Ryerson. A case of thoracoplasty for the removal of a large cicatrical fibrous growth from the interior of the chest, the result of an old empyema. *Med. Rec. (N.Y.),* 1893, **44,** 838-39

2158. Delorme, Edmond. Nouveau traitement des empyèmes chroniques. *Gaz. Hôp. (Paris),* 1894, **67,** 94-96

2159. Körte, Werner. Ueber Lungenresektion wegen bronchiektatischer Cavernen. *Verh. Berl. Med. Ges.,* (1908), 1909, **39,** 5-9

2160. Brunn, Harold. Surgical principles underlying one-stage lobectomy. *Arch. Surg.,* 1929, **18,** 490-515

2161. Nissen, Rudolph. Exstirpation eines ganzen Lungenflügels. *Zbl. Chir.,* 1931, **58,** 3003-3006

2162. Graham, Evarts Ambrose and Singer, Jacob Jesse. Successful removal of entire lung for carcinoma of the bronchus. *J. Am. Med. Assoc.,* 1933, **101,** 1371-74

2163. Lilienthal, Howard. Pneumonectomy for sarcoma of the lung in a tuberculous patient. *J. Thorac. Surg.,* 1933, **2,** 600-15

2164. Emerson, Charles Phillips. Pneumothorax; a historical, clinical, and experimental study. *Johns Hopk. Hosp. Rep.,* 1903, **11,** 1-450

2165. Pasteur, William. The Bradshaw Lecture on massive collapse of the lung. *Lancet,* 1908, **2,** 1351-55

2166. Barnard, William George. The nature of the "oat-celled sarcoma" of the mediastinum. *J. Pathol. Bact.,* 1926, **29,** 241-44

2167. Campbell, John Munro. Acute symptoms following work with hay. *Br. Med. J.,* 1932, **2,** 1143-44

2168. Maytum, Charles Koran. Tetany caused by functional dyspnea with hyperventilation: report of a case. *Proc. Mayo Clin.,* 1933, **8,** 282-84

2169. Killian, Gustav. Ueber directe Bronchoskopie. *Münch. Med. Wschr.,* 1898, **45,** 844-47

2170. Waters, Charles Alexander *et al.* Roentgenography of the lung; roentgenographic studies in living animals after intratracheal injection of iodoform emulsion. *Arch. Int. Med.,* 1917, **19**, 538-49

2171. Sicard, Jean Athanase and Forrestier, Jacques. L'exploration radiologique des cavités broncho-pulmonaires par les injections intra-trachéales d'huile iodée. *J. Méd. Franç.,* 1924, **13**, 3-9

2172. Kruse, Walther. Die Erreger von Husten und Schnupfen. *Münch. Med. Wschr.,* 1914, **61**, 1547

2173. *Dienes, Louis and Edsall, Geoffrey. Observations on L-organism of Klieneberger. Proc. Soc. Exp. Biol. (N.Y.), 1937, 36, 740-44*

2174. Neufeld, Fred and Haendel, Ludwig. Weitere Untersuchungen über Pneumokokken-Heilsera. III. Mitteilung. Über Vorkommen und Bedeutung atypischer Varietäten des Pneumokokkus. *Arb. k. GesundhAmte,* 1910, **34**, 293-304

2175. Heidelberger, Michael and Avery, Oswald Theodore. The soluble specific substance of pneumococcus. *J. Exp. Med.,* 1923, **38**, 73-79; 1924, **40**, 301-16

2176. Coutard, Henri. Un cas d'épithélioma spino-cellulaire de la région latérale du pharynx, avec adénopathie angulo-maxillaire, guéri depuis six mois par la röntgenthérapie. *Bull. Ass. Franç, Étude Cancer,* 1921, **10**, 160-68

2177. Macht, David Israel and Ting, Giu-Ching. A study of antispasmodic drugs on the bronchus. *J. Pharmacol.,* 1921, **18**, 373-98

2178. Hirsch, Samson. Klinische und experimentelle Beitrag zur krampflösenden Wirkung der Purinderivate. *Klin. Wschr.,* 1922, **1**, 615-8

2179. Camps, Percy William Leopold. A note on the inhalation treatment of asthma. *Guy's Hosp. Rep.,* 1929, **79**, 496-98

2180. Abreu, Manoel de. Röntgen-photographia. Processo e apparelho de röntgen-photographia. Tuberculose pulmonar. Cadastro social. Radiographia e radioscopia. Röntgen-photographia collectiva. *Rev. Assoc. Paul. Med.,* 1936, **9**, 313-24

2181. Evans, Gladys Mary and Gaisford, Wilfrid Fletcher. Treatment of pneumonia with 2-(*p*-aminobenzenesulphonamido) pyridine. *Lancet,* 1938, **2**, 14-19

2182. Reimann, Hobart Ansteth. An acute infection of the respiratory tract with atypical pneumonia: a disease entity probably caused by a filtrable virus. *J. Am. Med. Assoc.,* 1938, **111**, 2377-84

2183. Eaton, Monroe Davis *et al.* Studies on the etiology of primary atypical pneumonia. A filterable agent transmissible to cotton rats, hamsters, and chick embryos. *J. Exp. Med.,* 1944, **79**, 649-68

2184. Chanock, Robert Merritt. Growth on artificial medium of an agent associated with atypical pneumonia and its identification as a PPLO. *Proc. Nat. Acad. Sci. (Wash.),* 1962, **48**, 41-9

2185. Chanock, Robert Merritt *et al.* Recovery from infants with respiratory illness of a virus related to chimpanzee coryza agent (CCA). *Am. J. Hyg.,* 1957, **66**, 281-90

2186. Fraser, David William *et al.* Legionnaires' disease. Description of an epidemic of pneumonia. *New Engl. J. Med.,* 1977, **297**, 1189-97

2187. McDade, Joseph E. *et al.* Legionnaires' disease. Isolation of a bacterium and demonstration of its role in other respiratory diseases. *New Engl. J. Med.,* 1977, **297**, 1197-1203

2188. Churchill, Edward Delos and Belsey, Ronald Herbert Robert. Segmental pneumonectomy in bronchiectasis. The lingula segment of the left upper lobe. *Ann. Surg.,* 1939, **109**, 481-99

2189. Meade, Richard Hardaway. A history of thoracic surgery. Springfield, *C. C. Thomas,* 1961

2190. Müller, Franz Hermann. Tabakmissbrauch und Lungencarcinom. *Z. Krebsforsch.,* 1939, **49**, 57-85

2191. Doll, Sir William Richard Shaboe and Hill, Sir Austin Bradford. Smoking and carcinoma of the lung. Preliminary report. *Br. Med. J.,* 1950, **2**, 739-48; 1952, **2**, 1271-86; 1956, **2**, 1071-81; 1964, **1**, 1399-1410

2192. Wynder, Ernest Ludwig and Graham, Evarts Ambrose. Tobacco smoking as a possible etiologic factor in bronchogenic carcinoma. *J. Am. Med. Assoc.,* 1950, **143**, 329-36

2193. Bodington, George. Essay on the treatment and cure of pulmonary consumption. London. *Longmans & Co.,* 1840

2194. Forlanini, Carlo. A contribuzione della terapia chirurgica della tisi; ablazione de polmone? pneumotorace artificiale? *Gazz. Osp. Clin.,* 1882, **3,** 537, 585, 601, 609, 617, 625, 641, 657, 665, 689, 705. English translation in *Tubercle,* 1934–5, **16,** 61–87

2195. Cayley, William. A case of haemoptysis treated by the induction of pneumothorax so as to collapse the lung. *Trans. Clin. Soc. Lond.,* 1885, **18,** 278–84. Artificial pneumothorax by pleural incision in intractable haemoptysis. See also *Lancet,* 1885, **1,** 894–95

2196. Lowson, David. A case of pneumonectomy. *Br. Med. J.,* 1893, **1,** 1152–54

2197. Tuffier, Théodore. Chirurgie du poumon en particulier dans les cavernes tuberculeuses et la gangrène pulmonaire. Paris, *Masson,* 1897

2198. Macewen, Sir William. On some points in the surgery of the lung. *Br. Med. J.,* 1906, **2,** 1–7

2199. Brauer, Ludolph. Indications du traitement chirurgical de la tuberculose pulmonaire. *Congr. Ass. Franç. Chir.,* 1908, **21,** 569–74

2200. Parrot, Joseph. Recherches sur les relations qui existent entre les lésions des poumons et celles des ganglions trachéo-bronchiques. *C. R. Soc. Biol. (Paris),* 1876, sér. 6, **3,** 308–09

2201. Ghon, Anton. Der primäre Lungenherd bei der Tuberkulose der Kinder. Berlin and Wien. *Urban & Schwarzenberg,* 1912

2202. Sauerbruch, Ernst Ferdinand. Die Beeinflüssung von Lungenerkrankungen durch künstliche Lähmung des Zwerchfells (Phrenikotomie). *Münch. Med. Wschr.,* 1913, **60,** 625–26

2203. Jacobæus, Hans Christian. Endopleurale Operationen unter der Leitung des Thorakoskops. *Beitr. Klin. Tuberk.,* 1916, **35,** 1–35

2204. Vajda, Ludwig. Ob das Pneumoperitoneum in der Kollapstherapie der beiderseitigen Lungentuberkulose angewandt werden kann? *Z. Tuberk.,* 1933, **67,** 371–75

2205. Banyai, Andrew Ladislaus. Therapeutic pneumoperitoneum. A review of 100 cases. *Am. Rev. Tuberc.,* 1934, **29,** 603–27

2206. Freedlander, Samuel Oscar. Lobectomy in pulmonary tuberculosis. Report of a case. *J. Thorac. Surg.,* 1935, **5,** 132–42

2207. Semb, Carl Boye. Thoracoplasty with extrafascial apicolysis. *Acta Chir. Scand.,* 1935, Suppl. 37, pt. 2, 1–85

2208. Kayne, George Gregory, Pagel, Walter and O'Shaughnessy, Laurence. Pulmonary tuberculosis. Pathology, diagnosis, management and prevention. London, *Oxford Univ. Press,* 1939

2209. Mantoux, Charles. Intradermo-réaction de la tuberculine. *C. R. Acad. Sci. (Paris),* 1908, **147,** 355–57

2210. Calmette, Léon Charles Albert *et al.* Essai d'immunisation contre l'infection tuberculeuse. *Bull. Acad. Méd. (Paris),* 1924, 3 sér., **91,** 787–96

2211. Calmette, Léon Charles Albert *et al.* Sur la vaccination préventive des enfants nouveau-nés contre la tuberculose par le B.C.G. *Ann. Inst. Pasteur,* 1927, **41,** 201–32

2212. Heaf, Frederick Roland George. The multiple-puncture tuberculin test. *Lancet,* 1951, **2,** 151–53

2213. Griffiths, Margaret Isabel and Gaisford, Wilfrid Fletcher. Freeze-dried B.C.G. Vaccination of newborn infants with a British vaccine. *Br. Med. J.,* 1956, **2,** 565–8

2214. Feldman, William Hugh *et al.* The effect of promin (sodium salt of P.P'-diamino-diphenyl-sulfone-N, N'-dextrose sulfonate) on experimental tuberculosis: a preliminary report. *Proc. Mayo Clin.,* 1940, **15,** 695–99

2215. Schatz, Albert *et al.* Streptomycin, a substance exhibiting antibiotic activity against Gram-positive and Gram-negative bacteria. *Proc. Soc. Exp. Biol. (N.Y.),* 1944, **55,** 66–69

2216. Hinshaw, Horton Corwin and Feldman, William Hugh. Streptomycin in treatment of clinical tuberculosis: a preliminary report. *Proc. Mayo Clin.,* 1945, **20,** 313–18

2217. Lehmann, Jörgen. *Para-*aminosalicylic acid in the treatment of tuberculosis. *Lancet,* 1946, **1,** 15–16

2218. Domagk, Gerhard *et al.* Ueber eine neue, gegen Tuberkelbazillen in vitro wirksame Verbindungsklasse. *Naturwissenschaften,* 1946, **33,** 315

2219. Hart, Philip Montagu D'Arcy. Chemotherapy of tuberculosis. Researches during the past 100 years. *Br. Med. J.,* 1946, **2,** 805–10, 849–55

2220. Waksman, Selman Abraham and Lechevalier, Hubert Arthur. Neomycin, a new antibiotic active against streptomycin-resistant bacteria, including tuberculosis organisms. *Science,* 1949, **109**, 305–07

2221. Finlay, Alexander Carpenter *et al.* Viomycin, a new antibiotic active against mycobacteria. *Am. Rev. Tuberc.,* 1951, **63**, 1–3. Pp. 1–61 provide a series of papers on Viomycin

2222. Robitzek, Edward Heinrich *et al.* Chemotherapy of human tuberculosis with hydrazine derivatives of isonicotinic acid. (Preliminary report of representative cases.) *Q. Bull. Sea View Hosp.,* 1952, **13**, 27–51

2223. Rist, Noël *et al.* Experiments on the antituberculous activity of alpha-ethyl-thioisonicotinamide. *Am. Rev. Tuberc.,* 1959, **79**, 1–5

2224. Thomas, J. P. *et al.* A new synthetic compound with antituberculous activity in mice: ethambutol (dextro-2,2′-(ethylenediimino)-di-l-butanol). *Am. Rev. Resp. Dis.,* 1961, **83**, 891–3

2225. Atlas, E. and Turck, M. Laboratory and clinical evaluation of rifampicin. *Am. J. Med. Sci.,* 1968, **256**, 247–254

2226. Kunin, C. M., Brandt, D. and Wood, H. Bacteriologic studies of rifampin, a new semisynthetic antibiotic. *J. Infect. Dis.,* 1969, **119**, 132–137

2227. Verbist, L. and Gyselen, A. Antituberculous activity of rifampin *in vitro* and *in vivo* and the concentrations attained in human blood. *Am. Rev. Resp. Dis.,* 1968, **98**, 923–932

2228. Lorian, V. and Finland, M. *In vitro* effect of rifampin on mycobacteria. *Appl. Microbiol.,* 1969, **17**, 202–207

2229. Ehrlich, Paul (1956–60). See ref. 1777

2230. Wassermann, August von *et al.* Eine serodiagnostische Reaktion bei Syphilis. *Dtsch. Med. Wschr.,* Berlin, 1906, **32**, 745–46

2231. Schaudinn, Fritz Richard and Hoffmann, Erich. Vorläufiger Bericht über das Vorkommen von Spirochaeten in syphilitischen Krankheitsprodukten und bei Papillomen. *Arb. k. GesundhAmte,* 1905, **22**, 527–34

2232. Landsteiner, Karl and Mucha, Viktor. Zur Technik der Spirochaetenuntersuchung. *Wien. Klin. Wschr.,* 1906, **19**, 1349–50

2233. Ehrlich, Paul and Hata, Sahachiro. Die experimentelle Chemotherapie der Spirillosen (Syphilis, Rückfallfieber, Hühnerspirillose, Frambösie). Berlin, *J. Springer,* 1910

2234. Noguchi, Hideyo. A method for the pure cultivation of pathogenic Treponema pallidum (Spirochaeta pallida). *J. Exp. Med.,* 1911, **14**, 99–108

2235. Ehrlich, Paul. Ueber Laboratoriumsversuche und klinische Erprobung von Heilstoffen. *Chem. Ztg.,* 1912, **36**, 637–38

2236. Mahoney, John Friend *et al.* Penicillin treatment of early syphilis. A preliminary report. *Vener. Dis. Inform.,* 1943, **24**, 355–57; also in *Am. J. Publ. Hlth,* 1943, **33**, 1387–91

2237. Jacobs, Walter Abraham and Heidelberger, Michael. Chemotherapy of trypanosome and spirochete infections. Chemical series. I, N-phenylglycineamide-*p*-arsonic acid. *J. Exp. Med.,* 1919, **30**, 411–15

2238. Loevenhart, Arthur Salomon and Stratman-Thomas, Warren Kidwell. On the chemotherapy of neurosyphilis and trypanosomiasis. *J. Pharmacol.,* 1926, **29**, 69–82

2239. Domagk, Gerhard. Ein Beitrag zur Chemotherapie der bakteriellen Infektionen. *Dtsch. Med. Wschr.,* 1935, **61**, 250–53

2240. Tréfouël, J. *et al.* Activité du *p*-aminophénylsulfamide sur les infections streptococciques expérimentales de la souris et du lapin. *C. R. Soc. Biol. (Paris),* 1935, **120**, 756–58

2241. Whitby, Sir Lionel Ernest Howard. Chemotherapy of pneumococcal and other infections with 2-(*p*-amino-benzenesulphonamido) pyridine. *Lancet,* 1938, **1**, 1210–12

2242. Evans, Gladys Mary and Gaisford, Wilfrid Fletcher (1938). As ref. 2181 but p. 18

2243. Gsell, Otto. Chemotherapie akuter Infektionskrankheiten durch Ciba 3714 (Sulfanilamidothiazol). *Schweiz. Med. Wschr.,* 1940, **70**, 342–50

2244. Finland, Maxwell *et al.* Sulfadiazine. Therapeutic evaluation and toxic effects on four hundred and forty-six patients. *J. Am. Med. Assoc.,* 1941, **116**, 2641–47

2245. Macartney, Donald William *et al.* Sulphamethazine: clinical trial of a new sulphonamide. *Lancet,* 1942, **1**, 639–41

2246. Janbon, M., Chaptal, J., Vedel, A. and Schaap, J. Accidents hypoglycémiques graves par un sulfamidothiadiazol (le VK57 or 2254RP). *Montpell. Méd.* 1942, **21–22**, 441–444

2247. Loubatières, Auguste. Analyse du mécanisme de l'action hypoglycémiante de *p*-amino-benzène-sulfamido-isopropylthiodiazol (2254 RP). *C. R. Soc. Biol. (Paris)*, 1944, **138**, 766–7

2248. Loubatières, A. The hypoglycemic sulfonamides: history and development of the problem from 1942 to 1955. *Ann. N.Y. Acad. Sci.*, 1957, **71**, 4–11

2249. Franke, Hans and Fuchs, J. Ein neues antidiabetisches Prinzip. Ergebnisse klinischer Untersuchungen. *Dtsch. Med. Wschr.*, 1955, **80**, 1449–52

2250. Maske, Helmut. Über die orale Behandlung des Diabetes mellitus mit N-(4-Methyl-Benzol-sulfonyl)-N'Butyl-Harnstoff (D 860). *Dtsch. Med. Wschr.*, 1956, **81**, 823–46

2251. Dodd, Matthew Charles and Stillman, William Barlow. The in vitro bacteriostatic action of some simple furan derivatives. *J. Pharmacol.*, 1944, **82**, 11–18

2252. Bushby, S. R. M. and Hitchings, G. H. Trimethoprim, a sulphonamide potentiator. *Br. J. Pharmacol. Chemother.*, 1968, **33**, 72–90

2253. Bushby, S. R. M. Trimethoprim-sulfamethoxazole: *in vitro* microbiological aspects. *J. Infect. Dis.*, 1973, **128** Suppl., S442–462

2254. Kasanen, A., Sundquist, H. and Junnila, S. Trimethoprim in the treatment of acute urinary tract infection. *Curr. Ther. Res.* 1979, **25**, 202–209

2255. Mann, Ronald D. and Jones, Jacqueline L. Trimethoprim in the treatment of urinary tract infections. *Br. J. Pharm. Pract.*, 1980, **2**, 29–40

2256. Tyndall, John. The optical deportment of the atmosphere in relation to the phenomena of putrefaction and infection. *Phil. Trans.*, 1876, **166**, 27–74

2257. Emmerich, Rudolf and Löw, Oscar. Bakteriolytische Enzyme als Ursache der erworbenen Immunität und die Heilung von Infectionskrankheiten durch dieselben. *Z. Hyg. Infekt.-Kr.*, 1899, **31**, 1–65

2258. Fleming, Sir Alexander. Lysozyme. *Proc. R. Soc. Med.*, 1932, **26**, 71–84

2259. Fleming, Sir Alexander. On the antibacterial action of cultures of a penicillium, with special reference to their use in the isolation of *B. influenzae*. *Br. J. Exp. Pathol.*, 1929, **10**, 226–36

2260. Dubos, René Jules. Bactericidal effect of an extract of a soil bacillus on gram-positive cocci. *Proc. Soc. Exp. Biol. (N.Y.)*, 1939, **40**, 311–12

2261. Oxford, Albert Edward *et al.* Studies in the biochemistry of micro-organisms. LX. Griseofulvin, $C_{17}H_{17}O_6Cl$, a metabolic product of *Penicillium griseo-fulvum* Dierckx. *Biochem. J.*, 1939, **33**, 240–48

2262. Chain, Sir Ernst Boris *et al.* Penicillin as a chemotherapeutic agent. *Lancet*, 1940, **2**, 226–28

2263. Abraham, Sir Edward Penley and Chain, Sir Ernst Boris. An enzyme from bacteria able to destroy penicillin. *Nature (Lond.)*, 1940, **146**, 837

2264. Abraham, Sir Edward Penley *et al.* Further observations on penicillin. *Lancet*, 1941, **2**, 177–89

2265. Abraham, Sir Edward Penley *et al.* Penicillamine, a characteristic degradation product of penicillin. *Nature (Lond.)*, 1943, **151**, 107 (only)

2266. Hamilton-Miller, J. M. T. Penicillinacylase. *Bacteriol. Rev.*, 1966, **30**, 761–771

2267. Johnson, Balbina A. *et al.* Bacitracin: a new antibiotic produced by a member of the *B. subtilis* group. *Science*, 1945, **102**, 376–77

2268. Ainsworth, Geoffrey Clough *et al.* "Aerosporin," an antibiotic produced by *Bacillus aerosporus* Greer. *Nature (Lond.)*, 1947, **160**, 263

2269. Stansly, Philip Gerald *et al.* Polymyxin: a new chemotherapeutic agent. *Bull. Johns Hopk. Hosp.*, 1947, **81**, 43–54

2270. Ehrlich, John *et al.* Chloromycetin, a new antibiotic from a soil actinomycete. *Science*, 1947, **106**, 417

2271. Smadel, Joseph Edwin and Jackson, Elizabeth B. Chloromycetin, an antibiotic with chemotherapeutic activity in experimental rickettsial and viral infections. *Science*, 1947, **106**, 418–19

2272. Herrell, Wallace Edgar *et al.* Procaine penicillin G (duracillin); a new salt of penicillin which prolongs the action of penicillin. *Proc. Mayo Clin.*, 1947, **22**, 567–70

2273. Symposium. Aureomycin – a new antibiotic. *Ann. N.Y. Acad. Sci.*, 1948, **51**, 175–342

2274. Hanson, Frederick Reuben and Eble, Thomas Eugene. An antiphage agent isolated from *Aspergillus* sp. *J. Bact.*, 1949, **58**, 527–9

2275. Finlay, Alexander Carpenter *et al.* Terramycin, a new antibiotic. *Science,* 1950, **111,** 85
2276. Hazen, Elizabeth Lee and Brown, Rachel Fuller. Fungicidin, an antibiotic produced by a soil actinomycete. *Proc. Soc. Exp. Biol. (N.Y.),* 1951, **76,** 93–97
2277. Burton, H.S. and Abraham, Sir Edward Penley. Isolation of antibiotics from a species of *Cephalosporium.* Cephalosporins P$_1$, P$_2$, P$_3$, P$_4$ and P$_5$. *Biochem. J.,* 1951, **50,** 168–74
2278. McGuire, James Myrlin *et al.* "Ilotycin," a new antibiotic. *Antibiot. Chemother.,* 1952, **2,** 281–83
2279. Abraham, Sir Edward Penley *et al.* Purification and some properties of cephalosporin N, a new penicillin. *Biochem. J.,* 1954, **58,** 94–102
2280. Newton, Guy G.F. and Abraham, Sir Edward Penley. Cephalosporin C, a new antibiotic containing sulphur and D-α-aminoadipic acid. *Nature (Lond.),* 1955, **175,** 548
2281. Gold, W. *et al.* Amophotericins A and B, antifungal antibiotics produced by a streptomycete. *Antibiot. Ann.,* 1955–6, 579–586
2282. Umezawa, Hamao *et al.* Production and isolation of a new antibiotic, kanamycin. *J. Antibiot. Jpn. Ser. A,* 1957, **10,** 181–88
2283. Weinstein, Marvin Joseph *et al.* Gentamicin, a new antibiotic complex from *Micromonospora. J. Med. Chem.,* 1963, **6,** 463–4
2284. Office of Population Censuses and Surveys. Trends in mortality 1951–1975; Series DH1 No. 3. London, *HMSO,* 1978, Figure 1.5
2285. Ecclesiasticus xxxviii, 4
2286. Langley, John Newport (1905–6). As ref. 1390 but pp. 410–12
2287. Elliott, Thomas Renton. On the action of adrenalin. *J. Physiol. (Lond.).,* 1904, **31,** *Proc. Physiol. Soc.,* pp. xx–xxi
2288. Barger, George *et al.* An active alkaloid from ergot. *Br. Med. J.,* 1906, **2,** 1792
2289. Howell, William Henry. Vagus inhibition of the heart in its relation to the inorganic salts of the blood. *Am. J. Physiol.,* 1905–6, **15,** 280–94
2290 Hunt, Reid and Taveau, René de M. On the physiological action of certain cholin derivatives and new methods for detecting cholin. *Br. Med. J.,* 1906, **2,** 1788–91
2291. Dixon, Walter Ernest and Hamill, Philip. The mode of action of specific substances with special reference to secretin. *J. Physiol. (Lond.),* 1908–9, **38,** 314–36
2292. Windaus, Adolf and Vogt, Karl. Synthese des Imidazolyläthylamins. *Ber. Dtsch. Chem. Ges.,* 1907, **40,** 3691–95
2293. Barger, George and Dale, Sir Henry Hallett. Chemical structure and sympathomimetic action of amines. *J. Physiol. (Lond.),* 1910, **41,** 19–59
2294. Dale, Sir Henry Hallett and Laidlaw, Sir Patrick Playfair. The physiological action of β-iminoazolylethylamine. *J. Physiol. (Lond.),* 1910, **41,** 318–44
2295. Barger, George and Dale, Sir Henry Hallett. β-iminazolylethylamine a depressor constituent of intestinal mucosa. *J. Physiol. (Lond.),* 1911, **41,** 499–503
2296. Hunt, Reid and Taveau, René de M. On the relation between the toxicity and chemical constitution of a number of derivatives of choline and analogous compounds. *J. Pharmacol.,* 1909, **1,** 303–39
2297. Henry, Thomas Anderson. The plant alkaloids. London, *J. & A. Churchill,* 1913
2298. Dale, Sir Henry Hallett. The action of certain esters and ethers of choline, and their relation to muscarine. *J. Pharmacol.,* 1914, **6,** 147–90
2299. Ewins, Arthur James. Acetylcholine, a new active principle of ergot. *Biochem. J.,* 1914, **8,** 44–49
2300. Hunt, Reid. Vasodilator reactions. *Am. J. Physiol.,* 1918, **45,** 197–267
2301. Spiro, Karl and Stoll, Arthur. Ueber die wirksamen Substanzen des Mutterkorns. *Schweiz. Med. Wschr.,* 1921, **2,** 525–29
2302. Loewi, Otto. Ueber humorale Uebertragbarkeit der Herznervenwirkung. *Pflüg. Arch. Ges. Physiol.,* 1921, **189,** 239–42; 1922, **193,** 201–13; 1924, **203,** 408–12; **204,** 361–67, 629–40
2303. Loewi, Otto and Navratil, E. Ueber humorale Uebertragbarkeit der Herznervenwirkung. *Pflüg. Arch. Ges. Physiol.,* 1924, **206,** 123–40; 1926, **214,** 678–96
2304. Banting, Sir Frederick Grant and Best, Charles Herbert. The internal secretion of the pancreas. *J. Lab. Clin. Med.,* 1922, **7,** 251–66
2305. Cushny, Arthur Robertson. Biological relations of optically isomeric substances. Baltimore, *Williams & Wilkins,* 1926

2306. Hanzlik, Paul John. Actions and uses of the salicylates and cinchophen in medicine. *Medicine,* 1926, **5**, 197–373

2307. Trevan, J.W. The error determination of toxicity. *Proc. R. Soc. (Biol.),* 1927, **101**, 483–514

2308. Best, Charles Herbert *et al.* The nature of the vaso-dilator constituents of certain tissue extracts. *J. Physiol. (Camb.),* 1927, **62**, 397–417

2309. Dale, Sir Henry Hallett and Dudley, Harold Ward. Presence of histamine and acetylcholine in the spleen of ox and horse. *J. Physiol. (Lond.),* 1929, **68**, 97–123

2310. Clark, Alfred Joseph. The mode of action of drugs on cells. London, *E. Arnold & Co.,* 1933

2311. Feldberg, Wilhelm Siegmund and Gaddum, Sir John Henry. The chemical transmitter at synapses in a sympathetic ganglion. *J. Physiol. (Lond.),* 1934, **81**, 305–19

2312. Vialli, Maffo and Erspamer, Vittorio. Cellule enterocromaffini e cellule basigranulose acidofile nei vertebrati. (Ricerche istochimiche). *Z. Zellforsch. Mikr. Anat.,* 1933, **19**, 743–73

2313. Brown, Sir George Lindor *et al.* Reactions of the normal mammalian muscle to acetylcholine and to eserine. *J. Physiol. (Lond.),* 1936, **87**, 394–424

2314. Bovet, Daniel and Staub, Ann-Marie. Action protectrice des éthers phénoloques au cours de l'intoxication histaminique. *C. R. Soc. Biol. (Paris),* 1937, **124**, 547–9

2315. Gunn, James Andrew. The pharmacological actions and therapeutic uses of some compounds related to adrenaline. *Br. Med. J.,* 1939, **2**, 155–60, 214–19

2316. Euler, Ulf Svante von. A specific sympathomimetic ergone in adrenergic nerve fibres (sympathin) and its relations to adrenaline and nor-adrenaline. *Acta Physiol. Scand.,* 1946, **12**, 73–97

2317. Paton, Sir William Drummond Macdonald and Zaimis, Eleanor. Curare-like action of polymethylene *bis*-quaternary ammonium salts. *Nature (Lond.),* 1948, **161**, 718–19

2318. Rocha E Silva, Mauricio *et al.* Bradykinin, a hypotensive and smooth muscle stimulating factor released from plasma globulin by snake venoms and by trypsin. *Am. J. Physiol.,* 1949, **156**, 261–73

2319. Ahlquist, R.P. A study of adrenotropic receptors. *Am. J. Physiol.,* 1948, **153**, 586–600

2320. Katz, Sir Bernard. The release of neural transmitter substances. Liverpool, *University Press,* 1969

2321. Lands, A.M. *et al.* Differentiation of receptor systems activated by sympathomimetic amines. *Nature (Lond.),* 1967, **214**, 597–598

2322. Levy, B. and Wilkenfeld, B.E. An analysis of selective beta receptor blockade. *Eur. J. Pharmac.,* 1969, **5**, 227–234

2323. Choo-Kang, Y.F.J. *et al.* Response of asthmatics to isoprenaline and salbutamol aerosols administered by intermediate positive-pressure ventilation. *Br. Med. J.,* 1970, **4**, 465–468

2324. Black, James Whyte *et al.* Definition and antagonism of histamine H_2-receptors. *Nature (Lond.),* 1972, **236**, 385–390

8

Aspects of Modern Drug Use

Most people would now acknowledge that humane social attitudes and an environment produced by attention to the public health, are preventive of disease. The conditions of inner city life for many people, the numbers of persons unemployed, the somewhat feudal exposure of the employee to the employer, and other such factors, suggest that the accomplishment of the body politic has been limited. But compared with the previous century it has been real.

Plague is the most obvious example of a great and terrible disease the pathogenesis of which altered drastically in a way we cannot properly explain. Most of the great diseases seem influenced in their natural history by the social factors – and the killing cardiovascular and neoplastic lesions of today may be just as much affected by these factors as were the pandemic and infective diseases of the past. The relevant social issues must be assumed to change and our present concerns might reasonably include the dietary prevention of cardiovascular disease and the removal of toxic substances and known carcinogens from the environment. Perhaps no century since antiquity has so clearly recognized the importance of preventive medicine.

There have been surprising advances in the management of many of the diseases which remain important – but the advances have been unequal. They have also been associated with hazards and drug disasters that, before thalidomide, were so unexpected that there was no legislation to minimize or prevent them. As these hazards are important, it is worth recalling what was, in Europe, the first major drug disaster.

Thalidomide

The modern concepts of chemotherapy originated with the work of Paul Ehrlich on the organic arsenicals. With the introduction of arsphenamine in 1911 this work commenced the era of chemotherapy as we now know it. Almost a quarter of a century later the BPC of 1934, in its monograph on arsphenamine, observed that[2325]:

It was due to Ehrlich's hypothesis, that pentavalent arsenicals such as sodium aminarsonate are reduced in the body to the trivalent form, that the spirochæticidal power of the arsphenamines was realised. The therapeutic application of this research constitutes the greatest achievement yet made, not only in the treatment of syphilis but in the whole of chemotherapy.

Exactly half a century after the new era began another synthetic chemical drug – thalidomide – caused the unexpected tragedy of 1961. It is from this event that the whole complex mass of modern drug regulatory controls originates.

Between 1959 and 1962 the thalidomide disaster produced an estimated 10 000 deformed children born in those countries in which the drug was taken by women in the early stages of pregnancy. Speaking of this event in Britain, the Ministry of Health report of 1964 on *Deformities caused by thalidomide*[2326] said: 'The information obtained suggests that there are between 200 and 250 living children with limb deformities resulting from thalidomide and a further 50 with deformities other than those of the limbs. The extreme upper and lower limits for the total of children with limb deformities are given on differing assumptions as 430 and 150. The total foetal loss including abortion and stillbirth cannot be computed.'

Great efforts were made to relieve the lot of these malformed children. Special units where powered limbs were made available were set up at Roehampton, Oxford and Liverpool and charities were established to assist in rehabilitation and with the introduction of prostheses. Nevertheless, the same official report observed that: 'This tragic episode is shown to have involved fewer families than was feared at one time and the relief available to individual children has been improved. Yet each case was a personal disaster which no amount of subsequent help can wholly relieve.' As if to accompany this understatement, the report provides a plate (reproduced as Figure 144)[2327] showing a $4\frac{1}{2}$-year-old child with amelia of the upper limbs and phocomelia of the lower limbs; pneumatic upper limb prostheses have been fitted and the equipment includes rocker-ended pylon sockets of leather, these embracing both hips to give stability.

Thalidomide (α-phthalimidoglutarimide) is a fairly simple organic compound derived from glutamic acid and chemically unrelated to either the barbiturates or narcotic alkaloids. It was first synthesized by Kunz, Keller and Mückter (1956)[2328] in the laboratories of the German pharmaceutical company, Chemie Grünenthal. Some of the accounts which have been written of the subsequent events suggest that thalidomide was just another, and not very necessary, hypnotic whose only remarkable feature (prior to its human teratogenic effect becoming obvious) was its over-enthusiastic commercialization. Such a view overlooks the fact that, at the time, thalidomide seemed to be an important new drug which had quite real clinical advantages.

There was, and there still is, a need for an hypnotic which was so safe in overdose that its use would avoid the frequently lethal effect of accidental or deliberate barbiturate poisoning. The outstanding property of thalidomide, both in man and the animals in which it was tested, was that it produced sedation and, in higher doses, sleep. The important feature was that even substantial doses were not lethal. Thus, mice, which were well sedated with a dose of 50 mg per kg body weight orally, were able to tolerate single doses of 5000 mg per kg; similarly, dogs

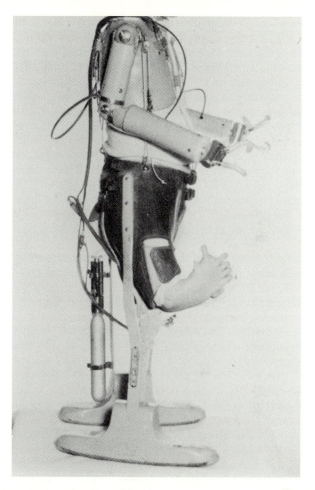

Figure 144 Thalidomide-induced amelia of the upper limbs and phocomelia of the lower limbs in a child of 4½ years fitted with pneumatic upper limb prostheses and additional equipment. [*From: Ministry of Health. Reports on public health and medical subjects, No. 112. HMSO (1964).*]

could tolerate 1000 times the sedative dose without ill effect. These findings provided a real reason for thinking that thalidomide might be important – and they explain its ready clinical acceptance.

Thalidomide had other useful properties: it was active by mouth but did not cause gastric irritation or vomiting; it was not contraindicated in patients with renal or hepatic disease; it seemed free from serious dependence-producing potential and could fairly easily be withdrawn from patients who had been taking for it long periods of time. Above all, clinical cases were recorded of survival after doses 16–160 times the sedative dose had been taken. Even in these cases, unconsciousness was of limited duration and recovery was complete.

The degree of safety in single massive doses may have been due to poor absorption of the relatively insoluble drug in solid dosage forms – but it was a characteristic which offered hope of a valuable hypnotic with which suicide would be almost impossible. In a drug which had no effect, even in sedative doses, on the heart rate, blood pressure or respiration, it made the introduction of the drug seem an interesting and promising event.

It may be of some importance that this introduction took place in the hands of an organization that was not part of the well-established German pharmaceutical industry. Chemie Grünenthal had been founded only in 1946 – and then as a subsidiary of a larger company whose products were soaps, detergents and cosmetics. In addition to this limitation of experience, it seems likely that the data behind the compound were less than fully adequate compared with the standards of the established pharmaceutical houses of the day. Finally, the existence, after the launch of the product, of errors of technical judgement is implied by the eventual legal settlements although these, in England, were not reached until July, 1973.

The remarkable thing is that the data, whatever their deficiencies, met the regulatory standards of the day – because there were none: in both Germany and Britain, in 1961, hardly more than 20 years ago, the population relied on the pharmaceutical industry to ensure that its medicines were effective and safe.

Having completed the animal work and clinical studies that they wished to undertake, Chemie Grünenthal marketed thalidomide in Germany in November, 1956. The first product (Grippex) was a fixed combination for the treatment of minor respiratory tract infections. The parent drug was made available as a sedative and hypnotic (Contergan) in October, 1957. The drug was heavily promoted and additional fixed combinations, often with substances such as aspirin, were used to expand the market. The success was such that other companies became interested and, in Britain, thalidomide – as the hypnotic, Distaval – was launched in April, 1958 by the Distillers Company whose subsidiary, Distillers Company (Biochemicals) Limited (DCBL), became the British manufacturers and licensees. In the United Kingdom the fixed combination dosage forms were given the names Asmaval, Tensival, Valgis and Valgraine – indicating the market segments in which it was expected that the drug would be useful.

The literature shows that there was at least one important point which was left outstanding before the drug entered clinical use in Britain: J. McC. Murdoch, of the Edinburgh University Department of Therapeutics, and his colleague, G. D. Campbell – equally a student of Professor Derrick Dunlop – published an article on the *Antithyroid activity of N-phthalyl glutamic acid imide (K 17)*[2329] in the *British Medical Journal* of January 11th, 1958. This study, reported 3 months before the drug was launched, was concerned with the effects of thalidomide on the thyroid uptake of radioactive iodine in nine euthyroid patients; it showed a mild but definite antithyroid effect when the drug was given in doses of 200 mg or more. The authors concluded that '. . . it would seem unjustifiable to use the drug for long-term sedative or hypnotic therapy, pending the results of a more detailed study of its long-term effects in a larger series of patients, and notably those suffering from mild or moderately severe hyperthyroidism.' In Germany the drug had been used in doses of 25–50 mg two to four times daily, as a day-time sedative, and in doses of 50–100 mg as a night-time hypnotic. German workers had already noted a marked reduction of the raised basal metabolic rate in mild and moderately severe cases of hyperthyroidism as a result of thalidomide therapy; Murdoch and Campbell's study was therefore undertaken to see if the effect on basal metabolic rate was related to depression of thyroid function, or to some other action. Their warning was quite clearly important in relationship to a drug likely to be used at doses not far remote from those they had studied and for long periods of time.

In the months that followed the British launch of April 1958, the drug was heavily promoted in Germany. Harvey Teff and Colin R. Munro, in their excellent study, *Thalidomide, the legal aftermath*[2330], of 1976, note that in August, 1958 Chemie Grünenthal circulated over 40000 doctors in Germany; on this occasion the covering letter to the material advertising the drug 'explicitly stated that Contergan "does not damage either mother or child". ' Teff and Munro add that, in Britain, as late as October, 1961, only a few weeks before the drug was withdrawn from the market, DCBL 'issued an advertisement which said: "Distaval can be given with complete safety to pregnant women and nursing mothers without adverse effect on mother or child." ' Behind this, now seemingly incredible statement, lay 5 years experience since the launch of the drug in Germany. From the accounts written it seems unlikely that the British licensees had, in the later period of their promotion of the drug, access to the totality of the adverse reactions data. Even so, it is clear that at the time it was printed this statement was unwise: earlier than 1961, with a number of drugs, including penicillin, it had been learnt that no usefully active drug can be given with *complete* safety to anyone – much less to pregnant women and nursing mothers. In the event, and in retrospect, this extravagant claim stands as part of the drug's indictment.

Sjöström and Nilsson (*Thalidomide and the power of the drug companies,* 1972)[2331], discussing the toxic effects of thalidomide, record that by late 1959, Chemie Grünenthal were receiving reports of the clinical occurrence of a poly-neuritic syndrome possibly due to the drug. It seems that there were also other reported side-effects for these authors say:

> Apart from the polyneuritis, severe symptoms of effects on the central nervous system often appeared. Involuntary twitchings of the facial muscles occurred, trembling of the muscles of the entire body, abnormal bodily sensations and severe disturbances of the ability to concentrate, together with speech difficulties, double vision and in some cases even epileptic seizures. In contrast to the peripheral neuritis type of damage, these effects on the central nervous system disappeared when the medication was stopped.

This is a striking statement, for thalidomide is not now commonly remembered as a drug producing central, as distinct from peripheral, nervous system adverse effects in clinical use – and in this paragraph these effects are said to have been severe and frequent. They included speech difficulties, double vision and convulsions. A long list of possible explanations can be drawn up but those that must have been considered, or would certainly now be considered, include:

(1) The symptoms being due to the psychiatric or physical illnesses likely to be treated with a new hypnotic and sedative.

(2) A formulation defect – perhaps due to different particle sizes affecting the batches of drug as, once the launch stocks were used up, subsequent batches were blended, as a means of economy, with material from the pilot and scale-up runs.

(3) The dose being too high – perhaps because the prelaunch clinical studies had been conducted in severely ill, hospitalized subjects who needed a bigger dose than the less severely ill patients seen in family practice and out-patient clinics once the drug was marketed.

(4) The patient population being different – maybe because the formal clinical trials were conducted on young or middle-aged patients whereas the drug, after launch, was most frequently given to older people whose capability for its metabolic handling was diminished.

(5) The data being misrepresented or the conclusions exaggerated (and the statement given above is not quantified – perhaps because its importance was not fully appreciated).

(6) The drug having a real and serious central nervous system toxicity in man – just as described in the paragraph quoted – and this being, perhaps, species specific so that there was no reason why the animal data should be anything other than reassuring.

(7) The drug having a different metabolic pathway in man than in the animal species used in the premarketing safety evaluation; man might therefore produce a toxic metabolite unseen in the animals.

(8) The breakdown of the drug in the liver or its excretory pathway through the kidney being critical so that, in widespread clinical use, it picks off those with damaged livers or kidneys and, in them only, throws up a pattern of serious side-effects.

(9) The occurrence of a drug interaction so that the new drug produces a marked adverse effect only in those few patients given another drug or class of drugs.

Today, assuming a reliable and sensitive assay for the drug in biological fluids and its use in a proper comparison of the metabolism of the drug in man and the animal species in which it was tested, some of these possibilities would have been excluded from the beginning; others would be excluded by contemporary good manufacturing practices and other advances. But it remains not uncommon for drugs to cause serious adverse effects which were not expected when they were launched. In 1961, sorting out the confusing picture presented by reports of central and peripheral side-effects must have seemed a very great puzzle indeed.

It would seem that the point of understandable difficulty was, in Germany, substantially earlier than 1961. Sjöström and Nilsson (1972) say that 'By the end of 1960 Chemie Grünenthal had received 1600 reports of various side-effects which had been connected with thalidomide, among which were over 100 cases of the severe polyneuritis.'[2332] Hesitation at this point is much harder to understand and the same authors continue: 'During the autumn Grünenthal learned that Distillers, the licensee in England, had received seven reports of effects on the nervous system ascribed to thalidomide. Mention of these side-effects was made in the Distillers' commercial literature. In August and December a circular letter was sent to over 20 000 doctors, which included a warning of the risk of peripheral neuritis . . .'

Apart from noting that the licensee in Britain seems to have acted far more promptly and on the basis of much less information than the drug's parent company, the account can be left with the comment by Teff and Munro (1976)[2333] that 'In the absence of an exhaustive inquiry with full disclosure of relevant documents, it is idle to speculate on the precise allocation of legal and moral responsibility for the tragedy.' Other writers have, perhaps understandably, been less restrained.

Situations similar to the confusing period with thalidomide's initially mixed picture of side-effects have occurred with other drugs in more recent years. They prompt two obvious questions: How does one avoid having to sort out this kind of problem while the drug is in the market-place and patients are being exposed in uncontrolled clinical use – a use enhanced by the drug's commercial promotion? Secondly, should a drug to which infrequent, but severe, adverse effects are being attributed remain in use for trivial indications? These questions are merely special expressions of the equation that relates benefit to risk. The difficulty is that benefit can be widespread and risk manifest itself in only a few.

In Britain there was a notable change in the problems presented to the profession by thalidomide when Dr A. Leslie Florence published, in the *British Medical Journal* of December 31st, 1960, the following historic letter[2334]:

Is Thalidomide to Blame?

SIR,—I feel that four cases which have occurred in my practice recently are worthy of mention, as they may correspond to the experience of other practitioners. They all presented in more or less the same way – each patient complaining of: (1) Marked paraesthesia affecting first the feet and subsequently the hands. (2) Coldness of the extremities and marked pallor of the toes and fingers on exposure to even moderately cold conditions. (3) Occasional slight ataxia. (4) Nocturnal cramp in the leg muscles. Clinical examination in each case has been essentially negative, and during this time I have not noticed similar cases in my practice.

It seemed to me to be significant that each patient had been receiving thalidomide ("distaval") in a dose of 100 mg at night, the period during which the drug had been given varying from eighteen months to over two years. Thalidomide is generally regarded as being remarkably free of toxic effects, but in this instance the drug was stopped. Three of the patients have now received no thalidomide for two to three months, and there has been a marked improvement in their symptoms, but they are still present. The fourth patient stopped taking the drug two weeks ago, and it is therefore too early to assess the effect of withdrawal.

It would appear that these symptoms could possibly be a toxic effect of thalidomide. I have seen no record of similar effects with this drug, and I feel it would be of interest to learn whether any of your readers have observed these effects after long-term treatment with the drug. I might add that I have found it otherwise to be a most effective hypnotic with no "morning hang-over" effect. It has been especially useful in patients with skin pruritus and discomfort. – I am, etc.,

Turriff, Aberdeenshire.   A. LESLIE FLORENCE.

The letter is a fine example of its kind: there were four cases, each with a well-characterized and unusual syndrome. All four patients had received long-term administration of the drug. Comparison with the absence of the syndrome in the rest of the practice made the suspicion that the 'symptoms could possibly be a toxic effect of thalidomide' singularly well based. The letter is a prime example of clinical alertness combined with restraint producing a valuable 'early warning'.

The suspicion was soon confirmed. Most of the events of real importance can be followed in the weekly editions of the *British Medical Journal* of 1961 – a few of the critical references appear elsewhere, especially in the *Lancet*, and in the German literature.

Dr Florence's letter was of the last day of 1960. It prompted Dr Denis Burley, of DCBL, to note, in January, 1961[2335], that for some while the literature supplied with thalidomide had mentioned that 'peripheral neuritis could be a toxic hazard, albeit a rare one...' It was recommended that 'a watch should be kept for changes in sensation in the peripheries should the drug be given over a period of months.'

'Five similar cases', apparently of peripheral sensory neuropathy, were reported from Edinburgh on January 28th, 1961[2336]. Two possible cases were reported from Burnley on March 18th and the appearances in the first of these patients suggested 'that the drug is capable of inducing the changes within a relatively short time'[2337]. The changes, paraesthesiae and numbness, had appeared in the hands following 9 weeks with a nightly dose of 100 mg in an elderly patient.

Soon after the 'early warning' in Britain and its tentative confirmation, three papers, each of importance, appeared in Germany. On May 6th, 1961 Dr H. Frenkel published an article (*Contergan-Nebenwirkungen*)[2338] in which he reviewed the side-effects of thalidomide in 21 patients and discussed the poly-neuritic syndrome. On May 12th, 1961, W. von Scheid and his colleagues, in their paper *Polyneuritische Syndrome nach längerer Thalidomid-Medikation*[2339], gave a full account of the polyneuritic illness that could follow long-term thalidomide administration. In the same edition of *Deutsche Medizinische Wochenschrift*, writing from a clinic at Essen, Hans von Raffauf, in a paper entitled *Bewirkt Thalidomid (Contergan) keine Schaden?*[2340], attempted to answer the question of whether or not thalidomide could cause damage.

By the beginning of June, 1961 there was no reasonable doubt that thalidomide was producing, in clinical use, an unexpected incidence of peripheral neuropathy. The only reasonable doubt was the dose and duration of treatment needed to produce the toxic effect, the true frequency with which it appeared, its clinical correlates, and its mechanism. But that it occurred had been admitted in the DCBL letter of January 14th, confirmed by suggestions in the English medical press, and fairly fully discussed in the German literature.

Nothing to compare with the substantial publications which had appeared in

Germany was published in England in the Spring or Summer of 1961 but the *British Medical Journal* of July 8th that year answered a question on the occurrence of purpura in patients taking thalidomide[2341] and, in its edition of September 2nd, carried a letter in which both neurological and purpuric features were reported in a woman of 28 who 'had been taking "asmaval" tablets (thalidomide 12.5 mg; ephedrine hydrochloride 20 mg) intermittently over a period of three to four months.'[2342] The *British Medical Journal* of September 30th, 1961 printed two items of greater substance. In an article on *Neuropathy after intake of thalidomide (Distaval)*[2343] Pamela Fullerton and Michael Kremer, of the Middlesex Hospital, London, described the neurotoxic effects of thalidomide in 13 patients they had studied. In these patients neurological symptoms had appeared in 2–18 months after beginning regular medication in doses varying from 50 to 400 mg nightly. The disease was reported as not being just a simple neuropathy and the authors added in their summary: 'The disorder was predominantly a sensory peripheral neuritis, but there was evidence of more widespread effects on the nervous system.' This important paper became the subject of an editorial in the edition in which it appeared. The editorial noted that Fullerton and Kremer 'were unable in the light of other investigations to explain the mechanism of the drug's toxic action'[2344]; it added that a 'significant feature of this series of thirteen patients is that none have shown much improvement in their symptoms or signs on withdrawal of the drug...'; it concluded that greater caution was needed in the use of the drug and it should not be prescribed 'for long periods except under regular and careful supervision'.

Letters reporting cases of neuropathy appeared on October 21st[2345] and 28th[2346]; the Journal's edition of November 4th[2347] brought out a report of a psychotic episode following treatment with thalidomide, an account of a patient in whom the drug caused impairment of glucose absorption, and a letter reporting a probable early case of peripheral neuritis in a man 75 years of age. November 11th[2348] produced a letter complaining that the advertising by Distillers no longer reflected the facts and a letter in which Dr Burley wrote: 'I feel that a rather one-sided view is being presented of this neuropathic complication of thalidomide administration...'. The letter advised that the company had, at that time, details of 40 cases of thalidomide neuropathy but in 17 of these the symptoms had remitted on withdrawing the drug. Other authors stated 'that sensory neuropathy at least does not resolve rapidly after withdrawal of thalidomide'[2348] and that, in the hope of avoiding the problem, they had reduced the 'nightly dosage from 100 mg to 50 mg, with little lessening of hypnotic effect'.

There were three more letters on thalidomide in the *British Medical Journal* of November 18th, 1961[2349]; one on November 25th[2350], and four on December 2nd[2351]. These four included one from the Managing Director of The Distillers Company (Biochemicals) Ltd. announcing the withdrawal from the market of thalidomide and its combinations because 'reports have been received from two overseas sources possibly associating thalidomide ("distaval") with harmful effects on the foetus in early pregnancy.'

The action of Distillers when faced with these reports of fetal abnormalities seems to have been immediate. The letter of December 2nd, 1961 represents the first indication to the profession of such abnormalities being due to the drug. It came almost exactly a year after Dr A. Leslie Florence had published his letter of

December 31th, 1960 alerting the profession in Britain to the problem of peripheral neuropathy; it was 6 months after the May, 1961 date by which it had become clear that neuropathy could be the result of thalidomide therapy.

Throughout 1961 little had been heard of the adverse central nervous system effects which had been earlier reported in Germany and it can probably be safely concluded that such effects are not a major part of the toxicity of thalidomide in man.

On December 16th, 1961 the *Lancet* published the first medical report[2352] in the British medical press indicating that thalidomide might be a human teratogen: this announcement, by Dr W. G. McBride, an obstetrician practising in Sydney, Australia, shortly preceded McBride's publication of a very similar text in the December 23rd, 1961 edition[2353] of the *Medical Journal of Australia* – but this is the *Lancet* version:

THALIDOMIDE AND CONGENITAL ABNORMALITIES

SIR,—Congenital abnormalities are present in approximately 1·5% of babies. In recent months I have observed that the incidence of multiple severe abnormalities in babies delivered of women who were given the drug thalidomide ('Distaval') during pregnancy, as an antiemetic or as a sedative, to be almost 20%.

These abnormalities are present in structures developed from mesenchyme – i.e., the bones and musculature of the gut. Bony development seems to be affected in a very striking manner, resulting in polydactyly, syndactyly, and failure of development of long bones (abnormally short femora and radii).

Have any of your readers seen similar abnormalities in babies delivered of women who have taken this drug during pregnancy?

Hurstville, New South Wales.   W. G. McBRIDE.

The first to detect and report this drug-related teratogenicity in man had been the German physician, W. Lenz, of the Universität-Kinderklinik at Hamburg-Eppendorf. At a meeting of paediatricians in Dusseldorf on November 18th, 1961, Dr Lenz had discussed his suspicions; on November 26th a newspaper article brought these anxieties to the attention of the general public. Dr Lenz then wrote to the *Lancet* to comment on the letter of McBride and, in his own letter of January 6th, 1962[2354], commented that 'I have seen 52 malformed infants whose mothers had taken "Contergan" in early pregnancy...'; Lenz also reported that since the November 18th conference he had received 'letters from many places in the German Federal Republic, as well as from Belgium, England, and Sweden, reporting 115 additional cases in which this drug was thought to be the cause'. The defects (amelia, phocomelia, certain forms of atresia and other abnormalities) were all striking because the specific limb deformities seen had, in all countries, previously been excessively rare; Lenz now estimated that the risk to the fetus of a mother taking Contergan during the fourth to eighth week after conception 'may be definitely higher than 20%'. Other workers, writing from Germany in the same edition of the *Lancet*, noted that in 1949–56 the incidence of congenital abnormalities now being associated with thalidomide had been 'less than 1 in every 5000 newborns'[2355].

Further correspondence preceded an important letter (*Thalidomide and congenital abnormalities; Lancet*, April 28th, 1962)[2356] in which Dr G. F. Somers, a pharmacologist of standing and member of DCBL, advising the results of laboratory work undertaken since the announcements by McBride and Lenz, said: 'Our first experiments in rats showed resorption sites but no malformations. Now we have succeeded in producing deformities in rabbits remarkably similar to those seen in humans.' The successful experiments had been carried out in New Zealand White rabbits, the mothers being given thalidomide 150 mg per kg body weight orally each day from day 8 to day 16 of pregnancy. The laboratory staff had never previously seen lesions of this kind in over 50 years' experience of rabbit breeding or in the breeding of over 1000 progeny in the rabbit colony concerned. Somers noted that full details of the experiments, and of other studies in mice, rats, and hens' eggs would be published and observed that 'As testing for teratogenic effects is not part of standard pharmacological screening procedure, experience in this field is very limited.' Despite this limitation, the report was available within some 4 months of McBride's announcement.

Somers, as most would now agree, had indeed been fortunate: he had not only demonstrated the effect but had hit upon one of the few species, other than man, in which it is readily and reliably demonstrable. His discovery was founded upon known but seldom applied methodology and led to a quite unfounded period of euphoria in which it was assumed, fairly widely, that animal teratogenicity testing, diligently applied, would produce clinically-protective results that could be easily interpreted.

Before discussing the mechanism of the teratologic effect of thalidomide another study which Somers undertook is worth noting. Knightley and his co-authors (1979)[2357] record that 'In his laboratory at Speke, Somers and three assistants carried out a series of tests with thalidomide in powder form compounded with sugar and other sweeteners. Grünenthal already had a liquid or suspension version of thalidomide on the market called Contergan Saft . . .' In England a similar attempt was being made to develop a liquid dosage form.

The results of this formulation work must have been disturbing: they showed that the liquid preparation of thalidomide was toxic to a degree quite unlike the tablets. It was suggested that 'Micro-fining' the material 'and mixing it with a sugar solution allowed it to be absorbed more easily, and once absorbed, it was poisonous'. Somers is quoted as writing: 'We do not therefore regard the formulated suspension as prepared by Grünenthal to be a safe preparation like the tablets and we are of the opinion that there is a very real danger of deaths occurring following overdosage.' Knightley (personal communication) places the date of these observations as January, 1960. This would suggest that throughout 1961, during the period when the evidence that the drug could cause peripheral neuropathy became overwhelming, there were unexplained facets of the pharmacokinetics that may have been clinically relevant. The alternative explanations are that there were unpublished data or that these aspects of the subject failed to interest the authors of the literature consulted.

The mechanism of the teratogenic effect of thalidomide remains elusive despite the amount of work done and the vast bibliography which has arisen. Even at the stage when McBride was developing his suspicions regarding thalidomide he entertained the idea that the drug might be an antimetabolite, a

607

folic acid antagonist. This idea was attractive to Håvard Skre who, in a study on *Thalidomide embryopathy and neuropathy* ... (1963)[2358], wrote that 'Clinical reports seem to have documented that thalidomide is an antimetabolite which has a teratogenic effect in man.' Skre considered his animal experiments as having provided confirmation of this theory and he noted that thalidomide could not only produce clinical appearances resembling acute B_2 avitaminosis or polyneuritis but that the embryopathy which followed its use morphologically resembled that which results from experimental B-avitaminosis in laboratory animals. From his exact and interesting studies Håvard Skre thought that it was unlikely that the mechanism of the phocomelia was the result of breakdown in the primary growth zones of the fetal limbs; the view was preferred that the damage was the result of obstructed differentiation or degenerative processes in an already preformed extremity.

Such concepts link the thalidomide story with the commonplace clinical knowledge of the time. It was well known that deficiencies of one or more of the vitamins of the B complex could lead to neuropathy and that deficiencies of thiamin, pantothenic acid, nicotinic acid or pyridoxine could cause symmetrical, mixed sensory and motor peripheral nerve lesions; vitamin B_{12} deficiency, subacute combined degeneration of the spinal cord was also understood and is characterized by demyelination affecting especially the posterior columns and corticospinal tracts of the cord.

Thus, the clinical knowledge of the time not only emphasized the importance of drug-related peripheral neuropathy, it also offered hypothetical links which McBride seems to have appreciated. Skre's 1963 publication concluded with the comment: 'Peripheral neuropathies may be thought to contribute to the formation of phocomelia, and degenerative nerve changes and pareses are seen in embryopathy produced by B_2-avitaminosis.'

In late 1959 and the 2 years that followed the fact that thalidomide caused peripheral neuropathy might well have led to hypotheses concerning B-avitaminosis; it would be improper to suggest that it would infer that teratogenicity tests should be undertaken. In retrospect it is perhaps different: the inference is that thalidomide may inhibit the effect of these vitamins in the organism and that this unfortunate property may underlie both the peripheral neuropathy and teratogenic potential in man.

A decade after Skre of Norway had published his findings, Janet McCredie (*Thalidomide and congenital Charcot's joints*, 1973)[2359] again sought some sort of unifying concept that would link peripheral neuropathy with teratogenic effects. McCredie was of the Royal Prince Alfred Hospital, Australia, and was able to study 12 sets of radiographs of Australian children referred for radiological opinion by McBride of Sydney and a second group of 80 cases seen in England at Chailey Heritage, Sussex and Queen Mary's Hospital, Roehampton. Both of these latter two institutes were much involved in the rehabilitative programme undertaken in the United Kingdom. McCredie's finding was that radiological analysis of the limbs of children with thalidomide deformities showed joint changes analogous to the classical X-ray signs of adult neuropathic (Charcot) joints. This finding suggested that embryonic sensory peripheral neuropathy was the mechanism of the thalidomide deformities. Entering on an extension of this hypothesis, McCredie proposed a general concept suggesting that an embryo might sustain damage to the neural crest while its autonomic nervous system or other neural-crest derivatives were evolving. The expression of this embryonic neuropathy would be incomplete or imperfect growth of the viscera supplied by the segment of the autonomic nervous system which was affected, or truncated formation of whatever other somatic structure is related to the segment of neural crest which had been damaged.

It is possible to seek this work as a mechanistic explanation and extension of the neurogenic theory of the thalidomide pathogenesis which had been put forward by Skre and, a little later, by others in England. The work, therefore, seems interesting.

A somewhat different emphasis was given by other workers who had noted that McBride's original report of 1961 had suggested that it is the mesenchyme, particularly the prospective bone tissue of the embryo, which is injured. Working at the Institute of Animal Genetics at Edinburgh, A. Jurand (*Early changes in limb buds of chick embryos after thalidomide treatment*, 1966)[2360] introduced thalidomide suspended in thin egg white into chicken eggs which had been pre-incubated for 64–68 hours; under these conditions the drug caused dilation of the axial limb-bud artery 24 hours after treatment. This injury, when present in extreme degree, almost completely destroyed the mesoblast leaving only a small group of mesoblast cells situated in the dorsal area of the limb bud.

These results suggested that the primary cause of thalidomide abnormalities is an injury to the endothelial lining of the axial limb artery. This forms the third of the more popular explanations of the pathogenesis or causative mechanism of thalidomide teratogenicity. It was followed up in studies conducted by David Poswillo (*Hemorrhage in development of the face*, 1975)[2361]. This worker, studying the Macaca irus monkey amongst other species, described animal models of hemifacial microsomia and thalidomide-induced otomandibular dysostosis. The work showed that the causal mechanism of the malformations seemed to be related to the formation of a haematoma at the time of development of the stapedial arterial systems. Thus, focal haemorrhages, developing early in embryogenesis, seemed to play a major part in the pathogenesis of the malformations.

There have been explanations closely related to the chemistry and metabolic handling of the drug. R. T. Williams (*Thalidomide – a study of biochemical teratology*, 1968)[2362] showed that thalidomide is unstable in solution and undergoes hydrolysis. He found that when this drug encounters a pH of greater than 6 in the body, its hydrolyses spontaneously – and at a rate which is pH dependent. Williams and his colleagues tested seven of the metabolites of thalidomide but were not able to demonstrate that any were, in fact, teratogenic. Kohler and his co-workers (1975) studied derivatives of 1,3-indandion and produced results suggesting that an intercalation of the flat purine-like molecular moieties of thalidomide and some of its analogues between base pairs of the DNA double helix might explain the embryotoxic and teratogenic effects observed[2363]. More recently Gordon and his associates (1981) returned to this subject and suggested, from studies in a novel *in vitro* assay, that a toxic arene oxide metabolite might be involved in the teratogenicity of thalidomide[2364].

McBride, following his original disclosures of the drug's human teratogenic effect, remained deeply concerned with the problem and, in studies of 1974[2365] and 1976[2366], showed that the drug damaged the neurons of the dorsal root ganglia of the rabbit fetus. His later work strongly suggests that destruction of the embryonic limb nerves appears to have an effect which is most marked on the preaxial side of the limb: this may lead to reduction deformities of the preaxial areas of the limb, more severe nerve destruction resulting in amelia.

It is clear that despite the great amount of work done and the long period of time which has passed since the thalidomide tragedy, we still lack an adequate explanation of the mechanism involved in this drug's ability to produce embryopathic and teratogenic effects in man. Writing in his book *Drugs as teratogens*[2367] in 1976, J. L. Schardein said that: 'Whatever the mechanism of thalidomide teratogenesis, we must ultimately decipher the fundamental processes of its specific action, if we are to fully understand the general nature of teratogenic insult.' It would seem clear that the situation has not changed and that, even in this narrow and specialized field, we are caused to act upon the problems of drug toxicity by the exercise of general principles. When it is impractical to withdraw a drug which produces an unexpected toxic effect and determine the mechanism of that effect before proceeding, the nature of those general principles remains of profound interest.

Somers was fortunate in finding, in the New Zealand White rabbit, an animal species in which he could demonstrate the teratogenic effect of thalidomide. Studies since then have shown that teratogenic effects due to this drug can be produced in other animal species, but not readily; a much more usual result is death and resorption of the fetus *in utero*.

There is no doubt that, well before the initial synthesis of thalidomide, it was known that external factors could produce human fetal malformation. This fact was established by N. M. Gregg and reported in an important paper on *Congenital cataract following German measles in the mother*[2368] which had been published in Australia in 1941. Gregg was the first to draw attention to the association of death, blindness, and deafness amongst the infants of 78 women who had been exposed to rubella during pregnancy. From the time of this communication the scientific community recognized that external and environmental factors could result in fetal death or malformation. This knowledge has, of course, received ample and unfortunate confirmation following subsequent outbreaks of German measles. Despite Gregg's findings and the widespread ingestion of drugs during pregnancy, there was no general anxiety regarding the effects of maternally-taken drugs on the fetus until the thalidomide tragedy taught its own sudden and sharp lesson. Before this the only governmental recommendation for testing the effect of drugs on the reproductive capability of animals was the so-called 'litter test' – a 6 week chronic toxicity test in male and female rodents which were followed over two pregnancies. The principal parameter measured was fetal survival and the test seemed designed to exclude the production of grossly impaired fertility, by gonadal damage, rather than anything else. Information on this test is given by Schardein (1976)[2367] who also provides the following comment on the inconsistency of the results of teratogenicity testing with thalidomide in animals[2369]:

Thalidomide, despite its profound teratogenic effect in humans, is markedly less potent in laboratory animals. To date, in approximately 10 strains of rats, 15 strains of mice, 11 breeds of rabbits, 2 breeds of dogs, 3 strains of hamsters, 8 species of primates, and in such other varied species as cats, armadillos, guinea pigs, swine, and ferrets in which thalidomide has been tested, teratogenic effects have been induced only occasionally. Effects similar to the phocomelic-type limb deformities observed in man have been produced consistently in only a few breeds of rabbits and in seven species of primates.

The present situation is bewildering: in excess of 2000 chemicals have been tested in laboratory animals and about *one-third* of them have been shown to be teratogenic in one or more species. Schardein (1976) gives data showing that of the 1930 compounds tested at that time, 580 were teratogenic in one or more species, 1200 were not teratogenic, and in 150 the results were equivocal or unknown[2370].

It might then be expected that many drugs would be teratogenic in man – but it is not so: apart from those which are predictably teratogenic the only drugs clearly shown to be teratogens in man are thalidomide, androgens, progestogens, aminopterin, methotrexate, and the antithyroid drugs (the latter producing a defect which is not strictly developmental). As the cells of the fetus are rapidly dividing they would be expected to be vulnerable to a predictable and obvious group of drugs, such as the alkylating agents, the antimetabolites and cytotoxic drugs, which dramatically affect dividing cells and thus become predictable teratogens. There are other suspect drugs – but the list of proven human teratogens remains small.

Thalidomide is, so far, in a class apart: a number of authors have shown that it induces malformations of the limbs (most frequently) and of the ears (less often) when it is given on days 21–36 following conception. This is not long after the first missed period and many women, thus exposed, may not realize they are pregnant.

The difficulty of predicting human risk from animal teratogenicity tests is illustrated by the facts that, although aspirin is a proven teratogen in the rat, mouse, guinea pig, cat, dog, and monkey[2371], it is also one of the substances which has been widely used by pregnant women and yet not been shown to produce any kind of characteristic malformation[2372].

If one attempts to summarize the points mentioned, the complexity of the subject becomes evident. Whilst it is clear that human teratogenicity can neither reliably be predicted, nor reliably excluded, on the basis of animal studies (which, at all events, produce many 'false positives') it is evident that it is possible to avoid misrepresenting the position. It is certainly wrong to think that, learning from the thalidomide disaster, steps have been taken to ensure that the pregnant woman is kept safe from harm: the difficulties involved in the science are such that even the most well-intentioned cannot provide that level of assurance.

The clinician, especially the general practitioner, and the patient, need to understand the limitations of the present methodology and accept the need for prudence in the giving or taking of drugs by the pregnant or possibly pregnant. There are certainly some drugs that have been so widely used that their human teratogenic potential, if any, must be so low that only an extreme view would exclude them when they are useful. It would seem that, at present, the responsibility must rest with the clinician to ensure that, in the pregnant or possibly pregnant, a drug is used only when it is essential and when, on an individual patient basis, its expected benefits clearly seem to outweigh the potential risk – and there are no pharmacologically active drugs for which the risk has been or, within practical limits, can be totally excluded.

This view is supported by the knowledge that teratogenicity is by no means the only harmful effect which drugs can produce in pregnancy, and some 200 drugs and environmental substances have been reported as causing adverse effects on the human fetus. Schardein, from whose indispensible book we have quoted extensively, comes to the conclusion that: '...it would seem wise to avoid the administration of drugs altogether during pregnancy, except where the health of the mother is in serious jeopardy. Still, a problem exists, because the critical stages of fetal development and drug risk occur before many women are even aware of their pregnancies.' It is perhaps a conclusion that the doctor needs to ensure that the female patient possessed of reproductive capacity understands.

We can conclude, firstly, that thalidomide caused two major side-effects in man and, secondly, the fact that it caused a serious and unusual peripheral neuropathy was clear several months before the announcement of its teratogenic effect. Neither of these effects had been predicted from the limited laboratory and clinical studies undertaken before marketing and, even today, there is no guarantee that the conventional preclinical and clinical programme would disclose either effect. However, such disclosure is likely – for more than one species is included in teratology and fertility testing and adequate numbers of patients followed for 1 or 2 years might be included in the clinical programme. The latter remains the weak point, for what some would consider adequate protection of the community exposed to a new drug cannot, as increasing experience shows, be obtained from the present requirements.

There remain two questions. Would the present drug registration requirements ensure the detection of the thalidomide problem before it reached the proportions of a major disaster? Secondly, if thalidomide had been promptly withdrawn for re-evaluation once it was clear that it was producing one major unexpected side-effect, would that have minimized the later disaster – and what might that imply in evaluating the adverse reactions data from other new drugs?

Drug regulatory requirements

There have always been two different classes of drugs: those used by the professions set apart to deal with disease, and those of folk medicine – the latter, in modern times, includes some of the proprietary medicines obtainable by the public from retail outlets. Even known poisons were widely available most of the way through the nineteenth century. In the United Kingdom control over the sale of poisons was, to all practical purposes, begun with the Arsenic Act of 1851 but the Pharmacy Act of 1868 provided the first real attempt to control the labelling and selling of poisons. The Poisons and Pharmacy Act of 1908 amended the 1868 Act but there was still no limitation on the provision of poisons or supply of dangerous drugs prescribed by a medical practitioner and such substances could be sold to people known to the pharmacist. It was not until the Defence of the Realm (Consolidation) Regulations of 1917 that the supply of barbitone, morphine, cocaine and similar drugs was restricted to patients for whom a physician had prescribed them.

The medical profession, in the late nineteenth and early twentieth centuries, showed itself concerned with the exploitation of the public by those who sold proprietary medicines. The British Medical Association organized the analysis of some of these patent medicines and, in *Secret Remedies, What they cost and what they contain* (1909)[2373], and in *More Secret Remedies, What they cost and what they contain* (1912)[2374], published the findings, comparing the cost of the actual ingredients with the claims made for the products.

This matter was formally investigated, resulting in the *Report from the Select Committee on Patent Medicines* . . . (1914)[2375]. The Select Committee had been appointed 'to consider and inquire into the question of the sale of Patent and Proprietary Medicines and Medical Preparations and Appliances, and Advertisements relating thereto . . .' Its meetings extended over three sessions of Parliament and involved 33 public sittings with 42 witnesses being asked 14 000 questions.

It found that while, at that time, the sale of medical preparations in the United States was regulated by the Food and Drugs Acts (1906, with an amending Act in 1912), the situation in Britain regarding the sale and advertisement of patent and proprietary medicines could be summarized in the following manner:

> For all practical purposes British law is powerless to prevent any person from procuring any drug, or making any mixture, whether potent or without any therapeutical activity whatever (so long as it does not contain a scheduled poison) advertising it in any decent terms as a cure for any disease or ailment, recommending it by bogus testimonials and the invented opinions and facsimile signatures of fictitious physicians, and selling it under any name he chooses, on the payment of a small stamp duty, for any price he can persuade a credulous public to pay.

The Select Committee gave many examples of the secret remedies they had investigated. Some of them had exotic claims puffed up from small contents:

> *"Mer-syren."* – "Composed of the active principles of certain rare plants which flourish in the valleys situated on the southern slopes of the Himalaya, between the immense gorge separating Nepaul from Bhutan on the East, and Almorah on the North-West." Recommended by "Dr. Pearson, late principal Medical Officer, North Bhangulpore, India." No place named Bhangulpore is mentioned in the Imperial Gazetteer of India. A cure for "dropsy, insanity, smallpox, angina pectoris, diphtheria, erysipelas." etc. No substance but potato starch could be detected by analysis.

Others were a quite different matter, offering toxic ingredients to susceptible populations:

> *"Steedman's Soothing Powders."* – These contain, according to the Government Chemist's report, 27.1 per cent. of calomel. The directions for use for children say: "One may be taken for three or four nights successively at any time when the child complains of being poorly". The powders vary in weight, and a child may thus get one grain of calomel for several nights in succession.

The text of the report includes the following examples of fraudulent claims, several other examples of which are given showing that the practice of making such claims was common:

> "The best remedy for consumption." (*Congreve's Elixir.*)
> "Cures Bright's disease." (*Munyon's Kidney Cure,* consisting of sugar only.)
> "It never fails to cure cancerous ulcers, syphilis, piles, rheumatism, gout, dropsy." (*Clarke's Blood mixture.*)
> "It will be sufficient to offer a few general remarks, and to indicate the method of cure [of syphilis], which is, beyond all, the question of supreme importance. Let it never be forgotten that even a slight delay in dealing with diseases of this type may be terribly fruitful of future trouble. In the first place, the advice of a properly qualified medical man is necessary, whatever the character of the disease, or whether it be hereditary or acquired. But the process of eradicating the poison from the system will be materially assisted by the aid of a perfectly safe, but reliable, searching, cleansing, purgative medicine; and nothing better for that purpose can be used than Beecham's Pills. They should be taken immediately, and continued for a considerable time after the cure is apparently complete." (*Beecham's Pills.*)

From some of the organizations whose products were investigated at that time, major pharmaceutical houses of excellence have arisen. This important and welcome change seems to have been a response not only to the establishment of scientific disciplines within the companies but also to the greatly increased expectations of the community. It was (perhaps surprisingly) not due to the implementation of the recommendations of the Select Committee – although some of the proposals now seem to underlie the provisions of the Medicines Act in force in the United Kingdom today. In their report the Committee recommended:

(1) That the administration of the law governing the advertisement and sale of patent, secret and proprietary medicines and appliances be coördinated and combined under the authority of one Department of State.

(2) That this administration be part of the functions of the Ministry of Public Health when such a Department is created, and that in the meanwhile it be undertaken by the Local Government Board.

(3) That a competent officer be appointed to this Department, with the duty of advising the Minister at the head of the Department concerned regarding the enforcement of the law in respect of these remedies.

(5) That there be established at the Department concerned a register of manufacturers, proprietors and importers of patent, secret and proprietary remedies, and that every such person be required to apply for a certificate of registration and to furnish (*a*) the principal address of the responsible manufacturer or representative in this country, and (*b*) a list of the medicine or medicines proposed to be made or imported.

(6) That an exact and complete statement of the ingredients and the proportions of the same of every patent, secret and proprietary remedy; of the contents other than wine, and the alcoholic strength of every

medicated wine, and a full statement of the therapeutic claims made or to be made; and a specimen of every appliance for the cure of ailments other than recognised surgical appliances, be furnished to this Department, such information not to be disclosed except as hereinafter recommended, the Department to control such statement, at their discretion, by analyses made confidentially by the Government Chemist.

(7) That a special Court or Commission be constituted with power to permit or to prohibit in the public interest, or on the ground of non-compliance with the law, the sale and advertisement of any patent, secret or proprietary remedy, or appliance, and that the commission appointed for the purpose be a judicial authority such as a Metropolitan Police Magistrate sitting with two assessors, one appointed by the Department, and the other by some such body as the London Chamber of Commerce.

(8) That the President of the Local Government Board (or Minister of Health) have power to institute the necessary proceedings to enforce compliance with the law, the sale and advertisement of any patent, secret or proprietary remedy or appliance.

(9) That a registration number be assigned to every remedy permitted to be sold, and that every bottle or package of it be required to bear the imprint "R.N. . ." (with the number), and that no other words referring to the registration be permitted.

(10) That in the case of a remedy the sale of which is prohibited, the proprietor or manufacturer be entitled to appeal to the High Court against the prohibition.

(11) That the Department be empowered to require the name and proportion of any poisonous or potent drug forming an ingredient of any remedy to be exhibited upon the label.

(12) That inspectors be placed at the disposal of the Department to examine advertisements and observe the sale of proprietary remedies and appliances.

(13) That an annual fee be payable in respect of every registration number issued.

The proposals for further legislation included:

(1) That the advertisement and sale (except the sale by a doctor's order) of medicines purporting to cure the following diseases be prohibited:–

cancer	diabetes	locomotor ataxy
consumption	paralysis	Bright's disease
lupus	fits	rupture (without operation
deafness	epilepsy	or appliance)

(2) That all advertisements of remedies for diseases arising from sexual intercourse or referring to sexual weakness be prohibited.

(3) That all advertisements likely to suggest that a medicine is an abortifacient be prohibited.

(4) That it be a breach of the law to change the composition of a remedy without informing the Department of the proposed change.

(5) That fancy names for recognised drugs be subject to regulation.

(6) That the period of validity of a name used as a trade mark for a drug be limited, as in the case of patents and copyrights.

(7) That it be a breach of the law to give a false trade description of any remedy, and that the following be a definition of a false trade description:— "A statement, design or device regarding any article or preparation, or the drugs or ingredients or substances contained therein, or the curative or therapeutic effect thereof, which is false or misleading in any particular." And that the onus of proof that he had reasonable ground for belief in the truth of any statement by him regarding a remedy, be placed upon the manufacturer or proprietor of such remedy.

(8) That it be a breach of the law—
   (a) To enclose with one remedy printed matter recommending another remedy
   (b) To invite sufferers from any ailment to correspond with the vendor of a remedy.
   (c) To make use of the name of a fictitious person in connection with a remedy. (But it should be within the power of the Department to permit the exemption of an old-established remedy from this provision.)
   (d) To make use of fictitious testimonials.
   (e) To publish a recommendation of a secret remedy by a medical practitioner unless his or her full name, qualifications and address be given.
   (f) To promise to return money paid if a cure is not effected.

For some curious reason there was no Recommendation number 4 amongst those numbered 1–13 above. And the tragedy – for the recommendations may have helped avoid the disaster of thalidomide and similar difficulties – is that the Report was 'Ordered, by The House of Commons, to be Printed, 4th August 1914'. This, by mischance, was the day that at the beginning of World War I, Britain declared war upon Germany – a coincidence which delayed the establishment of drug regulatory control.

After the War, biological substances, requiring biological standardization as neither their purity nor potency could be assessed by chemical means, created problems which led to the passing of the Therapeutic Substances Act of 1925. This Act, in effect, began modern concepts of drug safety. Its importance has been emphasized in a valuable review of *The state control of medicines: the first 3000 years*[2376], by R. G. Penn (1979).

Despite the Venereal Disease Act of 1917 and the Cancer Act of 1939 the situation remained that only the Therapeutic Substances Act (and its dependent regulations of 1925 and 1956) controlled drug safety in the mid-twentieth century, and these regulations affected only limited classes of drugs; no regulatory requirements existed that demanded a demonstration of drug efficacy at the time when thalidomide was developed and marketed. Although reputable drug houses tested both the safety and efficacy of their products and were genuinely concerned with product quality, their standards were internal and were their own. Thus, after the thalidomide disaster, in a debate in Parliament on May, 8th 1963, the responsible Minister, Kenneth Robinson, had this to say:

'I come to my last main topic which is the control and safety of drugs. This is of course a subject which was thrust to the fore both in this House and in the public press a year or so ago as a result of the thalidomide tragedy. The House and the public suddenly woke up to the fact that any drug manufacturer could market any product, however inadequately tested, however dangerous, without having to satisfy any independent body as to its efficacy and safety and the public was almost uniquely unprotected in this respect.'

Sir Frank Hartley (*The Medicines Act and the physician*, 1980)[2377] has noted that he and many others involved with these issues had, for a number of years, felt concern that the Pharmacy and Poisons Act 1933, the Pharmacy and Medicines Act 1941, and the Therapeutic Substances Act 1956 (revising and extending the original 1925 Act) 'provided inadequate means of dealing with the problems of safety and quality of substances and preparations that were not poisons in the ordinary meaning of that word. Nor were they biological substances in the sense expressed in the final Therapeutic Substances Act.' Sir Frank, in this passage, was looking back to the days before 1963 and the pronouncement of Kenneth Robinson on the thalidomide problem.

After thalidomide, on the advice of a committee under Lord Cohen of Birkenhead, a Committee on Safety of Drugs was established by the Health Ministers to deal, on a voluntary basis, with the problem of drug regulation until legislation could be enacted. This temporary measure was official only to the extent that the Health Ministers provided the accommodation, the finance, a limited secretariat, and a moral and practical sanction which was, in the event, of some consequence. The Association of the British Pharmaceutical Industry (ABPI, the trade association of the segment of the industry mainly concerned with the supply of prescription products) and the Proprietary Association of Great Britain (PAGB) undertook that their member companies would neither perform clinical trials of new drugs nor market new medicines without the advice of the Committee on Safety of Drugs.

This Committee operated under the chairmanship of Sir Derrick Dunlop whose personal contribution was immense. In a number of meetings and in numerous opportunities offered to those concerned with the problem, Dunlop taught that submissions to the Committee, itself of considerable academic standing, should be short and like those sent to a professional journal. The attempt to produce material which could be offered in the face of this instruction had a salutary effect upon industry and was, to no small extent, responsible for the rapid growth of industrial clinical pharmacology as a medical speciality.

Although the official language that conveyed its decisions at times spoke of submissions being 'approved' or 'not approved', the Dunlop Committee, in its professional contacts, gave its findings in the form of a double-negative. Few of its members had ever developed a drug or had responsibility for a major commercial venture and the Committee left the responsibility with those who proposed such undertakings. The decision, that the Committee 'did not object', enhanced the responsibility of those who had taken the decision to subject a drug to clinical trial or market it.

The Committee on Safety of Drugs was established in June, 1963 and on January 1st, 1964 began to assess drugs in accordance with its terms of reference:

'to advise whether a new drug should be submitted for clinical trial; to advise whether a drug should be released for marketing; and to study adverse reactions to drugs already in use'. It is to be noted that the Committee was not concerned with drug efficacy – although its understanding on this changed as time went by.

The first annual report covered the whole of 1964[2378] and emphasized that even the best of preparatory work was no substitute for 'prolonged experience of the use of the drug in practice'. It also showed that new formulations and the like would be treated as 'new drugs' and, to show the value of pressures other than the full force of the law, it included the following paragraph:

> The Committee have been gratified by the readiness of manufacturers to co-operate with them in ensuring that no new drug is put to clinical trial, or released for marketing, without the Committee's consent. In a circular which was sent to all doctors and dentists in the United Kingdom the Health Ministers undertook to inform prescribers of any cases of drugs being marketed or put to clinical trial without the Committee's approval. In the one or two cases which had to be reported to the Ministers it has been unnecessary to make an announcement of this sort because the manufacturers concerned have readily agreed to stop the marketing and promotion of the drug concerned pending the Committee's recommendation.

The second report, for 1965[2379], showed the changed emphasis leading to a consideration of the usefulness of a drug: the Committee had been challenged regarding their sometimes wanting evidence of the efficacy of a drug; the report said:

> The Committee however must consistently consider efficacy in relation to safety. If a drug likely to be ineffective is recommended for the treatment of a serious illness for which there is already a satisfactory treatment this constitutes an unacceptable risk to the patient. Similarly if a drug is likely to be quite ineffective in the treatment of even a trivial disease for which it is recommended and yet carried the slightest risk to the patient the Committee would regard it as unsafe for use as recommended.

Regarding 'me-too' drugs, the report for 1966[2380] expressed the 'concern that the Committee views the extent to which the drug houses have tended to flood the market with so many similar preparations.' Despite the acknowledged limitations of teratogenicity tests in animals the Committee noted that such tests should except 'in the most exceptional circumstances' be carried out before the drug was used in clinical trials in women of child-bearing age. Then the report noted that 'only a small percentage of the adverse reactions to drugs are actually reported' – a theme subsequently many times repeated.

The report for 1967[2381] directly addressed the public controversy and anxiety regarding the one specific drug side-effect then affecting fit, healthy young people; the Committee's view was given in the paragraph:

> Public interest in the relationship between the use of oral contraceptives and thrombo-embolic disorders is unabated. In 1966 the Committee co-operated with the Medical Research Council and the Royal College of General

Practitioners in retrospective studies of this subject. A preliminary report was published in the *British Medical Journal* on 6th May, 1967. A much more detailed report has been prepared and will be published early in 1968. It has been shown beyond reasonable doubt that there is a causal relationship between the taking of oral contraceptives and thrombo-embolic disorders. The Committee, however, does not consider it would be justified in recommending that oral contraceptives be withdrawn from the market as long as they remain obtainable on prescription only and doctors and the public are aware that their use involves some risk.

The 1968 report[2382] showed that one company had marketed products without submitting information on them to the Committee. As a result, 'The Ministers accordingly advised hospitals, doctors and pharmacists against using any of those products.' The same report showed the withdrawal from the market of an anti-arthritic agent due to serious adverse reactions, a rise in death rate of some 300% in asthmatics possibly associated with the use of pressurized aerosols and seemingly lessened by the precautions taken, and the issuance of the final report which showed 'that the use of oral contraceptives by a healthy non-pregnant woman increased the risk of pulmonary embolism and cerebral thrombosis.'

The Committee on Safety of Drugs issued a combined report for 1969 and 1970[2383], for its interim function was drawing to a close. The main Committee was now chaired by Professor E. F. Scowen who noted that 1969, the sixth complete year of operation by the Committee, had been expected to be its last; it continued during 1970 as it became clear that licensing under the Medicines Act, which had passed through Parliament in 1968, would be introduced somewhat later than expected. The combined report for 1969 and 1970 gave a very important, wide-ranging definition of 'drugs' and 'new drugs':

> "drug" has been interpreted as "any substance or mixture of substances destined for administration to man for use in the diagnosis, treatment, investigation or prevention of disease or for the modification of physiological function". In the category "new drug" the Committee includes new formulations of established drugs, drugs to be presented for a new use or existing substances not previously used as drugs.

(The definition includes, as it obviously must, oral contraceptives; as it stands, it must also include antiperspirants administered to man to lessen the physiological function of sweating.) The report then gave emphasis to a truism which those who take drugs need to recall:

> no drug which is pharmacologically effective is entirely without hazard. The hazard may be insignificant or may be acceptable in relation to the drug's therapeutic action. Furthermore, not all hazards can be known before a drug is marketed; neither tests in animals nor clinical trials in patients will always reveal all the possible side effects of a drug. These may only be known when the drug has been administered to large numbers of patients over considerable periods of time.

The hazards noted by the Committee, since its Adverse Reactions Register was established, included 'those following the use of preparations containing anti-arthritic drugs; the sudden death of asthmatics using certain pressurised aerosols; the incidence of haemolytic anaemia from a drug used for the treatment of hypertension; and the relationship between the use of oral contraceptives and death from thrombo-embolism. Reports on one occasion drew attention to adverse reactions from a suspected batch variation.'

Of more recent events the Committee noted that it had sent two warning letters to doctors about oral contraceptives (the first suggesting that sequential oral contraceptives appeared to be less effective than combined preparations but did not seem to have less risk of thromboembolism, and the second advising that, of those preparations which contained oestrogen, those containing only $50 \mu g$ of the hormone carried less risk of thromboembolic episodes than those with higher doses). Full details of the study on which the $50 \mu g$ warning was based were published in the *British Medical Journal* (1970)[2384]. The Committee's commissioned study on the *Rise and fall of asthma mortality in England and Wales in relation to use of pressurised aerosols*[2385] was published in the *Lancet* (1969). Finally, the Committee discussed its position on the problem of the renal toxicity of the very widely used drug, phenacetin:

> The danger of nephropathy associated with taking phenacetin attracted much attention during 1969 and 1970. The Committee discussed this potential hazard some years ago and commented on it in the Annual Report for 1966. The danger appears to arise only when the drug is used in excessive doses over a long period, generally through self-medication. It is the safety of drugs in normal usage that is the Committee's concern, and because all drugs have their hazards when abused, particularly by over-dosage, the Committee has not considered that it should take special action in connection with phenacetin. A statement was however made in 1966 by the Pharmaceutical Society of Great Britain advising retail pharmacists to be ready to give advice to people who bought products containing phenacetin, and this action was welcomed by the Committee.

It is clear that 6 years after it had started its work the Committee had good reason to be emphasizing that pharmacologically active drugs cannot be used without some measure of hazard, however limited, and that sometimes these hazards cannot be detected, despite the activities of an expert Committee, until long after the drugs have been marketed.

In May, 1969 Sir Derrick Dunlop resigned, having been Chairman of the Committee on Safety of Drugs since its formation in June, 1963; Sir Derrick then became the first Chairman of the Medicines Commission established by the Ministers to oversee the implementation of the Medicines Act. In June, 1970, a Committee on Safety of Medicines was appointed under the Act. Its functions became continuous with those of the previous Committee on Safety of Drugs but changed in the very material respect that it evaluated drugs in terms of efficacy, safety, and quality – efficacy now being a prime consideration and not limited to efficacy as an aspect of safety.

The Report for the year ended December 31st, 1971[2386] therefore saw the end of the Dunlop Committee, whose primary concern had been with drug safety, and the beginning of the activities of the Committee on Safety of Medicines, functioning in implementation of the Medicines Act 1968 and with a broader remit. The legislative power resides in the Licensing Authority (ultimately the Ministers) and, on September 1st, 1971, the first appointed day, the voluntary scheme of the Dunlop Committee ceased to function and (in the words of the report) 'the Committee on Safety of Medicines began to advise the Licensing Authority on the safety, efficacy and quality of new medicinal products.'

The 1971 report noted that 'Evidence came to the attention of the Committee that topical administration of corticosteroids to pregnant animals could cause abnormalities of foetal development.' It discussed the actions taken to advise the profession that 'while the relevance of the finding in animals to human beings had not been established, topical steroids should not be used extensively in pregnancy . . .' The same report reiterated the concern, expressed in many of the reports over the years of the life of the Committee, that only a small, and possibly decreasing, proportion of drug-related adverse effects were being reported.

The text and tables of the Dunlop Committee's annual reports provide the information summarized in Table 4 regarding the submissions made to the Committee and the actions it had taken. The figures reflect, in terms of the definitions used by the Committee and those who wrote its reports, the activity of the pharmaceutical industry in Britain from 1964 to 1971 – the time when it recovered from the thalidomide disaster and during which contemporary drug development techniques formalized and their output became subject to formal external scrutiny. The figures for the final eighth year of functioning are for the first 8 months of the year (up to August 31st, 1971), after which the new statutory Committee on Safety of Medicines commenced operation.

The number of new submissions started with 600 in 1964, reached its peak of 908 two years later, and then declined to 714 in the last full year, 1970. The Committee defined new indications, new formulations, new routes of administration, new ranges of dosing and the like, as new submissions. Only a small proportion were for new drugs, in the sense of new chemical entities. Between 1964 and 1970 (both years included) the average number of new chemical entities was 62.4 – the range (from 55 to 69) shows that this figure was surprisingly constant.

This mean figure for the number of new chemical entities coming forward each year has since declined – a subject of much controversy. Those who believe that regulatory activity from outside the drug industry fetters it, ascribe the decline to the drug regulatory process, pointing out that the decline came after the voluntary system ended and legislative controls were imposed with all of their pedantry. Others point out that the decline came once the industry had to show its products clinically effective and useful – that to make ten such potential new drugs a year is more use than to turn out 60 that are merely safe, or reasonably safe. Other views are that the seam of chemical drugs synthesized since Ehrlich began the process had begun to run dry, or that the methods by which drugs are investigated affect the ability to recognize useful drugs and lead to good medicines being discarded. Yet other views are that the industry has become so sunk in its own commercialism that it dissipates its creative energies on profit maximization, re-inventing the wheel to seek easier profit – or that the last decade is the lull before the new biotechnologies are applied. It must be observed that the number of worthwhile, clinically useful, new drugs never, even in the mid- and late-1960s, approached the number of new chemical entities. The issue that matters is

Table 4 Committee on Safety of Drugs (Dunlop Committee), 1964–1971

	1964	1965	1966	1967	1968	1969	1970	1971
Submissions handled								
In hand at beginning of the year:								
(i) Still under consideration	–	68	47	84	41	53	75	137
(ii) Referred back	–	99	49	39	43	34	47	68
New submissions received	600	874	908	765	791	848	714	554
Total	600	1041	1004	888	875	935	836	759
NCEs included among new submissions	55	69	66	56	56	66	69	?
Action taken on submissions								
Decisions given:								
(i) Approved	386	807	771	698	669	694	499	411
(ii) Not approved	15	19	24	36	36	33	53	38
Submissions withdrawn or not proceeded with	32	119	86	70	83	86	79	66
In hand at the end of the year:								
(i) Still under consideration	68	47	84	41	53	75	137	170
(ii) Referred back for further information	99	49	39	43	34	47	68	74
Total	600	1041	1004	888	875	935	836	759
Not approved } as % of	2.5	1.8	2.4	4.1	4.1	3.5	6.3	5.0
Not approved and withdrawn } total	7.8	13.3	11.0	11.9	13.6	12.7	15.8	13.7

Data derived from Committee on Safety of Drugs, annual reports 1–6, and Committee on Safety of Medicines, report for year ended December 31st, 1971

622

whether the number of new drugs of excellence has declined.

Over the life of the Dunlop Committee the number of applications 'not approved' started at 15 in 1964 and rose fairly steadily to its peak of 53 in 1970; over the period 254 (presumably separate) applications were turned down. As a proportion of the total applications in hand, between 1.8 and 6.3% were declined. Some of the applications 'withdrawn' were probably handled in this way by companies who realized that rejection of the submission was inevitable. Thus the number of 254 applications 'not approved' over the 8 years represents the minimum number of clinical trials or marketing proposals put forward by the industry and considered, on safety grounds only, unacceptable. Unless the Dunlop Committee was grossly over-cautious (and its handling of drug problems once drugs had been marketed does not suggest that it was) it must be assumed that these refusals not only protected the public but establish that an external drug regulatory agency is essential.

The latter conclusion is convincing: the Dunlop Committee, as a peer group, had reason to preserve its reputation for giving a balanced opinion and not, without compelling reasons, condemning a drug offered for clinical trial or marketing. The system it operated was voluntary and, while the Ministers could exert effective pressure on the few companies who transgressed, the Committee could not have continued to function if it antagonized the whole industry by being unnecessarily restrictive. Finally, the Committee was considering safety only. The number of 254 applications 'not approved' quantifies, therefore, a substantial hazard to the public. It seems likely that some of the applications 'withdrawn' would have been rejected if they had not been saved from continued scrutiny. Thus, even if only drug hazard is considered, there can be no doubt that a regulatory agency, external to the pharmaceutical industry, is essential to protect the public health – and this conclusion can be based on the protracted experience of the Dunlop Committee, as well as on the record of events like that which occurred with thalidomide.

The Medicines Act 1968 provides regulatory control of medicinal products by a system of licences and certificates. To undertake clinical trials of a new drug a clinical trial certificate (or the more recently introduced exemption) is necessary (unless the study is to be conducted in normal volunteers or subjects in whom the question of therapeutic benefit does not arise). To market a new drug a product licence must be obtained. Those making or assembling medicinal products must hold a manufacturer's licence and parties concerned with the distribution of drugs must hold a wholesale dealer's licence.

These licences are issued by the licensing authority, ultimately the Health and Agriculture Ministers of the United Kingdom; in practice, the licences for human medicinal products are dealt with by the Medicines Division of the Department of Health and Social Security.

The licensing authority is advised regarding the safety, efficacy and quality of medicinal products by the Committee on Safety of Medicines (which deals with new products, urgent safety matters, adverse reactions data, and the like) and by the Committee on Review of Medicines (which deals with the reappraisal of medicinal products). There are other specialist advisory committees, such as that on Dental and Surgical Materials, and there is a Veterinary products Committee, for the Act controls animal as well as human drugs.

In addition to these bodies there is an independent Medicines Commission which advises the Ministers on relevant matters of policy and acts as the final arbiter on appeals brought against certain decisions of the licensing authority.

It is apparent that within such a system clinical trial certificates, product licences and the like are granted by the licensing authority which is advised by Committees, of which the Committee on the Safety of Medicines is one. The common idea, frequently stated, that a medicinal product has the licence of the Committee on Safety of Medicines is in error.

The scope of the Medicines Act 1968 is potentially very wide. Section 130 of the Act defines 'medicinal product' in terms of medicinal purpose and says that the latter terms means:

> any one or more of the following purposes, that is to say—
> (a) treating or preventing disease;
> (b) diagnosing disease or ascertaining the existence, degree or extent of a physiological condition;
> (c) contraception;
> (d) inducing anaesthesia;
> (e) otherwise preventing or interfering with the normal operation of a physiological function, whether permanently or temporarily, and whether by way of terminating, reducing or postponing, or increasing or accelerating, the operation of that function or in any other way.

There are exclusions for certain situations, as when the drug is given under specified test conditions or in circumstances 'where the manufacturer has no knowledge of any evidence that those effects are likely to be beneficial to those human beings...' It seems reasonable to look upon these provisions as those of a broad enabling Act. The powers have been further extended by statutory orders which bring certain biological substances, some absorbable surgical materials, dental filling substances, contact lenses and contact lens fluids within the provisions. Thus, licensing applies to a wider range of substances than would usually be thought of as medicines but it does not apply to chemicals used to make ingredients nor usually to bulk ingredients used in the making of medicinal products.

There are some important exceptions from the Act. To take but two examples from the *Medicines Act Leaflet MAL 1*[2387]:

> A doctor or dentist is not required to hold a product licence for a product prepared to his prescription for administration to a particular patient; nor is he required to hold a manufacturer's licence in order to assemble or manufacture a product to his own prescription or that of another doctor or dentist for a particular patient.

Herbal medicines receive special consideration:

> A herbal remedy means a product made solely from plants by drying, crushing or any other process.
> Such a remedy may be sold, supplied, manufactured or assembled without a licence in a shop or consulting room, provided that the occupier of the premises

sells or supplies the remedy for administration to a particular person in that person's presence and after being requested to use his judgement as to the treatment required.

A limited class of herbal remedies is exempt from all licensing, if they are not imported. This consists of dried, crushed or powdered plants provided that the label simply describes the actual contents without any recommendation as to use, eg "Dried and crushed dandelion leaves".

The advertising of licensed medicinal products is extensively controlled by the Act. Recommending the product for uses and clinical indications which do not form part of the product particulars in the licence is forbidden and false or misleading advertisements are also an offence. Details of the permitted uses, dosage recommendations, known side-effects, and approved contraindications, precautions and warnings are, for each licensed product which is to be promoted to the profession, given in the 'Data Sheet' – and the form and layout of this vital document is stipulated in *The Medicines (Data Sheet) Regulations 1972* (SI 1972 No. 2076)[2388]. The Data Sheets are concise and straightforward guides to the prescriber and it is required by the regulations that, in respect of promoted products, a Data Sheet must be sent or delivered to any practitioner likely to see the advertisement unless it has been made available within the previous 15 months. An alternative is that advertisements may carry a prominent statement advising that a Data Sheet will be sent on application.

The use of the smallest possible number of different drugs, and a familiarity with the contents of the Data Sheet for each of the remedies included in the prescriber's personal pharmacopoeia, are probably two of the more important steps towards safe prescribing. The process is facilitated by the annual issuance of the *ABPI Data Sheet Compendium*. Participation in this Compendium is open to all companies making human medicinal products intended for use under medical supervision. The Compendium also contains the Code of Practice for the Pharmaceutical Industry.

The Medicines Act 1968 is a tortuous document containing a number of transitional provisions now long out of date; it is far too obscure in language and, with its dependent regulations, overly long and in need of a consolidating Act. But, from the medical point of view, its fulcrum comes in Section 19, clauses 1 and 2, where – considering factors relevant to determining the outcome of an application for a product licence – it says:

> **19.** (1) Subject to the following provisions of this Part of this Act, in dealing with an application for a product licence the licensing authority shall in particular take into consideration—
>
> (a) the safety of medicinal products of each description to which the application relates:
>
> (b) the efficacy of medicinal products of each such description for the purposes for which the products are proposed to be administered; and
>
> (c) the quality of medicinal products of each such description, according to the specification and the method or proposed method of manufacture of the products, and the provisions proposed for securing that the products as sold or supplied will be of that quality.

(2) In taking into consideration the efficacy for a particular purpose of medicinal products of a description to which such an application relates, the licensing authority shall leave out of account any question whether medicinal products of another description would or might be equally or more efficacious for that purpose:

Provided that nothing in this subsection shall be construed as requiring the licensing authority, in considering the safety of medicinal products of a particular description, in relation to a purpose for which they are proposed to be administered, to leave out of account any question whether medicinal products of another description, being equally or more efficacious for that purpose, would or might be safer in relation to that purpose.

Thus, the licensing authority is, by the Act, specifically debarred from considering comparative efficacy – although it can, in considering safety for a specific purpose, prefer the safer of equally effective drugs. It might seem remarkable that the Act makes no demand that new medicines shall be in any way better than the existing ones; nor does it do anything to inhibit 'me-too' drugs unless they are demonstrably more toxic than the existing licensed ones. The Medicines Act makes no attempt to invest in drugs of excellence or to improve existing standards to the benefit of the innovative segment of the industry, or anyone else. The situation is even more remarkable when there is no selected list of pharmaceutical products chosen for reimbursement within the National Health Scheme.

That a National Health Scheme should reimburse the cost of all and any drugs given by prescription for almost any purpose to the whole of the community appears a proposition which the expense alone, apart from the problems of adverse drug effects, will, in time, refute. Experience shows that a limited judgement only can be made before drugs are marketed and their usefulness and adverse effects explored in extensive clinical use. Thus, to give a licence on the basis of the premarketing safety, efficacy and quality data would seem to be all that can be done. Perhaps a second system, that selects the preferred drug and rewards the drug of excellence, should be considered as part of the process of reimbursement. Such a system might effect economies, not just on the cost of drugs but by fostering the most effective drug and lessening the hospital and other costs of iatrogenic disease.

The kind of prospective, monitored postmarketing study which would define the preferred drug suitable for inclusion in the pharmacopoeia of a National Health Scheme hardly exists, neither the hospital nor the general practitioner resources of the Scheme having been organized for the purpose. However, it is possible to look back and see examples of situations in which the ability to deny reimbursement to a drug of doubtful merit might have been useful, and might have contributed to patient-care.

One example arose from the *Study of fatal bone marrow depression with special reference to phenylbutazone and oxyphenbutazone*[2389] published by William H. W. Inman in the middle of 1977. Inman noted that, at the time, the Adverse Reactions Register of the Committee on Safety of Medicines included 513 reports of drug-induced fatal aplastic anaemia or agranulocytosis. The two drugs most frequently suspected of causing these deaths were phenylbutazone (188 deaths) and oxyphenbutazone (62 deaths). It should be remembered that neither of these two non-steroidal anti-inflammatory drugs is curative. Thus, Inman set out to investigate the problem from another approach and studied the histories of 269 patients who had suffered from aplastic anaemia or agranulocytosis but whose death certificates did not mention a drug. In this group of patients it was found that 83 of the 269 deaths had probably been caused by drugs, 'the most common cause of aplastic anaemia being treatment with phenylbutazone (28 deaths) and oxyphenbutazone (11 deaths). Thirteen out of 17 deaths from agranulocytosis were attributed to co-trimaxazole treatment.' Inman's discussion included the observation that:

> When compared with other anti-inflammatory drugs prescribed to a similar extent, phenylbutazone and oxyphenbutazone clearly account for a disproportionately large number of fatal blood dyscrasias – probably over one-third of all drug-induced blood dyscrasias in the United Kingdom (excluding cancer chemotherapy).

Although this finding – that, excluding cancer chemotherapy, these two drugs were probably causing one-third of all drug-induced fatal blood dyscrasias in the United Kingdom – was published in the widely-read *British Medical Journal*, the prescribing medical profession continued to use phenylbutazone and oxyphenbutazone on a scale which does not suggest that it was limited to serious situations where no alternative was available.

These findings, even when linked with the reported adverse effects of both drugs apart from blood dyscrasias, were insufficient to lead to the removal of the drugs from the market by the exercise of the powers conferred by the Medicines Act. The widespread acceptance and apparent usefulness of these drugs, although they were neither specific nor curative, seems to have been such that, for this benefit, the risk was accepted. What is not in dispute is that 'compared with other anti-inflammatory drugs prescribed to a similar extent, phenylbutazone and oxyphenbutazone clearly account for a disproportionately large number of fatal blood dyscrasias . . .' Had a means existed to drop such drugs that compared unfavourably, and in such an important respect, with alternative drugs then the outcome for a number of patients since 1977 might have been different.

Experience suggests that in the UK the refusal of a defective application or the removal from the market of a drug which is a cause of anxiety may be unduly difficult. The Act provides that the licensing authoirty may *not* refuse a licence on the grounds of safety, efficacy or quality without consulting an appropriate Committee. These include the Committee on Safety of Medicines and the Committee on Review of Medicines – the latter largely concerned with drugs already on the market and, in particular, with scrutiny of the Product Licences of Right granted, without scientific assessment, to products on the market when the Act became operative.

If the appropriate expert committee decides it cannot advise the licensing authority to grant the application, then the applicant can make oral or written representations to it. Should this appeal fail, the applicant will have a further right of appeal, this time to the Medicines Commission. Only when this entire process is exhausted can the licensing authority finally say, 'no'. Even then, if the authority decides that it wants to adopt a course of action different from that advised by the Medicines Commission, the applicant will have a right of appeal to 'a person appointed' for the purpose.

The applicant who pursues the full course, presumably in support of an application of such limited merit that great debate is needed, will have resisted the view of the licensing authority, rejected the recommendations of a peer group and expert committee of standing, and carried his case to the Medicines Commission. It is a personal view that patients, presumably expecting the safety and efficacy of licensed drugs to be fairly readily demonstrable, might prefer not to be exposed to products, or the claims for them, which acknowledged experts find it so difficult to permit.

The actions of the licensing authority seem equally inhibited by the provisions of the Medicines Act when it comes to limiting the use of a drug because of adverse experience after marketing. Section 28 of the Act gives the licensing authority power to suspend, vary or revoke a licence – but only in carefully defined circumstances. Perhaps the most important of these is given in section 28 (g):

> that medicinal products of any description to which the licence relates can no longer be regarded as products which can safely be administered for the purposes indicated in the licence, or can no longer be regarded as efficacious for those purposes.

But, even though the burden of proof regarding the problem of hazard seems, under these provisions, to lie with the licensing authority, it cannot, by the use of section 28, vary, suspend, or revoke a licence without consultation with the appropriate committee – and the applicant has all the previous double or triple rights of appeal.

There are additional, stronger powers – but they reside in the Ministers. Under section 62 of the Act 'the appropriate Ministers, where it appears to them to be necessary to do so in the interests of safety, may by order . . .' prohibit the sale or supply or importation of medicinal products but they must either consult the appropriate committee or the Medicines Commission or limit the order to a period of 3 months duration or less.

In practical terms the only evidence that can sustain this burden of proof is that of measured damage to patients. Patient exposure continues as long as it takes the reported data to reach the level which sustains the burden of proof. Here, the real need may be for the prescriber and dispenser to ensure that side-effect reporting is complete and reliable – and for those who license drugs to have a greater facility to restrict the number of patients exposed, if the data, as they accumulate, suggest that the benefit-to-risk ratio needs to be reconsidered. At all events it is clear that, as with some of the non-steroidal anti-inflammatory drugs, the present insensitive system requires too great an accumulation of patient harm before the scales tip against it.

The subject of drug regulation has always provoked a measure of controversy. Establishing his attitudes in considering *The effect of regulation on international drug development*[2390], D. C. Quantock (1980) said: 'That there is a need is beyond question. That there are advantages of independent assessment is axiomatic.' Yet he was speaking in a symposium entitled '*Risk and regulation in medicine – the fettered physician'* which shows its own prejudice. Much of the polarity hinges on the colossal costs involved, for Quantock goes on: 'Various observers have quoted costs of £5 million to £25 million during the last 3 years with an NCE (new chemical entity) taking as long as 10 years to develop into a new medicine.' Many see the regulatory process not as encouraging that part of industry which discovers and develops necessary new drugs, whilst inhibiting the 'me-too' and indifferent drug, but as a dead hand that quickens nothing and makes the process more time-consuming and costly.

A rich variety of positions are possible – but not one that says a licensing system can totally prevent hazards from drugs once they are marketed. The preclinical and clinical requirements of the American regulatory body are markedly more costly and extensive than those traditional in Europe. Yet they are not an adequate and complete protection and an experienced American commentator, William M. Wardell (1980), discussing postmarketing drug surveillance (PMS), has suggested that [2391]:

> The difficulty is that, as things now stand, the embattled regulator still has to make virtually an all-or-nothing decision on a drug, and is, therefore, naturally cautious, inclined to ask for ever more data and to defer a decision until all conceivable doubts are resolved. We need to render the decision less apocalpytic and hence easier to make; a greatly improved system of PMS that will quickly identify problems that arise after marketing would achieve this. The issue is so important that we should consider making graded or monitored release part of the PMS system in special circumstances if it is required.

The reason that discussion turns to new methods is that both experience and the simple arithmetic of the problem show that there is no way in which, from information on a few hundred patients comprising typical examples of a disease and treated with the investigational new drug only, the results of the use of that drug in many thousands of patients can be forecast – and this is especially true as the thousands of patients will include those with several diseases, on three or four drugs, and of younger and older age groups than those included in the clinical trials. If, then, the result cannot be forecast, marketing, especially on an explosive scale with intense promotion, is an uncontrolled experiment in which the patients given the drug in its earliest years will serve to quantify the risks – and give an impression of the benefit. It would seem that explosive marketing must always be a hazard and that, in some new way, the process of licensing should allow only progressive and measured patient exposure during which the benefit-to-risk ratio is assessed as new populations are added. It seems hard to deny that any such system can accept only a small number of drugs for evaluation and the less meritorious must fall by the way, just as those that are grossly toxic in animals, or pharmacologically unpromising, fall at an earlier stage. There must then be a *need* for a new drug, and it must appear to have real merit, if its development is to continue to the point of reimbursement by inclusion in a selected list. Such a process, if it is to permit drug innovation to survive, much less expand, has huge patent implications.

For the purpose of discussion it will, for the moment, be assumed that the protection of patients is more important than commercial gain; that the total cost to the community of the pharmaceutical industry is acceptable, and that a substantial proportion of prescribing is unsupported by appropriate objective evidence quantifying safety and efficacy.

The first of these assumptions seems self-evident. Its problem is that the only pharmaceutical industry to have created, throughout this century, worthwhile patient benefit is that industry which, without profit, would not exist. Thus, while the protection of patients is more important than commercial gain, this axiom requires the protection of profit. This is not to countenance the profit-maximization which plagues large segments of the industry to the degree that balanced management is eroded by the knowledge that those who do not 'grow' their divisions or companies by an imposed percentage (new products or not) are unlikely to survive more than three or four annual budgets. Patients are, in fact, threatened more by excessive commercial objectives than by any need for workable profit; industry predictably resists all forms of reform, protesting that change threatens essential profit when what is at risk is profit maximization.

The second of these assumptions – that the total current cost of the industry is acceptable – is often attacked. The proportion of gross national product to be devoted to health is a value judgement, and the selection of whatever part of the total health fund is to be spent upon drugs is a similar choice. The assumption that the present total cost is not to be challenged is made because present interest lies in discussing the use of the total fund set aside to go to the industry. In 1981, the United Kingdom pharmaceutical industry spent £130 million ($199 million) on promoting the sales of medicines to the National Health Scheme[2392]; of this sum, £106 million was allowed as an expense in assessing the price of NHS medicines. The sum spent on the promotion of drugs is of the order of the real research costs of the industry. It is this massive fund, now devoted to promotional spend, which some would wish to see made available for a totally different purpose. Those who hold this view seem to agree that a learned profession has no need to base its technical decisions upon information biased by the techniques of commodity advertising. Much of the vast sum spent on pharmaceutical detailing and the visits to prescribers and dispensers by drug industry representatives, and much of the lesser sum spent upon decorative but unscientific advertising, could be spent on a proper provision of information, the discovery of useful drugs, and those exercises which promise the selection of the preferred drug and the provision of better patient care.

The third of these assumptions – that most prescribing is unsupported by objective evidence of safety and efficacy – is offered as a truism because only a minority of patients attending family physicians suffer from the kinds of well-defined illnesses conventionally subjected to statistically meaningful clinical trials. Whilst it is clearly essential that the doctor should make available any drug which, with acceptable safety, can be confidently expected to provide the individual patient with benefit, it is clear that great resources are wasted on remedies unlikely to help the trivial conditions for which they are used; other patients are exposed to the full potential of the random side-effects of drugs from which they have only a small chance of receiving worthwhile help. Speaking of expectorants, for example, the *British National Formulary* (1982)[2393] says that the assumption that subemetic doses of the traditional drugs can 'promote expectoration is a myth. Thus there is no scientific basis for prescribing these drugs although a harmless expectorant mixture may have a useful role as a placebo.' Of the vastly more expensive mucolytics the BNF says 'Inhalation of steam or an aerosol of water is probably more effective for liquefying sputum.' It is not an unsafe assumption that a proportion of prescriptions could, with advantage, remain unwritten.

It must follow, unless it is desired to see the pharmaceutical industry in all its segments thrown into eclipse, that if drugs are to be used less and more rationally they must be proportionally more expensive. Some competition between candidate drugs may be necessary but the industry should be protected from the need to promote excessive drug use in order to flourish. And it is doubtful that, at the present margin of profit on the unit cost of drugs, the industry could survive if globally the use of its products was rational. Thus, if the third of these assumptions is accepted and it agreed that there is a considerable potential for reducing the number of drugs prescribed, there are financial implications which run counter to the common suggestion that drug costs should drop.

In the United Kingdom a material change to the practice of both the licensing authority and the industry was brought about by *The Medicines (Exemption from Licences) (Clinical Trials) Order 1981* (S.I. 1981, 164)[2394]. The new scheme provided a means by which companies were able to secure exemption from the need to hold a clinical trials certificate before studies in man in which therapeutic benefit was to be expected could be undertaken. The clinical trials certificate exemption (CTX) scheme was introduced after a long period of dissatisfaction during which it was felt that delays in obtaining the ordinary clinical trials certificate were inhibiting the development of new drugs in the UK and driving overseas the opportunities of new-drug clinical pharmacology. It is of importance that the new scheme was an addition to the existing provisions. A company refused a CTX could still apply for a clinical trials certificate in the usual way knowing that this would ordinarily be referred to the Committee on Safety of Medicines (or other appropriate committee), whereupon the usual rights of hearings and representations would exist.

To obtain a CTX the company had to make a notification in a prescribed form, provide summaries of the relevant technical and medical data, and enter into a series of defined undertakings. It is of interest that the notification had to be accompanied by what the Statutory Instrument describes as:

> a certificate signed by a doctor listing his medical and scientific qualifications who works within the United Kingdom and which states both that he is a medical adviser in the employment of, or consultant to, the supplier and that he has satisfied himself as to the accuracy of the summaries specified . . . and that, having regard to the contents of those summaries, he is of the opinion that it is reasonable for the proposed clinical trial to be undertaken.

This unique provision, within a scheme widely considered to have been a notable success, represents a philosophical achievement and provides perhaps the beginnings of a regulatory role exercised from within the scientific departments of the industry by accredited professional people.

From the operational point of view the scheme is efficient for the licensing authority has 35 days in which to consider the exemption and advise whether or not it objects to the proposed trial. It can, if needed, extend this period by a further 28 days. These provisions employ the 'double-negative approach' (of 'not objecting' to the proposal) characteristic of the Dunlop Committee on the Safety of Drugs – they leave, therefore, a considerable measure of responsibility in the hands of those who have given the certificates accompanying the notification.

An additional point with widespread implications is that the company concerned must formally undertake to immediately notify the licensing authority of 'any refusal to approve the clinical trial by a committee established or recognized by a health authority constituted under the National Health Service Act 1977 . . . or by the Medical Research Council, to advise on the ethics of research investigations on human beings.' The licensing authority made it known that it expected that in all instances independent ethical approval would be obtained. These requirements, carried in by statutory instrument well over a decade after the Medicines Act became law, show the increased concern with the ethical issues of clinical research that characterized the period.

Any new scheme relating to product licensing might, in a similar way to the CTX scheme, be additional to the present system. Its prime objective must be that it should be safer than the present system and better protective of patients given a new drug in its early years of marketing. Its second objective might be that it should reward the innovation of a valuable new drug or therapeutic advantage in a way that ensures that creative research can be fostered. A third objective might be that it should economize on the public purse by lessening the hospital and community costs of iatrogenic disease; it might also seek to avoid the intangible costs of the parasitism of the non-science based segments of the industry – segments which offer apparent, short-term savings that, by not tackling the unsolved problems of disease, are ultimately costly.

As biotechnology becomes more fully established and the present science expands it seems possible that drug regulation and drug development will have to become more interactive with the regulator moving towards a participative rather than a passive role. As projects have less and less in common, the usefulness of the set-piece preclinical exercises in animal safety evaluation seems likely to lessen, each project becoming more an independent exercise in science. An alternative pathway should perhaps allow new techniques in toxicology – especially as it has not been shown that the present, already formalized methods are satisfactorily predictive of subsequent human hazard and experience. While much of this difficulty is due to non-publication of the data, the methods themselves might seem worth scrutiny and revision. In toxicological studies it might, for example, be wished to give the drug at a frequency depending purely on its biological half-life so that the cells of the vulnerable skin, liver, kidney, bowel lining and haematopoeitic system are never, once toxified, allowed a phase of recovery. Such toxicology may give predictive results quicker and in fewer animals than the traditional methods of test. Today, experimental drugs tend to be given with little regard for the differences in their metabolism between species and the time allowed for the recovery of the target cells is seldom considered. An alternative route to drug licensing, one which looked upon each drug develop-ment programme as a unique exercise in science, might give increased scope to alternative methods – it might also prove more relevant to the task in hand if the spate of 'me-too' drugs is slowed down, so that there is a greater difference between the average run of drug development projects than there is now.

An essential feature of an addition to the present licensing system would seem to be its use of some form of structured or *phased release* allowing the earliest possible entry into man but ensuring that larger and larger patient populations are exposed only when the monitored benefit-to-risk relationships in the previous groups have been understood. The risk of developing a new drug is unlike what might be expected: it is small when less is known about the drug and its early clinical pharmacology is being worked out in a few chosen volunteers or patients studied under optimal conditions in experienced units. The intense monitoring that takes place under these conditions, and the very cautious moves made by way of titrating the dose and moving from single to multiple doses, makes the short-term risk curiously small. Possibly the real potential merit of a drug can best be worked out, without unnecessarily sacrificing animals, by moving the drug early into patients in whom the expectation of benefit is maximal and the risk controlled and monitored by appropriate clinical pharmacology.

As patient populations expand, this level of monitoring cannot be provided and the numerical likelihood of meeting the really troublesome, unpredictable lethal risks, such as aplastic anaemia and agranulocytosis, increases. It should perhaps be recognized that too many drugs are expanded into populations bigger than those in which their benefit-to-risk ratio is at best advantage. Certainly the accumulating experience of chemical drugs seems to suggest that some sort of graded, monitored release system – the drug being reviewed at the end of each phase – is essential. Hopefully, such a system would ensure that the benefit and risk were quantified at each stage and found acceptable.

The shape of the contemporary pharmacopoeia is to no small extent fashioned by the Patent Act: only in infrequent circumstances can a company afford to develop a drug that it cannot securely patent. Even with the present system, in which the drug, once licensed, is promoted as though all potential for hazard had been washed away, the time when the costs are recovered and a real taxable profit begins to be made is later than the prescriber might think. And the attempt has to be made to make a worthwhile profit while what is left of the patent lasts. It would seem quite impossible to add requirements for graded release associated with expensive monitoring without ensuring that therapeutic advantages, as well as molecules, are patentable and, equally or more importantly, that the whole period until the drug enters unqualified release is added to the patent-protected phase.

Such a graded-release licensing system associated with very extensive patent protection and the opportunity for the preferred drug (or the drug in its preferred indication) to gain great advantage in a selected drug reimbursement scheme would seem one possible ideal to be evaluated when the need for reform of the present situation is accepted. Those who do not accept the need for reform must live with the incidence of drug adverse effects to be mentioned shortly, and must watch the underfunding of university and industrial research without anxiety. Many of those who feel the need for improvement will envisage methods which are different from those presently suggested. But it would seem that the beginning of any worthwhile new or additional system must involve a 'need clause' in the Medicines Act or, outside the licensing system, the founding of a selected drug list which at least denies reimbursement to the 'me-too' drug which has demonstrated no useful advantage. Such a list would treat the ineffective 'medicines' for trivial illnesses in the same way – by denying them reimbursement – whilst permitting the prices of approved and essential drugs to rise in proportion. A second vital commitment is to end the present unacceptable risk that arises from the explosive promotion of a new drug as soon as it is licensed. Here, some sort of graded release system associated with a realistic extension of patent protection and preferential reimbursement for the preferred drug would seem essential. While the prime objective of any change is to minimize damage to patients the welfare of the community as a whole requires that the creative research of the industry and university scientific departments should be fostered on a scale better than the present – even if some of the funds come from the savings on those varieties of promotional material which a profession of accomplishment should be unwilling to accept.

The reimbursement issue is critical. It is only by its employment, and by making the 'me-too' drug a hazardous, unprofitable investment, that such drugs will drop away – thereby saving many animal lives, providing the doctor with fewer, better-known drugs, lessening the incidence of iatrogenic disease, and allowing the industry to devote its budgets to original research, instead of having them sequestered by management and marketing pressures on the easy 'me-too' option where a short-term return can readily be made. Similarly, while doctors wish to be free to prescribe what they judge best for their patients, there is no need for a National Health Scheme to pay for the privilege and reimburse the cost of unproven drugs.

Once a selected list of proven remedies has been created for the purposes of reimbursement, additions should perhaps be restricted to licensed drugs which, during phased release, have shown a useful therapeutic advantage or have established that, in a well-defined indication, they have become the drug of choice. The number of promising new chemical entities now coming forward each year is not more than can be passed through a graded release system, provided proper consideration is given to establishing comparative efficacy.

The curative, fully effective drug is, in many respects, at the opposite extreme from the 'me-too' drug which exists only for commercial reasons and has no real advantage over the drugs already available. Between them there is a considerable area of practical therapeutics in which, although in formal clinical trials two drugs may seem equally effective, some patients respond better to one drug than the other. In such situations neither drug is likely to be dramatically effective and the advantage, even in individual patients, of one drug over another is likely to be limited. Because small changes in molecular formula can produce unpleasant surprises in terms of toxicity, all drugs must normally go through the same development process. Very frequently the essential, really effective remedy, the 'me-too' compound, and the equi-efficacious alternatives cost exactly the same in terms of animal suffering and wastage, patient exposure, and total ethical cost. The fate of animals used at the higher dose levels in long-term toxicity, especially carcinogenicity, studies is disturbing – and we must perhaps be prepared to sacrifice some marginal advantage, and the ability to 'ring the changes' in therapy, in order to avoid or diminish this ethical cost. It is in this context that the entry to the market of 'me-too' drugs, devoid of convincing advantage and therefore justification, might seem to be a cause for reasonable concern.

A somewhat similar concern relates to the confidentiality of data generated during drug development programmes. It might be held that once animals are involved in the course of the experiments, the data have been generated at an ethical cost. In respect of a necessary drug this cost has to be paid – until or unless advancing knowledge provides non-animal methods. It is of the essence of science that data are published to advance knowledge. Not to publish data, especially those gathered at ethical cost, is to usher in a modern Dark Age. Except in the house of a drug regulatory body it is presently impossible to use the totality of the world's knowledge to advance understanding of structure–activity relationships or the predictive value of toxicological studies. We should not be obscure about this: a year after animal data are generated they should enter the public domain.

Recent years have seen intense discussion about the postmarketing surveillance of new drugs, systems such as 'record-linkage' often being favoured in an attempt to link the record of drug side-effects or drug-associated 'events' with the product prescriptions. The United Kingdom has some uncommon assets in this regard, for there are accurate, potentially available prescription data (the vast majority of prescriptions written by general practitioners being on the appropriate form of the National Health Scheme) and there is, since the days of the Dunlop Committee, the 'yellow card' system whereby doctors can notify the Committee on Safety of Medicines of adverse drug effects in individual patients; there is also a well-organized Royal College of General Practitioners with potential for reporting drug 'events'.

Many drug side-effects first come to light, as with thalidomide, from the reports of acute events, seemingly drug-related, which appear in the correspondence columns of the major medical journals. Few things are as essential and economical as the case reports of the individual clinician with a high index of suspicion. J. P. Griffin (1981), in a paper on *Post-marketing surveillance*[2395], wrote that:

> Certain methods of monitoring are relatively economical and effective, for example, product defect reporting systems, spontaneous adverse reaction reporting (yellow card) systems and literature surveillance. Some special studies to elucidate specific problems with specific drugs as has been operated in the Monitored Release exercise and intensive hospital monitoring studies have value in particular circumstances.

The same author went on to note that event monitoring systems involving large numbers of patients, perhaps 10 000 to 100 000, would not only involve largely untried methods but would also be extremely expensive.

The object of any system of postmarketing surveillance must be to characterize and quantify the adverse effects of a drug so that a decision, balancing the drug's toxicity against its usefulness, can be taken. An unfavourable verdict must lead to restrictions on the use of the drug or, in an extreme case, to its withdrawal. Every such withdrawal confirms yet again that the outcome in large populations cannot be satisfactorily predicted from the data presently adequate to provide the product with a licence.

A system of limited licensing, or phased release, is also expensive – the justification being that the cost of the exercise is part of the drug's development programme, that it is recouped and more if the drug is a success, and that a substantial part of the toxicity which indiscriminant release permits should be prevented. Postmarketing surveillance that measures the damage done but permits it to reach gross proportions before action is taken is something which, when it produces its result, does so too suddenly and too late. No system can prevent patient harm – but perhaps a prospective, gradual procedure might keep the harm to more acceptable proportions.

Attempts to limit the adverse effects of prescription drugs ought to include the much less frequent use of drugs, especially new drugs, and the recognition that the clinical use of drugs needs to be carefully monitored. The effects of drugs on the vulnerable target organs and tissues seldom happens suddenly – and some of the savings from prescribing less often or in the smallest possible dose or for the shortest possible period of time might, with advantage, be spent on the closer biochemical and haematological monitoring of those treated with new medicines or those known to cause serious side-effects.

Postmarketing surveillance that does not involve patient education and adjustments to prescribing habits may have its uses – but perhaps a more forward looking system that teaches, as successive groups of doctors become involved, how the drug can be used to keep the benefit-to-risk ratio maximal may achieve more – and produce less harm to measure. It appears likely that the incidence of the adverse effects of medicinal drugs results as much from their too frequent or overly prolonged use as from their intrinsic toxicity – and the patient, the prescriber, the dispenser (in respect of the vast numbers of non-prescription drugs used) join with the promotional activities of the pharmaceutical companies in producing excessive drug use.

Within a phased release system promoting cautious drug use there is nothing of a clinical nature that needs to be done that the medical practitioner cannot undertake. However, the doctor alone can provide the diagnosis and assessment needed if the patient is to be treated as a whole; thus, the doctor has to be responsible for the education of the patient whose disease is self-limiting, just as he or she has to be responsible for the care of the patient who needs repeated observation or measurement before there can be a full understanding of the disease and definitive treatment can begin. The history of medicine teaches the importance of the quality of doctoring as a clinical art, it also suggests that doctors have, throughout history, used the more profound skills of the profession to help patients recover, or find an acceptable quality of life in the presence of disease that cannot be cured, before specific medicinal remedies were known. It seems possible that some of the time of the doctor might be saved for these essential things by the assistance of a latter-day apothecary.

The pharmacist has a valuable knowledge of medicinal chemistry and pharmaceutical science and is perhaps better equipped to understand some aspects of drug absorption, distribution, metabolism, interaction and excretion than is the average clinician. This knowledge might be adapted for particular use by a postgraduate course designed to let the resulting apothecary watch over the use of drugs in the vulnerable patient groups (the young, the very old, the pregnant, those on long-term or multiple therapy, those on new or hazardous drugs, those with an atopic history, and the like). Such a licensed apothecary is also in a good position to understand the importance of the known side-effects of drugs – such as the anti-anabolic effects of the tetracyclines other than doxy-cycline; he or she can be particularly alert if an elderly person whose renal function is unknown is given a tetracycline for bronchitis: in the presence of appropriate monitoring, the uraemia due to the tetracycline, should this happen, would not be dismissed as a bronchopneumonia supervening on the bronchitis. This is not a complex situation but there are drugs which can interfere with the action of oral contraceptives producing an unwanted pregnancy – the latter risk is probably not very large but the range of adverse effects and interactions becomes, as more and more drugs are added, complex enough for the clinician to perhaps value support – releasing more time for the difficult and valuable parts of medical care and providing added security for the patient. Such apothecaries, working in group practice units of reasonable size, would seem likely to provide a nearly essential resource in research centres selected to provide data for the phased release of new drugs. In such situations when blood levels of drug may need to be monitored, routine haematological and biochemical tests undertaken, and the patient's acts of self-medication recorded, some facility for the purpose seems almost essential. For a number of very practical reasons, it seems likely that an apothecary trained for a role in modern practice, would lead to better therapeutics.

Some attempt might perhaps be made to summarize these proposals, recognizing that, apart from a few alkaloids, effective modern drug therapy is very young: its span is of some 60 or 70 years – one man's lifetime. The successes, in anaesthesia, tuberculosis, and many infectious diseases have been enormous; the results in the arthropathies, arterial degenerative disease, and neoplasia are meagre and make imperative the support of the university and industrial research which can tackle these problems. The experience of the drug disasters that began with thalidomide, and the experience of the problems that lead to drugs being withdrawn once they have been marketed, is substantially shorter – about 20 years. The latter experience is, in terms of personal judgement, unsatisfactory. The adverse experience to date suggests that events after a drug has been marketed *cannot*, with an acceptable degree of security, be predicted from the data required by the present licensing system. The exception is the obvious one: the present system is adequate in respect of countries which launch a drug when the human toxicology has been worked out in markets that launched the drug earlier and permitted its unrestricted promotion.

It has been widely recognized that pharmacologically-active, useful drugs are never totally free from risk. This is true even of penicillin, the drug that is curative in so many conditions and that so seldom causes anaphylaxis. Benzyl-penicillin, the first of the penicillins, remains the drug of choice for streptococcal, pneumococcal, gonococcal, and meningococcal infections and for actinomy-cosis, anthrax, diphtheria, gas-gangrene, syphilis, tetanus, and yaws. The side-effects are uncommon sensitivity reactions and the very rare cases of anaphylactic shock in hypersensitive patients. It is inactivated by bacterial penicillinases, the β-lactamases, but must surely have a usefulness and therapeutic ratio that divides history into the period since its discovery and the millennia during which virtually every one of the illnesses for which it remains the drug of first choice was a grave threat. There are only a handful of such drugs – and a larger number which seldom cure anything and have a benefit-to-risk ratio which the prudent might only seldom accept.

Despite a vast literature, there is only limited hard information on the incidence of iatrogenic disease. The doctor has little incentive to report adverse drug effects and every disincentive when it comes to telling patients or writing on death certificates that the prescribed treatment produced unwanted results. There is therefore gross under-reporting of drug side-effects. Even so, the limited reasonably reliable information which is on record is half-hidden: the statistics available as a result of the 'yellow card' system in the United Kingdom are not published in a convenient form or summarized in the medical journals and pharmaceutical houses are not required to provide such a summary when promoting their products to individual physicians.

Some of the studies which have appeared in the literature on the epidemiology of adverse drug reactions are summarized in Table 5. Fairly accurate generalizations seem to have appeared at a quite early date: Patrick F. D'Arcy (writing in D'Arcy and Griffin, *Iatrogenic diseases*, 1979)[2396] noted that 'it is clear that adverse reactions are becoming an increasingly important problem in drug treatment. In Britain, perhaps 5% of general hospital beds are occupied by patients suffering from their treatment (Dunlop, 1969). In the United States, an estimate has been given of one in seven hospital beds taken up by patients under treatment for adverse reactions caused by drugs (US Department of Health, Education and Welfare, 1969).'[2397]

Commenting on the proportion of patients admitted to hospital in the United States, D'Arcy observes[2398] that adverse drug reactions 'can be responsible, for example, for 1.0–3.5% of all admissions to general medical wards and for 0.3–1.0% of all general hospital admissions'. The same author provides the following comment on the incidence of iatrogenic disease once the patient has been admitted to hospital care[2399]:

> In-patient statistics also cause concern, 10–30% of all patients admitted to medical wards experience at least one ADR each during their stay in hospital. Drug-attributed deaths occur in 0·29% of hospitalized medical patients and perhaps 10 times as many patients suffer life-threatening and sometimes permanent side-effects from their drug therapy.

When these numbers are multiplied up to take into account the patient populations involved it is clear that they represent an epidemic of iatrogenic disease; taken in conjunction with the record of drug disasters and drugs withdrawn after marketing due to unacceptable adverse effects, these figures show the degree to which drug marketing and drug use is less than adequately controlled.

The magnitude of the problem is further shown by the fact that, in a written Parliamentary reply on November 13th, 1980, Sir George Young stated that in 1977, 120366 patients were discharged from or died in hospitals in the United Kingdom after suffering the adverse effects of medicinal agents (Hansard, cited D'Arcy, 1981)[2400]

Severe, life-threatening, or lethal side-effects form, as might be expected, only a small part of these totals. They are largely restricted to drugs of known hazard, the use of which is confined to patients already seriously ill. Part of the real problem may be that some of the drug reactions, even the severe ones, may be

Table 5 Incidence of adverse drug reactions during hospitalization, or as a cause for admission, or in general practice

Author	Year and site of study	Duration of survey	Total number of patients	Number of patients with drug reaction		Reaction rate %	Method of study
				During hospital stay	As cause for admission		
Schimmel[2410]	1960–61 Yale Univ. Service	8 months	1014	103	—	10.0	House-officer reports
McDonald and Mackay[2411]	1962 Vermont	1 year	9557	98	—	1.0	House-officer reports
Seidl et al.[2412]	1964 Johns Hopkins	3 months	714	97	—	13.6	Prospective surveillance
Reidenberg[2413]	1964–66 Five Philadelphia hospitals	2 years	86100	772 reactions	—	0.9	Report cards
Smith et al.[2414]	1965 Johns Hopkins	1 year	900	97	—	10.8	Prospective surveillance
Ogilvie and Ruedy[2415]	1965–66 Montreal	1 year	731	132	—	18.0	Report cards
Hoddinott et al.[2416]	1966 Ontario	59 days	104	16	—	15.0	Prospective surveillance
Borda et al.[2417]	1966–67 Boston	11 months	830	405 reactions	—	35.0	Prospective surveillance

Table 5 Continued

Author	Year and site of study	Duration of survey	Total number of patients	Number of patients with drug reaction		Reaction rate %	Method of study
				During hospital stay	As cause for admission		
Hurwitz and Wade[2418]	1965–66 Belfast	1 year	1 160	118	—	10.2	Prospective surveillance
Hurwitz[2419]	1965–66 Belfast	1 year	1 268	—	37	2.9	Prospective surveillance
Gardner and Watson[2420]	1969 Florida	3 months	939	99	— / 48	10.5 / 5.1	Pharmacist surveillance
Wang and Terry[2421]	1967–68 Milwaukee	1 year	8 291	128	—	1.54	Nurse observer
BCDSP[2422]	1966–72 Boston	6 years	9 900	3 600	—	36.4	Boston Collaborative Drug Surveillance Programme
Miller[2423]	1966–73 USA, Canada and Israel	7 years	11 526	3 240	—	28.1	Surveillance Programme
Mulroy[2424]	1973 Yorkshire General Practice	1 year	9 315 consultations	239 consultations	—	2.6	Prospective surveillance

Jick[2425]	1966–74 BCDSP, USA and overseas	8 years / 8 years	19 000 / 7 017	— / 260 reactions	30.0 / 3.0	Prospective surveillance
Caranosos et al.[2426]	1969–72 Florida	3 years	6063	117	2.9	Pharmacist surveillance
McKenney and Harrison[2427]	1974 Virginia, USA	2 months	216	17	7.9	Pharmacist surveillance
McKenzie et al.[2428]	Not given Florida	3 years	3 556	72 admissions	2.0	Prospective surveillance – paediatrics
Levy et al.[2429]	1969–76 BCDSP, Israel	4 years (1969–72) / 4 years (1973–76)	1608 / 1163	315 / 88	19.6 / 7.6	Prospective surveillance
Martys[2430]	1979 Derbyshire General Practice	2 years	817	336 non-hospitalized	41.0	Prospective surveillance

avoidable. Kenneth Melmon, in an article on *Preventable drug reactions – causes and cures* (1971)[2401], noted that: '18–30% of all hospitalized patients have a drug reaction, and the duration of their hospitalization is about doubled as a consequence. In addition, 3–5% of all admissions to hospitals are primarily for a drug reaction, and 30% of these patients have a second reaction during their hospital stay.' Melmon, from the Division of Clinical Pharmacology of the University of California Medical Center, went on to suggest that: 'classic reactions make up less than 20–30% of drug reactions; the remaining 70–80% are predictable. Most of these are preventable without compromise of the therapeutic benefits of the drug.'

In 1973, the Committee on Safety of Medicines in the United Kingdom made available to large hospitals and medical schools a two volume register of the 'yellow card' data on adverse reactions reported between June, 1964 and October, 1971. R. H. Girdwood, Professor of Therapeutics at Edinburgh, in a paper on *Death after taking medicaments* (1974)[2402] wrote that these data showed that the number of drugs reported to have possibly caused over 50 deaths in the $7\frac{1}{2}$ years concerned was small; it comprised:

Oral contraceptives	332
Phenylbutazone	217
Chlorpromazine	102
Corticosteroids	94
Isoprenaline	84
Phenacetin	77
Acetylsalicylic acid	72
Oxyphenbutazone	69
Indomethacin	68
Halothane	57
Amitriptyline	50

Girdwood observed that these numbers originated from the period before the low-oestrogen/progestogen oral contraceptives entered widespread use; the paper also notes the care which must be taken in interpretation of these data – even so, the number of deaths seemingly associated with the non-steroidal analgesics, phenylbutazone, oxyphenbutazone and indomethacin, and the other analgesics, phenacetin and aspirin, seems a cause for comment.

George J. Caranasos and his colleagues, in a study of *Drug-associated deaths of medical inpatients* (1976)[2403] found a more reassuring picture as far as patients under hospital care were concerned. These workers reported that of 7423 medical inpatients, 16 (0.22%) died of drug-associated causes; all 16 of these patients had been terminally or seriously ill before the fatal drug reaction occurred. Antineoplastic drugs, azathioprine, prednisone, and sodium heparin were the most frequently implicated drugs. A comparable picture emerged from a study involving seven countries conducted as part of the Boston Collaborative Drug Surveillance Program and reported by Jane Porter and Hershel Jick (*Drug-related deaths among medical inpatients*, 1977)[2404]. Jick and his colleagues found that among 26 462 carefully monitored medical inpatients, 24 (0.9 per thousand), were thought to have died as a result of a drug or group of drugs. Most of these patients were seriously ill prior to the fatal reaction. Six deaths – five from fluid overload and one from excessive potassium therapy – were considered possibly preventable. These results allowed the *British Medical Journal* (June 11th, 1977) to reach the comfortable conclusion that 'Few patients appear to die as a result of our therapeutic endeavours, and most of those who do have been treated with powerful drugs given to delay the progress of otherwise fatal disorders.' [2405]

The literature is clearly confusing – perhaps because experience does vary greatly in different units and because in many situations it is difficult to isolate drug effects from the manifestations of gross pathology. Many of the drugs in common use have an incidence of serious side-effects which is such that the average doctor will seldom see them. As would be expected, the risk to the community is greatest with a small range of toxic drugs which are widely used, and with new drugs, some of which have soon shown an unexpected potential for causing serious harm.

At the time of the publication of the *Register of Adverse Reactions* (Committee on Safety of Medicines, 1976), as cited by William H. W. Inman (*Monitoring for drug safety*, 1980) [2406], the most frequently reported 20 drugs in the period January, 1964 to June, 1976 were those shown in Table 6.

Table 6   The 20 most frequently reported drugs. Number of reports and percentage of them reporting fatalities; January, 1964 to June, 1976. From Inman (1980) citing Committee on Safety of Medicines (1976)

Drug	Number of reports	Percentage fatal
Oral contraceptives	7017	5
Sulphamethoxazole	1424	3
Phenylbutazone	1364	26
Ampicillin	1122	6
Practolol	1037	2
Paracetamol	859	9
Methyldopa	837	6
Nalidixic acid	811	1
Aspirin	709	23
Diazepam	698	11
Amitriptyline	689	10
Chlorpromazine	584	20
Frusemide	576	10
Chlordiazepoxide	567	13
Measles vaccine	559	2
Ibuprofen	546	4
Propranolol	530	5
Pertussis vaccine	528	2
Potassium chloride	496	8
Nitrazepam	477	9

The number of deaths thought to be related to drug administration and represented by Table 6 is considerable. It does, of itself, provide a reason for close scrutiny of the efficiency of the drug regulatory system. It provides a reminder that in considering the benefit-to-risk ratio, it is hard indeed to quantify the risk.

It bears little relationship to the experience of the individual practitioner – an experience limited to a practice of perhaps 1500–3000 patients, a relatively small proportion of which will be given any one drug. It also bears little relationship to the number of patients studied in an average drug development programme – for this is unlikely to be as large as the number of patients in a practice. The risk has to be quantified in terms of a numerator and a denominator: a number of side-effects, and a number of prescriptions; the former is usually grossly under-reported for the reasons already considered, the latter frequently dwarfs the number of patients who contributed data to the submission leading to a Product Licence or approved New Drug Application. The data in Table 6 provide one reason for suggesting that more rigorous control is needed of drugs which are capable of producing serious, idiosyncratic side-effects, such as some of the blood dyscrasias, and are, nevertheless, used in trivial, self-limiting conditions. Other problems – a number of drugs have had to be withdrawn after marketing due to unexpected adverse experience, and a small number of drugs taken into long-term clinical trial have subsequently been shown to be animal carcinogens – support the impression that additions to the present drug regulatory procedures may be advisable.

Some such suggestions have been made in this text – very few of them have been new. A vast literature has arisen since the thalidomide disaster on the philosophy and practicalities of drug regulation. It is not proposed to compare the present suggestions with this literature in any systematic way. However, a few comparisons seem appropriate.

An attractive, comprehensive review of the subject as it appeared exactly 10 years after the passing of the Medicines Act of 1968 is given by the study, *Controlling the use of therapeutic drugs, an international comparison,* which was edited by William M. Wardell and published in 1978. This over-view examines the situation at that time in the United States, Canada, the United Kingdom, Switzerland, West Germany, Sweden, Denmark, Norway, New Zealand and Czechoslovakia; in respect of the UK, even at that date, Cuthbert, Griffin and Inman make the following comment[2407]:

> The basic concept of the U.K. approach to drug regulation is that pre-marketing controls are not sufficient, since most serious adverse reactions are very rare events, unlikely to be detected in clinical trials involving a few hundred patients. In the U.K. view, extensive clinical trials are less useful than an effective postmarketing drug surveillance scheme.

The scientific basis of official regulation of drug research and development was of the same vintage; this study, edited by A. F. de Schaepdryver and others, recorded the proceedings of a satellite symposium of the 7th International Congress of Pharmacology. In it, W. H. W. Inman reviewed the proposals which had been made for postmarketing surveillance in the United Kingdom[2408]. These comprised procedures known as 'recorded release', 'registered release', 'restricted release', and a scheme proposed by the Association of the British Pharmaceutical Industry.

Recorded release, first proposed by Inman in 1976, depended on doctors being issued with 'prescription books' each of which had a unique identification number and contained a registration form (to be sent to a monitoring centre when the patient was enrolled), a number of prescriptions, and a follow-up form (to be completed after a predetermined interval). Inman himself accepted that it was too complicated for national acceptance.

Registered release was proposed by Dollery and Rawlins (1977)[2409]; drug companies would have to produce a cohort of perhaps 10000 patients in whom use of the drug had been monitored before the product could be released in the usual manner. The practical details of the scheme were, of necessity, fairly complicated and, as with most of these schemes, prescription habits would be affected as the doctor would have to decide in advance that the patient given the new drug was going to be monitored.

Restricted release was proposed by Lawson and Henry (1977)[2431]: patients would be identified when the prescription was handed in at a pharmacy, the pharmacist sending a registration form to the monitoring centre. This complication could be eliminated by the more frequent proposal that patients given the drug would be identified by the Pricing Bureau, an office which handles all NHS prescriptions.

The ABPI proposal (Wilson, 1977)[2432] was that the Pricing Bureau would isolate the prescription, so identifying the doctor, who would be sent a request for follow-up information. This scheme would not disturb prescribing habits but it might be biased if an appreciable proportion of the prescribers failed to provide the requested information on side-effects, or 'events' as a whole, during the individual patient's experience with the drug.

To some extent interest in these proposals arose from the then recent adverse experience with practolol – a drug which was, quite unexpectedly, shown to cause the oculomucocutaneous syndrome. The β-adrenergic receptor blocking agent, practolol, was first marketed in 1970 and, by the end of 1975, when the full extent of the problem with the drug became apparent, the compound had received some 300000 patient-years of use in the UK and about one million such years of use worldwide (Nicholls, 1977)[2433]. Interest in the need to monitor experience with drugs was re-awoken by the realization that such a widely used drug could cause a severe and previously unknown syndrome.

The interest led to the holding of a special symposium in London (*Journal of the Royal College of Physicians*, 1977)[2434] and to a gathering of experts in drug evaluation who met in Honolulu (Gross and Inman, *Drug monitoring*, 1977)[2435]. In the latter publication, J.M. Crawford, of the Australian Department of Health, summarized the Australian experience during 1976 with three drugs entered into a 'limited monitored release system'[2436]; Inman, in a paper on 'recorded release'[2437] emphasized that 'adverse events, rather than suspected adverse reactions (should) be recorded in all patients receiving a new drug until its safety in normal use had been established'; amongst the conclusions of this important meeting, there appeared the statement that 'the success of the medical record linkage system in Finland suggests that much would be gained by establishing similar facilities in other countries.'[2438]

Commenting on these proposals, the *British Medical Journal*[2439] noted that: 'Britain has ideal circumstances for record linkage, but the opportunities have been sadly neglected'; the same article summarized Inman's 'recorded release' proposals in the following terms:

Selected drugs would be given a provisional licence for use in recorded patients. Any doctor would be free to prescribe these drugs provided he was prepared to co-operate in the scheme. When a patient was given his first prescription the doctor would send a reply-paid form to the Committee on Safety of Medicines containing a copy of the prescription and basic clinical information. Suspected adverse reactions would be notified in the usual way, but after a suitable period the doctor would be asked to return a second form recording any ailments reported by the patient, with details of referrals or hospital admissions. This would allow estimation of the incidence of adverse events among patients receiving a drug and should lead to identification of a hazard before there was any suspicion that the drug was responsible. Every patient receiving the drug would be studied until sufficient evidence of safety had accumulated for the drug to be recommended for general release. But surveillance would not stop there. Delayed effects could be monitored with the help of the Office of Population Censuses and Surveys, which could tell the monitoring centre whenever recorded patients were notified to a cancer registry or certified as dead.

At the Honolulu International Workshop, D.C.G. Skegg, of Oxford, described a pilot study in which 20 general practitioners in England with 40 000 registered patients monitored their prescriptions (10 000 per month) over a 2-year period. This important paper not only described ways in which linked records could be used to monitor drugs prescribed in general practice but also contained the following passage referring to what is probably the greatest weakness of all voluntary reporting systems[2440]:

> Recent experience has emphasized that existing monitoring methods cannot be relied on to detect all adverse effects of drugs, even if these are serious and relatively common. The beta-adrenergic blocking agent, practolol, was used widely in several countries before its propensity to cause an oculomuco-cutaneous syndrome was recognized (Wright, 1975; *British Medical Journal*, 1975). Although four years elapsed from the marketing of this drug in the United Kingdom to the first warnings about the condition (Felix and Ive, 1974; Wright, 1974), the Committee on Safety of Medicines received reports of only two patients with eye complaints during that period (Inman, personal communication). There was, however, a flood of reports once the effects had been described. This episode illustrated the fundamental weakness of voluntary reporting systems: unwanted effects are never reported until doctors have suspected that they may be caused by a drug.

Voluntary reporting systems are bedevilled by the fact that doctors do not know they do not know. They, therefore, ascribe (unless gifted with critical genius) what they see to what is known – often ascribing the unexpected event to the disease. Thus, the community either has to take drug safety so seriously that it does away with voluntary systems, properly monitoring, perhaps in selected populations, all 'events' and examining them for correlations with drug usage – or it has to rely on the critical faculties of the clinician with a high index of awareness.

In 1978 the Committee on Safety of Medicines issued a formal consultation letter setting out details of the proposed 'recorded release' system which was to augment the 'yellow card' reporting system (*British Medical Journal*)[2441]. The profession exhibited concern that if a practising doctor knew that a particular drug was under special surveillance he might be at risk if the patient developed an unfavourable reaction. Some held the view that the patient would accuse the doctor of using an experimental drug without valid, informed consent. The Committee on Safety of Medicines then set out proposals[2442] for a modified scheme, the 'Retrospective Assessment of Drugs Safety' (RADS) in which the drug would be prescribed in the normal way and prescriptions would be isolated by the Prescription Pricing Authority. After a period, perhaps a year, the doctor would be asked to provide simple details from the patient's case-record forms. The scheme took advantage of two of the special features of potential benefit in the United Kingdom: that, due to the organization of the National Health Scheme, patients were registered with a doctor, so that reasonable continuity of medical data on each patient can be assumed to exist and, secondly, that there is a central authority handling all prescriptions. It is perhaps less clear how the scheme would provide for data on controls, so that the observed events could properly be related to the causative agent, but it is apparent that it could take into account the virtues of 'event recording' – if doctors could be trained to record events and not just their interpretations of them. In a paper which received widespread attention (*The case for recording events in clinical trials*, 1977)[2443] D. C. G. Skegg and Sir Richard Doll had emphasized that the value of clinical trials in detecting unwanted effects of new medicines would be enhanced if doctors recorded all adverse events experienced by patients, and not just those regarded as adverse reactions to drugs; these authors suggested that 'All events should be reported to the centre co-ordinating the trial and analysed in treated patients and controls.' They further suggested that this method might have revealed the ocular toxicity of practolol before the drug was marketed in 1970.

Another difficulty with formal postmarketing surveillance schemes is the numbers of patients needed and, as a consequence, the costs which are likely to arise. These numbers have been long appreciated, Samuel Shapiro and Dennis Slone, of the Boston University Medical Center, in 1977[2444], suggesting that if the background probability of agranulocytosis in a non-exposed population is set at 1 per 100 000 patient-years of surveillance, then if the event rate in a drug-exposed population is raised to 1 per 500 patient-years (a relative risk of 200), something like 4000 patients must be followed for 1 year in order to see the difference. This is with an uncommon, fatal condition which is likely to be diagnosed. These authors, in an article on *Post-marketing assessment of drugs*, provide the data reproduced in Table 7 in which favourable circumstances for the investigation pertain (α is set at 0.5, β is limited to 0.2, the non-exposed factor is infinite, and the ratio exposed to non-exposed is set at 1:100 000).

The hypothesis can be advanced that any method of postmarketing surveillance does affect prescribing. Certainly, methods in which the prescriber knows that the drug is under special observation seem likely to do so. A level of caution is introduced which is different than prescribing what the last visit from the last representative from the industry suggested. Even so, retrospective surveillance, whilst useful and providing data which form a proper basis for decision making, must rely upon quantifying a substantial amount of harm already done. Until the decision is taken, these methods only indirectly minimize this damage. In this sense they may be of less value than methods designed to affect prescribing –

*Table 7   Required person-years of follow-up to detect events occuring at a rate
exceeding 1 per 100 000 per year.* From Shapiro, S. and Slone, D. (1977)

Rate of event per year of exposure	Relative risk	Required person-years of follow-up
1: 500	200	3 965
1:1 000	100	8 010
1:5 000	20	43 495
1:10 000	10	96 929
1:20 000	5	245 376
1:50 000	2	1 570 875

$\alpha = 0.05$; $\beta = 0.2$; non-exposed $= \infty$; exposed/non-exposed ratio set at 1:100 000

reducing drug use to those circumstances in which the benefit-to-risk ratio seems optimal.

Interest in the subject has continued and Judith Jones, of the Food and Drug Administration, has described American efforts to facilitate reporting, with a pilot trial of a free phone system[2445]; the same group have set out to encourage side-effect reporting by providing feedback of appropriate information. The World Health Organization Group on Adverse Reaction Reporting has been in operation since 1968 and in 1981 was supported by participation from 23 countries. A number of pharmaceutical companies have established surveillance exercises of different designs to evaluate specific products; postmarketing surveillance facilities have also been established by the Royal College of General Practitioners in the United Kingdom. One of the major contributors to the subject has been William Inman, who has not only edited the first full-length study of the theme to be published (*Monitoring for drug safety*, 1980)[2406] – a work to which reference has already been made – but who has also established the Drug Surveillance Research Unit at Southampton University. This unit, designed to undertake what Inman has called 'prescription event monitoring' (PEM), has, since January, 1982, organized its first six pilot studies of specific drugs.

By far the largest studies involving intensive hospital monitoring have been those of the Boston Collaborative Drug Surveillance Program. These studies have left no doubt about the issues in the minds of those concerned and Hershel Jick, as early as 1977, recorded the following statement[2446]:

> Newly marketed drugs should be routinely and systematically monitored for toxicity through compulsory registration and follow-up study of the earliest users.

If these views are accepted then it cannot be claimed that the present system of terminal licensing followed by unrestricted and unmonitored marketing remains acceptable. The point that some sort of postmarketing control is needed to prevent drug toxicity problems has also been made by William M. Wardell and Louis Lasagna who, in 1975, wrote the following[2447]:

> When widespread catastrophic drug toxicity has occurred, it has only been after a drug has been marketed, and never in the early phases of development.

There is a tendency for episodes of this nature to be taken as evidence of laxity in the drug approval process; however, in the present regulatory era when pre-clinical tests are being used to – and possibly beyond – the limit of their useful-ness, it would be more correct to regard widespread toxicity as a failure of post-marketing surveillance than as a failure of premarketing screening.

Advocates of what might be termed 'phased release' have been fewer. Hubert Bloch, writing on *Toward better systems of drug regulation*[2448] in 1973, roughly a decade ago, specifically approaches the concept with the words 'some sort of gradual use of the drug as opposed to massive prescribing by every doctor . . .'. The concept is also inherent in the phased approach involved in the successful Clinical Trial Certificate Exemption scheme now in use in the United Kingdom. This scheme arose from the deliberations of a Working Party set up by the Committee on Safety of Medicines under the chairmanship of Professor Grahame-Smith and from a study group established by the Association of the British Pharmaceutical Industry (ABPI). Eric S. Snell, of ABPI has recently (1983) written[2449]:

> The Association of the British Pharmaceutical Industry (ABPI) set up a working party to tackle the first problem by studying the data requirements to see if they could be modified so as to allow clinical trials to be safely conducted on the basis of different data. It concluded that this could be done by a phased approach in which the numbers of patients and the duration of their exposure to drugs was limited initially depending on the results of early laboratory testing. Extension of the clinical work would then be possible as the laboratory safety data was extended. This would have several advantages including the acceleration of development. The numbers of animals used would be reduced as well as the costs and would allow a large number of candidate experimental compounds to be tested in patients.

The suggestion that the phased approach should be extended to the marketing period but associated with an extension of patent life so that the programme remains commercially viable appears less often in the literature.

The idea that some such programme, perhaps associated with formal monitored release for appropriate drugs, should be linked with a demand that the new drug be of proven advantage compared with the remedies already available, finds expression in the current practices of a number of countries. In all forms it demands the demonstration of therapeutic advantage and the assessment of comparative efficacy. The literature contains well thought out objections to such a proposal. Wardell (1981) argues that 'While relative efficacy and safety are key factors . . . the time of access to the market is not the appropriate point to apply them'[2450]; he provides the following three reasons:

(1) 'The imposition of a comparative efficacy requirement would have an immediate dampening effect on the number of drugs available for serendipitous discoveries.'

(2) 'The second problem with imposing hurdles of relative efficacy and safety on access to the market is that the scientific criteria – and even more so the regulatory criteria – are at present undefined.'

649

(3) 'The third problem is that the methodology for determining comparative safety and efficacy on a large scale is technically difficult.'

These three points are simple quotations and a less than adequate expression of the original text. All three points, as paraphrased, would however be admitted: serendipitous discovery has, for example, added important new indications to the uses of metronidazole and its relatives, and is of great moment. Whilst comparative efficacy can be assessed (and drugs have been registered by comparison against placebos and promoted by comparison with one another for many years) it may be that, for nations traditionally much involved in drug discovery, the moment to apply the findings of comparative tests is not the moment of marketing. Since 1928 Norway has had a 'medical need' clause in its regulatory process and this involves consideration not only of relative efficacy but also drug cost. But it does not follow that a 'need clause' in the Medicines Act in the United Kingdom, or its equivalent as a requirement in the New Drug Application in America, would benefit either country. The arguments against reimbursing the cost of all drugs, even the unnecessary and ineffective, seem convincing: one means might be to provide an 'assessment rate' of reimbursement during phased release and to provide, at the end of this period and only for the drug of proven comparative merit, a far more rewarding rate for the successful drug that obtained entry to a selected drug list of essential and proven remedies.

In the United Kingdom there is already a requirement that Product Licences be renewed every 5 years. Experience suggests that this opportunity is seldom made use of as a means of ending the life of even the most outdated and ineffective of products. The present proposal is clearly not so distant from this procedure, were it applied with due diligence to protect patients from medicines inferior to the best amongst those available – recognizing that, almost always, a reasonable range of reimbused alternatives will need to be entered into any formulary.

A final point to consider in the present context is the number of medical products which need to be regulated and the number of new chemical entities which need to be evaluated. In an interesting presentation of pan-European issues M. N. G. Dukes and I. Lund (1980) note that [2451]:

> The European Economic Community presents the familiar uneven picture. Three relatively large countries have a vast number of specialties on the market. The Italian figure of 13,700 needs no comment, but our estimates of 15,000 for Britain and 15,000 for the Federal Republic of Germany are lower than the semi-official figures; in fact, the number of provisional and definitive licences in Britain is some 25,000 and in Germany rather in excess of 100,000 but these figures include many products which only marginally qualify as specialties, especially drugs prepared and sold by only a single pharmacy (and, in the case of Germany, herbal teas). Alongside this group of countries with a high figure, we have a second group of four countries – Ireland, France, Luxemburg and Belgium – with some 7,000–8,000 marketed specialties. Finally, there is a group of EEC countries where the count is much lower – the Netherlands with 3,400 specialties on the market and Denmark with 2,100.

Countries where each dosage form has a separate Product Licence or its equivalent cannot be compared directly with those in which only each parent drug substance is licensed – but the implication, that the UK has a surfeit of pharma-ceutical products, seems clear. The number of drugs really necessary can perhaps be estimated as a small multiple of the number (209) of items contained in the main list of the 1979 edition of the World Health Organization's report on *'The selection of essential drugs.'*[2154]

The number of new chemical entities is surprisingly small: G. E. Diggle and J. P. Griffin (1982) have compared the number of such entities emerging in both the UK and USA during the period from 1974 to 1980/81 and have shown that this number is stable, either side of the Atlantic, at about 20 per year[2452]. It is, at a minimum, this number which has to be handled by some such process as phased release – and, hopefully, by means which will minimize the number of drug disasters and drug withdrawals due to toxicity.

Iatrogenic disease

In a slightly earlier paper describing *A survey of products licensed in the United Kingdom from 1971–1981*[2453], Griffin and Diggle (1981) showed that during the decade which they had examined the approximate number of 20 new chemical entities a year produced a total of 204 such compounds which were licensed and marketed. These are presumably the fruits of the industry's creative activity during the same decade was 3665 (4296 Product Licences were actually granted but 631 were allowed to lapse for commercial reasons, leaving the net total of 3665). NCEs licensed were therefore about 4.7% of total Product Licences in the 3665). NCEs licensed were therefore about 4.7% of total Product Licences in the 10 year period ending 1981.

The disappointing feature is that most of the new chemical entities entered therapeutic areas which were already over-subscribed. Griffin and Diggle (1981) show that in 1971, in the United Kingdom, aspirin, phenacetin, and seven other non-steroidal anti-inflammatory analgesics were already available – yet in the decade that followed a further 21 non-steroidal anti-inflammatory agents were introduced onto the British market. Before 1971 there was a total of 17 corti-costeroid substances and their various salts marketed in appropriate preparations – and yet, after that year, 19 new corticosteroid substances were licensed; 13 of these were new molecules and six were new salts of the previously available corticosteroids. In 1971, three β-adrenergic receptor blocking agents were already available in Britain; a further ten were licensed and eight marketed in the years of the study. Other over-subscribed areas represented the benzodiazepines, tricyclic antidepressants, penicillins and cephalosporins.

Apart from these areas in which industrial effort was intense, there were other segments of therapeutics in which there was little activity: Griffin and Diggle note that between 1971 and 1981 only one NCE inhalational anaesthetic agent was introduced and 'rather more sadly only one new chemical entity, namely oxamniquine, has been introduced for the treatment of schistosomiasis which is the world's commonest disease.' The same authors then comment that:

New therapeutic concepts have been few, the notable exception to this has been the introduction of H_2-receptor blocking agents for peptic ulceration.

Other new concepts worthy of note have been the development of selective enzyme inhibitors, for example, peripheral laevo-dopa decarboxylase inhibitors such as carbidopa and benserazide: the competitive inhibitor of 3β-hydroxysteroid dehydrogenase, trilostane, for the control of primary aldosteronism; and captopril, for the treatment of hypertension which exerts its action by inhibition of the angiotensin converting enzymes.

It is difficult to escape the conclusion that innovation is stifled by the need to achieve predictable commercial returns rather than being guided by therapeutic need or being creative of important new therapeutic concepts. Whilst we can hope that innovation, in the last two decades of the century, will produce drugs born of genetic engineering, it seems apparent that some relief from the need to make short-term profits must be linked with restrictions on profit maximization if the industry is to achieve more than a small part of its potential.

It is perhaps the desire for short-term commercial return, rather than the intrinsic toxicity of most drugs, which produces drug side-effects in their present epidemic proportions.

That these proportions are epidemic is suggested by the figures for the number of reports of suspected adverse reactions during the period 1975–1980 and given in the *Committee on Safety of Medicines Annual Report for 1980*[2454]:

Year	*No. of reports*
1975	5 052
1976	6 490
1977	11 255
1978	11 873
1979	10 840
1980	10 179

Each of these reports arises because a doctor considers the matter of sufficient importance to warrant submission of an appropriate notification (usually a 'yellow card'); some impression of the scale of the problem can be gained by multiplying the numbers by a factor which will allow for the considerable under-reporting which is known to occur.

Clearly, these reports arise from old and new drugs and reflect a combination of factors including idiosyncratic reactions by patients, errors of diagnosis, intrinsic drug toxicity, the results of over-prescribing and, amongst other causes, the consequences of precipitant marketing. The latter effect, and the consequent sudden exposure of a large patient population to a new drug, can be seen in greater isolation from the additional figure and footnote added to these data in the *Committee on Safety of Medicines Annual Report for 1981*[2455]:

Year	*No. of reports*
1977	11 255
1978	11 873
1979	10 840
1980	10 179
1981	13 032*

* This increase can mainly be attributed to a large number of reports on one drug.

The output from the 'yellow card' system of the Committee on Safety of Medicines in the United Kingdom is not inconsiderable. It includes the Annual Report, the Adverse Reactions Series of papers, the Current Problems circular, the Chairman's letters to doctors and pharmacists, and a small number of papers written by the professional secretariat of the Committee and published in the normal way in appropriate technical journals. The latter papers include important studies (*Adverse reactions to drugs – the information lag*, J. P. Griffin and P. F. D'Arcy, 1981[2456]; and its recent revision, *The information lag – has it improved?*, C. E. J. Twomey and J. P. Griffin, 1983[2457]) in which these authors examine the delay between particular side-effects becoming known and the profession being advised by means of the Committee's different means of communication.

Over the years, the Adverse Reactions Series (ARS) and Current Problems (CP) leaflets[2458], both of which are sent by mail to prescribers and which are issued on an occasional basis, have provided notable 'early warnings' of adverse drug effects. These have included the following:

February, 1964, (ARS)	Monoamine oxidase inhibitors	Liver damage Hypertensive crisis with pressor amines Interaction with pethidine and morphine
August, 1965 (ARS)	Phenylbutazone Oxyphenbutazone	Bone marrow depression Bone marrow depression
January, 1967 (ARS)	Chloramphenicol	Blood dyscrasias
June, 1967 (ARS)	Aerosols in asthma	Sudden death
December, 1969 (ARS)	Oral contraceptives (high dose oestrogen)	Pulmonary embolism
June, 1973 (ARS)	Erythromycin estolate	Jaundice
January, 1975 (ARS)	Practolol	Ocular damage
February, 1975 (ARS)	Prazosin	Sudden unconsciousness
June, 1975 (ARS)	Hormone pregnancy tests	Congenital defects
September, 1975 (CP)	Practolol Prazosin Ibuprofen Metoclopramide Tetracosactrin	Sclerosing peritonitis Loss of consciousness Bronchospasm Extrapyramidal effects Reactions
August, 1976 (CP)	Practolol and other β-blockers	(Repeat warning)

	Intravenous anaesthetics	
	Propanidid	Hypotension, urticaria, etc.
	Ketamine	Mental disturbances
	Alphadalone/Alphax-alone	Bronchospasm, hypotension
	Antibiotics	
	Clindamycin	Serious colitis
	Lincomycin	Serious colitis
	Phenformin	Lactic acidosis
	Maprotiline	Convulsions
May, 1977 (ARS)	Topical neomycin	Deafness
July, 1977 (ARS)	Perhexiline maleate	Peripheral neuropathy
		Abnormal liver function tests
		Hypoglycaemia
		Weight loss
February, 1978 (CP)	Emepronium bromide	Oesophageal ulceration
	Methyldopa	Hepatitis
	Metoclopramide	(Repeat warning)
	Nitrofurantoin	Hepatotoxicity
	Diazepam	Thrombophlebitis
	Tricyclic anti-depressants	Ileus
	Cotrimoxazole	Blood dyscrasia
	Benorylate	Transient deafness
	Alphadalone/Alphaxal-one	(Repeat warning)
April, 1979 (CP)	Clofibrate	Gallstones in treated group
	Nifedipine	Myocardial ischaemia
	Practolol	Intestinal obstruction
	Alphadalone/Alphaxa-lone	(Repeat warning)
	Phenothiazines	Tardive dyskinesia
	Diflusinal	Stevens–Johnson syndrome
June, 1979 (ARS)	Clindamycin	(Repeat warning)
	Lincomycin	(Repeat warning)
August, 1980 (ARS)	Clofibrate	(Repeat comment)
February, 1981 (CP)	Coumarin anticoagulants	Chrondrodysplasia punctata
	Topical agents for otitis externa	

654

	Chlorhexidine	Deafness
	Aminoglycoside antibiotics	Deafness
	Polymyxins	Deafness
	Triazolam	Psychotic effects
July, 1981 (CP)	Sodium valproate	Marrow hypoplasia
		Leukopenia
		Liver damage
		Hyperammonaemia
		Acute pancreatitis
	Cimetidine	Stomach cancer (drug may not be causative agent)
	β-adrenoceptor antagonists	Retroperitoneal fibrosis (association may be due to chance)
	Timolol eye drops	Bronchospasm
		Adverse cardiac reactions
	Sodium cromoglycate	Bronchospasm
	Debendox	(Causal relationship with congenital abnormalities has not been established)
December, 1981 (CP)	Mebhydrolin	Granulocytopenia or agranulocytosis
	Erythromycin	Liver damage – possibly due to any ester or the base
	Fluspirilene	Injection site nodules
	Cimetidine	Arthropathy
	Mianserin	Blood dyscrasias
August, 1982 Chairman's letter	Benoxaprofen	Gastrointestinal tract toxicity
		Liver toxicity
		Bone marrow toxicity
		Skin disorders
		Nail disorders
		Eye disorders
October, 1982 (CP)	Piroxicam	Gastrointestinal bleeding and perforation
		Precipititation of congestive cardiac failure

	Amiodarone	Pulmonary alveolitis
		Hepatitis
	Mianserin	Arthropathy
	Aminocaproic acid	Acute myopathy
	Quinidine	Granulomatous hepatitis
January, 1983 (CP)	Sodium valproate	Congenital abnormalities
April, 1983 (CP)	Mianserin	Severe blood dyscrasias
	Ketoconazole	Serious hepatic toxicity
	Latamoxef	Haemorrhagic diatheses
	Polyethoxylated castor oils	Anaphylactoid reactions
August, 1983 (CP)	Perhexiline maleate	Hepatotoxicity
		Neurotoxicity
	Zimeldine	Convulsions
		Liver damage
		Neuropathies
		Guillain–Barré syndrome
	Osmosin (controlled release indomethacin)	Gastrointestinal bleeding and perforation
October, 1983 (CP)	Bupivacaine (in Bier's block)	Fatalities during intravenous regional anaesthesia
	Isotretinoin	Human teratogenicity
	Flourescein (intravenous)	Fatal collapse
	Polyethoxylated castor oils	(Repeat warning)
	Oral contraceptives	Possible link with carcinoma of breast and cervix

As the 'Current Problems' series of leaflets has progressed it has served to issue a number of quite early warnings on serious adverse drug effects – sometimes at a stage before the statistics are convincing and whilst the profession can benefit from being alerted. Interest has increased on the means of validating 'early warnings' and this subject has been discussed by Geoffrey R. Venning (1982)[2459].

In respect of many of the apparent associations mentioned above, increased experience has eliminated all doubt and the drug in question has come to be regarded as causative of the side-effect mentioned; increased use, where this is permitted, serves only to quantify the incidence. Many of the adverse effects are rare and some are specific to man: they could not, therefore, be predicted from animal experiments, however prolonged, even if the numbers of animals conventionally used in such safety evaluations were increased. All of the adverse effects discussed in this list, derived from 'Current Contents', have manifested themselves after the drug has been marketed.

From time to time major drug disasters swell the numbers of observed side-effects and attract increased attention to the background pattern of the problem. Some of the early such events have been reviewed by J. O. Nestor (1975)[2460]; this author described the 'elixir of sulfanilamide' episode of 1933, which killed 108 persons, and the pronethalol episode of 1964, in which the drug was given to 90 humans in the USA (and more in other countries) before the Investigational New Drug exemption was closed because the compound had been found to be an animal carcinogen; he gives accounts of other difficulties with the drugs triparanol, hexobendine, triflocin, cinanserin, ethynerone, and chlormadinone acetate.

Some of the disasters have been quite puzzling: clioquinol, the halogenated hydroxyquinoline, was synthesized in Germany at the turn of the century; it achieved quite widespread use and by 1913 was marketed in Japan – and yet it was not until about 1955 that, in Japan, attention was drawn to an apparently increasing incidence of an unfamiliar neurological syndrome. This was gradually characterized as subacute myelo-opticoneuropathy. The close association of this very damaging illness with clioquinol has been excellently reviewed by M. N. G. Dukes (*The paradox of clioquinol and SMON*, 1981)[2461] – this author showing that, although there were only 60 confirmed cases in the whole of Japan up to and including 1961, in 1969 no less than 2340 new cases were reported. The Japanese Ministry of Health and Welfare prohibited the sale of clioquinol on September 8th, 1970. As Dukes comments: 'From 1971 onwards, new cases of SMON virtually ceased to occur in Japan.'

Other drug problems have produced equally new syndromes. The first descriptions of what has come to be known as 'tardive dyskinesia', perhaps one of the most distressing of iatrogenic diseases, appeared in Germany and France in 1957 and 1959. The syndrome is now recognized as being associated, in the vast majority of cases, with prolonged neuroleptic treatment. The severity of the syndrome and its personal and social consequences have seemed at times to challenge the usefulness of this group of drugs in the long-term management of the psychoses. A balanced appraisal is presented by P. G. Campbell (*Drug-induced disorders of central nervous function*, 1981)[2462] who comments that 'Psychiatrists familiar with the ravages of schizophrenia may continue to believe, on present evidence, that the probability of cumulative damage to the individual from that disease, if inadequately treated, outweighs the long-term hazards of tardive dyskinesia.'

Drug hazards have sometimes sought out the second generation in exhibiting their effects. In one instance this has involved the apparent causation of second-generation neoplasia. In the following passage this was summarized in a 'Chairman's letter' from the Committee on Safety of Medicines, May 1973[2463]:

> Over 80 cases of vaginal adenocarcinoma in young women attributed to their mothers' use of oestrogens during pregnancy have been discovered in the United States, including small epidemics reported in and around Boston and in New York State. Doses of at least 25 mg of stilboestrol a day had been taken by nearly all the patients' mothers. We have however failed to to find any similar cases in this country.

Practolol, an important cardioselective β-blocking agent with intrinsic sympathomimetic activity, became well established in the treatment of a number of cardiovascular disorders, particularly angina pectoris and cardiac arrythmias. Occasional rashes and the uncommon appearance of a syndrome akin to lupus erythematosus had been reported but then, in November 1974, Fclix, Ivc and Dahl gave an account of 21 patients suffering from practolol-induced rashes and seen over a period of 2 years[2464]; the rashes included 'a highly characteristic toxic erythematous psoriasiform eruption' and, in three patients, persistent ocular damage was a feature of the presenting clinical condition. In March 1975, Peter Wright, from Moorfields Eye Hospital, London, defined the condition in a paper on *Untoward effects associated with practolol administration: oculomuco-cutaneous syndrome*[2465]. The features of the illness comprised:

> Keratoconjunctivitis sicca, conjunctival scarring, fibrosis, metaplasia, and shrinkage developed in 27 patients as an adverse reaction to practolol. Rashes, nasal and mucosal ulceration, fibrous or plastic peritonitis, pleurisy, cochlear damage, and secretory otitis media also occurred in some cases. Three patients suffered profound visual loss though most retained good vision.

The impossibility of predicting such a syndrome from the premarketing data is shown by the fact that in June, 1975 the *British Medical Journal*, in an article on the *Side effects of practolol*[2466], said: 'the adverse effects should be kept in perspective as practolol has been widely used since 1970 (more than 200000 patient years)...' Practolol was withdrawn from general use and, at the subsequent meeting on postmarketing surveillance J. T. Nicholls reported that by November 20th, 1977 a total of 915 cases of the syndrome had been notified to Imperial Chemical Industries – the drug sponsor[2433]. Reviewing this symposium the *British Medical Journal* (in an article entitled *After practolol*)[2467] suggested that:

> At the end of the day, then, no magic solution had been found that could guarantee that future drugs would be free of serious, unexpected adverse effects. Closer attention to the recording of events (rather than side effects) in clinical trials would help, and there seemed an overwhelming case for some system of recording and storing details of the patients given each new drug as it comes on to the market.

The emphasis one might want to add to these words would relate to 'each new drug': the oculomucocutaneous syndrome, a virtually new illness, had arisen from a drug that was not the first of its therapeutic class or obviously different, in toxic effects, from the β-blocking agents already available and since entered into the market. There would seem to be a small, but nevertheless real, risk of producing adverse effects of this type with each new molecule entered into clinical practice.

Two of the most recent drug disasters have been somewhat different in that they have concerned a class of drugs long recognized as having a substantial potential for producing toxic effects of well-known varieties. The non-steroidal anti-inflammatory agent, benoxaprofen ('Opren'), was marketed in 1980 – approval was based on data from some 2000 patients who had taken the drug in the UK, USA, Canada and Mexico. It is reported that the efficacy of the drug was apparent and such that the drug was considered acceptable even though it was known to produce effects on the liver, kidney and gastrointestinal tract in animals (these effects being typical for a drug of its class); it was also known that the drug produced onycholysis and photosensitivity in man. The annual report of the Chief Medical Officer[2468] notes that: 'by July, 1981 the Committee were already concerned about its safety. In particular the Committee was concerned about the many reports of photosensitivity associated with the drug and about reports of gastrointestinal adverse reactions, including some serious and fatal cases.' Careful monitoring of progress was associated with appropriate precautionary measures but, by the end of July, 1982, 61 fatal cases had been reported in which benoxaprofen was suspected of causing adverse effects on various bodily systems, with liver damage as the most frequent cause of death. The Product Licences were suspended on August 4th, 1982 – and, once again, the perennial conclusion was reached:

> The story of *'Opren'* illustrates one of the main difficulties in drug regulation. Even when a drug has been carefully tested over a period of years in animals, and in carefully controlled clinical trials in man, rare adverse reactions may only be detected when the drug is in wide use. This underlines the importance of having a good system of adverse reaction monitoring, to supplement the testing which is required before a drug may be first marketed.

The other recent episode concerned the drug 'Osmosin' – indomethacin in a special formulation using an 'osmotic pump'. Reports of deaths during drug therapy do not necessarily indicate a causal link between the deaths and the drug, but the more frequent the association the more convincing it must seem. In a recent parliamentary reply the Health Minister gave the following data on deaths registered by the Committee on Safety of Medicines in respect of four recently withdrawn drugs. These figures concern 'suspected adverse reactions associated with the use of' the product in question:

Drug	Number of deaths
Zomax (zomepirac sodium)	7
Zelmid (zimeldine)	7
Osmosin (indomethacin, controlled release)	40
Flosint (indoprofen)	8

It must seem that, despite their vast usefulness, drugs have their dark side – not on a scale which will often throw its shadow across the path of the individual doctor, but on a scale which represents a real, and to some extent avoidable, risk to the community. There is ample evidence that the nature and extent of the risk of marketing a new drug cannot adequately be assessed from the techniques presently employed. The issue is whether, or not, the community is prepared to tolerate episodes such as those briefly described – or whether an addition to the present system is demanded in an attempt to minimize the nature and scale of the problem.

Recently, Lord Justice Lawton has spoken on the *Legal aspects of iatrogenic disorders*... (1983)[2469]. This is an issue which is clearly different in the USA than in the Royal Courts of Justice but, in respect of Britain, Lord Justice Lawton, talking of the hazards of treatment, said: 'If one patient in ten is likely to suffer, then there is such a risk – probably even when there is one patient in a hundred...' The risk is that of which the patient should be warned for consent to treatment to be likely to be judged valid in law. It might be noted that, at present, we do not have such quantified data relating to the real-life use of the drugs available.

What the doctor, even in the present state of knowledge, can do is (in a few instances) base treatment upon relative risk. The least toxic drug can be used first and the greater risk be taken only if necessary. This might seem particularly important in the use of non-curative drugs likely to be used for long periods of time and in vulnerable populations, like elderly people. A beginning in providing this kind of information has been made with papers of which that on the *Epidemiology of adverse reactions to non-steroidal anti-inflammatory drugs*[2470] by J. C. P. Weber (1982) form an example. Using criteria which make the comparison valid, Weber provides data of which Table 8 forms an illustration. In most circumstances the doctor would seem to be prudent if choosing, unless forced to do otherwise, the drug which, out of its class, least seldom produces adverse reactions. The table shows a very meaningful range of differences: even if the ranking is regarded as only a crude comparison between drugs, it is evident that the variations between them are considerable. At one end of the spectrum there are non-steroidal anti-inflammatory agents, such as feprazone, fenclofenac, and benoxaprofen, which, at the time of the study, were generating to the Committee on Safety of Medicines one adverse reaction report for every 200–400 prescriptions written. At the other end of the scale, diflunisal and piroxicam serve as examples of drugs which generate an adverse reaction considered serious enough to report only once in every 2300–3000 prescriptions. As these drugs do not differ markedly in overall efficacy, there has to be some good reason for choosing to treat an individual patient with one of the more troublesome drugs. The additional data provided by Weber show that, in terms of the ranked comparisons of the drugs included in the study, sulindac and diclofenac least seldom cause gastrointestinal haemorrhage or perforation; piroxicam markedly

Table 8   Total adverse rections. Ranked comparisons. From J. C. P. Weber (1982)

Drug	Ranks	Approximate number of prescriptions for one ADR report
Feprazone	1	200
Fenclofenac	2	280
Benoxaprofen	3	400
Diclofenac Azaproprazone	4	1200
Flurbiprofen Sulindac	5	1700
Diflunisal	6	2300
Piroxicam	7	3000

less often causes liver damage or blood dyscrasias. There is a much earlier paper on *Adverse reactions to anti-rheumatic drugs: some correlations with animal toxicity studies*[2471] by M. F. Cuthbert (1977) which shows the differences between some of these drugs in terms of the bodily systems most frequently involved in overall adverse reactions or fatal drug effects. It might seem that comparisons of this type are of importance in permitting a rational choice between the drugs available for prescription. In particular, the paper by Weber (1982) begins to look like a pioneer attempt to derive, from the accumulated adverse reactions data, quantified guidance towards patient care.

References

2325. BPC (1934). As ref. 120 but p. 164
2326. Ministry of Health, Reports on public health and medical subjects No. 112. Deformities caused by thalidomide. London, *HMSO,* 1964, p. iii
2327. Ministry of Health (1964). As ref. 2326 but Plate 4
2328. Kunz, W., Keller, H. and Mückter, H. *Arzneim.-Forsch.,* 1956, **6,** 426. See Jung, Herman. Klinische Erfahrungen mit einem neuen Sedativum. *Arzneim.-Forsch.,* 1956, **6,** 430–432
2329. Murdoch, J. McC. and Campbell, G. D. Antithyroid activity of N-phthalyl glutamic acid imide (K17). *Br. Med. J.,* 1958, **1,** 84–85
2330. Teff, Harvey and Munro, Colin, R. Thalidomide, the legal aftermath. Farnborough, *Saxon House,* 1976
2331. Sjöström, Henning and Nilsson, Robert. Thalidomide and the power of the drug companies. Harmondsworth, *Penguin,* 1972, p. 53
2332. Sjöström and Nilsson (1972). As ref. 2331 but p. 56
2333. Teff and Munro (1976). As ref. 2330 but p. xii
2334. Florence, A. Leslie. Is thalidomide to blame? *Br. Med. J.,* 1960, **2,** 1954
2335. Burley, Denis. Is thalidomide to blame? *Br. Med. J.,* 1961, **1,** 130
2336. Kuenssberg, E. V. *et al.* Is thalidomide to blame? *Br. Med. J.,* 1961, **1,** 291
2337. Shafar, J. Is thalidomide to blame? *Br. Med. J.,* 1961, **1,** 829
2338. Frenkel, H. Contergan-Nebenwirkungen. *Die Med. Welt,* 1961, **1(18),** 970–975
2339. Schied, W. von. *et al.* Polyneuritische Syndrome nach längerer Thalidomid-Medikation. *Dtsch. Med. Wschr.,* 1961, **86,** 938–941
2340. Raffauf, Hans Joachim von. Bewirkt Thalidomid (Contergan) keine Schäden? *Dtsch. Med. Wschr.,* 1961, **86,** 935–938
2341. Anonymous. Purpura associated with thalidomide. *Br. Med. J.,* 1961, **2,** 125
2342. Longstaff, J. H. Purpura associated with thalidomide. *Br. Med. J.,* 1961, **2,** 660
2343. Fullerton, Pamela M. and Kremer, Michael. Neuropathy after intake of thalidomide (Distaval). *Br. Med. J.,* 1961, **2,** 855–858
2344. Anonymous. Thalidomide neuropathy. *Br. Med. J.,* 1961, **2,** 876–877
2345. Heathfield, K. W. G. Neuropathy after thalidomide ('Distaval'). *Br. Med. J.,* 1961, **2,** 1084
2346. Powell-Tuck, G. A. Neuropathy after thalidomide ('Distaval'). *Br. Med. J.,* 1961, **2,** 1151
2347. Stevenson, J. S. K. Neuropathy after thalidomide ('Distaval'). *Br. Med. J.,* 1961, **2,** 1223
2348. Jewesbury, Eric C. O. Neuropathy after thalidomide ('Distaval'). *Br. Med. J.,* 1961, **2,** 1286
2349. Magrath, D. Neuropathy after thalidomide ('Distaval'). *Br. Med. J.,* 1961, **2,** 1359
2350. Hayman, D. J. Neuropathy after thalidomide ('Distaval'). *Br. Med. J.,* 1961, **2,** 1435
2351. Kremer, Michael and Fullerton, Pamela, M. Neuropathy after thalidomide ('Distaval'). *Br. Med. J.,* 1961, **2,** 1498. (See also p. 1499)
2352. McBride, W. G. Thalidomide and congenital abnormalities. *Lancet,* 1961, **4,** 1358
2353. McBride, W. G. Congenital abnormalities and thalidomide. *Med. J. Aust.,* 1961, (Dec. 23), 1030
2354. Lenz, W. Thalidomide and congenital abnormalities. *Lancet,* 1962, **1,** 45

2355. Pfeiffer, R.A. and Kosenow, W. Thalidomide and congenital abnormalities. *Lancet,* 1962, **1**, 45–46

2356. Somers, G.F. Thalidomide and congenital abnormalities. *Lancet,* 1962, **2**, 912–913

2357. Knightley, Phillip *et al.* Suffer the children: the story of thalidomide. London, *Andre Deutsch,* 1979

2358. Škre, Håvard. Thalidomide embryopathy and neuropathy, some correlations with embryology and teratology. Bergen, *Norwegian Univ. Press,* 1963

2359. McCredie, Janet. Thalidomide and congenital Charcot's Joints. *Lancet,* 1973, **4**, 1058–1061

2360. Jurand, A. Early changes in limb buds of chick embryos after thalidomide treatment. *J. Embryol. Exp. Morph.,* 1966, **16(2)**, 289–300

2361. Poswillo, David. Hemorrhage in development of the face. *Brith Defects: Original Article Series,* 1975, **XI(7)**, 61–81

2362. Williams, R. Teewyn. Thalidomide, a study of biochemical teratology. *Arch. Environ. Health,* 1968, **16**, 493–502

2363. Kohler, F. *et al.* Embryotoxicitat und Teratogenitat von Derivaten des 1,3-Indandion. *Arch. Toxicol. (Berl.),* 1975, **33(3)**, 191–197

2364. Gordon, G.B. *et al.* Thalidomide teratogenesis: evidence for a toxic arene oxide metabolite, *Proc. Natl. Acad. Sci. USA,* 1981, **78(4)**, 2545–2548

2365. McBride, W.G. Fetal nerve cell degeneration produced by thalidomide in rabbits. *Teratology,* 1974, **10**, 283–292

2366. McBride, W.G. Studies of the etiology of thalidomide dysmorphogenesis. *Teratology,* 1976, **14**, 71–87

2367. Schardein, James L. Drugs as teratogens. Cleveland, *CRC Press,* 1976

2368. Gregg, N. McAlister. Congenital cataract following german measles in the mother. *Trans. Ophthalmol. Soc. Aust.,* 1941, **3**, 35–46

2369. Schardein, James L. (1976). As ref. 2367 but p. 5

2370. Schardein, James L. (1976). As ref. 2367 but p. 6

2371. Robertson, Richard T. *et al.* Aspirin: teratogenic evaluation in the dog. *Teratology,* 1979, **20**, 313–320

2372. Layton, William M. An analysis of teratogenic testing procedures. In Janerich, D.T., Skalko, R.G. and Porter, I.H. (eds.) Congenital defects, New York, *Academic Press,* 1974, pp. 205–217

2373. Secret remedies, what they cost and what they contain. London, *British Medical Association,* 1909

2374. More secret remedies, what they cost and what they contain. London, *British Medical Association,* 1912

2375. Report from the Select Committee on patent medicines, together with the proceedings of the Committee, minutes of evidence, and appendices. London, *HMSO,* 1914

2376. Penn, Raymond G. The state control of medicines: the first 3000 years. *Br. J. Clin. Pharmac.,* 1979, **8**, 293–305

2377. Hartley, Sir Frank. The Medicines Act and the physician. In Harcus, A.W. (ed.) Risk and regulation in medicine – the fettered physician. London, *Association of Medical Advisers in the Pharmaceutical Industry,* 1980, pp. 9–23

2378. Committee on Safety of Drugs. Report of the Committee on Safety of Drugs for the year ended December 31st, 1964...London, *HMSO,* 1965

2379. Committee on Safety of Drugs. Report for the year ended December 31st, 1965 ...London, *HMSO,* 1966

2380. Committee on Safety of Drugs. Report for the year ended December 31st, 1966 ...London, *HMSO,* 1967

2381. Committee on Safety of Drugs. Report for the year ended December 31st, 1967 ...London, *HMSO,* 1968

2382. Committee on Safety of Drugs. Report for the year ended December 31st, 1968 ...London, *HMSO,* 1969

2383. Committee on Safety of Drugs. Report for 1969 and 1970. London, *HMSO,* 1971

2384. Inman, W.H.W. *et al.* Thromboembolic disease and the steroidal content of oral contraceptives. A report to the Committee on Safety of Drugs. *Br. Med. J.,* 1970, **2**, 203–209

2385. Inman, W. H. W. and Adelstein, A. M. Rise and fall of asthma mortality in England and Wales in relation to use of pressurised aerosols. *Lancet,* 1969, **2**, 279–285

2386. Committee on Safety of Medicines. Report for the year ended 31st December, 1971. London, *HMSO,* 1972

2387. Department of Health & Social Security. Medicines Act leaflet. A guide to the licensing system (MAL 1). London, *DHSS, Medicines Division,* 1976

2388. The Medicines (Data Sheet) Regulations 1972. S.I. 1972 No. 2076. London, *HMSO,* 1973

2389. Inman, William H. W. Study of fatal bone marrow depression with special reference to phenylbutazone and oxyphenbutazone. *Br. Med. J.,* 1977, **1**, 1500–1505

2390. Quantock, D. C. The effect of regulation on international drug development. In Harcus, A. W. (1980). As ref. 2377 but pp. 85–94

2391. Wardell, W. M. What is the proper role of a drug regulatory agency? In Harcus, A. W. (1980). As ref. 2377 but pp. 95–113

2392. *v.* Scrip No. 815, 1983, p. 1

2393. British National Formulary, Number 4 (1982). London, *British Medical Association and The Pharmaceutical Society of Great Britain,* 1982, p. 110

2394. The Medicines (Exemption from Licences) (Clinical Trials) Order 1981. S.I. 1981 No. 164. London, *HMSO,* 1981

2395. Griffin, John P. Post-marketing surveillance. In Wardell, W. M. and Velo, G. (eds.) Drug development, regulatory assessment, and postmarketing surveillance. New York, *Plenum,* 1981, pp. 241–249

2396. D'Arcy, Patrick Francis and Griffin, John Parry. Iatrogenic diseases. (2nd edn.), Oxford, *Univ. Press,* 1979. (1st edn., 1972)

2397. D'Arcy, Patrick F. and Griffin, John P. (1979). As ref. 2396 but p. 39

2398. D'Arcy, Patrick F. and Griffin, John P. (1981). As ref. 2396 but 'Update 1981', p. 10

2399. D'Arcy, Patrick F. and Griffin, John P. (1981). As ref. 2398, p. 10

2400. D'Arcy, Patrick F. and Griffin, John P. (1981). As ref. 2398 but p. 11

2401. Melmon, Kenneth L. Preventable drug reactions – causes and cures. *New Engl. J. Med.,* 1971, **284**, 1361–1368

2402. Girdwood, R. H. Death after taking medicaments. *Br. Med. J.,* 1974, **1**, 501–504

2403. Caranasos, George J. *et al.* Drug-associated deaths of medical inpatients. *Arch. Intern. Med.,* 1976, **136**, 872–875

2404. Porter, Jane and Jick, Hershel. Drug-related deaths among medical inpatients. *J. Am. Med. Assoc.,* 1977, **237**, 879–881

2405. Anonymous. Deaths due to drug treatment. (Editorial), *Brit. Med. J.,* 1977, **1**, 1492–1493

2406. Inman, William, H. W. In Inman, W. H. W. (ed.) Monitoring for drug safety. Lancaster, *MTP Press*, 1980, p. 15

2407. Cuthbert, M. F., Griffin, J. P. and Inman, W. The United Kingdom. In William M. Wardell (ed.) Controlling the use of therapeutic drugs, an international comparison. Washington, *American Enterprise Institute,* 1978, p. 133

2408. Inman, William H. W. Standpoint of the regulating agency in the U.K. In A. F. De Schaepdryver and others (eds.) The scientific basis of official regulation of drug research and development. Ghent, *Heymans Foundation*, 1978, p. 137

2409. Dollery, Colin T. and Rawlins, Michael D. Monitoring adverse reactions to drugs. *Br. Med. J.,* 1977, **1**, 96–97

2410. Schimmel, Elihu M. The hazards of hospitalization. *Ann. Intern. Med.,* 1964, **60**, 100–110

2411. MacDonald, Murdo G. and Mackay, Bruce R. Adverse drug reactions, experience of Mary Fletcher Hospital during 1962. *J. Am. Med. Assoc.,* 1964, **190**, 1071–1074

2412. Seidl, L. G. *et al.* Studies on the epidemiology of adverse drug reactions. III. Reactions in patients on a General Medical Service. *Bull. Johns Hopk. Hosp.,* 1966, **119**, 299–315

2413. Reidenberg, Marcus M. Registry of adverse drug reactions. Report of the Drug Reaction Registry Subcommittee of the Greater Philadelphia Committee for Medical-Pharmaceutical Sciences. *J. Am. Med. Assoc.,* 1968, **203**, 31–34

2414. Smith, Jay W. *et al.* Studies on the epidemiology of adverse drug reactions. V. Clinical factors influencing susceptibility. *Ann. Intern. Med.,* 1966, **65**, 629–640

2415. Ogilvie, R. I. and Ruedy, J. Adverse drug reactions during hospitalization. *Can. Med. Assoc. J.,* 1967, **97** 1450–1457

2416. Hoddinott, B. C. *et al.* Drug reactions and errors in administration on a medical ward. *Can. Med. Assoc. J.,* 1967, **97**, 1001–1006

2417. Borda, I. T. *et al.* (Boston Collaborative Drug Surveillance Program). Assessment of adverse reactions within a drug surveillance program. *J. Am. Med. Assoc.,* 1968, **205,** 645–647

2418. Hurwitz, Natalie and Wade, O. L. Intensive hospital monitoring of adverse reactions to drugs. *Br. Med. J.,* 1969, **1,** 531–536

2419. Hurwitz, Natalie. Admissions to hospital due to drugs. *Br. Med. J.,* 1969, **1,** 539–540

2420. Gardner, Pierce and Watson, L. Jeannine. Adverse drug reactions: a pharmacist-based monitoring system. *Clin. Pharmacol. Ther.,* 1970, **11,** 802–807

2421. Wang, R. I. H. and Terry, L. C. Adverse drug reactions in a Veterans Administration Hospital. *J. Clin. Pharmacol.,* 1971, **11,** 14–18

2422. Boston Collaborative Drug Surveillance Program. Adverse drug interactions. *J. Am. Med. Assoc.,* 1972, **220,** 1238–1239

2423. Miller, R. R. Drug surveillance utilizing epidemiologic methods: a report from the Boston Collaborative Drug Surveillance Program. *Am. J. Hosp. Pharm.,* 1973, **30,** 584–592

2424. Mulroy, R. Iatrogenic disease in general practice: its incidence and effects. *Br. Med. J.,* 1973, **2,** 407–410

2425. Jick, Hershel. Drugs – remarkably nontoxic. *New Engl. J. Med.,* 1974, **291,** 824–828

2426. Caranasos, G. J. et al. Drug-induced illness leading to hospitalization. *J. Am. Med. Assoc.,* 1974, **228,** 713–717

2427. McKenney, J. M. and Harrison, W. L. Drug-related hospital admissions. *Am. J. Hosp. Pharm.,* 1976, **33,** 792–795

2428. McKenzie, M. W. *et al.* Adverse drug reactions leading to hospitalization in children. *J. Pediatr.,* 1976, **89,** 487–490

2429. Levy, M. *et al.* Drug utilization and adverse drug reactions in medical patients. Comparison of two periods, 1969–72 and 1973–76. *Israel J. Med. Sci.,* 1977, **13,** 1065–72

2430. Martys, Cedrick R. Adverse reactions to drugs in general practice. *Br. Med. J.,* 1979, **2,** 1194–1197

2431. Lawson, D. H. and Henry, D. A. Monitored adverse reactions to new drugs: 'restricted release' or 'monitored release'? *Bri. Med. J.,* 1977, **1,** 691–692

2432. Wilson, A. B. Post-marketing surveillance of adverse reactions to new medicines. *Br. Med. J.,* 1977, **2,** 1001–1003

2433. Nicholls, J. T. The practolol syndrome – a retrospective analysis. In Post-marketing surveillance of adverse reactions to new medicines, report of a meeting held on 7 December 1977 under the chairmanship of Sir Richard Doll. MedicoPharmaceutical Forum, publication No. 7, 1977, pp. 4–11

2434. Anonymous. *Journal of the Royal College of Physicians,* 1977, **11,** cited by *Br. Med. J.,* 1977, **1,** 861–862

2435. Drug monitoring; proceedings of an International Workshop held in Honolulu from 24 to 28 January, 1977 and sponsored by Ciba-Geigy. eds. Gross, F. H. and Inman, W. H. W. London, *Academic Press,* 1977

2436. Crawford, J. M. (1977). As ref. 2435 but pp. 55–58

2437. Inman, W. H. W. (1977). As ref. 2435 but pp. 65–78

2438. Anonymous (1977). As ref. 2435 but p. 308

2439. Anonymous. New strategies for drug monitoring. *Br. Med. J.* 1977, **1,** 861–862

2440. Skegg, D. C. G. (1977) As ref. 2435 but p. 59

2441. Anonymous. New proposals on surveillance of drugs. *Br. Med. J.,* 1978, **1,** 588

2442. Anonymous. Postmarketing surveillance of drugs. *Br. Med. J.,* 1979, **1,** 1229

2443. Skegg, D. C. G. and Doll, Sir Richard. The case for recording events in clinical trials. *Br. Med. J.,* **2,** 1523–1524

2444. Shapiro, Samuel and Slone, Dennis. Post-marketing assessment of drugs. In ref. 2433 (1977) but pp. 19–26

2445. Jones, Judith K. (1981). As ref. 2395 but pp. 233–240

2446. Jick, Hershel. The discovery of drug-induced illness. *New Engl. J. Med.,* 1977, **296,** 481–485

2447. Wardell, William M. and Lasagna, Louis. Regulation and drug development. Washington, DC, *American Enterprise Institute for Public Policy Research,* 1975, p. 105

2448. Bloch, Hubert. Toward better systems of drug regulation. In Regulating new drugs, ed. Landau, Richard L. Chicago, *Univ. of Chicago Center for Policy Study,* 1973, p. 263

2449. Snell, Eric S. Regulatory authorisation of clinical trials. *Br. J. Clin. Pharmac.,* 1983, **15,** 625–627

2450. Wardell, William M. (1981). As ref. 2395 but pp. 3–4

2451. Dukes, M. N. G. and Lunde, I. (1980). As ref. 2377 but pp. 180–181

2452. Diggle, Geoffrey E. and Griffin, John P. Licensing times in granting marketing authorizations for medicines – a comparison between the U.K. and U.S.A. *Pharmacy Int.,* 1982, **3,** 230–236

2453. Griffin, John P. and Diggle, Geoffrey E. A survey of products licensed in the United Kingdom from 1971–1981. *Br. J. Clin. Pharmac.,* 1981, **12,** 453–463

2454. Annual reports for 1980 of Medicines Commission, Committee on Safety of Medicines, etc. London, *HMSO,* 1981

2455. Annual reports for 1981 of Medicines Commission, Committee on Safety of Medicines, etc. London, *HMSO,* 1982

2456. Griffin, John P. and D'Arcy, P. F. Adverse reactions to drugs – the information lag. In Side effects of drugs annual, ed. Dukes, M. N. G. Amsterdam, *Excerpta Medica*, pp. xv–xxiv

2457. Twomey, C. E. J. and Griffin, John P. The information lag – has it improved? *Pharmacy Int.,* 1983 (March), 57–61

2458. Current Problems, Number 1. Committee on Safety of Medicines. London, *HMSO,* 1975 (Sept.). No. 2, August 1976; No. 3, February 1978; No. 4, April 1979; No. 5, February 1981; No. 6, July 1981; No. 7, December 1981; No. 8, October 1982; No. 9, January 1983; No. 10, April, 1983; No. 11, August 1983; No. 12, October 1983

2459. Venning, Geoffrey R. Identification of adverse reactions to new drugs. I. What have been the important adverse reactions since thalidomide? *Br. Med. J.,* 1983, **286,** 199–202. (Then parts:) II, ibid, pp. 289–292; II (cont.) ibid, pp. 365–368; III ibid, pp. 458–460; IV ibid, pp. 544–547

2460. Nestor, J. O. Results of the failure to perform adequate preclinical studies before administering new drugs to humans. *S. A. Med. J. (Suppl. S.A. J. Lab. Clin. Med.),* 1975, **49,** 287–290

2461. Dukes, M. N. G. The paradox of clioquinol and SMON. In D'Arcy and Griffin. As ref. 2396 but *Update* 1981, pp. 105–113

2462. Campbell, P. G. Drug-induced disorders of central nervous function. In D'Arcy and Griffin. As ref. 2396 but pp. 114–136

2463. Committee on Safety of Medicines. CSM/AR/18C, May 1973

2464. Felix, R. H. *et al.* Cutaneous and ocular reactions to practolol. *Br. Med. J.,* 1974, **4,** 321–324

2465. Wright, Peter. Untoward effects associated with practolol administration: oculomucocutaneous syndrome. *Br. Med. J.,* 1975, **1,** 595–598

2466. Anonymous. Side effects of practolol. *Br. Med. J.,* 1975, **1,** 577–578

2467. Anonymous. After practolol. *Br. Med. J.,* 1977, **2,** 1561–1562

2468. Department of Health and Social Security. On the state of the public health. The Annual Report of the Chief Medical Officer . . . for the year 1982. London, *HMSO,* pp. 122–123

2469. Lawton, The Right Hon. Lord Justice. Legal aspects of iatrogenic disorders: discussion paper. *J. R. Soc. Med.,* 1983, **76,** 289–291

2470. Weber, J. C. P. Epidemiology of adverse reactions to non-steroidal anti-inflammatory drugs. In Side-effects of anti-inflammatory analgesic drugs, eds. Rainsford, K. D. and Velo, G. New York, *Raven Press,* 1984, Vol. 6, pp. 1–7

2471. Cuthbert, M. F. Adverse reactions to anti-rheumatic drugs: some correlations with animal toxicity studies. In Current approaches in toxicology, ed. Ballantyne, Bryan. Bristol, John Wright, 1977, pp. 279–288

Conclusion

The whole experience of modern drug use covers a period of not much more than three-quarters of a century. The history of medicine dwarfs this short period and it is perhaps not surprising that the final result is something less than the consistent and rational outcome that some would like to believe it to be. Much of the information which best shows its inconsistencies is only slowly and irregularly entering the scientific domain. The period during which this book has been written and printed has seen a marked change in this respect, important data on drug side-effects and adverse experience having been recently published in response to political questioning as well as scientific activity.

The present-day inconsistencies are such that whilst the great achievements – the understanding of the autonomic nervous system, the discovery of antibiotics, the development of antituberculosis chemotherapy, and so on – look to be completely secure, we can be fairly certain that the almost indiscriminate use of the non-steroidal anti-inflammatory agents, for example, will in retrospect seem less of an accomplishment.

The proportions of the inconsistency can be measured by the curative effects of the antibiotics contrasted with the fact that in 1983 the non-steroidal anti-inflammatory agents accounted for about 25% of the total of 12689 drug side-effects reported to the Committee on Safety of Medicines[2472].

The great difference between the pharmacopoeias of roughly 100 years ago and those of today is the transition from a herbal to a chemical pharmacopoeia. Even so, some of the contents of the contemporary pharmacopoeia have direct links with the botanical medicines of the earliest times. Obvious examples are acetylsalicylic acid and the willow tree and its use in classical times; the poppy, and the first-century description of the preparation of opium by Scribonius Largus; the foxglove, and the discovery of digitalis by William Withering. We are now almost exactly 200 years from the first appearance of Withering's *An account of the foxglove*... (1785)[1053] – a book, beginning modern clinical pharmacology, which makes one wonder how far the use of this herb and its essential glycoside reaches back into folklore. Many of the medicinal remedies that have now been discarded and replaced by less toxic drugs, but were in the pharmacopoeias of even 50 years ago, were also derived from plants: the

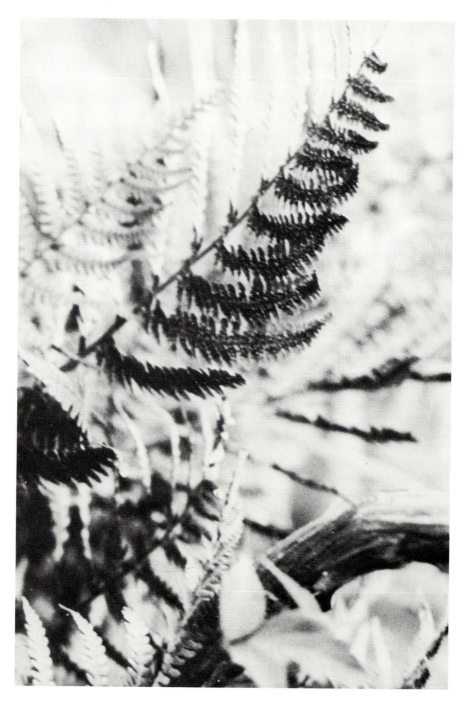

Figure 145 *Dryopteris filix-mas* (the male fern).

anthelmintic Extract of Male Fern from *Dryopteris filix-mas* (Figure 145), and the different preparations of aconite, from *Aconitum napellus,* the Monkshood or Wolfsbane (Figure 21), form obvious examples.

Amongst the most interesting of these examples is the family Salicaceae, which includes both *Salix alba*, the White or European Willow, and *Salyx nigra*, the Black American Willow. The natural habitat of the White Willow is central and southern Europe and in Britain its thin green shoots of new wood are visible in March; it flowers in April and May, the bark being easily separable throughout the summer, and forms a large tree with a rough, greyish bark, the stems being characteristically brittle at the base. It is the bark which provides both tannins and salicin. The Black Willow is said to have a natural habitat in New York State and Pennsylvania; it is usually 15–25 feet high and is most frequent on the banks of rivers and streams. The synonym is Pussy Willow, a term used as a country name to describe the European Willow (Figure 146) in its typical appearance.

Salicin (BPC 1954) is the crystalline β-glucoside obtained from the bark of young shoots of various species of *Salix* and *Populus*, especially *Salix fragilis*. Salicylic acid (*ortho*-hydroxybenzoic acid) was prepared from salicin by Raffaele Piria in 1838[1659]; it was also prepared from oil of gaultheria (wintergreen) by August André Cahours in 1845[2473]. Acetylsalicylic acid (*ortho*-acetoxybenzoic acid, salicylic acid acetate) was made by Charles Frédéric Gerhardt, Professor of Chemistry at Strasbourg, but the synthesis, which was reported in 1853[2474], aroused no interest.

It is perhaps curious that this substance has, as 'aspirin', become today's most widely used drug. From this simple synthesis in the mid-nineteenth century the story of the salicylates reaches back to the botanical remedies of antiquity. The Willow itself forms part of the botany of the Bible, whose commentators used to refer to *Salix octandra, Salix Aegyptiaca* and *Salix Babylonica*. In Ezekiel (xvii, 5) the willow appears in the parable of the two eagles and the vine; in Job[2475] the prophet finds:

> The shady trees cover him with their shadow;
> the willows of the brook compass him about.

However, any real knowledge of the antipyretic, analgesic, and other actions of aspirin, including its usefulness in acute rheumatism, arose much later, the current studies of the clinical significance of the effects of the drug upon platelet behaviour being still incomplete.

One of the first to define the therapeutic activity of the willow in near-modern terms was the Revd. Edward Stone. This author's report[2476] appears in the *Philosophical Transactions . . .* of 1763 in the following terms:

XXXII. *An Account of the Succefs of the Bark of the Willow in the Cure of Agues. In a Letter to the Right Honourable* George *Earl of* Macclesfield, *Prefident of R. S. from the Rev. Mr.* Edward Stone, *of* Chipping-Norton, *in* Oxfordfhire.

My Lord,

Read June 2d, 1763.

Among the many useful difcoveries, which this age hath made, there are very few which, better deferve the attention of the public than what I am going to lay before your Lordfhip.

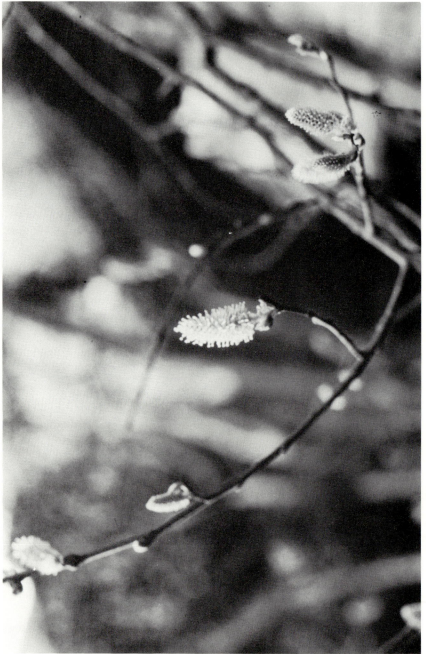

Figure 146 Salix alba (the White or European Willow).

There is a bark of an Englifh tree, which I have found by experience to be a powerful aftringent, and very efficacious in curing aguifh and intermitting diforders.

About fix years ago, I accidentally tafted it, and was furprifed at its extra-ordinary bitternefs; which immediately raifed me a fufpicion of its having the properties of the Peruvian bark. As this tree delights in a moift or wet foil, where agues chiefly abound, the general maxim, that many natural maladies carry their cures along with them, or that their remedies lie not far from their caufes, was fo very appofite to this particular cafe, that I could not help applying it; and that this might be the intention of Providence here, I muft own had fome little weight with me.

The exceffive plenty of this bark furnifhed me, in my fpeculative difquifitions upon it, with an argument both for and againft thefe imaginary qualities of it; for, on one hand, as intermittents are very common, it was reafonable to fuppofe, that what was defigned for their cure, fhould be as common and as eafy to be procured. But then, on the other hand, it feemed probable, that, if there was any confiderable virtue in this bark, it muft have been difcovered from its plenty. My curiofity prompted me to look into into the difpenfatories and books of botany, and examine what they faid concerning it; but there it exifted only by name. I could not find, that it hath, or ever had, any place in pharmacy, or any fuch qualities, as I fufpected afcribed to it by the botanifts.

However, I determined to make fome experiments with it; and, for this purpofe, I gathered that fummer near a pound weight of it, which I dryed in a bag, upon the outfide of a baker's oven, for more than three months, at which time it was to be reduced to a powder, by pounding and fifting after the manner that other barks are pulverized.

It was not long before I had an opportunity of making a trial of it; but, being an entire ftranger to its nature, I gave it in very fmall quantities, I think it was about twenty grains of the powder at a dofe, and repeated it every four hours between the fits; but with great caution and the ftricteft attention to its effects: the fits were confiderably abated, but did not entirely ceafe. Not perceiving the leaft ill confequences, I grew bolder with it, and in a few days encreafed the dofe to two fcruples, and the ague was foon removed.

It was then given to feveral others with the fame fuccefs; but I found it better anfwered the intention, when a dram of it was taken every four hours in the intervals of the paroxifms.

I have continued to ufe it as a remedy for agues and intermitting diforders for five years fucceffively and fuccefsfully. It hath been given I believe to fifty perfons, and never failed in the cure, except in a few autumual and quartan agues, with which the patients had been long and feverely afflicted; thefe it reduced in a great degree, but did not wholly take them off; the patient, at the ufual time for the return of his fit, felt fome fmattering of his diftemper, which the inceffant repetition of thefe powders could not conquer: it feemed as if their power could reach thus far and no farther, and I did fuppofe that it would not have long continued to reach fo far, and that the diftemper would have foon returned with its priftine violence; but I did not ftay to fee the iffue: I added one fifth part of the Peruvian bark to it, and with this fmall auxiliary it totally routed its adverfary. It was found neceffary likewife, in one or two obftinate cafes, at other times of the year, to mix the fame quantity of that bark with it; but thefe were cafes where the patient went abroad imprudently, and caught cold, as a poft-chaife boy did, who, being almoft recovered from an inveterate tertian ague, would follow his bufinefs, by which means he not only neglected his powders, but, meeting with bad weather, renewed his diftemper.

One fifth part was the largeft and indeed the only proportion of the quinquina made ufe of in this compofition, and this only upon extraordinary occafions: the patient was never prepared, either by vomiting, bleeding, purging, or any medicines of a fimilar intention, for the reception of this bark, but he entered upon it abruptly and immediately, and it was always given in powders, with any common vehicle, as water, tea, fmall beer and fuch like. This was done purely to afcertain its effects; and that I might be affured the changes wrought in the patient could not be attributed to any other thing: though, had there been a due preparation, the moft obftinate intermittents would probably have yielded to this bark without any foreign affiftance: And, by all I can judge from five years experience of it upon a number of perfons, it appears to be a powerful abforbent, aftringent, and febrifuge in intermitting cafes, of the fame nature and kind with the Peruvian bark, and to have all its properties, though perhaps not always in in the fame degree. It feems likewife to have this additional quality, viz. to be a fafe medicine; for I never could perceive the leaft ill effect from it, though it had been always given without any preparation of the patient.

The tree, from which this bark is taken, is ftiled by Ray, in his Synopfis, Salix, alba, vulgaris, the common white Willow. Hæc omnium nobis cognitarum maxima eft, et in fatis craffam et proceram Arborem adolefcit.

It is called in thefe parts, by the common people, the willow, and fometimes the Dutch willow; but, if it be of a foreign extraction, it hath been fo long naturalized to this climate, that it thrives as well in it as if it was in its original foil. It is eafily diftinguifhed by the notable bitternefs and the free running of its bark, which may be readily feparated from it all the fummer months whilft the fap is up. I took it from the fhoots of three or four years growth, that fprung from Pollard trees, the diameters of which fhoots, at their biggeft end, were from one to four or five inches: it is poffible, and indeed not improbable, that this cortex, taken from larger or older fhoots, or from the trunk of the tree itfelf, may be ftronger; but I have not had time nor opportunities to make the experiments, which ought to be made upon it. The bark, I had, was gathered in the northern parts of Oxfordfhire, which are chiefly of dry and gravelly nature, affording few moift or moory places for this tree to grow in; and therefore, I fufpect that its bark is not fo good here as in fome other parts of the kingdom. Few vegetables are equal in every place; all have their peculiar foils, where they arrive to a greater perfection than in any other place: the beft and ftrongeft Muftard-feed is gathered in the county of Durham; the fineft Saffron-Flowers are produced in fome particular fpots of Effex and Cambridgefhire; the beft Cyder-apples grow in Herefordfhire, Devonfhire and the adjacent counties; the roots of Valerian are efteemed moft medicinal, which are dug up in Oxfordfhire and Glocefterfhire: And therefore why may not the Cortex Salignus, or Cortex Anglicanus, have its favourite foil, where it may florifh moft, and attain to its higheft perfection? It is very probable that it hath; and perhaps it may be in the fens of Lincolnfhire, Cambridgefhire, Effex, Kent, or fome fuch like fituations; and, though the bark, which grew in the county of Oxford, may feem in fome particular cafes to be a little inferior to the quinquina, yet, in other places, it may equal, if not exceed it.

The powders made from this bark are at firft of a light brown, tinged with a dufky yellow, and the longer they are kept, the more they incline to a cinnamon or lateritious colour, which I believe is the cafe with the Peruvian bark and powders.

I have no other motives for publifhing this valuable fpecific, than that it

672

may have a fair and full trial in all its variety of circumftances and fituations, and that the world may reap the benefits accruing from it. For thefe purpofes I have given this long and minute account of it, and which I would not have troubled your Lordfhip with, was I not fully perfuaded of the wonderful efficacy of this Cortex Salignus in agues and intermitting cafes, and did I not think, that this perfuafion was fufficiently fupported by the manifold experience, which I have had of it.

I am, my Lord,

with the profoundeft fubmiffion and refpect,

Chipping-Norton,
Oxfordshire,
April 25, 1763.

your Lordfhip's moft obedient
humble Servant

Edward Stone.

There are scores of other examples of botanical items which once formed part of medicine, its folklore, and its therapeutics. Solomon's Seal (*Polygonatum multiflorum*; Figure 147), of the Liliaceae, is a close relative of the Lily-of-the-Valley and has a long medicinal tradition. In Galen's time its distilled water is said to have been used as a cosmetic and for cleansing the skin. Mrs Grieve[2477] quotes Gerard as writing that the name *Sigillum Solomons* was given to the root of the plant 'partly because it bears marks something like the stamp of a seal, but still more because of the virtue the root hath in sealing and healing up green wounds, broken bones and such like, being stamp't and laid thereon.' These same cleansing and healing properties led to the plant being called 'Lady's Seal' or 'St. Mary's Seal' (*Sigillum Sanctae Mariae*) by different writers.

Rosemary (*Rosmarinus officinalis*), of the Labiatae, is still widely used for culinary purposes. It used to be called *Rosmarinus coronarium* because it was an ancient emblem of affection. Its Old French name was *Incensier* because it provided an inexpensive source of incense. It still has minor medical uses: it is the source of Rosemary Oil (BPC) which is said to be carminative and mildly irritant; it is an ingredient of Soap Liniment BPC, many medicinal hair lotions, and Eau-de-Cologne. William Woodville (1810)[2478], describes the most potent source of the aromatic principles of the plant in the following passage:

> Rosemary is a native of the South of Europe and the Levant. It is commonly cultivated in our gardens, where it usually flowers in April and May.
> The ancients were well acquainted with this plant, as it is mentioned by Dioscorides, Galen, and Pliny. It grows wild in some of the southern parts of France, but more abundantly in Spain and Italy. Its cultivation in this country, like many other plants which we have had occasion to mention, is probably of ancient date, but now cannot be traced beyond the time of Gerard.
> Rosemary has a fragrant aromatic smell, and a bitterish pungent taste. The leaves and tops of this plant are the strongest in their sensible qualities: the flowers, which are also directed for use by the College, are not to be separated from their cups or calyces, as the active matter principally, if not wholly, resides in the latter.

The Pine (*Pinus*, various species; Figure 149), of the Pinaceae, is the source of

673

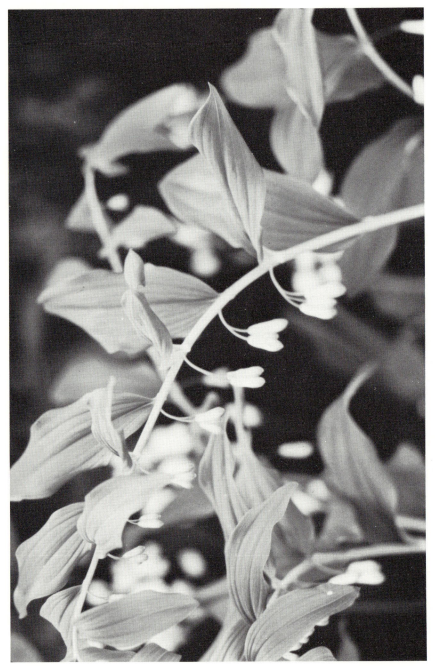

Figure 147   Polygonatum multiflorum (Solomon's Seal).

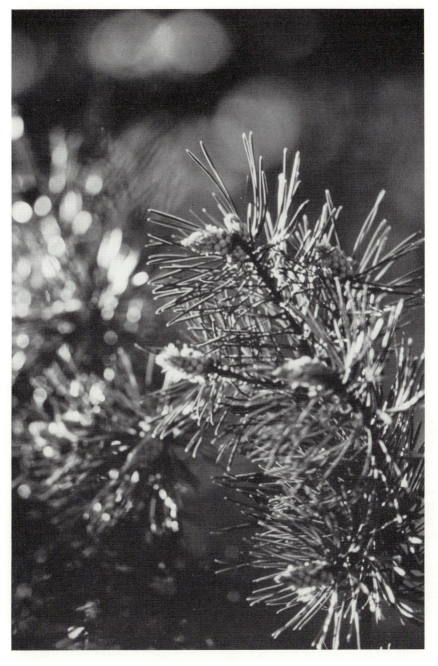

Figure 148 *Pinus sylvestris* (the Wild Pine).

Turpentine, the oleoresin obtained as an exudate from many species of the tree; it is also the source of Turpentine Oil (BP), the oil obtained by distillation and rectification from turpentine. Turpentine oil is still widely used as a rubefacient and ingredient of liniments for rheumatic pain and stiffness. These uses are very old and Celsus (*De medicina*)[2479] alludes to the Stone Pine (*Pinus pinea*), pine kernels being given in honey for cough and internally to relieve inflammation of the kidney and the symptoms of liver disease. The resin was given as a suppurative, erodent and epispastic in external use; the pitch was commonly used in plasters and as an emollient. Thus, while turpentine oil finds now no internal use, its external application is not unlike some of the uses of first-century Rome.

Eucalyptus globulus, and its many related species of the Myrtaceae, is indigenous to Australia and Tasmania where many specimens provide some of the tallest trees of the world. Synonyms are the Blue Gum Tree and Stringy Bark Tree or Fever Tree – the latter name deriving from the fact that as the tree grows it dries and drains swampy soil, so forming a natural eradicant of malaria. It has been widely introduced in the south of Europe, Algeria, Egypt, South Africa, India and California; the specimen shown in Figure 149 is typical of the species which readily thrive in southern Britain. Medicinal Eucalpytus Oil is frequently considered to be the most powerful antiseptic agent of its class; it is obtained by rectifying the oil distilled from the fresh leaves and terminal branches of various species of *Eucalyptus* and contains a large proportion of cineole (eucalyptol) and a little phellandrene with other pinenes and terpenes. Its vapour is inhaled to relieve the congestion of bronchitis and upper respiratory tract infections but like most of these essential oils it is, when swallowed or absorbed in large quantities, more toxic than its traditional uses might lead one to suspect. Deaths have been recorded from doses varying from 3.5 to 21 ml of the oil[2480].

Poisoning by plant substances produces alarming clinical conditions, sometimes the subject of conflicting reports. Amanda Bramley and Roy Goulding, in a short report on *Laburnum 'poisoning'*[2481] quote an official bulletin which says that, 'After the yew tree, the laburnum is the most poisonous tree grown in Britain...' The beautiful appearance of the tree (*Laburnum anagyroides*; Figure 150) would not lead to the suspicion that 'all parts of it are toxic, the wood, bark and roots being consistently so throughout the year...' Bramley and Goulding reported 49 cases in which patients had consumed small numbers of laburnum seeds or pods – none came to serious harm. In a subsequent letter[2482] Professor H. Ippen of Göttingen pointed out that the toxic component of laburnum is 'cytisine, also known as baptitoxine, sophorine, or ilexine...' The study serves as a reminder that the evil reputation of some plant substances seems not to be validated by objective reports.

The eclipse of medical botany today seems to be almost complete. A comparison of Jonathan Pereira's splendid *The elements of materia medica* of 1839–40[1108] and a modern pharmacopoeia shows little trace of the subject. Its remnant lies in the many, completely unproven, polypharmaceutical herbal remedies which are publicly available, and in the practice of the professional herbalist. Contemporary comment can be represented by the recent book, *Green pharmacy, a history of herbal medicine* (1981) by Barbara Griggs. This book, eminently readable, has the merit of research which has unearthed much valuable material unlikely to be familiar to the orthodox practitioner. The book does more

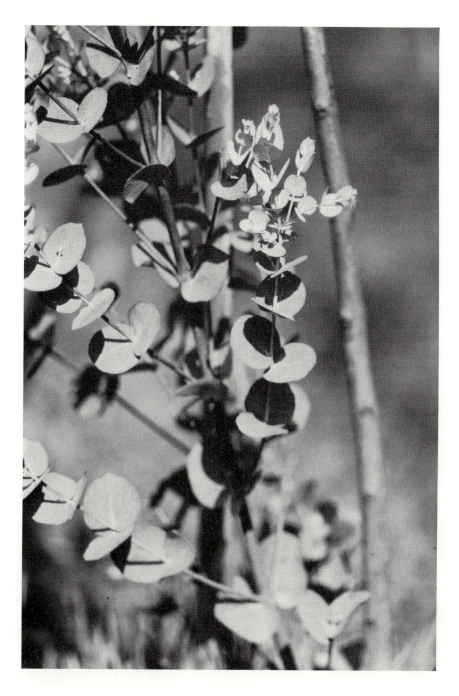

Figure 149 Eucalyptus globulus (the Blue Gum Tree, var.).

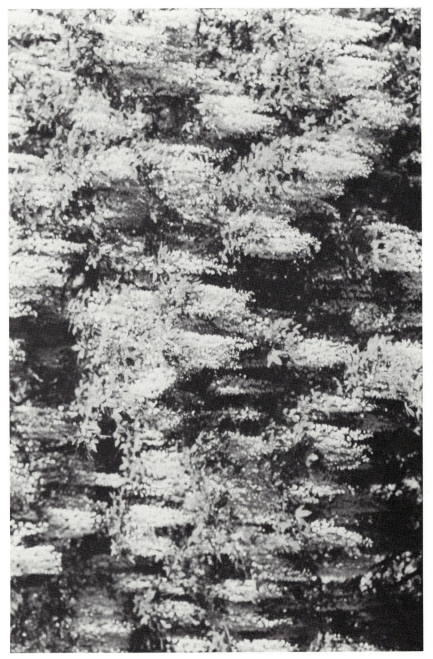

Figure 150 Laburnum anagyroides (the Common Laburnum).

to attack orthodoxies than prove the safety and efficacy of herbal remedies – it is, nevertheless, critical and refreshing. Despite these virtues, this work cannot save its subject from disgrace: perhaps the strongest evidence in favour of any one herbal product relates to a drug development project which was planned, from the outset, to be 'as super-efficient and as scientifically "respectable" '[2483] as it could possibly be made. References numbered 6–10 are then cited – the first is a set of 'double-blind trials with 123 mentally retarded children . . .'; the second is a study of the 'protective action on the fertility of white mice receiving X-ray treatment . . .'; the third is a programme in which 'sixty medical practitioners assessed the effect of each of the . . . preparations on 1140 patients . . .'; the fourth refers to the testing 'in a commercial laboratory both for chronic toxicity and for possible teratogenic (fetus-damaging) effect' (importantly, 'No adverse effects were seen in any of the preparations in any of the tests'); the fifth of these references is concerned with 'a double-blind trial . . . carried out on patients convalescing from surgery, and receiving radiation therapy'. The first of these references is cited, with appropriate details, as an 'unpublished report'; the second is not clinical; the third is of two pages; the fourth is an item in the London *Observer*, the fifth is an 'unpublished paper'. Of the sponsor of these studies it is said: '. . . he set about organizing a series of clinical trials which would leave nobody in any doubt of the worth of his product. The results of some of these were startling, to put it mildly.'

The product, or group of products, concerned in these tests may well be safe, effective, and of good quality: the present remarks are not concerned with these issues. The point of interest is the general one that in the study *Green pharmacy* . . . this seems to be the product for which the strongest formal evidence available is cited. The fact that formal double-blind clinical studies have been undertaken with a herbal remedy is important; the additional fact that conventional animal safety evaluation tests have been used in assessing such a remedy is of almost equal interest. It is perhaps disappointing that the data entered into the public domain and reviewed in a book which treats of its subject at length are such that without access to the personal communications concerned one cannot learn from the conclusions.

By and large, the available published data on herbal remedies are, to the scientist, everywhere equally disappointing.

There are many possible explanations: the herbal drugs may be neither safe, nor effective, nor of any reasonable quality; the tests that would examine these parameters have not yet been done, or the results not yet entered into the public domain; or the philosophy of the herbalist renders the tests irrelevant. The latter possibility is interesting for, if the practitioner considers each patient unique and chooses a drug judged to be specifically appropriate to that patient, then the techniques of the controlled study become inapplicable and the herbalist seeks, in effect, exemption from any legislation which imposes an inappropriate philosophy.

Such a position means that the reassurance involved in the consultation, the placebo effect of the drug, and any real activity of the drug in objective terms cannot be separated and assessed. The position would disappoint those who believe that valuable medicines remain to be discovered among the herbal remedies of repute; it would also be a cause for concern were such remedies assumed, without testing, to be safe. Patients do perhaps need to understand that the suggestion 'It seems reasonable to assume that any plant drug with a centuries-long reputation for being perfectly safe as well as effective has probably earned that reputation'[2484] overlooks what is known of the carcinogenic, mitogenic, and chronic toxic effects of some not uncommon plants.

The subject provides, to the orthodox practitioner, some unexpected examples of active plant substances. An example is the Elecampane (*Inula helenium*, of the Compositae), which has been famous for centuries, and is also known as Scabwort, Elf Dock, The Wild Sunflower, Horseheal, and Velvet Dock. It is one of the traditional healing drugs, the wort (OE *wyrt* etc.) being a plant, herb or vegetable used for food or medicine. Because of these associations the word forms the second element of various plant names, such as colewort, liverwort, and scabwort. Inulin BP is the polysaccharide granules obtained from the tubers of *Dahlia variabilis, Helianthus tuberosus,* and other genera of the family Compositae; the substance is well known as it is rapidly removed from the bloodstream following intravenous administration and predominantly eliminated in the urine by glomerular filtration – it is not subject to enzymic degradation and, as a result of these characteristics, inulin is used as a diagnostic agent to measure the glomerular filtration rate. But there is another substance, alantolactone, or Helenin (also known as Alant camphor, Elecampane camphor, or Inula camphor) which is a terpene obtained from the roots of *Inula helenium*. Alantolactone has been used as an anthelmintic but it has a curious place in the history of late nineteenth century medicine.

Mrs Grieve (*A modern herbal...*, 1931) says of the elecampane that 'In herbal medicine it is chiefly used for coughs, consumption and other pulmonary complaints...'; in the same article on the plant it is said that: 'Of late years', modern scientific research has proved that the claims of Elecampane to be a valuable remedy in pulmonary diseases has a solid basis'[2485]:

> One authority, Korab, showed in 1885 that the active, bitter principle, Helenin, is such a powerful antiseptic and bactericide, that a few drops of a solution of 1 part in 10,000 immediately kills the ordinary bacterial organisms, being peculiarly destructive to the Tubercle bacillus. He gave it successfully in tubercular and catarrhal diarrhœas, and praised it also as an antiseptic in surgery.

Koch announced the discovery of the tubercule bacillus[1515] in 1882 and, guided by the passage quoted from Mrs Grieve, it can be found that de Korab published a paper on the *Action exercée par l'hélénine sur les bacillus de la tuberculose* in that same year[2486]; he reached the following conclusion, and at a time when antituberculous drugs, of clinical application, were far into the future:

> Ces faits semblent indiquer que l'on pourra se servir de l'hélénine pour combattre les bacillus, notamment ceux de la tuberculose; et, s'il est vrai que les bacillus soient les véhicules de cette maladie, les propriétés éminemment toxiques de l'hélénine, à l'égard de ces organismes, trouveraient peut-être quelques applications heureuses.

The contemporary book, *Healing plants, a modern herbal,* edited by the physician William A. R. Thomson (1978)[2487] provides an excellent illustration of

Inula helenium and notes that the plant 'was formerly cultivated for use as a dyeing agent and for medicinal purposes'; Tyler, Brady and Robbers (*Pharmacognosy*, 1981)[2488], like Thomson, discuss the availability of inulin and its properties without at the same time referring to the work of de Korab or its subsequent exploration. Jean-Luc Stampf and his colleagues (1982)[2489] have shown that helenin is a potent sensitizer for guinea-pigs, as are alantolactone and isoalantolactone, the two main constituents of helenin; in other present-day studies Dalvi and McGowan (1982) have reported on *Helenin inhibition of liver microsomal enzymes*[2490]. Most interestingly of all, Kowalewski, Kedzia and Koniar, in a paper on the *Action of helenin on microorganisms* (1976)[2491], show that the substance is a natural, moderately potent, antibiotic with an unusually broad spectrum of activity against various genera of bacteria, yeasts and dermatophytes; these authors note that 'Helenin is not toxic for the human body and has long been employed therapeutically in doses of over 100 mg as an expectorant, cholagogue, cholerrhetic drug and to stimulate intestinal secretion' – they cite also the report of 1962 by Benigni, Capra and Cattorini on the anti-tuberculosis activity of helenin.

Thus, it is possible that therapeutic concentrations might be attained in man. If so, then the literature seems to have known of an antituberculosis antibiotic of herbal origin since the year Koch discovered the tubercule bacillus.

There are, as is well known, many associations between the botanical medicines of the past and those of today. An example, already mentioned, is *Chondodendron tomentosum* (pareira), of which Lewis and Elvin-Lewis (*Medical botany, plants affecting man's health,* 1977)[2492] say that it is 'A chief ingredient of South American Indian arrow poisons or curare'; they note it 'contains the neurologically active bis-isoquinoline alkaloid tubocurarine'. Without any idea that it might contain this neuromuscular blocking agent, which is so important, with its pharmacologically similar relatives, in modern anaesthesia, the ancients knew the same plant. It appeared in the writings of later authors, including Sir Benjamin Brodie – who did important work on physiology before he turned surgeon. In Brodie's day the plant was known as *Cissampelos pareira*, the *Pareira brava,* or Velvet Leaf and was widely used in diseases of the urinary bladder. Jonathan Pereira (*The elements of materia medica*, 1839–40)[2493] says of its history and uses:

HISTORY.—The root of this plant was first mentioned by Piso (*Hist. Nat. Brasil,* 94) in 1648, under the name of *Caapéba.* It was introduced into Paris, in 1688, by M. Amelot, the French ambassador at Portugal (Murray, *App. Med.* i. 499).

It is usually termed *Pareira* (Parreyra) *brava,* which means, literally, *wild vine,* on account of its supposed resemblance to the root of the wild vine. The Germans call it *Grieswurzel* (*i.e.* gravel root), on account of its beneficial effects in stone or gravel.

PHYSIOLOGICAL EFFECTS.—I am unacquainted with any experiments made to determine the effects of this root in the healthy state of the body. From its taste, botanical affinities, and effects in diseases, it appears to possess a tonic power, and occasionally to act as a diuretic. Furthermore, its efficacy in certain maladies of the urinary organs induces us to ascribe an almost specific influence to this root over the mucous membrane lining the urinary passages. It certainly does appear to have the power of altering the quality of the urinary secretion. Large doses prove aperient.

USES.—It was originally introduced into medicine as a lithontriptic. Its powers in this way were at one time highly vaunted, and Helvetius even went so far as to assert that calculi, the size of an olive, had disappeared under its use, and that the operation for lithotomy was no longer necessary! We now employ it almost solely *in discharges from the urino-genital mucous membrane.*—It has been used in gonorrhœa, leucorrhœa, and chronic inflammation of the bladder. In the latter of these diseases Sir B. Brodie (*Lond. Med. Gaz.* i. 300) states, that he has seen more good done by this root than by the Uva-ursi. "I am satisfied," says this eminent surgeon, "that it has a great influence over the disease which is now under consideration, lessening very materially the secretion of the ropy mucus, which is itself a very great evil, and, I believe, diminishing the inflammation and irritability of the bladder also." He recommends it to be taken in the form of a concentrated decoction, to which may be added some tincture of hyoscyamus; and in these cases, in which there is a deposit of the triple phosphates, muriatic or diluted nitric acid may be added.

Brodie would have been surprised to learn of the uses, by injection, which later surgeons would find for the active principle of the plant which he preferred, in treating bladder disease, to Uva-ursi (*Arctostaphylos Uva-ursi, Arbutus Uva-ursi*, The Bear-berry).

Many plants contain active principles about which only a limited amount is yet known – and the potential uses of which are largely unexplored. *Hibiscus rosa-sinensis*, the China rose plant, is a common Indian garden plant and is widely distributed. In the Ayurvedic literature the flowers of this species are credited with contraceptive properties. This tradition and other references stimulated Singh and co-workers (1982)[2494] to study the antifertility activity of various extracts of *Hibiscus rosa-sinensis* in female albino rats. It was found that the ether soluble portion of the water insoluble fraction of a benzene extract showed significant anti-implantation and abortifacient activities.

A different type of hormone or hormone-like activity arising in plants and potentially capable of affecting man has been reviewed by H. R. Lindner in an essay on the *Occurrence of anabolic agents in plants and their importance* (1976)[2495]. Linder noted that more than 40 plant species had been shown to contain substances active in biological assays for oestrogenic activity. These phyto-oestrogens are widely distributed among the plants which serve as animal fodder or are grown for direct human consumption. It is clear that in excessive amounts herbal oestrogens can adversely affect reproductive performance in sheep and form residues in the animal carcass. While these substances present no known serious risk to man, improved knowledge of their ecological importance seems essential.

In the present state of the subject it does perhaps seem likely that the systematic exploration of identified plant active principles will be far more fruitful than the study of highly variable pieces or complex residues of plants. However, one example of the usefulness of subjecting complex extracts or residues to conventional clinical trials is the report by Wright and Burton (*Oral evening-primrose-seed oil improves atopic eczema*, 1982)[2496]. This double-blind cross-over study evaluated various doses of oral evening-primrose oil in 99 patients and showed a significant clinical improvement when the preparation was taken in high dosage; side-effects were not noted.

In recent years the incidence of iatrogenic disease and the reports of drug disasters and drugs withdrawn from the market due to unexpected toxic effects, has motivated something of a revival of interest in medical botany and alternative medicine, including herbal medicine. This has affected, in the Western civilization, only a minority of orthodox practitioners, few of whom could recognize the items of the materia medica about which Jonathan Pereira wrote so well in 1839 and 1840. There are, however, huge segments of the world population to which herbal or indigenous remedies are virtually the only form of medical care available on a routine basis. It is important, therefore, that these remedies should be as useful as possible – and that more should be known about them.

For this reason the 31st World Health Assembly in 1978 adopted a resolution calling for an inventory of the medicinal plants used throughout the world. Dr Giuseppe Penso, previously director of the WHO unit for the study of medicinal plants, as a result, compiled a list of some 21 000 medicinal plants from 91 countries and the writings of Ayurvedic and Unani medicine. This list, the *Index plantarum medicinalium*, has recently been published in Milan.

The careful recording of some aspects of the herbal tradition might seem equally important: whilst it is highly unlikely that much will come of the generalized and usually meaningless claims made for the polypharmaceutical herbal gatherings from what might have been the Culpeper wheelbarrow, a steady tradition suggesting that a simple mixture or even single herb produces a readily verifiable effect is a different matter. Jenner may have discovered smallpox vaccination from such a tradition: if the milkmaids were the only young women not pocked by the smallpox he might well have noticed, and wondered what protected them. Withering might have discovered digitalis in the same way: the dropsy either was, or was not, relieved by the herb his examination of the tradition taught him to prescribe. In the same way, claims for a herbal contraceptive are so soon refuted that an ineffective drug would equally soon lose its reputation.

To the orthodox scientist or practitioner in the Western hemisphere much of the revival of interest must lie in the developments which have changed classical, descriptive pharmacognosy into the newer science of phytochemistry and natural product chemistry. The change can be seen in the altered contents of the successive editions of *Pharmacognosy*[2497], the study by Trease and Evans which is now widely regarded as the standard British work on its subject. The first edition of this book was published 50 years ago, in 1934; the 12th edition appeared in 1983. The contemporary approach in its practical aspects has been summarized in a valuable series of four papers by J. David Phillipson and Linda Anderson of the School of Pharmacy, London. The first of these papers, *Pharmacologically active compounds in herbal remedies* (1984)[2498], emphasizes that the pharmacological effects of herbal remedies in man are poorly documented, so that toxic adverse effects or drug interactions can result. It is clear that more information on such interactions is needed and is of interest to both the herbalist and orthodox practitioner alike.

In recent decades the knowledge of plant chemistry has been advanced by refined laboratory techniques which have made is possible to isolate compounds in extremely small quantities and undertake the structural analysis of highly complex substances. These techniques are common to many branches of chemistry and biology and provide a basis for multidisciplinary teamwork. As an example of the fruits of such work, Kurt Torssell, in his *Natural product chemistry, a mechanistic and biosynthetic approach to secondary metabolism* (1983)[2499], describes recent developments in the area of chemical communication among insects as 'a stunning example of the opening of new frontiers in science...' The complex mechanisms of nature frequently seem to involve molecules of an order of potency and acting at dilutions that were unmeasurable not many years ago. Of the natural plant products, Alfred Burger, for whom the American Chemical Society named its Award in Medicinal Chemistry, writes of 'Polyacetylenes from Compositae (which) are toxic to mosquito larvae. One of these, α-terthienyl, is more potent than DDT in insects exposed to light.' Later in his book, *A guide to the chemical basis of drug design* (1983)[2500], Burger looks back and speaks of the great era, already possibly past, of chemical new drug development:

> The years 1928–1962 have been called the golden age of medicinal science. Even World War II could not interrupt the exuberant developments in medicinal chemistry and in the experimental biochemical and biomedical sciences, with a concomitant revolutionary upturn in all branches of medicine. Although the period will prove not to have been unique, it certainly constituted an unprecedented emergence of new methods and new drugs. Medicinal chemistry contributed to these developments by furnishing hundreds of thousands of these compounds for biological evaluation. The most active areas were the antimalarials, antituberculous agents, sulfonamide drugs, antihistaminics, antipsychotic drugs, centrally acting analgetics, antihypertensive agents, oral antidiabetics, steroids, and antibiotics. Towards the end of the golden-age period, nonsteroidal antiinflammatory agents, antidepressants, antianxiety agents, semisynthetic penicillins, and the first potent anticancer drugs became the leaders in research efforts.

It is of course naïve to think that all of the complex molecules of nature are benign – or to imagine that plant substances, apart from the well-known poisonous plants and mushrooms, are innocuous. We do not yet know much about the long-term harmful effect of mutagens in man – but it is clear that the potential hazard from mutated male gametes is substantially greater than the danger from female sexual cells that have undergone mutation. Unless we are indifferent to the care of our genetic material, we should note with some concern that Lewis and Elvin-Lewis, as early as 1977[2501], listed 14 mutagens derived from plants – and, of these, aflatoxin B_1 (from *Aspergillus flavus* and other sources), cycasin (the glycoside from *Cycas circinalis* and *Cycas revoluta*), and retrosine (from *Senecio*, groundsel or ragwort) are also known to be carcinogenic. The same authors list 37 plant-derived teratogens capable of deforming the offspring of animals, if not man.

From the McArdle Laboratory at Wisconsin, James A. Miller and Elizabeth C. Miller (1983)[2502] wrote that 'A small (~ 30) but varied group of organic and inorganic compounds appear to be carcinogenic in both humans and experimental animals. A much larger number and wider variety of chemical carcinogens, primarily synthetic organic compounds, are known for experimental animals. These agents include a small (~ 30) and varied group of metabolites of green plants and fungi. Many more of these carcinogens must exist in the living world.' Many of these substances have been discussed in a number of publications; these include: *Food additives and cancer* (Fairweather and Cheryl A. Swann, 1981)[2503]; *Natural carcinogenic products of plant origin* (Iwao Hirono, 1981)[2504] – who says 'It is now clear from epidemiologic data that most human cancers are induced by environmental causes'; *Naturally occurring carcinogens* (G. N. Wogan, 1974)[2505]; and, an article on *Carcinogens occurring naturally in foods*, by Miller and Miller (1976)[2506]. The latter authors conclude their paper with the comment 'Reduction of the amounts of carcinogenic natural products in human dietaries may eventually constitute a useful weapon in the prevention of important human cancers'; they also provide the following table showing the chemicals recognized as human cancer-causing agents:

Chemicals recognized as carcinogens in the human as well as in experimental animals

Carcinogen	Targets in the human
2-Naphthylamine, benzidine, 4-aminobiphenyl, 4-nitrobiphenyl	Urinary bladder
N,N-bis(2-Chloroethyl-2-naphthylamine	Urinary bladder
bis(2-Chloroethyl) sulfide	Respiratory tract
Diethylstilbestrol	Vagina
Chloromethyl methyl ether, bis(chloromethyl) ether	Lungs
Vinyl chloride	Liver
Certain soots, tars, oils	Skin, lungs
Cigarette smoke	Lungs, other tissues
Betel nuts	Buccal mucosa
Chromium compounds	Lungs
Nickel compounds	Lungs, nasal sinuses
Asbestos	Lungs, pleura
Arsenic compounds	Skin, lungs

Another problem easily avoided is the ingestion of known mitogens, such as Poke root. As the root of *Phytolacca decandra*, this substance appeared in the BPC (1934)[2507] where it found the following uses:

Action and Uses.—Phytolacca has emetic, purgative and mildly narcotic properties, but is rarely used in medicine. The powdered drug is a powerful sternutatory. It has been employed in chronic rheumatism, usually in the form of tincture (1 in 10) or liquid extract (1 in 1).

Because of this benign early association, the substance is still found in a few complex herbal remedies.

Poke root also appears as the root of *Phytolacca americana*, synonym *P. decandra*, all parts of which are toxic except the segments growing above the ground early in the spring. Lewis and Smith (1979)[2508] reported a case of Poke root poisoning and noted that 'In May 1979, the Herb Trade Association issued a policy statement to its members requesting that because of its toxicity, poke root should not be sold as an herbal beverage or food.' The scientific work on the ability of certain plant seed proteins (lectins) to activate resting or dormant cells in the circulatory system of the human, and transform them to an active growth state, has been reviewed in an essay on *Pokeweed and other lymphocyte mitogens* by Alexander McPherson (1979)[2509].

If it is important to identify environmental carcinogens and possible genetic toxins, and avoid them in the expectation of lessening the 'carcinogen load', and so lowering the incidence of cancer, it is also important to note that the natural environment contains anticancer as well as cancer-inducing or procancerous agents. Plants have been used in the treatment of cancer for 3500 years or more, but it was only in 1959 that a systematic effort to screen crude plant extracts for their inhibitory activity against animal tumour systems began – and then under the care of the American National Cancer Institute. By the time this programme was reviewed by G. A. Cordell (*Recent experimental and clinical data concerning antitumor and cytotoxic agents from plants*) in 1977[2510], over 180 000 plant extracts from 2500 genera had been passed through this screen for potential anti-cancer activity.

The antileukaemic activity of helenalin, brusatol, bruceantin and their esters in experimental *in vivo* systems has been discussed by Iris H. Hall and colleagues (1981)[2511] – and the significance of some of the chemical configurations involved in these structures has been explored by the same group of workers from the University of North Carolina in a further publication of the same year[2512]. The two alkaloids, vincaleukoblastine (vinblastine) and leurocristine (vincristine), from the Madagascan periwinkle, *Catharanthus roseus*, are two of the most important plant anticancer agents in current clinical use. Their early history and later development has been reviewed in the essay *Anticancer agents from plants* contributed by Geoffrey A. Cordell to the interesting study *Progress in phytochemistry* (1978)[2513].

We have now a number of anticancer agents derived from botanical sources. These include several antibiotics which interfere with nucleic acids and act as cell cycle non-specific agents. Amongst these there is actinomycin D, from *Streptomyces chrysomallus* and *S. antibioticus*; bleomycin, obtained by the growth of *Streptomyces verticillus* or by other means; daunorubicin, produced by *Streptomyces coeruleorubidus* or *S. peucetius*; doxorubicin, isolated from *Streptomyces peucetius* var. *caesius*; mithramycin, produced by the growth of

Streptomyces argillaceus, S. plicatus and *S. tanashiensis*; mitomycin, which is derived from *Streptomyces caespitosus*; streptozocin (also classed as a nitrosourea), produced by synthesis or by the growth of *Streptomyces achromogenes* in variant forms; and zinostatin, which is obtained from *Streptomyces carzinostaticus*.

Some of the plant alkaloids used as antineoplastic agents, and acting as cell-cycle stage-specific agents, include vindesine (a synthetic vinca alkaloid derived from vinblastine sulphate) as well as vinblastine itself and vincristine, both of which have been already mentioned. There are, in addition, etoposide and teniposide, derived from podophyllotoxin; and mitopodozide, which is derived from podophyllin.

Although many of these agents are highly toxic and provide handling difficulties and major problems with side-effects, these and similarly active antineoplastic agents are used in the primary treatment of choriocarcinoma, leukaemia, myeloma, and some other conditions in which surgery or radiotherapy is impossible. The outstanding point is that it has been convincingly shown that permanent remissions are possible in choriocarcinoma and in acute lymphoblastic leukaemia. Varying degrees of remission or palliation can sometimes be obtained in other malignancies when these agents are used alone, in combination, or in conjunction with surgery or radiotherapy.

Thus, the plant sources have produced, in the contemporary pharmacopoeia, a substantial number of useful drugs. Perhaps the most conspicuous of these are the antibiotics – for these range in the spectrum of their effects from the ability to inhibit or destroy a wide variety of pathogenic microbial cells to an ability to attack and sometimes eradicate the malignant cell itself.

It is clear that, until the present century, the history of therapeutics was very largely the history of herbal medicine. It is easy to forget how big a part herbal remedies played in even the most orthodox forms of medicine in the first few decades of the present century. The situation has now dramatically changed and herbals, as such, are now of interest only to the herbalist and a small but perhaps growing minority of patients who turn to the herbal practitioner for medical care. It must seem unfortunate that the herbalist, perhaps through no fault of his own, has declined or been unable to apply contemporary methodology to the demonstration of the safety and efficacy of his remedies. Not unjustifiably, the consensus view has become that these remedies have no place in the management of those varieties of serious disease for which orthodox medicine has anything useful to offer.

It might be concluded that the great strides being made in pharmacognosial science, phytochemistry, and natural plant chemistry are profoundly more interesting than the current activities in herbalism. These sciences are in the vanguard of the users of contemporary laboratory technology; the molecules that they disclose can be isolated, analysed, and in some cases synthesized. It would seem that these sciences fill the hiatus left by the loss of the tradition of medical botany – and that their products, like those of the medicinal chemist, can be evaluated in the pharmacological and toxicological screens which, in the laboratory, indicate their potential usefulness, or the lack of it. Thus, it would appear that there is a real need to ensure that studies in these subjects are adequately and properly funded and that, as in the biotechnological sciences, the necessary people are trained and the products protected by appropriate types of patent – allowing them to become commercially viable medicines.

The short span

Compared with the long period during which plant medicines have been used and primitive superstition has slowly lessened its hold, the entire span of modern medicine has been quite brief. It was preceded by the recapture of the spirit of the writings of classical Greece, the intellectual adoption of the fact-based structure of science and, latterly, by the development of the experimental method. Nevertheless, the growth of modern medicine cannot be dated much before the appearance of the first edition of Laennec's *De l'auscultation médiate* . . . [1130] in 1819. It was this work, as representative of the French school of medicine of the time, which first brought together the findings of morbid anatomy and the clinical manifestations of disease. It was soon followed by the achievements of Bright, Addison, and Hodgkin in London.

The preparation of the first modern medicines can be dated from just a little earlier: from 1805, when Serturner reported [1649] the isolation of morphine. The remaining great landmarks of the nineteenth century were the development of the cell and germ theories, as epitomized by the . . . *Untersuchungen* . . . (1839) of Theodor Schwann [1200], the *Die cellularpathologie* . . . (1858) of Rudolf Virchow [1263], and the vitally important *Mémoire sur les corpuscles organisés qui existent dans l'atmosphère* . . . by Pasteur in 1861 [1490].

During this same century physiology was much advanced by the novel work of Claude Bernard and, to the meagre means of therapeutics then available, Morton [1468] added ether in 1846, Sir James Young Simpson [1473] added chloroform in 1847 – these two advances providing the miracle of inhalational anaesthesia – and, in 1867, Lord Lister [1561] introduced antiseptic surgery. The end of the century was marked by Koch's discovery of the tubercule bacillus [1515] in 1882 and Röntgen's discovery [1695] of X-rays in 1895.

The ability of the doctor to directly affect the course of disease remained strikingly limited: to today's physician the best things in the first *British Pharmacopoeia* of 1864 [1672] might seem to be digitalis, opium, atropine, a salt of morphine, quinine sulphate, ether, chloroform, ferrous sulphate, iodine, sodium bicarbonate, salt, a few household remedies, and the sources of some of the vitamins (none of which had yet been described); to this list we would want to add Jenner's vaccine. The BP itself contained, in addition to these useful materials, a fairly substantial range of toxic plant and mineral substances.

A glance through the *British Pharmaceutical Codex* of 1934, a volume [120] of exactly 50 years ago, will show how long many of the items in use in earlier centuries survived; this BPC, of just before World War II, does of course exclude all of the anbtibiotics and most of the medicines in contemporary use. The difference between the BPC of 1934 and the last one [78], of 1973, typifies the fact that, in the twentieth century, in many departments of knowledge, progress has been exponential; this has certainly been so in therapeutics. In other areas of medicine, especially in the understanding and treatment of the arteriosclerotic

688

degenerations of the great vessels and the many forms of malignancy, progress has been much less assured.

Perhaps one of the most convenient ways to recapture the medicine of the turn of the century, at its best, is to re-read Osler's *The principles and practice of medicine*...[2010], of which the first edition was published in 1892, the seventh edition (the last done by Osler alone) was produced in 1909, and the ninth edition was dated 1920. The work was marked by a clear literary style which attracted readers other than professional physicians and their students and, because of its celebrated readership, it became influential in establishing many of the Rockefeller benefactions to medicine. Osler started his descriptions of diseases with a definition and a historical note – and many of these notes are still of great value. He followed a clear plan in describing each illness and made a judicious use of statistics. As an example we can take, from his account of the aetiology of typhoid fever, the comment[2514] that: 'In the South African War the British army, 557 653 officers and men, had 57 684 cases of enteric fever, with 8225 deaths..., while only 7582 men died of wounds received in battle.' That 10.3% of this army suffered enteric fever and that 14.3% of those who contracted this illness died of it remains as memorable, from Osler's account – it is also a fact that the disease was a greater killer under active service conditions than was combat.

In 1967, reprints of selected sections of the book, with contemporary expert commentaries, were made available in a volume (*Osler's textbook revisited*)[2515] edited by A. McGehee Harvey and Victor A. McKusick. Both of these authors are of the Johns Hopkins University School of Medicine, Baltimore, where in 1889 Osler achieved the singular honour of being elected the first Professor of Medicine. At Baltimore, Osler produced, in what were perhaps the greatest years of his life, the first organized clinical unit of its kind in any Anglo-Saxon country: he taught small groups of students at the bedside and allowed detailed clerking of the patients by the students, as in the English tradition, and linked the wards with the clinical laboratories, after the German model. His therapeutics reflects that of the time: even in Edwardian England the physicians had available, as specific remedies, only quinine for malaria; emetine, active in amoebic dysentery; and mercury, used at the cost of great toxicity, in syphilis.

Erhlich's introduction[2233] of the arsenical compound 606 or 'Salvarsan', in 1911, forms the landmark which began antimicrobial chemotherapy. There was then a gap, despite all expectations, of almost 25 years before, in 1935, Domagk announced the introduction of prontosil red[2239], so beginning the sulphonamide era. During this long period, from shortly before World War I to shortly before World War II, the chemotherapeutic agents which were available seemed to attack only the protozoal parasites and the causative agent of syphilis. The sulphonamides were far more widely useful and the studies of Domagk showed that prontosil red could protect mice experimentally infected with streptococci – so beginning the era in which it has been possible to treat, with specific or directly-acting agents, microbial infections due to many of the common pathogenic cocci and bacilli.

Without doubt the greatest medical discovery of the century was the recognition, in 1928, by Sir Alexander Fleming, of the antibacterial action of a *Penicillium*[2259]. The subsequent isolation, in Oxford, of penicillin by Sir Ernst Chain and Lord Florey led to the demonstration in 1940[2262] of the therapeutic action of penicillin – this epoch-making demonstration beginning the modern era of effective antibiotic therapy.

Other great achievements which have contributed to the evolution of the modern pharmacopoeia can be represented by Walter Gaskell's *The involuntary nervous system* (1916)[1387], John Langley's *The autonomic nervous system* (1921)[1391], the work of George Barger and Sir Henry Dale on ergot and the isolation of histamine[2295], and the part played by Sir Frederick Banting and Charles Best in the discovery of insulin[2304] and its physiological effects in and about 1922. More modern history would note the fundamental part played by Sir James Whyte Black in the discovery and development of both the β-adrenergic blocking agents[2153] and the drugs able to block the histamine H_2-receptors[2324].

Studies which have introduced other drugs, important in their own right or important as beginning a new class of drugs, can be represented by the paper of Eisleb and Schaumann (1939)[2516], reporting the synthesis of pethedine, and that of Courvoisier and his colleagues (1953)[2517] on chlorpromazine. The latter became the lead drug of the phenothiazines which, despite problems of tardive dyskinesia and other adverse effects, have made such a vast difference to the treatment of many of the psychoses. Further examples are the report by Gregory Pincus and Chang Min Chueh[2518] who, in 1953, provided the first practical demonstration of the use of an oral contraceptive, and the publication by Lowell Randall and others[2519] which in 1960 introduced 'Librium', methamino-diazepoxide, so beginning the era of the 'tranquillizers'.

Any attempt to quantify the improvements brought about by modern drug therapy is difficult, if not impossible. Beneficial drug effects cannot be separated from those due to improvements in nutrition, housing, hygiene, clean water, the wider availability of better food storage, antenatal and infant welfare care, greater economic security, improved education – and a host of such factors, including the changing patterns of the natural history of disease. Perhaps the benefit is most obvious in tuberculosis: there is little doubt that effective chemotherapy has emptied many sanatoria and converted others to new uses – and much of this must be put down to the benefits of chemotherapy, even if the social factors mentioned have also conspired to lessen the numbers needing admission to such institutions. The same is true of the mental hospitals: as a result of drug therapy many patients who would previously have become institutionalized have been restored to the community. In respect of the overall mortality due to infective illnesses, Figure 143 speaks eloquently of the change between 1951 and 1973 – and it would be nihilistic to pretend that modern prophylactic and therapeutic agents have not been of substantial importance in effecting this massive change.

Regrettably, there has been a darker side. An anxiety is sometimes expressed regarding the ecological effects on both present and future generations of the endless introduction of chemical and biological entities which are unknown in nature. We have no means of knowing the effects of some of these substances on several generations of man, or upon his means of support. A number of difficulties are possible – amongst them the risk that a wide range of harmful genetic changes could arise as a result of the mutagenic action of chemicals. It is accepted that the genetic variation in man is such that the cumulative effects of additional mutations may take many generations to become manifest. In order to guard against these risks *Guidelines for the testing of chemicals for mutagenicity* (1981)[2520] have been authoritatively issued. These propose test procedures which 'when combined with studies of exposure to and metabolism of the chemicals in question, should enable an evaluation of the genetic hazards of the use of chemicals to be made.' As the same report notes, 'This should eventually enable realistic assessments of risk and benefit to be made in order to minimize any potential increase in population levels of hereditary disease.' Similar guidelines relating to carcinogenic risk have been published. While it is certainly necessary to maintain perspective regarding these remote risks, it seems equally necessary to insist that the protective tests get done, and under conditions in which the results enter the scientific domain.

Drug-induced hereditary or neoplastic disease may still be virtually unknown – but chemicals that are certain mutagens or animal carcinogens are by no means rare. The risks of these agents and of factors such as therapeutic irradiation have been discussed by several workers. Their publications include *Induced disease – drug, irradiation, occupation* (1980)[2521] edited by Leslie Preger and R. E. Steiner, and *Drug-induced pathology*[2522], edited by E. Grundmann and also of 1980. The latter authors comment that: 'The number of iatrogenic cancers among the overall cancer incidence in man is very low, but carcinogenic drugs are often used in the treatment of certain diseases.'

Few subjects have engendered such intense discussion as to the use of animals in drug development. The subject of animal experimentation came alive in the middle of the Victorian era and the resulting public debate culminated in the 1876 Cruelty to Animals Act. Rodney Deitch[2523] has summarized the recent United Kingdom parliamentary debate involving the *Laboratory Animals Protection (H.L.) Bill*[2524], introduced by The Earl of Halsbury and ordered to be printed 16th July 1979, and the competing *Protection of Animals (Scientific Purposes) Bill*[2525], presented by Mr Peter Fry and ordered, by The House of Commons, to be printed on 27th June 1979. Most seem agreed that the 1876 Act is no longer adequate in view of the great advances in research over the past century but Mr Fry and his associates seemed to consider the Halsbury Bill as 'little more than a vivisectionists' charter'. Following protracted European debate, the British Government proposals for new legislation to replace the Act of 1876 eventually appeared in the White Paper, *Scientific procedures on living animals*, published in May 1983 and summarized in the *Biologist*[2526] of that year.

Much of the debate has centred upon the design of alternative methods which avoid the use of animals and more than one conference has made it clear that progress has been slow and alternatives are unlikely ever to be the complete answer; it is also clear that they will be expensive. Illustrations of the type of unfortunate animal experiments which motivate those who oppose such studies appeared in the *BMA News Review*[2527] of April 1982 – but the literature of science continues to accumulate publications which record discomforting animal experiments for which adequate justification is lacking.

It is also worrying that it remains possible to put forward justifications, other than those of absolute biological or human need, for *repetitive* animal or human experimentation. The cost and time taken to do such repeat studies does, of course, protect a drug innovator from the copyist – but this, if the existing data are adequate for all reasonable scientific purposes, provides grossly inadequate justification for further animal sacrifice. There is always some justification, for a repeated experiment must always have some chance of adding to knowledge – but it is doubtful if the protection of commercial interest can, of itself, justify animal wastage. One would therefore disagree with a Director of Patents and Trade Marks who, in a paper on the *Confidentiality of Registration Data* (1979)[2528], suggested that second parallel experimentation 'finds its justification not only in avoiding damage to the first applicant, but also and no less in added scientific knowledge'. The 'first applicant' is, of course, the drug innovator and his application is for marketing approval for his product.

A test, the LD_{50}, which has become a mandatory requirement in the acute toxicity evaluation of new compounds, has been much criticized, not only for its great waste of animals but also for its imprecision. Dietrich Lorke (*A new approach to practical acute toxicity testing*, 1983)[2529] has recently suggested an alternative, using far fewer animals. An innovative approach to developing alternatives to the use of living animals, and with the obvious advantages of using a human and widely available living tissue, has been discussed in the recent work, *Placenta – a neglected experimental animal*[2530], by Peter Beaconsfield and Claude Villee (1979). Societies, such as FRAME, have been established to consider alternatives to the use of animals – and their activities have resulted in the valuable symposium, *Animals and alternatives in toxicity testing*[2531] (1983). Thus, there are many attempts being made to find scientifically viable alternatives to the ever-increasing volume of experimental animal use.

The fact remains that, for many essential purposes, we have at present no real alternative: there is, at this time, no way of determining if a chemical is a putative human carcinogen, other than by dose-related, life-time studies in animals and studies of the handling and metabolism of the chemical in man and the experimental species in which it is evaluated.

Three suggestions might perhaps be made: firstly, that as all toxicity testing in animals is undertaken at ethical cost, in order that all such studies should be fully utilized and unnecessary repetitions should be avoided, all studies which have used animals should rapidly enter the scientific domain, even if this is at the cost of vested interests; secondly, chemicals and drugs, because their prudent introduction into man or the environment can only take place after evaluation in animals, should be developed in response to a social need and not, with the minimum of testing, to satisfy commercial imperatives; thirdly, those who attack animal testing should not tilt at the wrong windmill: the organizations which waste animal lives are the developers of the non-essential drug, or chemical. The people who want to lessen animal suffering must be prepared to forego the possibly real advantages of the copyist drug, with its improvements. The essential need is perhaps for investment into the research which, at molecular level, will disclose the mechanisms of carcinogenesis and co-carcinogenesis, so permitting the new and predictive tests to be designed which will make the whole-animal tests that now seem essential look simplistic and primitive.

The more immediate cause for concern is that there is, in the community, an unacceptable incidence of iatrogenic, or doctor-induced, disease. Geoffrey R. Venning (1983)[2459] provides a table showing that the number of fatal reports notified on 'yellow cards' or death certificates between 1964 and 1980, and due to 12 types of adverse reaction; this amounts to 1759 persons and not one of the drugs concerned is an anticancer drug or agent specifically designed for the terminally ill. It seems likely that a proportion of these 1759 patients would not have died from their disease and might well have survived on alternative therapy.

The information on adverse reactions to drugs is of two principal types: firstly, that which tells the prescriber of a particular drug what are its most likely side-effects; and secondly, information, relating to each symptom, and indicating the most likely causative drug.

The first type of information is readily available but in an unquantified way. The *Physician's desk reference* or (to a lesser extent) the *British National Formulary*, or the individual-product *Data Sheet*, lists the side-effects reported with the particular drug. This information, although it would be more useful if it were ranked to disclose incidence, enables the prescriber to watch out for likely side-effects; it also enables tests to be undertaken to detect likely adverse effects at an early stage.

The second type of information is harder to come by: it enables the clinician, faced with a symptom or illness of obscure cause, to determine, in order of probability, the most likely causative drug if, in fact, the lesion is iatrogenic.

In the United Kingdom the Committee on Safety of Medicines possesses a *Register of Adverse Reactions* which has been built up, since the days of the Dunlop Committee, from data submitted as 'yellow cards' by individual medical practitioners. This data base is unique in both duration and extent. Its basis is the opinions of clinicians who have attended the patients who have suffered the drug reactions: it is therefore as fallible, and as reliable, as the judgements of doctors regarding their own patients. At autopsy (the process often regarded as the final arbiter of fact) the pathologist has to make up his mind whether, for example, the patient has died *with* or *of* a pulmonary embolism. Some subjectivity creeps into this decision, and a good deal more into any decision-making that relates to the living. But there is not, and there is not likely to be, a firmer data base regarding drug side-effects than the voluntary adverse reaction reports of the patient's physician.

Even so, the inclusion of a side-effect in the *Register of Adverse Reactions* does not necessarily mean that it has been caused by the drug: other drugs may have been taken, the patient may have suffered more than one side-effect, the so-called 'adverse effect' may have been due to the underlying disease or have been fortuitous to treatment or, in some other way, the doctor may have been wrong. Large numbers of reports are not likely to be due to such causes and, unless there are only a few reports, such causes are not likely to invalidate comparisons between drugs – other things being equal.

A computer print-out with the code number FO6S is supplied to the medical and dental professions on request; it lists, by its generic or non-proprietary name, the drug indicated by the reporting doctor as the one most likely to have been responsible for suspected reaction. Only the most important reaction in the individual patient is listed in this print-out, which has obvious problems in relation to combination products: in the case of oral contraceptives, for example, thrombotic events are usually listed against the oestrogen rather than the progestogen. Nevertheless, the doctor who includes a drug in his personal pharmacopoeia and is not familiar with the current FO6S cannot regard himself as fully informed.

Numerical comparisons between reactions associated with different drugs cannot be considered reliable unless special precautions are taken. It is necessary to consider not only the incidence of a particular reaction with a specific drug over unit time (the numerator) but also the relevant volume of prescriptions, as an indicator of patient exposure (the denominator). Even this fraction may need restrictions so that drugs are compared only with others in the same therapeutic class and comparison is made between their adverse reactions profile during a comparable stage after marketing: with non-steroidal anti-inflammatory drugs, for example, J. C. P. Weber (1984)[2470] has shown that the rate of reporting increases usually towards the end of the second calendar year of marketing and thereafter declines.

An alternative presentation of the data from the *Register of Adverse Reactions* of the Committee on Safety of Medicines is exemplified in Tables 9–14 inclusive[2532]. The master Tables (FO5SM) from which these abbreviated Tables were derived have certain characteristics: only the drug suspected of causing the reaction is included. If the patient was having more than one drug then the reporting physician or specialist medical assessor has decided which was the one most likely to have caused the reported side-effect. Only the most important adverse reaction is included. Reports were discarded if the most important reaction started before the suspect drug was commenced. Deaths considered to be due to the drug are included in both the 'reports' and 'deaths' columns. Data for the whole period 1964–1978 are given in one column, then those of the separate years from 1979 to 1984 (cut-off point, 16 February, 1984), then there is a total for the whole period of data collection, 1964–1984.

In the abbreviated Tables 9–14 the drug has been omitted if, for the total period 1964–1984, the number of reports is less than ten or the number of attributed deaths less than two. This not only shortens the Tables, it cuts out many of the 'background' factors. In addition, the individual years between 1979 and 1984 are represented by the data for 1983, the last complete year and the one best showing the present pattern of side-effects. The abbreviated Tables retain the original totals for the reaction, as in the master Tables, and the total number of drugs in the master Tables is shown as '*n*'.

The doctor faced with deciding the most probable cause of an extrapyramidal disorder due to a drug might note, from Table 9, that metoclopramide is by far the most commonly reported if the whole period 1964 to 1984 is considered; however, in 1983, only 37 reports (of which two were fatalities) were received for this condition.

From Table 10 it can be noted that roughly two-thirds of the 916 apparent drug-related cases of aplastic anaemia that have been reported over the 20 years of data collection have been fatal; this condition, when it does occur, is one of the greatest killers – phenylbutazone was by far the most frequently associated drug and was considered to account for 223 deaths.

Agranulocytosis, as shown in Table 11, has been reported as being caused by drugs somewhat less often – on 647 occasions; of these, something like 40% were fatal, but again phenylbutazone was the most frequent cause of both reports and drug-attributed deaths. In 1983, however, mianserin was the most frequently reported cause of agranulocytosis.

Table 9 Extrapyramidal disorders

Drug name	1964–1978 Reports	1964–1978 Deaths	1983 Reports	1983 Deaths	1964–1984 Reports	1964–1984 Deaths
Prochlorperazine	49	0	3	0	62	0
Perphenazine	46	0	0	0	50	0
Trifluoperazine	19	0	0	0	22	0
Thiethylperazine	7	0	0	0	10	0
Fluphenazine	56	1	0	0	62	2
Flupenthixol dihydrochloride	13	0	6	0	26	0
Thioridazine	9	0	0	0	10	0
Haloperidol	45	1	6	2	53	3
Metoclopramide	246	1	9	0	329	1
Diazoxide	12	0	0	0	12	0
$n = 134$						
Totals for reaction*	669	3	37	2	886	7

*Totals for reaction are those for all 134 drugs listed on the master table – see text for explanation.

Table 10 Aplastic anaemia

Drug name	1964–1978		1983		1964–1984	
	Reports	Deaths	Reports	Deaths	Reports	Deaths
Phenobarbitone	6	4	0	0	6	4
Methaqualone	5	4	0	0	5	4
Methoin	4	4	0	0	4	4
Phenytoin	8	6	2	0	10	6
Troxidone	3	2	0	0	4	3
Pheneturide	2	2	0	0	2	2
Chlorpromazine	3	2	0	0	3	2
Trifluoperazine	2	2	0	0	3	3
Diazepam	6	5	0	0	6	5
Amitriptyline	7	5	0	0	7	5
Mianserin	0	0	1	0	4	3
Dextropropoxyphene	3	2	0	0	3	2
Phenylbutazone	268	213	1	0	287	223
Oxyphenbutazone	93	69	1	1	98	73
Piroxicam	0	0	1	1	4	4
Acetylsalicylic acid	3	2	0	0	3	2
Aurothiomalate Sod.	16	13	0	0	19	14
Fenoprofen Calcium	4	2	0	0	9	5
Benoxaprofen	0	0	0	0	9	6
Flurbiprofen	1	1	1	0	5	3
Ibuprofen	7	6	0	0	11	10
Naproxen	7	5	2	2	13	10
Flufenamic acid	2	2	0	0	2	2
Indomethacin	26	23	2	0	35	28
Carbamazepine	9	4	0	0	16	7
Methyldopa	8	8	0	0	8	8
Oxprenolol	5	3	0	0	5	3
Digoxin	4	3	0	0	4	3
Diphenhydramine	2	2	0	0	2	2

Carbimazole	4	4	0	0	4	4
Chlorpropamide	5	4	0	0	6	5
Acetazolamide	3	3	1	1	4	4
D-penicillamine	7	5	4	2	13	7
Ampicillin	4	3	0	0	4	3
Streptomycin	4	2	0	0	4	2
Chloramphenicol	30	26	0	0	31	26
Tetracycline	5	2	0	0	5	2
Oxytetracycline	5	5	0	0	5	5
Sulphasalazine	7	4	0	0	10	5
Co-trimoxazole	21	17	1	1	29	22
Aminosalicylate Sod.	3	2	0	0	3	2
Influenza vaccine (Inactivated)	2	2	0	0	2	2
Methotrexate	5	5	0	0	7	7
Azathioprine	6	5	0	0	8	7
Thiotepa	6	4	0	0	6	4
Busulphan	6	6	0	0	8	8
Chlorambucil	4	3	0	0	4	3
Cyclophosphamide	9	7	0	0	9	7
Bleomycin sulphate	1	1	0	0	2	2
n = 166						
Totals for reaction	759	560	30	8	916	642

Table 11 Agranulocytosis

Drug name	1964–1978		1983		1964–1984	
	Reports	Deaths	Reports	Deaths	Reports	Deaths
Methaqualone	8	3	0	0	8	3
Nitrazepam	6	2	0	0	6	2
Phenytoin	5	2	1	0	7	2
Promazine.	11	5	0	0	12	6
Chlorpromazine	31	20	3	1	39	25
Fluphenazine	2	2	0	0	2	2
Thioridazine	8	5	2	2	14	9
Diazepam	6	4	0	0	6	4
Mianserin	1	0	10	1	32	3
Clomipramine	1	1	1	1	4	2
Amiphenazole	4	2	0	0	4	2
Dipyrone	6	3	0	0	6	3
Phenylbutazone	61	37	2	2	67	40
Oxyphenbutazone	32	11	0	0	34	12
Aurothiomalate Sod.	2	2	1	1	3	3
Benoxaprofen	0	0	1	1	6	4
Mefenamic acid	2	2	0	0	3	3
Feprazone	1	1	0	0	2	2
Indomethacin	10	4	1	0	12	4
Methyldopa	6	2	0	0	7	2
Propranolol	3	2	0	0	3	2
Phenindione	7	3	0	0	8	3
Methylthiouracil	3	2	0	0	3	2
Carbimazole	25	8	2	1	33	12
Chlorpropamide	3	3	0	0	3	3
Hydrochlorothiazide	2	2	0	0	2	2
Bendrofluazide	2	2	0	0	3	2
Ethacrynic acid	3	2	0	0	4	3

D-penicillamine	8	2	0	0	12	3
Penicillin N.O.S.	3	2	0	0	3	2
Chloramphenicol	7	5	0	0	7	5
Sulphasalazine	16	7	5	2	33	13
Sulphadimidine	4	3	0	0	5	3
Sulphametropyrazine	3	1	0	0	5	2
Co-trimoxazole	26	8	1	1	39	12
Sulphonamide N.O.S.	3	3	0	0	3	3
Dapsone	6	3	4	2	12	6
Methotrexate	3	3	0	0	4	4
Azathioprine	6	4	1	0	8	4
Thiotepa	7	4	0	0	7	4
Cyclophosphamide	3	3	0	0	5	5
Totals for reaction	461	206	54	21	647	265

$n = 134$

699

Table 12   Jaundice

Drug name	1964–1978 Reports	Deaths	1983 Reports	Deaths	1964–1984 Reports	Deaths
Halothane	224	81	6	2	242	83
Methaqualone	11	1	0	0	11	1
Sodium valproate	4	2	2	0	10	2
Chlorpromazine	203	33	4	0	220	34
Prochlorperazine	8	0	1	0	10	0
Trifluoperazine	9	1	0	0	11	1
Thioridazine	9	0	0	0	11	0
Chlordiazepoxide	10	0	0	0	11	0
Diazepam	11	0	0	0	12	0
Imipramine	19	2	0	0	20	2
Amitriptyline	29	0	1	0	31	0
Mianserin	4	0	4	0	16	0
Iprindole	38	0	0	0	38	0
Dothiepin	7	0	0	0	10	0
Zimelidine hydrochloride	0	0	10	0	16	0
Phenoperidine	7	2	0	0	7	2
Dextropropoxyphene	28	0	0	0	34	0
Phenylbutazone	27	0	1	0	32	0
Oxyphenbutazone	11	0	0	0	12	0
Benoxaprofen	0	0	2	1	33	10
Ibuprofen	12	0	0	0	12	0
Ibufenac	26	2	0	0	26	2
Diclofenac Sodium	0	0	0	0	11	0
Feprazone	2	0	0	0	15	0
Indomethacin	23	2	1	0	25	2
Sulindac	10	0	3	0	21	0
Carbamazepine	18	0	0	0	32	0
Methyldopa	72	2	0	0	76	2

Cimetidine	9	1	1	0	28	1
Ethinyloestradiol	66	1	0	0	70	1
Mestranol	34	0	0	0	34	0
Human Antihaemophilic fraction	3	0	1	0	11	0
Frusemide	8	1	1	0	12	1
Fusidic acid	27	0	8	1	50	1
Rifampicin	43	2	1	0	53	2
Erythromycin	7	1	2	0	16	1
Erythromycin estolate	53	0	2	0	62	0
Co-trimoxazole	54	0	1	0	64	0
Isoniazid	14	0	0	0	14	0
Nitrofurantoin	13	0	1	0	16	0
Ketoconazole	0	0	11	0	21	0
Estramustine	0	0	0	0	4	4
$n = 302$						
Totals for reaction	1562	156	98	5	2029	179

Table 13 Melaena

Drug name	1964–1978		1983		1964–1984	
	Reaction	Deaths	Reaction	Deaths	Reaction	Deaths
Phenylbutazone	24	1	1	0	27	1
Piroxicam	0	0	16	0	97	1
Acetylsalicylic acid	18	1	0	0	21	1
Diflunisal	13	1	0	0	28	1
Benorylate	7	0	0	0	13	0
Ketoprofen	32	1	8	2	50	3
Fenoprofen Calcium	15	0	2	1	19	1
Benoxaprofen	0	0	0	0	33	2
Indoprofen	0	0	9	0	15	0
Flurbiprofen	8	0	4	1	25	1
Ibuprofen	14	0	1	0	28	0
Diclofenac Sodium	1	0	6	1	19	1
Naproxen	34	0	7	0	59	0
Indomethacin	33	1	28	1	74	2
Sulindac	9	1	0	0	10	1
Zomepirac	0	0	3	0	18	0
Azapropaxone	9	0	2	0	18	0
Tiaprofenic acid	0	0	4	0	10	0
Anticoagulant N.O.S.	2	2	0	0	2	2
Corticosteroids N.O.S.	3	3	0	0	3	3
Totals for reaction	273	15	99	6	659	25

n = 80

Table 14 Haematemesis

Drug name	1964–1978		1983		1964–1984	
	Reaction	Deaths	Reaction	Deaths	Reaction	Deaths
Caffeine	9	2	0	0	9	2
Phenylbutazone	51	9	1	1	52	10
Piroxicam	0	0	22	1	85	4
Acetylsalicylic acid	31	12	5	0	48	12
Diflunisal	20	2	0	0	34	3
Benorylate	4	0	0	0	8	2
Ketoprofen	32	3	11	2	55	6
Fenoprofen Calcium	13	3	1	0	20	3
Fenbufen	0	0	6	0	10	0
Benoxaprofen	0	0	2	0	23	0
Indoprofen	0	0	14	1	17	1
Flurbiprofen	13	1	6	2	34	5
Ibuprofen	27	2	6	0	51	3
Diclofenac Sodium	0	0	5	0	17	1
Fenclofenac	0	0	1	0	11	1
Naproxen	47	2	9	1	84	6
Indomethacin	37	12	40	7	99	24
Sulindac	7	0	0	0	11	0
Zomepirac	0	0	1	0	19	1
Azapropazone	11	2	8	0	31	3
Analgesics N.O.S.	6	5	0	0	6	5
Phenindione	3	2	0	0	3	2
Anticoagulant N.O.S.	6	6	0	0	6	6
Cortisone	2	2	0	0	2	2
Prednisone	5	4	0	0	5	4
Prednisolone	5	2	0	0	5	2
Corticosteroids N.O.S.	18	16	0	0	18	16
n = 123						
Totals for reaction	438	98	159	18	916	142

Table 12 summarizes the data as they relate to drug-attributed jaundice. Over the 20 years there have been over 2000 reports of this condition and almost 9% of these have been fatal. No less than 302 drugs have been involved, halothane and chlorpromazine being most frequently reported. The place of both zimelidine hydrochloride and ketoconazole in these figures in 1983 is to be noted.

Melaena, as a seemingly drug-related event (Table 13) has been reported 659 times – about as often as agranulocytosis. The non-steroidal anti-inflammatory agents have been by far the commonest cause, piroxicam (97 reactions), indomethacin (74 reactions), naproxen (59 reactions) and ketoprofen (50 reactions) predominating.

Table 14 shows 916 reports of haematemesis over the 20-year period with 142 deaths. In 1983, indomethacin was the cause of 40 reports with seven deaths, piroxicam led to 22 reports with one death, indoprofen caused 14 reports with one death, and ketoprofen caused 11 reports with two deaths – again the non-steroidal anti-inflammatory agents were conspicuous.

The data contained in Tables 9–14, representative of only a very small segment of the information contained in the *Register of Adverse Reactions*, exemplify the value of the 'yellow card' reporting system; the Tables also illustrate the guidance to prescribers that can now be derived from the accumulated and analysed statistics. The available numbers imply, as might be expected, that potent drugs are seldom, if ever, safe enough to be used on any basis other than a careful benefit-to-risk appraisal in the individual patient.

It might be noted how little of this information has, in the past, entered the public domain – a situation which is now rapidly changing. The restricted way in which these figures have been used is striking – and especially as there has been much information on therapeutics in general. The quantitative content of the *British Medical Journal* over the 2.5 year period from 3 January, 1981 to 25 June, 1983 was, for example, as follows:

Leading articles: total 596, of which 100 (16.8%) were mainly on drugs.
Original papers: total 2085, of which 629 (30.2%) were largely on drugs.
Questions: total 500, of which 146 (29.2%) emphasized drugs.
Letters: total 3484, of which 636 (18.3%) were on drug subjects.
Book reviews: total 748, of which 46 (6.1%) were concerned with books on drugs and drug subjects.

During the whole of this period there was no regular display of data summarizing the content of the *Register of Adverse Reactions*.

Recent events have emphasized the difficult adverse reactions experience resulting from widespread use of the non-steroidal anti-inflammatory agents. It has been reported[2533] that in the last 5 years the total number of reports received on 'yellow cards' by the Committee on Safety of Medicines amounted to the following:

1979	10 840 reports
1980	10 179
1981	13 032
1982	10 922
1983	12 689

These numbers show that iatrogenic disease has reached substantial proportions; the probability that there is gross under-reporting of drug side-effects adds weight to this suggestion. In 1983, 3154 (about 25%) of the total of 12 689 yellow card reports were associated with the non-steroidal anti-inflammatory agents. The number of adverse effects attributed to this group of drugs has risen over the recent years, as is shown by the following figures on the number of 'yellow card' reports, the number of reports received from industry, and the number from other sources – the data[2534] being given in response to a recent parliamentary question:

Year	Yellow-card report	Industry report	Others	Deaths
1964	84	15	20	21
1965	409	36	50	51
1966	184	37	24	49
1967	171	21	46	46
1968	190	27	44	47
1969	203	43	35	46
1970	188	29	32	40
1971	139	44	43	45
1972	215	38	51	51
1973	236	42	19	46
1974	433	75	54	67
1975	274	61	95	99
1976	472	84	49	54
1977	1 072	84	60	61
1978	1 679	242	69	61
1979	1 812	314	106	63
1980	2 309	594	84	55
1981	4 017	309	182	88
1982	3 021	255	309	111
1983	3 154	336	276	127

While these reports do not necessarily establish a causal relationship between the adverse reaction and the drug concerned, each report must represent such a suspicion in the mind of the attending physician – and none can be in a better position to know. In a further parliamentary reply[2534] it was advised that the number of reactions and deaths recorded since 1964 and in which phenylbutazone or oxyphenbutazone was the suspect drug came to the following:

	Total reports registered	Deaths
Phenylbutazone	1 693	445
Oxyphenbutazone	508	131

It seems likely that the total number of deaths quoted above was important in the decisions which, in the United Kingdom, have recently restricted the use of phenylbutazone to the treatment of ankylosing spondylitis and the distribution of the drug to hospitals only. It is only when these numbers are viewed against the undoubted analgesic activity of the drug and its vast use over a long period of time that the difficulties of such a decision are apparent. In the United Kingdom *The Medical Directory 1983* contains more than 100 000 entries[2535] – and the number of deaths thought to be due to phenylbutazone has to be spread over the prescribing activities throughout something like two decades of a profession approaching this size. It is perhaps not surprising that the individual practitioner reacts with hostility to a corporate decision made on the basis, or much influenced by, an inapparent global number – the total of reported deaths.

The epidemiological or community hazard is inapparent to the prescriber and Weber (1984)[2470] has made the point that both the proportionate approach (the number of reactions as a function of the number of prescriptions) and the absolute number of reactions may need to be considered by a Drug Regulatory Authority. The same is, of course, true for a pharmaceutical company. Weber then comments on the following theoretical example:

> A drug which causes the death of one patient during one year in which 100 000 prescriptions have been written, and which continues to do this at the same prescribing rate, will not constitute a serious epidemiological hazard. However, if the rate of prescribing is 2 000 000 prescriptions per year, there will be 20 deaths. After 2 years, a very short period in the marketing life of most drugs, there will be 40 deaths, and this, as an absolute total, may be unacceptable.
>
> In assessing this situation, a Drug Regulatory Authority will need to consider: (a) the severity and prognosis of the clinical condition the drug is used to treat; (b) the clinical efficacy of the drug; and (c) the availability and efficacy of alternative therapy.

Two further things follow. In a recent review[2536], *Postmarketing surveillance of adverse reactions to drugs*, Professor Michael D. Rawlins (1984), after revisiting the relevant studies so far undertaken and noting their size, comments that in future 'such studies are likely to be worthwhile ... only if they enrol at least 10 times the number of patients in the premarketing trials and include a reasonable comparative control group. They will therefore need to include at least 10 000 patients and 10 000 controls, and the cost will be substantial. Yet they will detect, with 95% confidence, only those events occurring in one in 3000 patients.' Other workers[2551, 2552] have given detailed consideration to the numbers needed in these studies.

Thus, it would seem that postmarketing surveillance could not monitor the 2 000 000 prescriptions for 2 years that would have produced 40 deaths likely to lead to regulatory action in Weber's example – nor could it be relied on to detect the ratio of the 445 phenylbutazone-attributed deaths, for these are likely to be less than 1 in 3000 patients during any practical monitoring period. Information is available showing the number of deaths each year from 1964 to 1983 and in which phenylbutazone was the suspect drug[2534]; of the 442 deaths considered, the mean annual number of deaths was 22.1 (range 4–48 in any 1 year). The 48 deaths were reported in 1975 (when there was a special study in progress) and the number of prescriptions was approximately 3 200 000.

The second point is that even the best of individual practitioners can have, from personal experience, no inkling of the problem: a practice of 3000 patients, even if a tenth of them are on the same drug, could be studied for a near infinite period without detecting an event that happens at a ratio of only 1 in 3000. And yet, if the event concerned is death, a ratio of 1 in 3000 is likely to be totally unacceptable: it means 100 deaths in 300 000 treated patients – and the latter number represents small-volume usage.

The problems of making the difficult decisions concerned with restricting the use of drugs once they have been marketed, or of removing them from the market altogether, are obvious: the ratio of severe reactions to the number of patients exposed to the drug may be unacceptable, or the absolute number of severe reactions may be intolerable, or both factors may combine to precipitate a decision. The difficulties do perhaps lend some support to the suggestion that drugs for general use should be those upon a selected list from which, for the purposes of reimbursement, they are displaced as alternative remedies are shown, during phased or graduated release, to be safer or more effective. It is a personal opinion, and that only, that drugs should be added to such a list only on the basis of demonstrated need and comparative advantage. The ranking of those alternatives within such a list might then reflect the whole weight of recorded experience, indicating to the individual prescriber the safest of the alternatives as the preferred choice with which to begin treatment.

Another option is that the doctor evaluates the alternatives himself, building a personal pharmacopoeia and including only those drugs found to be essential and which become well-known. Especial care needs to be taken to appreciate the problems of drugs used in the elderly, in association with other drugs, or given for any length of time. To build and maintain such a knowledge the prescriber needs the fullest possible information about the chosen drugs – and the greatest reluctance to add new drugs. To help with the choice – of great advantage to the sponsor of the preferred drug – the consumer-type advertising and detailing-aids might be replaced with summaries of the totality of the data and convenient presentations of the recorded drug side-effects, these being seen as a function of time and the volume of relevant prescriptions.

Whatever view is taken, controversy disappears when discussion urges the improved reporting of adverse reactions experience. Both the *Annual Report for 1982* and that for *1983*[2533] of the *Committee on Safety of Medicines* mention the important initiatives taken as a result of the Working Party established under the chairmanship of Professor Grahame-Smith to consider the role of the Committee in adverse drug reaction monitoring. The subject is the practitioner's individual responsibility: clinical acumen and alertness are clearly indispensable in detecting new and unknown aspects of drug efficacy or hazard, and differentiating these from the events of the diseases being treated; in just the same way, improvements in the techniques of reporting suspected adverse drug reactions must seem an essential contribution to the safe and effective use of medicines.

Phenylbutazone has, from many points of view, been a special case; it gives little or no indication of the threshold of harmful experience at which a drug regulatory authority, or pharmaceutical company, or both in consultation, will take action – and either severely limit the use of the drug to improve the benefit-to-risk ratio, or take it off the market altogether. Perhaps because it was the lead drug of its class, because it could be quite dramatic in some acute cases of gout and very useful in long-term use in some patients with severe osteoarthritic lesions, its risks – which were considered well understood – were tolerated. The toleration assumes that the practitioner can guard against the problem that he understands – but there is no proof, in respect of uncommon, fatal lesions of the gut or blood forming organs, that he can do that. By 1979 the profession was well aware of the problem – and yet, even though the number of prescriptions fell inexorably, the deaths fell only in proportion to the lesser usage of the drug. The profession was not more effective in preventing these deaths, except to the extent that it stopped using the drug.

Thus, the incidence of reported deaths per million prescriptions for phenylbutazone and oxyphenbutazone up to 1982 (the latest year for which full prescription figures are available)[2537] was as follows:

	Phenylbutazone	Oxyphenbutazone
1979	7.1	9.6
1980	3.9	6.1
1981	4.2	8.2
1982	6.1	4.4

The incidence of deaths reported as suspected adverse reactions associated with the use of *all* non-steroidal anti-inflammatory drugs over this same 4-year period was[2537]:

Year	Number
1979	4.1
1980	3.5
1981	5.2
1982	6.9

Some of the non-steroidal anti-inflammatory agents contributing to the last set of figures have provided experience which does, perhaps better than phenylbutazone, indicate the threshold at which there is an authoritative response.

Information about drugs withdrawn for safety reasons after marketing is available from a number of sources. In December, 1983 a *Consolidated list of products whose consumption and/or sale have been banned, withdrawn, severely restricted or not approved by governments* was issued after preparation by the United Nations Secretariat[2538]. There is also a report, *OPE Study 68*[2539], which was prepared for the Office of Planning and Evaluation of the United States FDA. The report shows that a total of 614 new chemical entities were introduced in the United States and United Kingdom during the period from January, 1960 to December, 1982. 367 of these drugs were introduced into the USA and 514 into the UK. There were therefore 881 entries on the combined markets. 133 of these

881 introductions were discontinued, 18 of them (eight in the USA and ten in the UK) for reasons of safety. The withdrawals of zomepirac (from both markets) and of zimeldine and indoprofen (the latter two in the UK only) took place after the closing date of the study. This brings the total of safety discontinuations in the United Kingdom to 13.

Of these 13 drugs withdrawn for safety reasons in the UK, five have been withdrawn fairly recently; these comprised one agent for the treatment of severe depression and four non-steroidal anti-inflammatory agents (the latter exclude phenylbutazone and oxyphenbutazone which underwent very gross restrictions and remain under review at the time of writing).

The antidepressant was Zelmid (zimeldine). It was introduced in the United Kingdom in 1982. In August, 1983 the Committee on Safety of Medicines reported[2540] that although there had been fewer than 100 000 prescriptions for the drug, over 300 reports of adverse reactions associated with it had been received. Of these, more than 60 were serious and included convulsions, liver damage, neuropathies, and cases of the Guillain–Barré syndrome. Deaths in which zimeldine was the suspect drug were seven[2472]. The manufacturers withdrew the product from the market in September, 1983 and surrendered the Product Licence.

The four non-steroidal anti-inflammatory agents which have been withdrawn from the UK market following concern about their safety during the last 5 years are Opren, Zomax, Osmosin, and Flosint.

Opren (benoxaprofen) is the subject of a fairly extensive summary in the Chief Medical Officer's annual report *On the state of the public health* for 1982[2541]. This points out that in August, 1982, the Product Licence for Opren was suspended on the grounds of safety after the Committee on Safety of Medicines had received over 3500 reports of adverse reactions associated with the drug, including 61 deaths. Following this suspension the manufacturer withdrew the drug worldwide and shortly afterwards surrendered the UK Product Licences.

The drug had been licensed in February, 1980 on the basis of data relating to some 2000 patients; it was known to cause a small number of cases of both onycholysis and photosensitivity but the efficacy was such that the 'benefit of the drug against its risk was acceptable'. Following the launch in 1980 the Committee became concerned about the number of reports of photosensitivity and severe gastrointestinal reactions being received and associated with the use of benoxaprofen. In May, 1982 the Committee, with the adverse reactions profile of the drug under close review, recommended that the dosage in elderly patients should, as a precaution, be halved. The evidence considered by the Committee included the important paper by Hugh McA. Taggart and Joan Alderdice (1982)[2542] reporting five patients over 80 years of age who had been taking benoxaprofen and had developed jaundice and had died.

The paper by Taggart and Alderdice and subsequent reports in the medical literature of liver and kidney damage thought to be due to the drug were followed by a rapid increase in the number of adverse reaction reports received by the Committee on Safety of Medicines. By the end of July, 1982, benoxaprofen had become the suspect drug in 61 fatal cases; various lesions of the gastrointestinal tract, liver, kidney and bone marrow had been reported, with liver damage the most frequent cause of death.

Parliamentary questions elicited the facts that the product was marketed for 22 months and that about 1 500 000 prescriptions were issued for it[2543]; as a result of the review of the non-steroidal anti-inflammatory agents and benoxaprofen in particular, the Committee indicated that from January, 1985 data on the effects of a new drug in the elderly would, in specified circumstances, have to be provided before new drugs were licensed[2544].

There are three points of outstanding medical interest that relate to benoxaprofen and go some way to explain its tragic story. Firstly, Taggart and Alderdice[2542] drew attention to work showing that in a dose of 600 mg daily the drug had a half-life of 111 hours at mean age 82 years compared with its much shorter half-life of 29 hours at a mean age of 41 years. Secondly, the same authors reported that in the three of their cases which came to necropsy, there was a canalicular cholestatic type of jaundice and 'A striking feature of all these cases was the rapidly fatal course after the onset of jaundice despite the immediate withdrawal of the drug. This was associated with acute renal failure in at least four of the patients.' The third point relates to the large number of serious adverse reaction reports which seem to have been received fairly shortly before the drug was withdrawn. One theory is that the paper of Taggart and Alderdice[2542], which appeared in the *British Medical Journal* in May, 1982, so much increased awareness of the problem that it prompted more reports. Even if this is correct, a second and much more significant factor is likely to have operated for J. P. Griffin (1984)[2545] has shown that the fatal cases of the benoxaprofen hepatorenal syndrome had received the drug for an average of 8.5 (SE ± 1.2, range 1–24) months, and the non-fatal cases for a mean of 6.9 (SE ± 1.9, range 0.5–15) months; similarly, fatal cases of liver damage alone had received the drug for an average period of 10.6 (SE ± 1.75, range 1.5–17) months and fatal cases of renal failure had been treated with benoxaprofen for a mean period of 6.2 (SE ± 2.4, range 1–26) months. Thus, treatment periods have to be prolonged before the hepatorenal syndrome becomes manifest. It is therefore highly unlikely that short-term studies would detect this syndrome or that it would show up convincingly in any postmarketing surveillance scheme unless this included long treatment periods. Very recently, Professor R. N. MacSween[2546] of the Department of Pathology, University of Glasgow, has exhibited, in a lecture given by Professor Sir Abraham Goldberg, histopathological specimens showing the hepatic and renal damage detected in a study of 22 patients treated with benoxaprofen. In 21 of these 22 patients, there was diffuse hepatocellular and canalicular cholestasis; some specimens show pathognomonic laminated concretions, of a rather unique and unusual appearance, in the bile ducts or canaliculi or renal tubules.

The work of Hamdy and his colleagues (1982)[2548] and Kamal and Koch (1982)[2549], showing a substantially prolonged half-life of over 100 hours for benoxaprofen in elderly subjects, has been re-examined by Hosie and Stevenson (1984)[2550]. These workers, in nine patients aged between 66 and 75 years, found that the mean elimination half-life of the drug in their elderly patients approximated to only 50 hours. They comment that their patients were generally healthier than those in the earlier reports, which had included mainly hospital in-patients many of whom appeared to have had impairment of renal function. It seems that it may be these factors, including general debility rather than just extreme age alone, which alter the pharmacokinetics of benoxaprofen and, in the presence of other still-unidentified factors, slowly produces the hepatorenal syndrome – a clinical picture, sometimes rapidly fatal once it is manifest, in which the laminated concretions described by MacSween sometimes form such a dramatic feature and in which the time-course of the illness, as described by Griffin (1984)[2545], is so important.

The second of the four non-steroidal anti-inflammatory agents recently withdrawn for safety reasons was Zomax (zomepirac sodium). This drug was removed from the market by the manufacturer following a similar withdrawal in the USA after five deaths due to severe allergic reactions associated with the drug had been reported in that country[2533]. At the time of withdrawal in the UK a total of 512 adverse reactions, including five deaths (none due to allergy) had been reported to the Committee on Safety of Medicines[2533]. Later information given in Parliament showed that by 22 February, 1984 a total of seven deaths had been reported in which zomepirac was the suspect drug[2472]. The pattern of reports was unremarkable, apart from the frequency of allergic states. The product was marketed for 23 months and some 900 000 prescriptions were issued for it[2543].

The third of these drugs was Osmosin, a sustained-release preparation of the well-known non-steroidal anti-inflammatory agent, indomethacin. It first reached the UK market in December, 1982. The number of reports soon caused concern for these added to the usual problems of indomethacin, lower intestinal perforation. In August, 1983, the Committee on Safety of Medicines, by means of *Current Problems, Number 11*[2540], commented on the supposed method of action of the formulation 'by an osmotic pump action as the tablet passes along the gut'; the Committee also noted the two reports of intestinal perforation, distal to the duodenum, which had been received and observed that 'this is an unusual site for damage with non-steroidal anti-inflammatory drugs'. Apart from this, it was noted that about 200 'yellow card' reports had been received although only a little over 400 000 prescriptions had been written for the product: this 'represents a high rate of reporting, even for a newly introduced product.' The product was withdrawn from the world market in September, 1983 and the Product Licence was surrendered in January, 1984[2533]. The information provided in response to Parliamentary Questions showed that Osmosin was marketed for 10 months; the number of prescriptions quoted remained at 400 000[2543]. The total of deaths in which Osmosin was the suspect drug was 40[2472].

The fourth of this group of drugs was Flosint (indoprofen), first marketed in the UK in September, 1982 and the subject of information, not previously available to the Committee on Safety of Medicines, relating to serious and fatal toxic effects of the drug, particularly gastrointestinal events[2533]. The product was marketed for 12 months and was the subject of approximately 120 000 prescriptions[2543]. The Product Licence was suspended by the Licensing Authority and eight deaths were notified in which indoprofen was the suspect drug[2472].

The information given above includes the duration of marketing of each of these four drugs, the number of prescriptions written during that period, and the number of deaths attributed to the use of the drug. Calculating the number of prescriptions equivalent to one death provides the following:

Product	Marketing period (months)	Deaths	Prescriptions for one death
Opren	22	61	24 590
Zomax	23	7	128 571
Osmosin	10	40	10 000
Flosint	12	8	15 000

These products are of the same therapeutic class, and probably drew their patients from the same universe in terms of diseases treated, age incidence, sex distribution, duration of therapy, and such factors. It is notable that when unsuspected grave toxicity has led to their withdrawal from the market it has done so within 2 years of marketing. The *OPE Study 68*[2539], already noted, found the same thing and commented 'The majority of documented safety discontinuations (14 of 18) occurred within 2 years of introduction and the exceptions tend to be somewhat unusual.'

All of these drugs are symptomatic remedies only, their major use being as analgesics; they are not curative of severe, life-threatening diseases – and it is doubtful if any level of proven mortality, unless this be an idiosyncratic and very rare event, is acceptable. The figures given above would, therefore, support the withdrawal decisions.

Zomax stands out as something of a special case, its potential for causing serious allergy being unusual. The ratio of prescriptions to one death for the other three drugs varies only from 10 to 25 000 in round terms. We cannot know how many patients received these prescriptions – but it seems unlikely that the diagnostic power of postmarketing surveillance could be relied upon to establish the presence of the adverse effects that led to the withdrawal decisions. Professor Paul Turner[2547], writing of Prescription Event Monitoring, which many would now view as a preferred form of postmarketing surveillance, has recently observed that:

> An independent, impartial facility for postmarketing surveillance now exists in the United Kingdom, and the CSM should consider restricting product licences on more new drugs and formulations until the results of PEM studies demonstrate acceptable safety. PEM is relatively cheap compared with most other methods of drug surveillance, and Inman anticipates that it should identify adverse drug reactions which have an incidence of one in 3000 or greater. Important reactions with a lower incidence will probably still depend on Yellow Card reporting to identify them.

The difficulty is that the important decisions may be, of necessity, made in respect of very serious events which do have an incidence of less than one in 3000 – this one in 3000 figure needs considerable modification, even as a working approximation, if the natural incidence of the adverse effect is not zero. It would seem a safe over-all conclusion that exercises such as Prescription Event Monitoring are, in the present circumstances, valuable adjuncts to the Yellow Card (or other spontaneous reporting) system.

In the examples discussed, the best case was (among the three drugs which seemed comparable) Opren with roughly 24 500 prescriptions for one death; it was withdrawn after 22 months of marketing. The next best case was Flosint, with 15 000 prescriptions for one death – and it went down very much quicker, in 12 months. The worst case was Osmosin, with a ratio of only 10 000 prescriptions for one death – and that was withdrawn most quickly of all, in 10 months. It might seem then that the withdrawals are taking place at a rate which responds to the hazard (however, it must be noted that this inference is based upon small numbers and must be further qualified by the fact that, with one of these drugs, a post-marketing surveillance exercise was helpful in identifying the problem).

The difficult part of the discussion is that by the time of drug withdrawal quite unacceptable damage has been done. Within the present system the most obvious way of lessening this is by increasing the rate of 'yellow card' reporting so that proof of a harmful effect, if there is one, will be obtained more quickly and with much less patient exposure. The real consequences of under-reporting, which merely serves to preserve a public hazard, are obvious.

Nevertheless, it must seem that the information in the public domain does establish that the nature and incidence of drug adverse effects is unacceptable – and that unpredictable drug withdrawals are taking place in a way which proves the present system to be inadequate. There may therefore be a place for additions to the system. The two most obvious hazards are the uncontrolled new product launch – which exposes a patient population so vast compared with the data submitted for Product Licence approval that the results are a guessing game – and the widely used drug, with its own massive patient population, and a data base of decades ago and probably not even excluding mutagenicity. A possible answer to the former problem is phased release, as has been discussed previously, so that patient populations are only slowly increased as the documented benefit-to-risk ratio in the earlier populations becomes known. The answer to the second problem is that the renewal of each Product Licence, as required by the existing Medicines Act in the United Kingdom, should be made something more meaningful.

A more prudent demand for drugs by patients and their more cautious prescription use, if linked with requirements such as phased release, better support for adverse reactions reporting, a selected drugs list from which drugs of real value obtain full reimbursement, would, if there are to be new remedies for the unconquered diseases, need great changes in the structure of drug pricing and the patent protection offered to drug innovators who do establish new therapeutic uses or bring out products that prove their right to a place in the pharmacopoeia.

One wonders if Heberden would not have looked at some of our more toxic and non-curative drugs, or our untested traditional drugs, as he looked upon mithridatium and theriac, about which he said[935]:

If our objections stopped here, and these grand antidotes were only good for nothing; it would hardly be worth while to censure or take any notice of them: but we may justly fear that their use is attended with a good deal of danger.

One must also wonder what he would have said about anaesthetics, Jenner's vaccine, vitamins, the antituberculous drugs, insulin, the antibiotics, and the other things he would have gladly added to the *Commentaries*.

It seems likely that we would have left him with a far bigger book – and, with his critical look, he would have offered us a slimmer pharmacopoeia.

References

2472. Hansard (Commons), 1984, Feb. 23, 632/633; Mar. 6, 565/569; Mar. 7, 631

2473. Cahours, August André. Recherches sur l'huile de Gaultheria procumbens. *J. Pharm. Chim.*, 1843, **3**, 364–8

2474. Gerhardt, Charles Frédéric. Untersuchungen über die wasserfreien organischen Säuren. *Leibig's Ann.*, 1853, **87**, 149–79

2475. Job xl, 22 (AV)

2476. Stone, *Revd. Mr* Edmund. An account of the success of the bark of the willow in the cure of agues. *Philosophical Transactions, giving some account of the present undertakings, studies, and labours, of the ingenious, in many considerable parts of the world.* 1763, **53**, 195–200

2477. Grieve, Mrs M. (1931). As ref. 124 but p. 749

2478. Woodville, William (1810). As ref. 129 but Vol. II, p. 330

2479. Celsus (Spencer edn. of 1938). As ref. 241 but Vol. II, p. xlvii

2480. Martindale (1977). As ref. 1 but p. 1018

2481. Bramley, Amanda and Goulding, Roy. Laburnum 'poisoning'. *Br. Med. J.*, 1981, **283**, 1220–1

2482. Ippen, H. Laburnum 'poisoning'. *Br. Med. J.*, 1981, **283**, 615

2483. Griggs, Barbara. Green pharmacy, a history of herbal medicine. London, *Norman & Hobhouse,* 1981, p. 305–6; 359

2484. Griggs, Barbara (1981). As ref. 2483 but pp. 297–8

2485. Grieve, Mrs M. (1931). As ref. 124 but p. 281

2486. Korab, M. de. Action exercée par l'hélénine sur les bacillus de la tuberculose. *Compt. Rend. Acad. d. Sc., Par.*, 1882, **95**, 441–3. Also: *Gaz. de Hôp., Par.*, 1882, **55**, 866–7

2487. Thomson, William A. R. Healing plants, a modern herbal. London, *Macmillan*, 1978, p., 75

2488. Tyler, Varro E., Brady, Lynn, R. and Robbers, James, E. Pharmacognosy. (8th edn.) Philadelphia, *Lea & Febiger*, 1981, p. 39

2489. Stampf, Jean-Luc, *et al.* The sensitizing capacity of helenin and of two of its main constituents, the sesquiterpene lactones alantolactone and isoalantolactone: a comparison of epicutaneous and intradermal sensitizing methods in different strains of guinea pig. *Contact Dermatitis*, 1982, **8**, 16–24

2490. Dalvi, R. R. and McGowan, C. Helenin inhibition of liver microsomal enzymes. *J. Agric. Food Chem.*, 1982, **30**, 988–9

2491. Kowalewski, Zdzislaw *et al.* Action of helenin on microorganisms. *Arch. Immunologiæ et Therapiea Exp.*, 1976, **24**, 121–5

2492. Lewis, Walter, H. and Elvin-Lewis, Memory P. F. Medical botany, plants affecting man's health. New York, *Wiley*, 1977, p. 29

2493. Pereira, Jonathan (1839–40). As ref. 1108 but Vol. II, p. 1327, 1329

2494. Singh, M. P. *et al.* Anti-fertility activity of a benzene extract of Hibiscus rosa-sinensis flowers on female albino rats. *Planta Medica*, 1982, **44**, 171–4

2495. Lindner, H. R. Occurrence of anabolic agents in plants and their importance. *Environmental Quality and Safety,* 1976, Pt. 5, Suppl., 151–8

2496. Wright, S. and Burton, J. L. Oral evening-primrose-seed oil improves atopic eczema. *Lancet*, 1982, **2**, 1120–2

2497. Trease, George Edward and Evans, William Charles. Pharmacognosy. (12th. edn.), London, *Baillière Tindall,* 1983

2498. Phillipson, J. David and Anderson, Linda A. Pharmacologically active compounds in herbal remedies. *Pharm. J.*, 1984, **232**, 41–4

2499. Torssell, Kurt B. G. Natural product chemistry, a mechanistic and biosynthetic approach to secondary metabolism. Chichester, *John Wiley,* 1983

CONCLUSION

2500. Burger, Alfred. A guide to the chemical basis of drug design. New York, *John Wiley*, 1983
2501. Lewis, Walter, H. and Elvin-Lewis, Memory P. F. Medical botany, plants affecting man's health. New York, *John Wiley*, 1977, pp. 92–4
2502. Miller, James A. and Miller, Elizabeth C. The matabolic activation and nucleic acid adducts of naturally-occurring carcinogens: recent results with ethyl carbamate and the spice flavors safrole and estragole. *Br. J. Cancer*, 1983, **48**, 1–15
2503. Fairweather, Frank, A. and Swann, Cheryl A. Food additives and cancer. *Proc. Nutr. Soc.*, 1981, **40**, 21–30
2504. Hirono, Iwao. Natural carcinogenic products of plant origin. In Critical Reviews in Toxicology. (ed: Leon Goldberg), Boca Raton, Florida, *CRC Press*, 1981, pp. 235–77
2505. Wogan, G. N. Naturally occurring carcinogens. In The Physiopathology of Cancer, Vol. 1: Biology and Biochemistry. Basel, *Karger*, 1974, pp. 64–109
2506. Miller, James, A. and Miller, Elizabeth C. Carcinogens occurring naturally in foods. *Fed. Proc.*, 1976, **35**, 1316–21
2507. BPC (1934). As ref. 120 but p. 803
2508. Lewis, Walter H. and Smith, Peter R. Poke root herbal tea poisoning. *J. Am. Med. Assoc.*, 1979, **242**, pp. 2759–60
2509. McPherson, Alexander. Pokeweed and other lymphocyte mitogens. In Toxic Plants, (ed: A. Douglas Kinghorn). New York, *Columbia Univ. Press*, 1979, pp. 83–102
2510. Cordell, G. A. Recent experimental and clinical data concerning antitumor and cytotoxic agents from plants. In New Natural Products and Plant Drugs with Pharmacological, Biological or Therapeutical Activity. Proceedings in Life Sciences (eds: Wagner & Wolff), 1977, pp. 54–81
2511. Hall, Iris H. *et al.* Antitumor agents, XLII: Comparison of antileukemic activity of helenalin, Brusatol, and bruceantin and their esters on different strains of P-388 lymphocytic leukemic cells. *J. Pharm. Sci.*, 1981, **70**, 1147–50
2512. Lee, Kuo-Hsiung *et al.* Antitumor agents. 44. Bis(helenalinyl) esters and related derivatives as novel potent antileukemic agents. *J. Med. Chem.*, 1981, **24**, 924–7
2513. Cordell, Geoffrey A. Anticancer agents from plants. In Progress in Phytochemistry, (eds: L. Reinhold, J. B. Harborne and T. Swain) Oxford, *Pergamon Press*, 1978, Vol. 5, pp. 273–316
2514. Osler, Sir William. As ref. 2010 but 7th edn. (1909), p. 58
2515. (Osler, Sir William) Osler's textbook revisited, reprint of selected sections with commentaries. (eds: A. McGehee Harvey and Victor, A. McKusick). New York, *Meredith*, 1967
2516. Eisleb, O. and Schaumann, O. Dolantin, ein neuartiges Spasmolytikum und Analgetikum. (Chemisches und pharmakologisches.) *Dtsch. Med. Wschr.*, 1939, **65**, 967–69 967–69
2517. Courvoisier, S. *et al.* Propriétés pharmacodynamiques du chlorhydrate de chloro-3(diméthyl-amino-3'propyl)-10 phénothiazine (4.560 R.P.). *Arch. Int. Pharmacodyn.*, 1953, **92**, 305–61
2518. Pincus, Gregory Goodwin and Chang Min Chueh. The effects of progesterone and related compounds on ovulation and early development in the rabbit. *Acta. Physiol. Latinoamer.*, 1953, **3**, 177–83
2519. Randall, Lowell Orlando, *et al.* The psychosedative properties of methaminodiazepoxide. *J. Pharmacol.*, 1960, **129**, 163–71
2520. Department of Health and Social Security. Guidelines for the testing of chemicals for mutagenicity. Report on Health and Social Subjects Number 24. London, *HMSO*, 1981, p. 5
2521. (Preger, Leslie and others). Induced disease, drug, irradiation, occupation. (ed: Leslie Preger), New York, *Grune & Stratton*, 1980
2522. Grundmann, E. and others). Drug-induced pathology. (ed: E. Grundmann). Heidelberg, *Springer-Verlag*, 1980
2523. Deitch, Rodney. Animal cruelty or science? *Lancet*, 1980, **1**, 887–8
2524. Laboratory Animals Protection (H. L.) Bill. The Earl of Halsbury. 16th July, 1979. London, *HMSO*
2525. Protection of Animals (Scientific Purposes) Bill. Mr Peter Fry. June 27, 1979. London, *HMSO*
2526. Editorial. *Biologist*, 1983, **30**, (4), 209–10

2527. Merry, Peter. Experiments on animals: are the protests valid? *BMA News Review*, 1982 (April), 12–20

2528. Mathez, Maurice. Confidentiality of registration data. In IFPMA Symposium on International Drug Registration. Zurich, *IFPMA,* 1979, pp. 147–53

2529. Lorke, Dietrich. A new approach to practical acute toxicity testing. *Arch. Toxicol.*, 1983, **54,** 275–87

2530. (Beaconsfield, Peter and Villee, Claude). Placenta, a neglected experimental animal. (eds: Peter Beaconsfield and Claude Villee). Oxford, *Pergamon Press*, 1979

2531. (Balls, Michael and others). Animals and alternatives in toxicity testing. (eds: Michael Balls, Rosemary J. Riddell and Alastair N. Worden). London, *Academic Press,* 1983

2532. Committee on Safety of Medicines – personal communication

2533. Committee on Safety of Medicines, Annual Report for 1983. London, *HMSO*

2534. Hansard (Commons), 1984. As ref. 2472 but c. 567

2535. The Medical Directory 1983 (139th. edn.) Harlow, *Churchill Livingstone*, 1983

2536. Rawlins, Michael D. Postmarketing surveillance of adverse reactions to drugs. *Br. Med. J.,* 1984, **288,** 879–80

2537. Hansard (Commons), 1984, Feb. 15, c. 235

2538. Anonymous. Consolidated list of products whose consumption and/or sale have been banned, withdrawn, severely restricted or not approved by Governments. Prepared by the United Nations Secretariat in response to General Assembly resolution 37/137. 30 December, 1983

2539. Anonymous. OPE Study 68. Office of Planning and Evaluation, Food and Drug Administration 1984 (March)

2540. Committee on Safety of Medicines. Current Problems, Number 11, 1983, August. London, *HMSO*

2541. Department of Health and Social Security. On the state of the public health. The Annual Report of the Chief Medical Officer... 1982. London, *HMSO*

2542. Taggart, Hugh McA. and Alderdice, Joan M. Fatal cholestatic jaundice in elderly patients taking benoxaprofen. *Br. Med. J.,* 1982, **284,** 1372

2543. Hansard (Commons), 1984, March 7, c. 631

2544. Hansard (Commons), 1983, Dec. 13, c. 441–2

2545. Griffin, John P. The advantages and limitations of drug orientated schemes for monitoring ADR's – Voluntary reporting (1984, in press)

2546. Macsween, R. N. 1984, personal communication

2547. Turner, Paul. Long-term assessment of drug safety and efficacy. *J. R. Soc. Med.,* 1984, **77,** 93–4

2548. Hamdy, R. C. *et al. Eur. J. Rheumatol. Inflam.,* 1982, **5,** 69

2549. Kamal, A. and Koch, I. M. *Eur. J. Rheumatol. Inflam.,* 1982, **5,** 76

2550. Hosie, J. and Stevenson, I. H. Benoxaprofen pharmacokinetics in elderly patients. 1984, in press

Appendix

The materia medica of the 1789 Pharmacopoeia:

Botanical Materials

1789 Listing *1931 or later Listing*	*Modern country name* *Representative synonyms*	*Part used*
Artemisia Abrotanum Artemisia abrotanum	Southernwood Old Man, Lad's Love, Boy's Love	leaf
Artemisia maritima Artemesia maritima	Sea Wormwood Old Woman	top
Artemisia Absinthium Artemisia absinthium	Common Wormwood Green Ginger	herb
Rumex Acetosa Rumex acetosa	Garden Sorrel Green Sauce, Sour Sauce, Cuckoo Sorrow	leaf
Aconitum Napellus Aconitum napellus	Aconite Monkshood, Blue Rocket, Friar's Cap	herb
Allium sativum Allium sativum	Garlic Poor Man's Treacle	root
Aloe perfoliata Aloe vera etc.	Aloes (The chief varieties of Aloes are Curacao or Barbados, Socotrine (including Zanzibar) and Cape)	—
Althaea officinalis Althaea officinalis	Marsh Mallow Mallards, Mauls, Schloss Tea, Cheeses, Mortification Root	root and leaf
(Amygdala amara) Amygdalus communis var. amara	Bitter Almond	nut

1789 Listing 1931 or later Listing	Modern country name Representative synonyms	Part used
(Amygdala dulcis) Amygdalus communis var. dulcis	Sweet Almond	nut
Ammoniacum Dorema ammoniacum	Ammoniacum Gum Ammoniac	gum-resin
Anethum graveolens Peucedanum graveolens	Dill Anethum graveolus. Fructus anethi	seed
Angelica Archangelic Angelica Archangelica	Angelica Garden Angelica, Archangelica officinalis	root, stem, leaf, seed
Pimpinella Anisum Pimpinella anisum	Anise	seed
Mimosa nilotica Acacia senegal	Acacia Gum Arabic, Gummi Mimosae	—
Arnica montana Arnica montana	Arnica Mountain Tobacco, Leopard's Bane	herb, flower, root
Arum maculatum Arum maculatum	Cuckoo-Pint Lords and Ladies, Arum, Starchwort, Adder's Root, Bobbins, Friar's Cowl, Kings and Queens, Parson and Clerk, Quaker, Wake Robin	fresh root
Ferula Assafoetida Ferula foetida	Asafetida Food of the Gods, Devil's Dung	gum resin
Asarum Europaeum Asarum Europaeum	Asarabacca Hazelwort, Wild Nard	leaf
Avena sativa Avena sativa	Oats Groats, Oatmeal	—
Citrus Aurantium (hispalense)	Sweet Orange	
Citrus Aurantium var. dulcis	Citrus vulgaris, Citrus bigaradia, Citrus Aurantium amara, Bigaradier, Bigarade Orange, Bitter Orange, Seville Orange, Citrus dulcis	leaf, flower, juice and rind of the fruit
Pinus Balsamea	Canada Balsam	—

1789 Listing 1931 or later Listing	Modern country name Representative synonyms	Part used
Pinus balsamea	Abies canadensis, Abies balsamea, Balsam Fir, Balm of Gilead Fir, Perusse, Hemlock Spruce	
Copaifera officinalis Copaifera Langsdorffi	Copaiba Copaiva, Balsam Copaiba, Copaiba officinalis	—
Myroxylon peruiferum Myroxylon Pereirae	Balsam of Peru Toluifera Pereira, Myrosperum Pereira	—
Toluifera Balsamum Myrospermum Toluiferum	Balsam of Tolu Balsamum Tolutanum, Tolutanischer Balsam	—
Arctium Lappa Arctium lappa	Burdock Lappa, Fox's Clote, Thorny Burr, Beggar's Buttons, Cockle Buttons, Love Leaves, Philanthropium	root
Veronica Beccabunga Veronica beccabunga	Brooklime Water Pimpernel, Beckly Leaves, Cow Cress, Housewell Grass, Limewort, Limpwort, Wall-ink	herb
Styrax Benzoë Styrax benzoin	Benzoin Gum Benzoin, Gum Benjamin, Siam Benzoin, Sumatra Benzoin	resin
Polygonum Bistorta Polygonum bistorta	Bistort Osterick, Oderwort, Snakeweed, Easter Mangiant, Adderwort, Twice Writhen	root
Acorus Calamus Acorus calamus	Sweet Sedge Calamus, Sweet Flag, Sweet Root, Sweet Rush, Sweet Cane, Gladdon, Sweet Myrtle, Myrtle Grass, Myrtle Sedge, Cinnamon Sedge	root root
Laurus Camphora Cinnamonum camphora	Camphor Laurel Camphor, Gum Camphor	—
Canella alba Canella alba	White Cinnamon Canella, White Wood, Wild Cinnamon, Canellae Cortex	bark

1789 Listing *1931 or later Listing*	*Modern country name* *Representative synonyms*	*Part used*
Cardamine pratensis Cardamine pratensis	Meadow Cress Lady-smock, Cuckoo-flower	flower
Amomum repens Elettaria Cardamomum	Cardamoms Amomum Cardamomum, Cardamomum minus, Amomum repens, Ebil, Capalaga, Ilachi, Ailum	seed
Centaurea benedicta Carbenia benedicta	Holy Thistle Blessed Thistle, Cnicus benedictus, Carduus benedictus	herb
Ficus Carica Ficus carica	Common Fig	—
Carum Carui Carum Carvi	Caraway Caraway Seed	seed
Caryophyllus aromaticus Eugenia caryophyllata	Cloves Eugenia aromatica	Cloves and their essential oil
Dianthus Caryophyllus Caryophyllus aromaticus	Caryophyllum rubrum Clove-pink, Carnation	flower
Cascarilla Croton Eleuteria	Cascarilla Sweetwood Bark, Bahama Cascarilla, Elutheria, Cascarillae Cortex, Aromatic Quinquina, False Quinquina	bark
Cassia Fistula Cassia fistula	Purging Senna Purging Cassia, Cassia Stick, Pudding Pipe-Tree, Alexandrian Purging Cassia	fruit
Mimosa Catechu Uncaria Gambier	Catechu Pale Catechu, Gambir	—
Gentiana Centaurium Erythraea centaurium	Centaury Centaury Gentian, Century, Red Centaury, Filwort, Centory, Christ's Ladder, Feverwort	top
Anthemis nobilis Anthemis nobilis	Common Chamomile Manzanilla, Maythen	flower
Conium maculatum Conium maculatum	Hemlock Herb Bennet, Spotted Corobane, Musquash Root, Beaver Poison, Poison Hemlock, Poison Parsley, Spotted Hemlock, Kex, Kecksies	herb, flower, seed
Cynara Scolymus Cynara Scolymus	Globe Artichoke	leaf

1789 Listing 1931 or later Listing	Modern country name Representative synonyms	Part used
Laurus Cinnamomum Cinnamomum zeylanicum	Cinnamon Laurus Cinnamomum	bark and its essential oil
Cochlearia officinalis Cochlearia officinalis	Scurvy Grass Spoonwort	herb
Colchicum autumnale Colchicum autumnale	Meadow Saffron Naked Ladies	fresh root
Cucumis Colocynthis Cucumis colocynthis	Colocynth Citrullus colocynthis, Bitter Apple, Colocynth Pulp, Bitter Cucumber	pith of fruit
Colomba Jateorhiza columba	Calumba Columba, Cocculus palmatus	root
Dorstenia Contrajerva Dorstenia contrayerva	Contrayerva Dorstenia Houstoni	root
Coriandrum sativum Coriandrum sativum	Coriander	seed
Crocus sativus Crocus sativus	Saffron Crocus, Karcom, Krokos	stigma of flower
Piper Cubeba Piper cubeba	Cubebs Tailed Pepper	—
Momordica Elaterium Echallium elaterium	Squirting Cucumber Momordica Elaterium, Wild Cucumber	fresh fruit
Cuminum Cyminum Cuminum cyminum	Cumin Cumino aigro	seed
Curcuma longa Curcuma longa	Turmeric Curcuma, Curcuma rotunda, Amomum curcuma	root
Pyrus Cydonia Pyrus Cydonia	Quince Cydonia vulgaris	apple and its seed
Rosa canina Rosa canina	Dog Rose	hip, the fruit
Daucus Carota Daucus carota	Wild Carrot Birds' Nest and Bees' Nest	seed
Digitalis purpurea Digitalis purpurea	Foxglove Witches' Gloves, Dead Men's Bells, Fairy's Glove, Gloves of Our Lady, Virgin's Glove, Fairy Caps, Folk's Glove, Fairy Thimbles	herb
Amyris Elemifera Canarium luzonicum	Elemi Manila Elemi	resin

1789 Listing 1931 or later Listing	Modern country name Representative synonyms	Part used
Enula Helenium Inula helenium	Elecampane Scabwort, Elf Dock, Wild Sunflower, Horseheal	root
Eryngium maritimum Eryngium maritimum	Sea Holly Eryngium campestre, Sea Hulver, Sea Holme	root
Polypodium Filix mas Dryopteris felix-mas	Male Fern Aspidium Filix-mas, Male Shield Fern	root
Anethum Foeniculum Foeniculum vulgare	Fennel Fenkel, Sweet Fennel, Wild Fennel	seed

Trigonella Foenum
   Graecum
Trigonella foenum-
   graecum.
	Fenugreek
	
	Bird's Foot, Greek Hay-seed
		seed

Bubon Galbanum Ferula Galbaniflua	Galbanum	gum-resin
Galla Gall	Gall Excrescences on the twigs of Quercus infectoria, resulting from the local effects of the gall- wasp, Adleria gallae-tinctoriae	—
Gambogia Garcinia Hanburyii	Gamboge Gutta gamba, Gummigutta, Tom Rong, Gambodia, Garcinia Morella	gum-resin
Spartium scoparium Cytisus scoparius	Broom Broom tops, Irish Tops, Basam, Bisom, Green Broom	top, the seed
Gentiana lutea Gentiana lutea	Yellow Gentian	root
Panax quinquefolium Panax quinquefolium	Ginseng Aralia quinquefolia, Five fingers, Tartar Root, Red Berry, Man's Health	root
Glycyrrhiza glabra Glycyrrhiza glabra	Liquorice	root
Punica Granatum Punica granatum	Pomegranate Grenadier, Cortex granati	flower and rind of fruit
Gratiola officinalis Gratiola officinalis	Hedge Hyssop	herb

1789 Listing 1931 or later Listing	Modern country name Representative synonyms	Part used
Guaiacum officinale Guaiacum officinale	Guaiacum Lignum Vitae	wood, bark and gum-resin
Helleborus foetidus Helleborus foetidus	Bearsfoot	leaf
Veratrum album Varatrum album	White Hellebore Veratrum Lobelianium, Veratrum Californicum	root
Helleborus niger Helleborus niger	Black Hellebore Christe Herbe, Melampode, Christmas Rose	root
Hordeum distichon Hordeum distichon	Barley Pearl Barley, Perlatum	
Hypericum perforatum Hypericum perforatum	St. John's Wort	flower
Jalapium Convolvulus jalapa	Jalap Bindweed Ipomea purga, Ipomea Jalapa	root
Ipecacuanha Psychortia ipecacuanha	Ipecacuanha Cephaelis Ipecacuanha, Uragoga ipecacuanha, Matto Grosso	root
Iris florentina Iris florentina	Iris Orris Root – derived from I. Germanica, I. pallida and I. Florentina	root
Juglans regia Juglans nigra	Walnut Carya, Jupiter's Nuts	unripe fruit
Juniperus communis Juniperus communis	Juniper Berries Genévrier, Ginepro, Enebro	berry and top
Gummi Gambiense Pterocarpus marsupium	Kino East Indian, Malabar, Madras, or Cochin Kino	resin
Cistus creticus Cistus Creticus	Ladanum Ladanum or Labdanum – the resin of Cistus Creticus, the European Rock Rose	resin
Lavandula Spica Lavandula spica	Spike Lavender Latifolia	flower
Laurus nobilis Laurus nobilis	Laurel Sweet Bay, True Laurel, Bay, Roman Laurel, Noble Laurel, Laurier Sauce	leaf and berry
Haematoxylum Campechianum	Logwood	

| 1789 Listing
1931 or later Listing | Modern country name
Representative synonyms | Part used |
|---|---|---|
| Haematoxylon
  Campeachianum | Haematoxylon Lignum, Lignum Campechianum, Peachwood, Bloodwood | |
| Citrus Medica
Citrus limonum | Lemon
Citrus medica, Citronnier, Limoun, Limone | juice, rind and essential oil |
| Linum usitatissimum
Linum usitatissimum | Flax
Linseed | seed |
| Oxalis Acetocella
Oxalis acetosella | Wood Sorrel
Wood Sour, Sour Trefoil, Stickwort, Fairy Bells, Hallelujah, Three-leaved Grass, Stubwort | leaf |
| Origanum Majorano
Origanum marjorana | Sweet Marjoram
Knotted Marjoram, Marjorana hortensis | herb |
| Malva sylvestris
Malva sylvestris | Blue Mallow
Common Mallow | leaf and flower |
| Manna
Manna | Manna
The juice from the stems of the European flowering ash, Fraxinus ornus | — |
| Marrubium vulgare
Marrubium vulgare | White Horehound
Hoarhound | herb |
| Teucrium Marum
Teucrium Marum | Cat Thyme
Marum | herb |
| Pistacia Lentifous
Pistacia Lentiscus | Mastic
Mastich, Lentisk | resin |
| Melissa officinalis
Melissa officinalis | Balm
Sweet Balm, Lemon Balm | herb |
| Mentha piperita
Mentha piperita | Peppermint
Brandy Mint | |
| Mentha spicata
Mentha viridis | Spearmint
Garden Mint, Mentha Spicata, Our Lady's Mint, Green Mint, Spire Mint, Sage of Bethlehem | herb |
| Daphne Mezereum
Daphne mezereum | Mezereon
Mezerei Cortex, Mezerei officinarum, Dwarf Bay, Flowering Spurge, Spurge Olive, Spurge Laurel | bark of the root |

1789 Listing 1931 or later Listing	Modern country name Representative synonyms	Part used
Morus nigra Morus nigra	Common Mulberry	fruit
Myrrha Myrrh	Myrrh Oleo-gum-resin from the stem of Commiphora molmol	gum-resin
Sisymbrium Nafturtium aquaticum Nasturtium officinale	Watercress	fresh herb
Nicotiana Tabacum Nicotiana tabacum	Tobacco Tabaci Folia	leaf
Myristica Mofchata Myristica fragrans	Mace Myristica officinalis Myristica moschata (The fruits of Myristica fragrans resemble a pear and contain a single erect seed, the nucleus being the wrinkled 'nutmeg', and the fleshy, irregular covering, which is scarlet when fresh but dries yellow, is the 'mace'.)	the essential oil, the expressed oil 'commonly called oil of mace', and mace – 1789 version
Juniperus lycia Boswellia thurifera	Frankincense Olibanum	gum-resin
Olea europoea Olea Europaea	Olive Olea Oleaster, Olea gallica, Olea lancifolia	oil
Pastinaca Opopanax Opopanax chironium	Opoponax Pastinaca Opoponax	gum-resin
Origanum vulgare Origanum vulgare	Wild Marjoram	herb
Papaver somniferum Papaver somniferum	White Poppy Opium Poppy, Mawseed	head
Papaver Rhaeas Papaver rhaeas	Red Poppy Corn Rose, Corn Poppy	flower
Cissampelos pareira Chondodendron tomentosum	Pareira Pereira Brava, Cissampelos Pareira, Velvet Leaf, Ice Vine (The chloride of (+)-tubocurarine is obtained from extracts of the stems of Chondodendron tomentosum.)	root
Parietaria officinalis Parietaria officinalis	Pellitory-Of-The-Wall Lichwort	herb

1789 Listing 1931 or later Listing	Modern country name Representative synonyms	Part used
Potentilla reptans Potentilla reptans	Five-Leaf Grass Cinquefoil, Five Fingers, Sunkfield	root
Cinchona officinalis Cinchona succirubra	Peruvian Bark Red Bark, Jesuits' Powder, Cinchona Bark	bark
Apium Petrofelinum Carum petroselinum	Parsley Apium petroselinum, Petroselinum lativum, Persely, Persele	root and seed
Myrtus Pimenta Pimento officinalis	Allspice Pimento, Jamaica Pepper	berry
Capsicum annuum Capsicum annuum var. minimum	Capsicum Chillies, Capsici Fructus, Paprika	fruit capsule
Piper longum Piper longum	Long Pepper	fruit
Piper nigrum Piper nigrum	Pepper Black Pepper, Piper	berry
Pix Burgundica Burgundy Pitch	Burgundy Pitch Pix Burgundica, White Pitch – a resinous extract from the Norway spruce, Picea abies	—
Tar Tar	Tar Pix Liquida, Pine Tar, Pix Pini – from the destructive distillation of the wood of the Scots pine, Pinus sylvestris	—
Prunus domestica Prunus domestica	Prunes Plum Tree	—
Prunus spinosa Prunus spinosa	Blackthorn Sloe	—
Mentha Pulegium Mentha pulegium	Pennyroyal Pulegium, Run-by-the-Ground, Pudding Grass, Lurk-in-the- Ditch	herb and flower
Quassia amara Picraena excelsa	Quassia Bitter Wood, Jamaica Quassia, Bitter Ash, Quassia Amara, Quassia Lignum	wood, bark, root
Quercus Robur Quercus robur	Common Oak Tanner's Bark	bark

1789 Listing 1931 or later Listing	Modern country name Representative synonyms	Part used
Cochlearia Armoracia Cochlearia armoracia	Horseradish Mountain Radish, Great Raifort, Red Cole	root
Rheum palmatum Rheum palmatum	Turkey Rhubarb East Indian Rhubarb, China Rhubarb	root
Ribes nigrum Ribes nigrum	Black Currant Quinsy Berries, Squinancy Berries	fruit
Ribes rubrum Ribes rubrum	Red Currant Ribs, Risp, Reps	fruit
Ricinus communis Ricinus communis	Castor Oil Plant Palma Christi, Castor Oil Bush	seed
Rosa centifolia Rosa centifolia	Cabbage Rose Hundred-leaved Rose	flower leaf
Rosa Gallica Rosa gallica	Red Rose Provins Rose	flower leaf
Rosmarinus officinalis Rosmarinus officinalis	Rosemary Polar Plant, Compass-weed, Compass Plant, Rosmarinus coronarium	top and flower
Rubia tinctorum Rubia tinctorum	Madder Krapp, Robbia, Dyer's Madder	root
Rubus idaeus Rubus idaeus	Raspberry Hindberry, Bramble of Mount Ida	fruit
Ruta graveolens Ruta graveolens	Rue Herb-of-Grace, Herbygrass, Garden Rue	herb
Juniperus Sabina Sabina cacumina	Savine Savine Tops – fresh dried tops of *Juniperus Sabina*	leaf
Saccharum non purificatum Saccharum bis coctum	Sugar, Double-refined sugar, Sucrose, Cane-sugar, Refined Sugar, Saccharose, Saccharum, Sucrosum – obtained from the juice of the sugar-cane (a woody grass, *Saccharum officinarum*) or the white-rooted varieties of the Sugar-beet, especially variety *Rapa*	

1789 Listing 1931 or later Listing	Modern country name Representative synonyms	Part used
Sagapenum	Sagapenum A foetid resin from *Ferula persica*	gum-resin
Salvia officinalis Salvia officinalis	Common Sage Sawge, Garden Sage, Red Sage, Broad-leaved White Sage, Narrow-leaved White Sage, Salvia salvatrix	leaf
Sambucus nigra Sambucus nigra	Elder Black Elder, Common Elder, Pipe Tree, Bore Tree, Bour Tree, Hylder, Hylantree, Eldrum	interior bark, flower and berry
Sanguis draconis	Dragon's Blood – the red exudate from the Dragon-tree, *Dracaena draco*	resin
Pterocarpus Santolinus Pterocarpus santalinus	Red Saunders Pterocarpi Lignum, Santalum rubrum, Lignum rubrum, Red Sandalwood, Rubywood, Rasura Santalum Ligni, Sappan	wood
Artemisia Santonicum Artemisia cina	Santonin/Levant Wormseed Sea Wormwood, Santonica, Semen Sanctum, Semen Cinae, Semen Contra, Semen Santonici, Artemisia Lercheana, Artemisia maritima, var: Stechmanniana, Artemisia maritima, var: pauciflora, Artemisia Chamaemelifolia, Santonin – obtained from the dried unexpanded flowerheads of *Artemisia cina* and other species of *Artemisia*	seed
Sarcocolla	Sarcocolla – a Persian gum from Astragalus or other plants	gum-resin
Smilax Sarsaparilla Aralia nudicaulis	Wild Sarsaparilla Bamboo Brier, Smilax sarsaparilla	root
Laurus Sassafras Sassafras officinale	Sassafras Sassafras varifolium, Laurus Sassafras, Sassafrax, Sassafras radix	wood, root and bark of root
Convolvolus Scammonia Convolvulus Scammonia	Syrian Bindweed Scammony	gum-resin

1789 Listing 1931 or later Listing	Modern country name Representative synonyms	Part used
Scilla maritima Urginea scilla	Squill Maritime Squill, Scilla maritima, Urginea maritima, Urginea Indica, White Squill, Red Squill	root
Teucrium Scordium Teucrium scorodonia	Sage-leaved Germander Wood Sage, Large-leaved Germander, Hind Heal, Ambroise, Garlic Sage	herb
Cassia Senna Cassia acutifolia	Senna Alexandrian Senna, Nubian Senna, Cassia Senna, Cassia lentiva, Cassia Lanceolata, Cassia officinalis, Cassia angustifolia, Egyptian Senna, Tinnevelly Senna, East Indian Senna	leaf
Polygala Senega Polygala Senega	Senega Snake Root, Senegae Radix, Seneca, Seneka, Polygala Virginiana, Senega officinalis, Milkwort, Mountain Flax, Rattlesnake Root	root
Aristolochia Serpentaria Aristolochia serpentaria	Snakeroot Aristolochia reticulata, Serpentary Rhizome, Serpentary Radix, Virginian Snakeroot, Aristolochia officinalis, Aristolochia sagittata, Snake- weed, Red River or Texas Snakeroot, Pelican Flower, Virginia Serpentaria, Radix Viperina, Snagrel, Sangrel, Sangree	root
Quassia Simarouba Simaruba amara	Simaruba Simaruba officinalis, Dysentery Bark, Mountain Damson, Bitter Damson, Slave Wood, Stave Wood, Quassia Simaruba	bark
Sinapis nigra Brassica nigra	Black Mustard Sinapis nigra, Brassica sinapioides	seed
Sium nodiflorum Sium latifolium	Water Parsnip Water Hemlock	herb
Spigelia marilandica	Pink Root	root

1789 Listing 1931 or later Listing	Modern country name Representative synonyms	Part used
Spigelia Marylandica	Indian Pink, Maryland Pink, Wormgrass, Carolina-, Maryland-, American-Wormroot, Starbloom	root
Rhamnus catharticus Rhamnus cathartica	Common Buckthorn Rhamnus, Bacca Spinae, Cervinae, Nerprun, Waythorn, Highwaythorn, Hartsthorn, Ramsthorn	berry
Delphinium Staphisagria Delphinium staphisagria	Stavesacre Lousewort	seed
Styrax officinalis Liquidambar orientalis	Storax Liquidambar imberbe, Styrax Praeparatus, Prepared Storax, Styrax liquidus, Balsam Styracis	resin
Tamarindus Indica Tamarindus Indica	Tamarinds Tamarindus officinalis, Imlee	fruit
Tanacetum vulgare Tanacetum vulgare	Tansy Buttons	flower and herb
Leontodon Taraxacum Taraxacum officinale	Dandelion Priest's Crown, Swine's Snout	root and herb
Terebinthina vulgaris Turpentine	Turpentine Turpentine – the oleoresin obtained as an exudate from various species of *Pinus*	—
Frankincense (already listed)		
Tormentilla erecta Potentilla Tormentilla	Tormentil Septfoil, Thormantle, Biscuits, Bloodroot, Earthbank, Ewe Daisy, Shepherd's Knot, English Sarsaparilla	root
Astragalus Tragacantha Astragalus gummifer	Tragacanth Gum Tragacanth, Syrian Tragacanth, Gum Dragon	gum
Menyanthes trifoliata Menyanthes trifoliata	Bogbean Buckbean, Marsh Trefoil, Water Trefoil, Marsh Clover	herb
Tricticum hybernum Tricticum spp.	Wheat	flower and starch
Tussilago Farfara Tussilago farfara	Coltsfoot Coughwort, Hallfoot, Horsehoof, Ass's Foot, Foalswort, Fieldhove, Bullsfoot, Donnhove	herb

730

1789 Listing 1931 or later Listing	Modern country name Representative synonyms	Part used
Valeriana officinalis Valeriana officinalis	Valerian Phu (Galen), All-heal, Great Wild Valerian, Amantilla, Setwall	root
Viola odorata Viola odorata	Sweet Violet Sweet-Scented Violet	fresh flower
Vitis vinifera Vitis vinifera	Vine Grape Vine	—
Raisins	Raisin (Dried Grape)	—
Wine	Wine (Fermented juice of grapes)	—
Ulmus campestris Ulmus campestris	Common Elm Ulmi cortex, Broad-leaved Elm, Ulmus suberosa	interior bark
Urtica dioica Urtica dioica	Greater Nettle Common Nettle, Stinging Nettle	herb
Arbutus Uva ursi Arctostaphylos Uva-Ursi	Bearberry Arbutus Uva-Ursi	leaf
Kaempferia rotunda Curcuma Zedoaria	Zedoary Turmeric, Zitterwurzel	root
Amomum Zingiber Zingiber officinale	Ginger	root

1789 Listing – animal materials

Adeps suilla	Hog's lard
Castoreum Russicum	Russian Castor. Castor is the dried preputial follicles and their secretion from the Beaver, *Castor* spp.
Cera flava	Yellow Beeswax – the secretion of the hive bee, *Aspis mellifera*
Cera alba	White Beeswax – bleached beeswax
Cornu cervi	Hartshorn – the antler of the red deer, *Cervidae* spp.
Isinglass	Isinglass – the dried swimming bladder of the sturgeon, *Acipenser huso* and other species of *Acipenser*
Mel	Honey – elaborated by bees from the nectar of flowers
Oniscus	Millepede – myriapods of the class, *Chilognatha*
Moschus	Musk – the strong-smelling substance obtained from the male musk-deer, *Moschus moschiferus*
Sevum ovillum	Mutton suet, fat of the sheep – the beardless woolly animal (Ovis) of the goat family
Spermaceti	Spermaceti – a waxy matter obtained mixed with oil from the head of the sperm whale of the *Odontoceti*

Spongia officinalis	Sponge – a member of the phylum Porifera, sessile aquatic animals with a single cavity in the body, with numerous pores
Ostrea edulis	Oyster-shells – from the bivalve shellfish, *Ostrea*
Meloe vesicatorius	Cantharides, Spanish Fly – the dried beetle *Cantharis vesicatoria* or other spp.
Cancer Pagurus	Crabs claws – from any of the Brachyura or short-tailed decapod crustaceans
Coccinella	Cochineal – scarlet dye-stuff consisting of the dried bodies of a Coccus insect gathered from a cactus in Mexico (Sp. cochinilla)
Ovum gallinaceum	Egg

1789 Listing – chemical materials

Acidum vitriolicum	Vitriolic acid – oil of vitriol, concentrated sulphuric acid
Argilla vitriolata	Alum – double sulphate of aluminium and potassium, with 24 molecules of water
Antimonium Sulphuratum	Antimony sulphate
Argentum	Silver
Natron impurum	Barilla – impure sodium carbonate got by burning certain seaside plants
Natron boracitatum	Borax – mineral hydrated sodium tetraborate
Lapis calcareus purus	Quicklime – unslaked lime, calcium oxide
Kali impurum	Pearl ashes – the prickly saltwort, *Salsola kali*, or glasswort, its ash
Creta	Chalk
Cuprum	Copper
Aerugo	Verdigris – basic cupric acetate; popularly, the green coating of basic cupric carbonate that forms in the atmosphere on copper, brass, or bronze
Cuprum vitriolatum	Blue Vitriol – crude copper sulphate
Ferrum	Iron
Ferrum vitriolatum	Green Vitriol – crude ferrous sulphate
Hydrargyrus	Quicksilver, mercury
Hydrargyrus sulphuratus	Cinnabar – sulphide of mercury, called vermilion when used as a pigment
Kali nitratum	Nitrum – crude sodium carbonate
Bitumen Petroleum	Petroleum
Plumbum	Lead
Cerussa	Cerusse – ceruse, white lead; cerusite, native lead carbonate
Lithargyrus	Litharge – lead monoxide, as obtained in refining silver
Magnesia vitriolata	Sal amarus, Bitter or Epsom salt – epsomite, a mineral, hydrated magnesium sulphate. Epsom salt, originally from springs at Epsom, Surrey
Isis nobilis	Red Coral – the calcareous internal skeleton of *Corallium rubrum*; it consists mainly of carbonate of lime principally coloured with oxide of iron
Ammonia muriata	Sal ammoniac – ammonium chloride
Natron muriatum	Common salt – sodium chloride

Sapo ex oleo olivae and natro confectus	Soap – an alkaline salt of a higher fatty acid: especially, such a compound of sodium (hard soap), or potassium (soft soap)
Stannum	Tin
Succinum	Amber – a yellowish fossil resin
Sulphuris flores	Flowers of sulphur (Sulphur, brimstone), Sublimed sulphur
Tartarum	Tartar, crude. Argol, chiefly acid potassium tartrate (with calcium tartrate etc.)
Crystals of tartar	Purified tartar
Acetum	Vinegar – dilute impure acetic acid
Zincum	Zinc
Lapis calaminaris ustus	Calamine – zinc carbonate
Tutty	Tutty – crude zinc oxide
Zincum vitriolatum	White Vitriol – crude zinc sulphate

1789 Listing – a partly identified material

Opium	The Apothecary who prepared the 1789 translation provided the following footnote on opium:

There has been no true botanical description of the species of poppy from which opium is made in Arabia. The most judicious of those who have observed the cultivation of opium of my acquaintance differ very much in opinion from Linnè, who probably never saw the plant. It is singular however that the College should not have followed the common opinion of authors. It is a mark of their care not to mislead. There has no writer given any tolerable account of the preparation of opium from the poppy.

Name Index

Subject Index

753